Handbook of Oncogenomics

Handbook of Oncogenomics

Editor: Zena Murray

AMERICAN
MEDICAL PUBLISHERS
www.americanmedicalpublishers.com

AMERICAN
MEDICAL PUBLISHERS
www.americanmedicalpublishers.com

Cataloging-in-Publication Data

Handbook of oncogenomics / edited by Zena Murray.
p. cm.
Includes bibliographical references and index.
ISBN 978-1-63927-251-8
1. Oncogenes. 2. Cancer--Genetic aspects. 3. Cancer--Molecular aspects. 4. Genomics. I. Murray, Zena.
RC268.42 .H36 2022
616.994 042--dc23

American Medical Publishers,
41 Flatbush Avenue,
1st Floor, New York,
NY 11217, USA

ISBN 978-1-63927-251-8 (Hardback)

Contents

Preface

The world is advancing at a fast pace like never before. Therefore, the need is to keep up with the latest developments. This book was an idea that came to fruition when the specialists in the area realized the need to coordinate together and document essential themes in the subject. That's when I was requested to be the editor. Editing this book has been an honour as it brings together diverse authors researching on different streams of the field. The book collates essential materials contributed by veterans in the area which can be utilized by students and researchers alike.

The accumulation of DNA mutations and epigenetic variations that leads to uncontrolled cell proliferation and formation of neoplasm refers to cancer. It is a genetic disease. The sub branch of genomics that deals with the study of cancer related genes is known as oncogenomics. The primary goal of the discipline is to recognize new tumor suppressor genes and oncogenes that may lead to new insights in the diagnosis of cancer, help predict the clinical outcome of different cancers and identify new targets for cancer therapies. It uses the techniques of transciptomes, genome sequencing, bioinformatics and functional analysis of oncogenes etc. The field is also concerned with personalizing cancer treatment by identifying and targeting mutations in an individual patient. The book elucidates the concepts and innovative models around the prospective developments with respect to oncogenomics. The various studies that are constantly contributing towards advancing technologies and evolution of this field are examined in detail. This book, with its detailed analyses and data, will prove immensely beneficial to professionals and students involved in this area at various levels.

Each chapter is a sole-standing publication that reflects each author's interpretation. Thus, the book displays a multi-facetted picture of our current understanding of application, resources and aspects of the field. I would like to thank the contributors of this book and my family for their endless support.

Editor

1

Genotype-phenotype associations in neurofibromatosis type 1 (NF1): an increased risk of tumor complications in patients with *NF1* splice-site mutations?

Adila Alkindy[1], Nadia Chuzhanova[2], Usha Kini[3], David N Cooper[4] and Meena Upadhyaya[4*]

Abstract

Neurofibromatosis type 1 (NF1) is a complex neurocutaneous disorder with an increased susceptibility to develop both benign and malignant tumors but with a wide spectrum of inter and intrafamilial clinical variability. The establishment of genotype-phenotype associations in NF1 is potentially useful for targeted therapeutic intervention but has generally been unsuccessful, apart from small subsets of molecularly defined patients. The objective of this study was to evaluate the clinical phenotype associated with the specific types of *NF1* mutation in a retrospectively recorded clinical dataset comprising 149 *NF1* mutation-known individuals from unrelated families. Each patient was assessed for ten NF1-related clinical features, including the number of café-au-lait spots, cutaneous and subcutaneous neurofibromas and the presence/absence of intertriginous skin freckling, Lisch nodules, plexiform and spinal neurofibromas, optic gliomas, other neoplasms (in particular CNS gliomas, malignant peripheral nerve sheath tumors (MPNSTs), juvenile myelomonocytic leukemia, rhabdomyosarcoma, phaechromocytoma, gastrointestinal stromal tumors, juvenile xanthogranuloma, and lipoma) and evidence of learning difficulties. Gender and age at examination were also recorded. Patients were subcategorized according to their associated *NF1* germ line mutations: frame shift deletions (52), splice-site mutations (23), nonsense mutations (36), missense mutations (32) and other types of mutation (6). A significant association was apparent between possession of a splice-site mutation and the presence of brain gliomas and MPNSTs ($p = 0.006$). If confirmed, these findings are likely to be clinically important since up to a third of NF1 patients harbor splice-site mutations. A significant influence of gender was also observed on the number of subcutaneous neurofibromas (females, $p = 0.009$) and preschool learning difficulties (females, $p = 0.022$).

Keywords: Neurofibromatosis type 1, Genotype-phenotype correlation, Malignant peripheral nerve sheath tumors, Brain glioma, Increased cancer susceptibility, Splice-site mutations, *NF1* gene, Gender effect

Introduction

Neurofibromatosis type 1 (NF1) (MIM #162200) [1] is a common familial cancer syndrome with a prevalence of 1 in 2,500 [2] and an autosomal dominant inheritance pattern; it is fully penetrant by 5 years of age. NF1 is a complex disorder that affects many cell types and involves multiple body systems [3]. The clinical phenotypic expression in NF1 is characterized by marked intra and interfamilial variability with many NF1 individuals only relatively mildly affected and their disease is limited to cutaneous involvement. Most NF1 patients also have mild learning difficulties. About a quarter of NF1 cases eventually develop one or more serious clinical multisystemic complications that lead to the significant morbidity and increased mortality characteristic of this disorder [4]. The many NF1-related clinical complications include neurological, cardiovascular, gastrointestinal, endocrine and orthopedic features. The overall risk of malignancy in NF1 is 5% to 15% higher than in the general population, the age of onset being earlier and with a poorer

* Correspondence: upadhyaya@cardiff.ac.uk
[4]Institute of Medical Genetics, Cardiff University, Heath Park, Cardiff CF14 4XN, UK

prognosis [5]. This increased incidence of malignancy primarily involves tumors of the CNS and connective tissue [5-7].

Neurofibromin, the *NF1* gene product, is a large (2,818 amino acids) [8] ubiquitously expressed protein present at low levels in most tissues, with the highest concentration found in the CNS [3,8]. The most inactivating *NF1* germ line mutations result in neurofibromin haploinsufficiency which seriously impairs its key role as a GTPase-activating protein that down-regulates most Ras protein activity in the cell [9-11]. Since Ras has a pivotal role in up-regulating cell proliferation, differentiation, survival and cell death, any functional loss of neurofibromin will result in the inappropriate and sustained activation of the Ras/Raf/ERK pathway. It is this cellular dysregulation that explains much of the NF1 clinical phenotype, especially the increased risk of benign and malignant neoplasms evident in NF1.

NF1 is however noted for the considerable inter and intrafamilial variation observed in the clinical phenotype even in patients who share the same germ line mutation. As a result, any decisions on surveillance tailored to some of these potentially treatable complications can be difficult to implement in the clinic. Successful genetic counseling is also hampered by clinical complications that are unpredictable both in severity and progression even within the same family [4]. This is particularly important in prenatal genetic counseling where the actual disease risk to the unborn infant is difficult to predict and where prenatal diagnosis creates difficulties in reproductive decision making for the families involved [4,12]. Hence, given such disease prediction and management problems, comprehensive genotype-phenotype studies are warranted.

Unfortunately, attempts to correlate the many and varied germ line *NF1* gene mutations with specific clinical features of NF1 have been largely unsuccessful [13], mainly due to the marked inter and intrafamilial variability in disease expression and the extent of the allelic heterogeneity underlying the disease. Two potential genotype-phenotype correlations that involve small subgroups of NF1 individuals have nevertheless been reported [3,14]. At least 1,347 different *NF1* gene mutations have been identified [15], many being unique to a specific individual or family [4,16]; fewer than 20% of *NF1* gene lesions are recurrent. As might be expected from the high mutation rate observed for the human *NF1* gene, almost half of all identified mutations occur *de novo* [16]. Given the marked clinical phenotypic variation associated with NF1 even in individuals carrying the same *NF1* mutation, it has been suggested that feature-specific modifier genes which are unlinked to the *NF1* locus itself, epigenetic alterations or other environmental factors may also contribute to such variable expression in NF1 [17,18].

The present retrospective study has attempted to assess whether any associated genotype-phenotype correlations could be identified in a large cohort ($N = 149$) of clinically well-characterized (but unrelated) NF1 patients with known pathogenic *NF1* mutations.

Methods

Patients

The present study is a retrospective analysis of the clinical data obtained from a cohort of NF1 patients collected for a previous Welsh study that characterized the *NF1* germ line mutations in patients referred from UK-wide medical genetic centers [19]. This new study was approved by the local ethical committee, with participants giving their informed consent. The study cohort comprised 149 unrelated *NF1* germ line mutation-positive patients whose associated clinical data were obtained from medical records over the past two years. The phenotypic information from each patient was generally recorded in a standardized way. This study actively excluded all patients known to harbor either a large genomic deletion [14] or the *NF1* 3-bp in-frame deletion in exon 17 [3], because both these mutation types have previously been found to have a tendency to be associated with a specific NF1 clinical phenotype.

Patient demographics

The patient cohort was characterized by an equal gender distribution, an ethnic origin that was predominantly Caucasian, and an age distribution which ranged from 1 day old to 71 years of age (mean age, 24 years). Most patients (137, approximately 92%) were clinically diagnosed as NF1 according to the National Institutes of Health (NIH) criteria [20]; three of these patients had concurrent diagnosis of other growth and developmental syndromes; five patients (approximately 3%) were diagnosed as NF1/Noonan syndrome (MIM #601321), four (approximately 3%) with NF1, familial spinal (MIM #162210) syndrome and three (2%) with Watson syndrome (MIM #193520). Seven patients (approximately 5%) did not meet the strict NIH clinical diagnostic criteria for NF1 when first tested for *NF1* mutations, whereas 49 patients (approximately 33%) had a positive family history of NF1, 90 patients (60%) were sporadic and 10 (approximately 7%) had an unknown family history. All patient data collected were anonymized prior to analysis.

Clinical features and associated mutations

Ten major NF1 clinical features were recorded for each patient, alongside patient age and gender, and the associated *NF1* germ line mutation. For the purposes of this analysis, patients were divided into three age groups: <6, 6 to 19 and >19 years. The germ line *NF1* mutations were recorded in terms of the type and specificity of the mutation, its genic location, and the predicted protein change. These mutations were further subdivided into five categories (see Figure 1): frame shift mutations (52 patients), splice-site mutations (23 patients), nonsense mutations (36 patients), missense mutations (32 patients) and six other less frequent types of mutation, including in-frame deletions (2), insertion/deletion (indel) mutations (1), single exon deletions (2) and intragenic multi-exonic deletions (1). The recorded clinical details included two numerical features: (1) the number of café-au-lait (CAL) spots, with four subgroups identified *viz.*, those with no CALs (ten patients), those with CALs of sizes 1 to 5 mm (11 cases), patients with CALs of sizes 6 to 99 mm (117) and four cases with large CALs (>111 mm); and (2) the number of cutaneous neurofibromas (CNFs) and subcutaneous neurofibromas (SCNFs), with patients subgrouped into those with no neurofibromas, those with only 2 to 5 CNFs, cases with 6 to 99 CNFs and SCNFs, those with 100 to 500 CNFs and SCNFs and those with >500 CNFs. Seven additional binary (presence or absence) clinical features were also examined, including skin freckling, Lisch nodules of the iris, plexiform neurofibromas (PNF), spinal neurofibromas (SpNF), optic gliomas, rare tumors known to be commonly associated with NF1 (including CNS gliomas, malignant peripheral nerve sheath tumors (MPNSTs), juvenile myelomonocytic leukemia (JMML), rhabdomyosarcoma, phaechromocytoma, gastrointestinal stromal tumors (GIST), juvenile xanthogranuloma and lipoma) and any other type of tumor recorded, and evidence of preschool learning difficulties.

Results

A multinomial logistic regression analysis was performed using mutation type, age group and gender as covariates, and the absence of clinical features as a reference (control) category. The results of this analysis, following removal of outliers, revealed a highly significant effect of the mutation type (specifically splice-site mutations) on the number of CALs, both with 1 to 5 CALs ($p = 1.8 \times 10^{-27}$) and 6 to 99 CALs ($p = 8.5 \times 10^{-43}$), as well as for skin freckling ($p = 0.028$) and neoplasms ($p = 0.006$). CNS gliomas and MPNST contributed to almost half of this group of neoplasms (see Table 1).

For the 6 to 19 years age group, a significant association was noted between the presence of a splice-site mutation and both CNF and SCNF numbers (6 to 99) ($p = 0.002$ and $p = 0.004$ respectively) and the presence of preschool learning difficulties ($p = 0.005$). A significant gender effect (female) was also observed with respect to SCNF number (6 to 99) (female, $p = 0.009$) and preschool learning difficulties ($p = 0.022$). This study therefore indicates a potential novel NF1 genotype-phenotype correlation, with *NF1* splice-site mutations being significantly associated ($p = 0.006$) with the tendency to develop tumors mostly composed of MPNSTs and CNS gliomas.

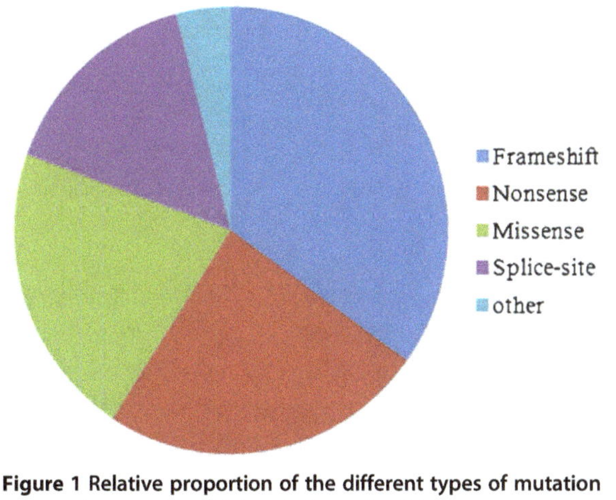

Figure 1 Relative proportion of the different types of mutation among the germ line *NF1* mutations identified.

Unusual cases

Several patients did not fulfill the strict NIH diagnostic criteria for NF1 even although they had been found to harbor *NF1* gene mutations. The NIH diagnostic criteria remain the 'gold standard' for NF1 diagnosis, the isolated occurrence of many of the NF1 features and complications being thought to be simply sporadic events [4,21]. Thus, *NF1* mutation testing is not routinely carried out unless there is a high index of suspicion of the disorder. Our findings indicate that such *NF1* gene testing, which

Table 1 Prevalence of neoplasms in a cohort ($N = 149$ with known NF1 mutation) of clinically well-characterized NF1 patients

Type of neoplasm	Number of neoplasms[a] reported (%)	
CNS gliomas (excluding optic gliomas)	12	8
Malignant peripheral nerve sheath tumor	8	5.5
Rhabdomyosarcoma (prostate)	1	0.7
Medullary thyroid carcinoma	2	1.3
Gastrointestinal stromal tumors	2	1.3
Multiple internal neurofibromas	3	2
Phaechromocytoma	3(1B/L)	2
Colorectal carcinoma at 71 years	1	0.7
Breast cancer - ductal type at 34 and 40 years	2	1.3
Glomus tumor	2	1.3
Xanthogranuloma	2	1.3
Lipoma	4	2.7
Juvenile myelomonocytic leukemia	0	0

[a]Some of the patients were found to have more than one type of tumor.

usually serves to confirm the clinical diagnosis in >95% of cases [4,16], should also be considered in the context of atypical cases. Some examples from the present patient cohort with identified *NF1* mutations include the following:

(1) An 18-year-old female presenting with an MPNST of the breast but with no other characteristic NF1 features or complications. Several of her family members were also reported to have had breast cancer but they lacked other features of NF1.

(2) A 10-year-old boy with a unilateral optic glioma, a few small CALs and mild learning difficulties but with a negative family history of NF1.

(3) NF1 patients with hypertrophic cardiomyopathy (HCM). In the study cohort, two cases of a father and his 29-year-old son and a 71-year-old male were noted to have symptomatic HCM which was diagnosed by echocardiogram and manifested as cardiovascular-associated NF1 complications. Echocardiographic findings of a septal to posterior left ventricular free wall ratio greater than 1.5 (suggestive of hypertrophic cardiomyopathy) were noted in at least 4% of NF1 patients [22,23] in one study. However, none of the 2,322 NF1 individuals retrospectively assessed for cardiovascular malformation in the National Neurofibromatosis Foundation International Database had HCM [24], suggesting that routine echocardiography should form part of the surveillance regimen in NF1. At least four other single reports of the cooccurrence of HCM and NF1 [25-28] have appeared in the literature. Cardiac hypertrophy is the most common risk factor contributing to cardiovascular mortality and morbidity in NF1 patients [29]. Congenital heart disease and cardiomyopathy are also a common accompaniment of several growth and development syndromes affecting the RASopathies [30,31]. Cardiomyopathy in these syndromes arises from increased signaling through Erk1/2 and mTOR complex 1 [29]. Neurofibromin is known to act in modulating the epithelial-mesenchymal transformation and proliferation in the developing heart by down-regulating RAS activity. In the absence of functional neurofibromin, mouse embryonic hearts develop an over-abundance of endocardial cushion which may obstruct blood outflow in some cases as a result of cellular hyperproliferation and a lack of apoptosis [32-34]. The cardiac-specific *Nf1* knockout mice, combined

Table 2 Summary of clinical features and germ line *NF1* mutation type in 18 patients lacking peripheral neurofibromas

Patient ID	Sex/age (years)	Mutation type	NIH	CNF/ SCNF	PNF	SpNF	6-99 CALs	Skin freckling	Other NF1 features/ complications
S149	F/24	Missense K1423E	Y	0	0	0	Y	B/L axilla	Low grade MPNST
S174	M/adult	Missense W1931R	Y	0	0	0	Y	B/L axilla	none
462	F/43	Missense F1193C	Y	0	0	0	Y	B/L axilla	Offspring-same phenotype
482	F/39	Missense W837R	Y	0	Y	0	Y	B/L axilla	GIST tumor
2198	M/22	Missense M11491	N	0	0	0	Y	N	Mild learning difficulties/ CALs only[a]
2444	M/24	Missense L1812P	Y	0	0	0	Y	B/L axilla/groin	CNS glioma
2483	F/29	Nonsense R1748X	Y	0	0	0	Y	extensive	none
2512	M/22	Nonsense R416X	Y	O	Y	0	Y	Submammary	none
2070	F/19	Nonsense R461X	Y	0	0	0	Y	B/L axilla	Unilateral optic glioma
2133	M/51	Nonsense K1517X	N	0	0	0	Y	N	CALs only[a]
2199	F/27	Frameshift c.6403insGA	N	0	0	0	Y	N	Mild learning difficulties/ CALs only[a]
2277	F/34	Frameshift c.3721-3722 ins A	Y	0	Y	0	Y	N	none
2278	M/39	Frameshift c.7892-7893delAA	Y	0	0	0	Y	B/L axilla	Mild learning difficulties
1663	M/25	Frameshift c.495delTGTT	Y	0	0	0	Y	B/L axilla	none
26445	F/18	Frameshift c.5406insT	Y	0	0	0	Y	Extensive	Mild learning difficulties
870	F/18	Frameshift c.6219 delT	Y	0	0	0	Y	B/L axilla/trunk	Bilateral optic glioma
2276	F/20	Frameshift c.6791insA	Y	0	0	0	Y	B/L axilla	none
2023	F/22	Splice-site c.589-2 A > G	?	0	0	0	Y	?	Severe learning difficulties

[a]Some of the patients were found to have more than one type of tumor.

with genetic rescue, suggest that neurofibromin is an important regulator of Ras signaling in cardiac myocytes, and that Ras activation can lead to progressive cardiac hypertrophy with associated pathological changes in adult mice [32,35,36].

(4) NF1 patients with absent CNF and SCNF. In the study cohort, 18 (12%) unrelated adult patients lacked peripheral and spinal neurofibromas, and only three patients had identifiable plexiform neurofibromas (see Table 2). All patients fulfilled the strict NIH diagnostic criteria for NF1 except for three patients who manifested only CALs and mild learning difficulties. In general, all these patients exhibited pigmentary changes of NF1 with very few NF1-related complications and had a milder clinical phenotype [3,4]. The types of mutations reported in this group were missense (six patients), nonsense (four) and microdeletions/microinsertions (seven). Only a single patient had a splice-site mutation and severe learning difficulties. Our finding is consistent with the previous observations, suggesting that the clinical phenotype of deceased NF1 patients is characterized by fewer CALs (albeit nonsignificant) and significantly more neurofibromas [6].

Discussion

NF1 patients with germ line *NF1* splice-site mutations were found to have an increased tendency to develop MPNSTs and CNS gliomas by comparison with patients harboring other mutation types, e.g. microinsertions, microdeletions, nonsense and missense mutations. Up to 30% of all NF1 patients carry germ line *NF1* splice-site mutations, and such mutations often lead to the synthesis of a truncated form of neurofibromin [4,16]. In the present NF1 patient cohort, however, only 23 individuals (15%) carried splice-site mutations. This comparatively low frequency could be explained by the fact that the current analysis was performed on genomic DNA (rather than cDNA), and some of the underlying splicing mutations (resulting from deep intronic mutations) could have been missed if they did not occur in the immediate vicinity of a splice site. Moreover, some of the missense or nonsense mutations identified could have exerted an effect on splicing. Despite the small patient number, our analyses identified a significant correlation between the presence of a splice-site mutation and the occurrence of neoplasms ($p = 0.006$), mostly brain and connective tissue tumors. This initial finding clearly merits further clinical investigation in a much larger mutation-known NF1 patient population. A multicenter study and prospective data collection, based on comprehensive clinical examination, would be necessary to substantiate this finding. If our initial conclusion is supported by further analysis, it could imply that the wider application of RNA-based analyses in NF1 patient screening (in order to detect splice-site mutations with high efficiency) [33] might be helpful in predicting which patients would benefit the most from regular clinical surveillance.

Of all the characteristic features of NF1, the presence of benign and malignant neoplasm contributes the most to the morbidity and mortality experienced by many NF1 individuals; indeed, the overall cancer risk associated with NF1 has been reported to be higher than in the general population in several NF1 studies [5-7], owing to markedly increased risks of brain and connective tissue tumors. Indeed, malignancy, alongside other tumor-related neurological complications, is the most frequent cause of death in NF1 patients, resulting in a reduced life expectancy of some 8 to 15 years as compared to the general population [5,7,27]. The predominance of cancer among causes of death in NF1 is consistent in most studies [5-7,34,37] and contributes disproportionately to the mortality in younger age groups (less than 40 years). This increased risk of malignancy in NF1 individuals is a cause of major concern for families and is difficult to address during genetic counseling.

If our finding of an association between the possession of an *NF1* splice-site mutation and the likelihood of tumor occurrence is borne out by future work, this group of patients should undergo rigorous clinical surveillance in order to facilitate early diagnosis and permit early management of any tumor-related complications as they arise. Although the types of tumors observed in our patient cohort were heterogeneous, they were similar to the spectrum of tumors reported in many NF1 patients, being mainly brain gliomas and MPNSTs [5-7,38] which comprised almost half of the neoplasms in our cohort. The prevalence of types of tumors other than the brain gliomas and MPNSTs reported in this cohort was very low, as noted in other studies [7]. A moderately increased susceptibility to develop breast cancer in female NF1 patients before the age of 50 years has previously been documented [39]. However, only 2/74 female (2.7%) cases in our cohort developed ductal type breast cancer between the ages of 34 and 41 years. Phaechromocytomas and catecholamine-secreting tumors of the neural crest are rare tumors in the general population and occur in 0.1% to 5.7% [40] of patients with NF1. In a recent study, a higher prevalence of 14.7% was noted [41]. At least three patients (2%) in our cohort had phaechromocytoma, whereas two patients had medullary thyroid cancer, one of these in association with bilateral phaechromocytoma as part of multiple endocrine neoplasia type 2A (MEN2A). The coexistence of MEN2A and NF1 (the neurocristopathies) has rarely been reported, suggesting that NF1 patients with phaechromocytoma should be thoroughly examined for clinical evidence of other phaechromocytoma-related syndromes. All three cases reported in the literature (including our own case) had identifiable germ line mutations in the *NF1* gene, but not in the *RET* proto-oncogene which is a known cause of MEN2A [42]. Colorectal carcinomas have been previously noted as a cause of death in NF1 [7]. Only one case of adenocarcinoma of the colon at the age of 71 was noted in our cohort and this could be a sporadic occurrence. GIST are mesenchymal tumors of the gastrointestinal tract and are commonly associated with NF1 and usually with a good prognosis [43,44]. We report two such tumors in our cohort. Glomus tumors are small, benign but painful tumors and are usually associated with NF1 and considered as part of the tumor spectrum of NF1 [45]. Two cases of multiple glomus tumors were reported in our cohort. Rhabdomyosarcomas are pediatric neoplasms which are more common in children with NF1 than in the general population [46]. One case of a child with rhabdomyosarcoma of the prostate was noted in the study cohort. Multiple subcutaneous lipomas [47] have been noted in one patient with NF1. However, solitary lipomas are also frequent in the general population, and the presence of these isolated lipomas in four of our patients could be purely coincidental. The presence of xanthogranulomas in pediatric NF1 cases may be related to the possible development of JMML [48], but none of the patients in our cohort had JMML. The prevalence of xanthogranulomas in the general population of normal children is quite high (1% to 2%), but these are rarely associated with systemic manifestations [48].

Our observation of a gender effect in NF1 has not been previously reported; despite the very similar sex distribution in our patient cohort, a disproportionate number of females exhibited learning difficulties ($p = 0.022$). Female NF1 patients were also found to be significantly more likely to manifest SCNFs ($p = 0.009$). This observation may relate to the differential effect that female steroid hormones appear to have on the development of CNFs and SCNFs, as previously noted in the peri-pubertal and pregnant subpopulations of affected NF1 individuals [49,50]. Peripheral neurofibromas have also been reported to express progesterone receptors [49,50] and this could explain the observed gender effect. SCNFs rarely transform into malignant tumors, but their presence could be an expression of a more aggressive disease [5,51]. A disproportionate number of SCNFs in a cohort of NF1 female patients could indicate a worse prognosis in females in comparison to males, as indicated in some studies [7,34,51].

Conclusions

Our study suggests a novel potential NF1 genotype-phenotype correlation, with *NF1* splice-site mutations being associated with an increased tendency to develop neoplasms, mostly composed of CNS gliomas and MPNSTs. This finding appears to constitute a novel genotype-phenotype correlation that has the potential to be clinically useful. Since up to one third of all NF1 patients harbor splice-site mutations, the early detection of this type of lesion might be helpful in predicting which patients would benefit the most from regular clinical surveillance, thereby improving their survival. Our study also supports previous observations of a gender effect on mortality and morbidity associated with NF1; significantly, more female patients exhibited learning difficulties and were found to be more likely to possess subcutaneous neurofibromas than their male counterparts.

Competing interests

The authors declare that they have no competing interests.

Authors' contributions

AA collected the clinical data and wrote the first draft of this paper. NC performed the bioinformatic data analysis, UK provided cinical data, DNC helped with the writing of the manuscript and MU provided the mutational data, helped with the writing of manuscript. All authors read and approved the final manuscript.

Acknowledgments

We are grateful to Dr. Debbie Shears (Oxford), Dr. Sue Holder (Kennedy Galton, London), Dr. Susan Huson (Manchester) and all other clinicians who have helped us to collect patient data. We thank all patients and their families for their kind cooperation.

Author details

[1]Clinical Genetics Department, Sultan Qaboos University Hospital, P.O. Box 39, Al-Khod, Muscat 123, Sultanate of Oman. [2]School of Science and Technology, Nottingham Trent University, Clifton LaneNottingham NG11 8NS, UK. [3]Department of Clinical Genetics, Churchill Hospital, Old Road Headington, Oxford OX3 7LJ, UK. [4]Institute of Medical Genetics, Cardiff University, Heath Park, Cardiff CF14 4XN, UK.

References

1. *Online Mendelian Inheritance in Man Database - Entry #162200.* http://www.omim.org/entry/162200.
2. Upadhyaya M, Cooper DN(E): *Neurofibromatosis Type 1: From Genotype to Phenotype.* Oxford: BIOS Publishers; 1998.
3. Upadhyaya M, Huson SM, Davies M, Thomas N, Chuzhanova N, Giovannini S, Evans DG, Howard E, Kerr B, Griffiths S, Consoli C, Side L, Adams D, Pierpont M, Hachen R, Barnicoat A, Li H, Wallace P, Van Biervliet JP, Stevenson D, Viskochil D, Baralle D, Haan E, Riccardi V, Turnpenny P, Lazaro C, Messiaen L: **An absence of cutaneous neurofibromas associated with a 3-bp inframe deletion in exon 17 of the *NF1* gene (c.2970-2972 del AAT): evidence of a clinically significant NF1 genotype-phenotype correlation.** *Am J Hum Genet* 2007, **80:**140–151.
4. Upadhyaya M: **Neurofibromatosis type 1 NF1): diagnosis and recent advances.** *Exp Opin Med. Diagn* 2010, **4:**307–322.
5. Rasmussen SA, Yang Q, Friedman JM: **Mortality in neurofibromatosis 1: an analysis using U.S. death certificates.** *Am J Hum Genet* 2001, **68:**1110–1118.
6. Zöller M, Rembeck B, Akesson HO, Angervall L: **Life expectancy, mortality and prognostic factors in neurofibromatosis type 1. A twelve-year follow-up of an epidemiological study in Goteborg, Sweden.** *Acta Derm Venereol* 1995, **75:**136–140.
7. Walker L, Thompson D, Easton D, Ponder B, Ponder M, Frayling I, Baralle D: **A prospective study of neurofibromatosis type 1 cancer incidence in the UK.** *Br J Cancer* 2006, **95:**233–238.

8. Marchuk DA, Saulino AM, Tavakkol R, Swaroop M, Wallace MR, Andersen LB, Mitchell AL, Gutmann DH, Boguski M, Collins FS: **cDNA cloning of the type 1 Neurofibromatosis gene: complete sequence of the *NF1* gene product.** *Genomics* 1991, **11**:931–940.
9. Daston MM, Ratner N: **Neurofibromin, a predominantly neuronal GTPase activating protein in the adult, is ubiquitously expressed during development.** *Dev Dyn* 1992, **195**:216–226.
10. Martin G, Viskochil D, Bollag G, McCabe PC, Crosier WJ, Haubruck H, Conroy L, Clark R, O'Connell P, Cawthon RM, Innis MA, McCormick F: **The GAP-related domain of the neurofibromatosis type 1 gene product interacts with ras p21.** *Cell* 1990, **63**:843–849.
11. Cichowski K, Jacks T: ***NF1* tumor suppressor gene function: narrowing the GAP.** *Cell* 2001, **104**:593–604.
12. Ferner RE, Huson SM, Thomas N, Moss C, Willshaw H, Evans DG, Upadhyaya M, Towers R, Gleeson M, Steiger C, Kirby A: **Guidelines for the diagnosis and management of individuals with neurofibromatosis 1.** *J Med Genet* 2007, **44**:81–88.
13. Castle B, Baser M, Huson SM, Cooper DN, Upadhyaya M: **Evaluation of genotype-phenotype correlations in neurofibromatosis type 1.** *J Med Genet* 2003, **40**:e109.
14. Kayes LM, Riccardi VM, Burke W, Bennett RL, Stephens K: **Large *de novo* DNA deletion in a patient with sporadic neurofibromatosis 1, mental retardation, and dysmorphism.** *J Med Genet* 1992, **29**:686–690.
15. *The Human Gene Mutation Database*. http:/www.hgmd.org.
16. Messiaen L, Wimmer K: **Neurofibromatoses**. In *Neurofibromatoses: NF1 mutational spectrum*, Basel:Monogr Hum Genet. Edited by Kaufmann D. Basel, Karger:; 2008, 16:63–77.
17. Easton DF, Ponder MA, Huson SM, Ponder BA: **An analysis of variation in expression of neurofibromatosis (NF) type 1 (NF1): evidence for modifying genes.** *Am J Hum Genet* 1993, **53**:305–513.
18. Sabbagh A, Pasmant E, Laurendeaul Parfait B, Barbarot S, Guillot B, Combemale P, Ferkal S, Vidaud M, Aubourg P, Vidaud D, Wolkenstein P, NF France Network: **Unravelling the genetic basis of variable clinical expression in neurofibromatosis 1.** *Hum Mol Genet* 2009, **18**:2768–2778.
19. Griffiths S, Thompson P, Frayling I, Upadhyaya M: **Molecular diagnosis of neurofibromatosis type 1: 2 years experience.** *Fam Cancer* 2007, **6**:21–34.
20. NIH: **National Institutes of Health Consensus Development Conference Statement: neurofibromatosis. Bethesda, Md., USA, July 13–15, 1987.** *Neurofibromatosis* 1988, **1**:172–178.
21. Jett K, Friedman JM: **Clinical and genetic aspects of neurofibromatosis 1.** *Genet Med* 2010, **12**:1–11.
22. Tedesco MA, Di Salvo G, Natale F, Pergola V, Calabrese E, Grassia C, Ratti G, Iarussi D, Iacono A, Calabrò R, Lama G: **The heart in neurofibromatosis type 1: an echocardiographic study.** *Am Heart J* 2002, **143**:883–888.
23. Lin AE, Birch PH, Korf BR, Tenconi R, Niimura M, Poyhonen M, Armfield Uhas K, Sigorini M, Virdis R, Romano C, Bonioli E, Wolkenstein P, Pivnick EK, Lawrence M, Friedman JM: **Cardiovascular malformations and other cardiovascular abnormalities in neurofibromatosis 1.** *Am J Med Genet* 2000, **95**:108–117.
24. Friedman JM, Arbiser J, Epstein JA, Gutmann DH, Huot SJ, Lin AE, McManus B, Korf BR: **Cardiovascular disease in neurofibromatosis 1: report of the NF1 Cardiovascular Task Force.** *Genet Med* 2002, **4**:105–111.
25. Hamilton SJ, Allard MF, Friedman JM: **Cardiac findings in an individual with neurofibromatosis 1 and sudden death.** *Am J Med Genet* 2001, **100**:95–99.
26. Fitzpatrick AP, Emanuel RW: **Familial neurofibromatosis and hypertrophic cardiomyopathy.** *Br Heart J* 1988, **60**:247–245.
27. Elliott CM, Tajik AJ, Giuliani ER, Gordon H: **Idiopathic hypertrophic subaortic stenosis associated with cutaneous neurofibromatosis: report of a case.** *Am Heart J* 1976, **92**:368–372.
28. Sachs RN, Buschauer-Bonnet C, Kemeny JL, Amouroux J, Lanfranchi J: **Cardiomyocardiopathie hypertrophique et maladie de von Recklinghausen.** *Rev Med Interne* 1984, **5**:154–156.
29. Prada CE, Zarate YA, Hagenbuch S, Lovell AM, Saal HM, Schorry EK, Hopkin RJ: **Lethal presentation of neurofibromatosis and Noonan syndrome.** *Am J Med Genet A* 2011, **155A**:1360–1366.
30. Tidyman WE, Rauen KA: **The RASopathies: developmental syndromes of Ras/MAPK pathway dysregulation.** *Curr Opin Genet Dev* 2009, **19**:230–236.
31. Zenker M: **Genetic and pathogenetic aspects of Noonan syndrome and related disorders.** *Horm Res* 2009, **72**:57–63.
32. Zhongjie S: **Overview of recent advances in molecular cardiology.** *Can J Cardiol* 2006, **22**:235–240.
33. Ars E, Serra E, García J, Kruyer H, Gaona A, Lázaro C, Estivill X: **Mutations affecting mRNA splice site are the most common molecular defects in patients with neurofibromatosis type 1.** *Hum Mol Genet* 2000, **9**:237–247.
34. Duong TA, Sbidian E, Valeyrie-Allanore L: **Mortality associated with neurofibromatosis 1: a cohort study of 1895 patients in 1980–2006 in France.** *Orphanet J Rare Dis* 2011, **6**:18.
35. Gelb BD, Tartaglia M: **RAS signaling pathway mutations and hypertrophic cardiomyopathy: getting into and out of the thick of it.** *J Clin Invest* 2011, **121**:844–847.
36. Xu J, Ismat FA, Wang T, Lu MM, Antonucci N, Epstein JA: **Cardiomyocyte-specific loss of neurofibromin promotes cardiac hypertrophy and dysfunction.** *Circ Res* 2009, **105**:304–311.
37. Evans DG, O'Hara C, Wilding A, Ingham SL, Howard E, Dawson J, Moran A, Scott-Kitching V, Holt F, Huson SM: **Mortality in neurofibromatosis 1: in North West England: an assessment of actuarial survival in a region of the UK since 1989.** *Eur J Hum Genet* 2011, **19**:1187–1191.
38. Upadhyaya M: **Genetic basis of tumorigenesis in NF1 malignant peripheral nerve sheath tumours.** *Front Biosci* 2011, **16**:937–951.
39. Sharif S, Moran A, Huson SM, Iddenden R, Shenton A, Howard E, Evans DG: **Women with neurofibromatosis 1 are at a moderately increased risk of developing breast cancer and should be considered for early screening.** *J Med Genet* 2007, **44**:481–484.
40. Erem C, Onder EH, Ukinç K, Hacihasanoglu A, Alhan E, Cobanoğlu U, Koçak M, Erdöl H: **Neurofibromatosis type 1 associated with pheochromocytoma: a case report and a review of the literature.** *J Endocrinol Invest* 2007, **30**:59–64.
41. Zinnamosca L, Petramala L, Cotesta D, Marinelli C, Schina M, Cianci R, Giustini S, Sciomer S, Anastasi E, Calvieri S, De Toma G, Letizia C: **Neurofibromatosis type 1 (NF1) and pheochromocytoma: prevalence, clinical and cardiovascular aspects.** *Arch Dermatol Res* 2011, **303**:317–325.
42. Gkaliagkousi E, Erlic Z, Petidis K, Semertzidis P, Doumas M, Zamboulis C, Neumann HP, Douma S: **Neurofibromatosis type 1: should we screen for other genetic syndromes? A case report of co-existence with multiple endocrine neoplasias 2A.** *Eur J Clin Invest* 2009, **39**:828–832.
43. Miettinen M, Fetsch JF, Sobin LH, Lasota J: **Gastrointestinal stromal tumors in patients with neurofibromatosis 1: a clinicopathologic and molecular genetic study of 45 cases.** *Am J Surg Pathol* 2006, **30**:90–96.
44. Miettinen M, Lasota J: **Histopathology of gastrointestinal stromal tumor.** *J Surg Oncol* 2011, **104**:865–873.
45. Brems H, Park C, Maertens O, Pemov A, Messiaen L, Upadhyaya M, Claes K, Beert E, Peeters K, Mautner V, Sloan JL, Yao L, Lee CC, Sciot R, De Smet L, Legius E, Stewart DR: **Glomus tumors in neurofibromatosis type 1: genetic, functional and clinical evidence of a novel association.** *Cancer Res* 2009, **69**:7393–7401.
46. Cecen E, Ince D, Uysal KM, Ozer E, Cetingoz R, Ozguven AA, Cakmakci H, Sarialioglu F, Olgun N: **Soft tissue sarcomas and central nervous system tumors in children with neurofibromatosis type 1.** *Childs Nerv Syst* 2011, **27**:1885–1893.
47. Oktenli C, Gul D, Deveci MS, Saglam M, Upadhyaya M, Thompson P, Consoli C, Kocar IH, Pilarski R, Zhou XP, Eng C: **Unusual features in a patient with neurofibromatosis type 1: multiple subcutaneous lipomas, a juvenile polyp in ascending colon, congenital intrahepatic portosystemic venous shunt, and horseshoe kidney.** *Am J Med Genet A* 2004, **127A**:298–301.
48. Raygada M, Arthur D, Wayne A, Rennert OM, Toretsky JA, Stratakis CA: **Juvenile xanthogranuloma in a child with previously unsuspected neurofibromatosis type 1 and juvenile myelomonocytic leukemia.** *Pediatr Blood Cancer* 2010, **54**:173–175.
49. Overdiek AWU, Mayatepek E, Rosenbaum T: **Schwann cells from human neurofibromas show increased proliferation rates under the influence of progesterone.** *Pediatr Res* 2008, **64**:40–43.
50. Roth TM, Petty EM, Barald KF: **The role of steroid hormones in the NF1 phenotype: focus on pregnancy.** *Am J Med Genet A* 2008, **146A**:1624–1633.
51. Khosrotehrani K, Bastji-Garin S, Riccardi VM, Birch P, Friedman JM, Wolkenstein P: **Subcutaneous neurofibromas are associated with mortality in neurofibromatosis type one: a cohort study of 703 patients.** *Am J Med Genet* 2005, **132**:49–53.

2

Comparative study and meta-analysis of meta-analysis studies for the correlation of genomic markers with early cancer detection

Zoi Lanara[1,2†], Efstathia Giannopoulou[3†], Marta Fullen[4], Evangelos Kostantinopoulos[2], Jean-Christophe Nebel[4], Haralabos P Kalofonos[3], George P Patrinos[2] and Cristiana Pavlidis[2*]

Abstract

A large number of common disorders, including cancer, have complex genetic traits, with multiple genetic and environmental components contributing to susceptibility. A literature search revealed that even among several meta-analyses, there were ambiguous results and conclusions. In the current study, we conducted a thorough meta-analysis gathering the published meta-analysis studies previously reported to correlate any random effect or predictive value of genome variations in certain genes for various types of cancer. The overall analysis was initially aimed to result in associations (1) among genes which when mutated lead to different types of cancer (e.g. common metabolic pathways) and (2) between groups of genes and types of cancer. We have meta-analysed 150 meta-analysis articles which included 4,474 studies, 2,452,510 cases and 3,091,626 controls (5,544,136 individuals in total) including various racial groups and other population groups (native Americans, Latinos, Aborigines, etc.). Our results were not only consistent with previously published literature but also depicted novel correlations of genes with new cancer types. Our analysis revealed a total of 17 gene-disease pairs that are affected and generated gene/disease clusters, many of which proved to be independent of the criteria used, which suggests that these clusters are biologically meaningful.

Keywords: Cancer, Meta-analysis, Gene, Association, Interaction, Single-nucleotide polymorphism, Alleles, Clustering

Introduction

Cancer is the result of a complicated process that involves the accumulation of both genetic and epigenetic alterations in various genes [1]. The somatic genetic alterations in cancer include point mutations, small insertion/deletion events, translocations, copy number changes and loss of heterozygosity [2]. These changes either augment the action and/or expression of an oncoprotein or silence tumour suppressor genes. Single-nucleotide polymorphism (SNP) is the most common form of genetic variation in the human genome. Although common SNPs for disease prediction are not ready for widespread use [3], recent genome-wide association studies (GWASs) using high-throughput techniques have identified regions of the genome that contain SNPs with alleles that are associated with increased risk for cancer such as *FGFR2* in breast cancer [4-7].

The knowledge on gene mutations that predispose tumour initiation or tumour development and progress will give an advantage in cancer patients' treatment. Despite the complexity and variability of cancer genome, numerous studies have examined the correlation of genome variation with cancer development and progression [8]. However, ambiguous results have been generated from the attempt to link genome variants with cancer prediction or detection. A literature search revealed that even among several meta-analyses, there were unclear results and conclusions.

We have, therefore, conducted a thorough meta-analysis of meta-analysis studies previously reported to correlate the random effect or predictive value of genome variations in certain genes for various types of cancer. The aim of the overall analysis was the detection of

* Correspondence: chpavlidou@upatras.gr
†Equal contributors
[2]School of Health Sciences, Department of Pharmacy, University of Patras, University Campus, Rio, Patras 26504, Greece

correlations (1) among genes whose mutation might lead to different types of cancer (e.g. common metabolic pathways) and (2) between groups of genes and types of cancer.

Methods

We performed a thorough field synopsis by studying published meta-analysis studies involving the association of various types of cancer with SNPs located in certain genomic regions. For each published meta-analysis included in our study, we also investigated the number of patients (cases) and controls, date, type of study, study group details (e.g. gender, race, age, etc.), measures included, allele and genotype frequency and also the outcome of each study, i.e. if there was an association or not, the interactions noticed in each of these studies, etc.

We have meta-analysed 150 meta-analysis articles (Additional file 1), which included 4,474 studies, 2,452,510 cases and 3,091,626 controls (5,544,136 individuals in total). The meta-analyses that have been meta-analysed included various racial groups, e.g. Caucasians, Far Eastern populations (Asian, Chinese, Japanese, Korean, etc.), African-American and other population groups (native Americans, Latinos, Aborigines, etc.). Three types of studies were included: (1) pooled analysis, (2) GWAS and (2) other studies, e.g. search in published reports. Collected data consisted of a list of genes, genomic variants and diseases with a known genotype-phenotype association (whether or not a given variation has an impact on susceptibility to a given disease). The principle of our study was to use data mining techniques to find groups (referred to as clusters hereafter) of genes or diseases that behave similarly according to related data. Such groupings will make it possible to find different cancer types susceptible to similar genotypes as well as different genes associated to similar cancer types. Furthermore, our approach would facilitate predicting whether susceptibility to one type of cancer may be indicative of predisposition to another cancer type. Moreover, the association between a group of genes and a given phenotype may suggest that these genes interact or belong to the same biochemical pathway. In order to allow data mining analysis, genotype-phenotype associations had to be classified within a fixed set of categories, i.e. yes/small yes/may/no. Moreover, genes or diseases with fewer than two entries were not considered in our analysis since their clustering would not be meaningful.

Then, data were processed using a state-of-the-art general purpose clustering tool, CLUTO [9]. Data analysis consisted in finding the tightest and most reliable groupings. Since CLUTO offers a wide range of methods, and many different scoring schemes can be used to estimate similarity between genotypes or phenotypes, cluster reliability was assessed by their robustness to clustering criteria (details are provided in Additional file 1). As a consequence, each putative association has been qualified as either 'highly consistent' or 'moderately consistent'. The biological significance of those clusters was, first, evaluated using the Search Tool for the Retrieval of Interacting Genes/Proteins (STRING) [10,11], a biological database and web resource of known and predicted protein-protein interactions. The STRING database contains information from numerous sources, including experimental data, computational prediction methods and public text collections. It is widely accessible, and it is regularly updated. Second, literature research was performed to complete this initial evaluation.

Results and discussion

In this study, we performed a meta-analysis of published meta-analysis studies to investigate possible correlations among genes and SNPs and various types of cancer, as well as among gene-gene and/or gene-environmental interactions. Furthermore, an advanced literature research was applied in order to evaluate our results obtained from our meta-analysis. Our data were not only consistent with previously published literature but we have also depicted novel correlations of genes with new types of cancer. Our analysis showed a total of ten cancer-related genes that are affected (Table 1).

Correlation of SNPs' genes with various types of cancer

The association highlighted by our meta-analysis between the *CYP2E1* gene and colorectal cancer (CRC), head and neck cancer (HNC) and liver cell carcinoma (LLC) is supported by published data [33-39,44,121]. An additional literature search to evaluate our initial results revealed novel correlations of the gene combination *CYP2E1* and *GSTM1* with prostate cancer (PC) susceptibility, lung cancer (LC) and bladder cancer (UBC) as shown in Table 2 [126-128]. A similar correlation was found in CRC using a knockdown model [32,40,41]. Studies not only confirm the possibility of association between the *CCND1* gene and breast cancer (BC) [25] but also suggest involvement with squamous cell carcinoma (SCC), oesophageal cancer (EC), oral cancer (OC) and malignant glioma (MG), as arisen from the interaction between the *CCND1* and *CCND3* genes [26,122-124]. This is further corroborated in mouse model studies that show association of *CCND1* with BC [25,27-31,153] and PC [125].

Moreover, as far as the *ERCC2* is concerned along with the association of *ERCC1* gene with BC and LC which is already confirmed [14-17,21,22], we have also identified from our further literature search on humans the existence of an association with OC [26] and with HNC [129-131]. There were no similar mouse studies that could confirm or overrule our findings.

Our findings regarding the *GSTP1* gene are confirmed by the published literature [39,46-55]. Furthermore, we

Table 1 Summary of genes and SNPs identified by meta-analysis to be positively correlated with various cancers

Gene	Cancer type	SNPs		References	Supporting references
		rs number	Other name		
ERCC2	BC	rs13181	p.K715Q	[12,13]	[14-17]
ERCC2	BC	rs1799793	p.D312N	[12,18]	[14-16]
ERCC2	LC	rs13181	p.K751Q	[19,20]	[17,21,22]
ERCC2	LC	rs1799793	p.D312N	[23]	[17,21,22]
CCND1	BC	rs603965	c.870G>A	[24]	[25-31]
CYP2E1	CRC	rs3813867	NA	[32]	[32-41][a]
CYP2E1	HNC	rs3813867	NA	[42,43]	[44]
CYP2E1	HNC	rs6413432	NA	[42]	[44]
GSTP1	CRC	rs1695	p.I105V	[45]	[39,46-55]
IL6	BC	rs1800795	c.-174G>C	[56,57]	
MTHFR	GC	rs1801131	c.1298A>C	[58]	[59,60][b]
MTHFR	BC	rs1801131	c.677C>T, c.1298A>C	[61,62]	[63,64]
SOD2	BC	rs4880	p.V16A, p.A9V	[62,65,66]	
TGFB1	BC	rs1800469	NA	[67-69]	
TGFB1	BC	rs1800470	NA	[67,70-73]	
TGFB1	BC	rs1982073	NA	[74]	[64,75-77]
TP53	BC	rs1042522	p.R72P	[78,79]	[80-94]
TP53	UBC	rs1042522	p.R72P	[95]	[96-100]
TP53	CRC	rs1042522	p.R72P	[78,101-103]	[104-108]
TP53	CRC	rs17878362	NA	[78]	[104-108]
TP53	EC	rs1042522	p.R72P	[109,110]	[111]
TP53	LC	rs1042522	p.R72P	[78]	[112-117]
TP53	LC	rs17878362	NA	[78]	[112-117]
VEGFA	BC	rs3025039, rs699947	c.936C>T, c.-2578C>A	[20,45,118,119]	[120]

These findings are supported by the published literature. [a]For a different SNP (rs1329149); [b]for c.677C>T and c.1298A>C. *NA* not available.

have noticed an association with PC derived from the combination of *GSTM1* and *CYP1A1* [126,128,132,133]. Likewise, previous experimental evidence supports the association we found between the *MTHFR* gene and BC, basal cell carcinoma (BCC) [63,134] and gastric cancer (GC) [59,60]. An association was also found between *MTHFR* gene with other types of cancer, such as acute lymphoblastic leukaemia (ALL) [135,136,154], LC [137], UBC coming from interaction between *CTH* and *GSTM1* [138], CRC [139], non-Hodgkin's lymphoma (NHL) [140,141], BC [64] and HNC [142]. Specifically, in the case of NHL, the gene combination of *MTHFR* and *TYMS* might influence the susceptibility to *NHL* [140,141].

Concerning *TGFB1*, apart from the BC [64] that was confirmed from the results of our further literature search on humans and on mouse model [75,76], we have noticed also the following associations with gastric dysplasia, LC, pancreatic cancer (PanC) and BC [77,143-146]. Also, an association of *TGFB1* with CRC was found using a mouse model [147].

In addition for *TP53* gene, we have observed in the results of our meta-analysis that it is associated with BC, UBC, CRC, EC and LC [80-87,96-100,104-108,111-113,149]. We have observed also that *TP53* gene might be associated with OC [88,148], too. Concerning the literature research on knockout mice, we have confirmed the associations with BC [89-94] and LC [114-117], and we have found also associations with ovarian cancer (OVCa) [150], GC [151] and OC [152]. Moreover for the *VEGFA* gene, based on further literature *TGFB1* research, we have confirmed the association with BC [120], but we had not found any other evidence supporting the association with other types of cancer.

Correlations between groups of genes and various types of cancer

We have examined and confirmed the highly consistent gene clustering results over further literature search via STRING. Our search revealed additional types of cancer, except from the types that we have studied in our meta-analysis that seems to be related with pair of genes.

Table 2 Summary of genes and SNPs identified by further literature search as positively correlated with various cancers

Gene	Cancer type	SNPs		References
		rs number	Other name	
CCND1	OC	rs603965	c.870G>A	[26,122-124]
CCND1	PC	rs603965	c.870G>A	[125]
CYP2E1	PC	NA	NA	[126]
CYP2E1	LC	NA	NA	[127]
CYP2E1	UBC	NA	NA	[128]
CYP2E1	OC	NA	NA	[40]
ERCC2	OC	rs1799793, rs13181	p.D312N, p.K751Q	[23]
ERCC2	HNC	rs1799793, rs13181	p.D312N, p.K751Q	[129-131]
GSTP1	PC	rs1695	p.I105V	[126,128,132,133]
MTHFR	BCC	rs1801131	c.677C>T, c.1298A>C	[134]
MTHFR	ALL	rs1801131	c.677C>T, c.1298A>C	[59,135,136]
MTHFR	LC	rs1801131	c.677C>T, c.1298A>C	[137]
MTHFR	UBC	rs1801131	c.677C>T, c.1298A>C	[138]
MTHFR	CC	rs1801131	c.677C>T, c.1298A>C	[139]
MTHFR	NHL	rs1801131	c.677C>T, c.1298A>C	[140,141]
MTHFR	HNC	rs1801131	c.677C>T, c.1298A>C	[142]
TGFB1	GC	rs1982073	c.+29C>T	[143]
TGFB1	LC	rs1982073	c.+29C>T	[144]
TGFB1	PC	rs1982073	c.+29C>T	[145]
TGFB1	PC	rs1982073	c.+29C>T	[146]
TGFB1	CRC	rs1982073	c.+29C>T	[147]
TP53	EmCa	rs1042522/rs17878362	p.R72P	[148]
TP53	PC	rs1042522/rs17878362	p.R72P	[114,149]
TP53	OVCa	rs1042522/rs17878362	p.R72P	[150]
TP53	GC	rs1042522/rs17878362	p.R72P	[151]
TP53	OC	rs1042522/rs17878362	p.R72P	[152]

NA not available.

STRING database reports binding interaction between *GSTP1* and *GSTM1* genes, activating interaction between *MMP2* and *EGF* genes, between *VEGFA* and *IL1B* genes and between *MMP-9* and *IL8* genes (Table 3). The application of our machine learning method has highlighted that those pair of genes have similar association profiles and, therefore, might be involved in the same pathways. The genes that do not appear in the associations do not probably correlate with the presence of a certain type of cancer.

First, in our meta-analyses, we observed that the interaction between *IL6* and *TGFB1* genes was associated to the following types of cancer: BC, CRC, GC, LC and PC as shown in Table 4. Although further literature search on humans could not validate our highly consistent results, we discovered that these interactions are associated to additional types of cancer, such as HNC [187], CRC [158], renal cancer (RC), small cell lung cancer

Table 3 Putative gene-gene associations with various cancer types

Gene associations		Considered phenotypes	Comments	STRING confirmation	Literature confirmation
Gene 1	Gene 2				
GSTP1	*GSTM1*	4		Binding interaction	[Reference]: study type
TGFB1	*IL6*	5	4 of 5 based on 'yes'		
MMP2	*EGF*	3	Based on 'yes'	Activating interaction	
VEGFA	*IL1B*	2		Activating interaction	
MMP9	*IL8*	4	Based on 'may'	Activating interaction	KEGG: same process
MMP1	*MMP3*	5	Based on 'may'		

Table 4 Summary of gene-gene interactions and the corresponding SNPs in these genes

Gene 1	Gene 2	Cancer type	SNP's gene 1		SNP's gene 2		References (gene 1)	References (gene 2)	Supporting references
			rs number	Other name	rs number	Other name			
IL6	*TGFB1*	BC	rs1800795	c.-174G>C	rs1800469, rs1800470	c.-509C>T, p.T29C	[56]	[67-70,72-74]	[155-157]
IL6	*TGFB1*	CRC	rs1800795	c.-174G>C	rs1800470	p.T29C	[57]	[71]	[158]
IL6	*TGFB1*	GC	rs1800795	c.-174G>C	rs1800470	p.T29C	[57]	[71]	
IL6	*TGFB1*	LC	rs1800795	c.-174G>C	rs1800470	p.T29C	[57]	[71]	
IL6	*TGFB1*	PC	rs1800795	c.-174G>C	rs1800470	p.T29C	[57]	[71]	[159]
MMP2	*EGF*	LC	rs2438650	c.-1306C>T	rs4444903	c.61A>G	[160]	[161]	[162]
MMP2	*EGF*	BC	rs2438650	c.-1306C>T	rs4444903	c.61A>G	[160]	[161]	[163-165]
MMP2	*EGF*	GC	rs2438650	c.-1306C>T	rs4444903	c.61A>G	[160]	[161]	
VEGFA	*IL1B*	BC	rs3025039	c.936C>T	rs114327	NA	[166-169]	[170]	[171]
VEGFA	*IL1B*	BC	rs699947	c.-2578C>A	rs1143634	NA	[172]	[170]	[171]
VEGFA	*IL1B*	BC	NA	NA	rs16944	NA	NA	[170]	[171]
VEGFA	*IL1B*	GC	rs3025039	c.936C>T	rs3087258	NA	[45]	[173]	
VEGFA	*IL1B*	GC	rs699947	c.-2578C>A	NA	IL1B-31-ami	[95]	[173]	
MMP9	*IL8*	BC	rs3918242	c.-1562C>T	rs4073	c.-251A>T	[160]	[174]	[171]
MMP9	*IL8*	CRC	rs3918242	c.-1562C>T	rs4073	c.-251A>T	[160]	[174]	
MMP9	*IL8*	GC	rs3918242	c.-1562C>T	rs4073	c.-251A>T	[160]	[175]	
MMP9	*IL8*	LC	rs3918242	c.-1562C>T	rs4073	c.-251A>T	[160]	[174]	
MMP1	*MMP3*	BC	rs1799750	c.-1607 1G>2G	rs3025058	c.-1171 5A>6A	[176]	[176]	
MMP1	*MMP3*	CRC	rs1799750	c.-1607 1G>2G	rs3025058	c.-1171 5A>6A	[176]	[176]	
MMP1	*MMP3*	HNC	rs1799750	c.-1607 1G>2G	rs3025058	c.-1171 5A>6A	[176]	[176]	
MMP1	*MMP3*	LC	rs1799750	c.-1607 1G>2G	rs3025058	c.-1171 5A>6A	[176]	[176]	[177,178]
MMP1	*MMP3*	OVCa	rs1799750	c.-1607 1G>2G	rs3025058	c.-1171 5A>6A	[176]	[176]	
GSTP1	*GSTM1*	CRC	rs1695	p.I105V	rs1065411	GSTM1 present/null	[45]	[179]	
GSTP1	*GSTM1*	BC	rs1695	p.I105V	rs1065412	GSTM1 present/null	[180]	[181]	[182,183]
GSTP1	*GSTM1*	OVCa	rs1695	p.I105V	rs1065413	GSTM1 present/null	[184]	[184]	
GSTP1	*GSTM1*	UBC	rs1695	p.I105V	rs1065414	GSTM1 present/null	[185]	[186]	

These were identified in our meta-analysis. Their correlation with various cancer types is also shown. *NA* not available.

[188], malignant melanoma (MM) [189-192] and OVCa [193]. Additionally, regarding our further research on the interaction between *IL6* and *TGFB1* genes on mouse models, we have confirmed our initial results principally for BC [155-157] and PC [159] and have noticed associations with epithelial cancer [194], skin tumour [195], LC [196], OVCa and cervical cancer (CC) [197,198] and HNSCC [199]. Second, we found that the interaction between *MMP-2* and *EGF* was associated with LC, BC and GC (Table 4). Subsequently with a further literature search, we confirmed the association with BC osteolysis [163,164] and also found new associations with EC [200], LC, RC and PC [162]. Furthermore, in some cases, we have observed the association of the aforementioned genes with OSCC [201]. In this study, *EGF* induced *MMP-1* expression that is required for type I collagen degradation. In addition, *MMP-1* is also associated with human papillomavirus [202] and BC [165].

Another interesting interaction that was revealed from our analysis was between the *VEGFA* and *IL1B* genes that were associated with BC and GC (Table 4). After proceeding with a further literature search, we have not found similar results - except from one report [171] - but we have identified additional associations with HNC, ALL, laryngeal carcinoma and MM [203-206]. For *MMP-9* and *IL8* interaction, there was no study confirming our initial results for BC, CRC and GC on neither humans nor mouse models. We have observed though that there was evidence for an association with nasopharyngeal carcinoma [171], LC [177,178] and UBC [207]. Similarly, we could not find any study that could support the interactions between *MMP-1* and *MMP-3* and *GSTP1* with *GSTM1*, although two studies confirmed that *GSTP1* and *GSTM1* interactions could be associated with BC [182,183] (Table 4).

Indications from further literature search on human models revealed associations for *MMP-1* and *MMP-3* with

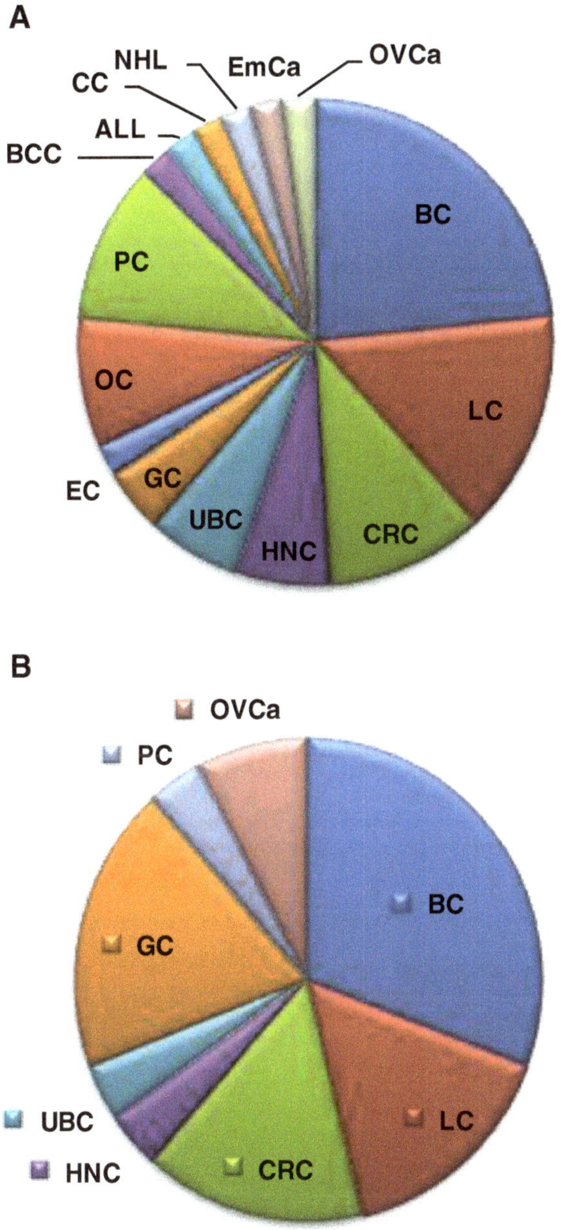

Figure 1 The distribution of various cancer types. According to (**A**) the number of SNPs per cancer type and (**B**) the number of genes or gene correlations per cancer type. By extrapolating the data in Tables 1, 2, 3 and 4, it seems that the number of genome variations and genes is profoundly bigger in BC, probably indicating that this type of cancer is not a single disease but, most likely, a spectrum of related disease states.

types of cancer such as BCC, metatypical cancer of the skin [208], colorectal adenoma and RC [209,210], and for *GSTP1* and *GSTM1*, endometrial cancer (EmCa) [211], LC [212], multiple myeloma (observed no significant association to prostatic adenoma and adenocarcinoma) [213], PC [133,214], ALL [215], chronic myeloid leukaemia [216] and PanC [217].

We have then attempted to depict the various types of cancers according to the number of SNPs and genes and/or gene clusters found from our meta-analysis to be meaningfully associated with certain cancer types. Our data indicate that BC is correlated more often than the other types of cancer both with the number of SNPs (Figure 1A) as well as with the number of genes or gene clusters (Figure 1B). This observation underlies the heterogeneity of BC, indicating that it is, most likely, not a single disease but a spectrum of related disease states.

Conclusions

In essence, our meta-analysis study generated clusters of genes and diseases, many of which proved to be independent of the criteria used, which suggests that these clusters are most likely biologically meaningful. Preliminary study of some clusters and of our results shows that indeed these genes interact. As regards the associations, with a further literature analysis on human and mouse models, we have also found meaningful gene associations related to other cancer types not previously reported in the literature, an observation that warrants further investigation.

Competing interests

The authors declare that they have no competing interests.

Authors' contributions

ZL carried out the data collection, result analysis and participated in the manuscript preparation. EG participated in the manuscript preparation and data analysis. MF participated in the result and statistical analysis and manuscript revision. EK participated in the data collection and manuscript revision. JCN carried out the result and statistical analysis and participated in the manuscript preparation. HPK participated in the manuscript preparation. GPP participated in the design of the study, data analysis and manuscript preparation. CP conceived of the study, participated in its design and coordination as well as manuscript preparation. All authors read and approved for the final manuscript.

Acknowledgements

This study was conducted to fulfil the requirements of an undergraduate thesis, jointly with the Universities of Trieste, Italy and Patras, Greece. This work was partly funded by the University of Patras research budget and a European Commission grant (GEN2PHEN; FP7-200754) to GPP.

Author details

[1]Faculty of Mathematical, Physical and Natural Sciences, Department of Biological Sciences, University of Trieste, Trieste 34128, Italy. [2]School of Health Sciences, Department of Pharmacy, University of Patras, University Campus, Rio, Patras 26504, Greece. [3]Clinical Oncology Laboratory, Division of Oncology, Department of Medicine, University of Patras, Rio, Patras 26504, Greece. [4]School of Computing and Information Systems, Faculty of Science, Engineering and Computing, Kingston University, London SW15 3DW, UK.

References

1. Lea IA, Jackson MA, Li X, Bailey S, Peddada SD, Dunnick JK: **Genetic pathways and mutation profiles of human cancers: site- and exposure-specific patterns.** *Carcinogenesis* 2007, **28**(9):1851–1858.
2. Dutt A, Beroukhim R: **Single nucleotide polymorphism array analysis of cancer.** *Curr Opin Oncol* 2007, **19**(1):43–49.
3. Chung CC, Chanock SJ: **Current status of genome-wide association studies in cancer.** *Hum Genet* 2011, **130**(1):59–78.
4. Rae JM, Skaar TC, Hilsenbeck SG, Oesterreich S: **The role of single nucleotide polymorphisms in breast cancer metastasis.** *Breast Cancer Res* 2008, **10**(1):301.
5. Teraoka SN, Bernstein JL, Reiner AS, Haile RW, Bernstein L, Lynch CF, Malone KE, Stovall M, Capanu M, Liang X, Smith SA, Mychaleckyj J, Hou X, Mellemkjaer L, Boice JD Jr, Siniard A, Duggan D, Thomas DC, WECARE Study Collaborative Group, Concannon P: **Single nucleotide polymorphisms associated with risk for contralateral breast cancer in the women's environment, cancer, and radiation epidemiology (WECARE) study.** *Breast Cancer Res* 2011, **13**(6):R114.
6. Inaki K, Liu ET: **Structural mutations in cancer: mechanistic and functional insights.** *Trends Genet* 2012, **28**(11):550–559.
7. You JS, Jones PA: **Cancer genetics and epigenetics: two sides of the same coin?** *Cancer Cell* 2012, **22**(1):9–20.
8. Lopez-Lazaro M: **A new view of carcinogenesis and an alternative approach to cancer therapy.** *Mol Med* 2010, **16**(3–4):144–153.
9. Rasmussen MD, Deshpande MS, Karypis G, Johnson J, Crow JA, Retzel EF: **wCLUTO: a Web-enabled clustering toolkit.** *Plant Physiol* 2003, **133**(2):510–516.
10. Szklarczyk D, Franceschini A, Kuhn M, Simonovic M, Roth A, Minguez P, Doerks T, Stark M, Muller J, Bork P, Jensen LJ, von Mering C: **The STRING database in 2011: functional interaction networks of proteins, globally integrated and scored.** *Nucleic Acids Res* 2011, **39**(Database issue):D561–D568.
11. *Search Tool for the Retrieval of Interacting Genes/Proteins.* www.string-db.org.
12. Jiang Z, Li C, Xu Y, Cai S, Wang X: **Associations between XPD polymorphisms and risk of breast cancer: a meta-analysis.** *Breast Cancer Res Treat* 2010, **123**(1):203–212.
13. Qiu LX, Yao L, Zhang J, Zhu XD, Zhao XM, Xue K, Mao C, Chen B, Zhan P, Yuan H, Hu X-C: **XPD Lys751Gln polymorphism and breast cancer susceptibility: a meta-analysis involving 28,709 subjects.** *Breast Cancer Res Treat* 2010, **124**(1):229–235.
14. Wang HC, Liu CS, Wang CH, Tsai RY, Tsai CW, Wang RF, Chang CH, Chen YS, Chiu CF, Bau DT, Huang CY: **Significant association of XPD Asp312Asn polymorphism with breast cancer in Taiwanese patients.** *Chin J Physiol* 2010, **53**(2):130–135.
15. Han W, Kim KY, Yang SJ, Noh DY, Kang D, Kwack K: **SNP-SNP interactions between DNA repair genes were associated with breast cancer risk in a Korean population.** *Cancer* 2012, **118**(3):594–602.
16. Hussien YM, Gharib AF, Awad HA, Karam RA, Elsawy WH: **Impact of DNA repair genes polymorphism (XPD and XRCC1) on the risk of breast cancer in Egyptian female patients.** *Mol Biol Rep* 2012, **39**(2):1895–1901.
17. Yin J, Vogel U, Wang C, Liang D, Ma Y, Wang H, Yue L, Liu D, Ma J, Sun X: **Hapmap-based evaluation of ERCC2, PPP1R13L, and ERCC1 and lung cancer risk in a Chinese population.** *Environ Mol Mutagen* 2012, **53**(3):239–245.
18. Yao L, Qiu LX, Yu L, Yang Z, Yu XJ, Zhong Y, Hu XC: **The association between ERCC2 Asp312Asn polymorphism and breast cancer risk: a meta-analysis involving 22,766 subjects.** *Breast Cancer Res Treat* 2010, **123**(1):227–231.
19. Zhang J, Gu SY, Zhang P, Jia Z, Chang JH: **ERCC2 Lys751Gln polymorphism is associated with lung cancer among Caucasians.** *Eur J Cancer* 2010, **46**(13):2479–2484.
20. Zhan P, Wang Q, Wei SZ, Wang J, Qian Q, Yu LK, Song Y: **ERCC2/XPD Lys751Gln and Asp312Asn gene polymorphism and lung cancer risk: a meta-analysis involving 22 case–control studies.** *J Thorac Oncol* 2010, **5**(9):1337–1345.
21. Yin J, Vogel U, Ma Y, Qi R, Wang H, Yue L, Liang D, Wang C, Li X, Song T: **HapMap-based study of a region encompassing ERCC1 and ERCC2 related to lung cancer susceptibility in a Chinese population.** *Mutat Res* 2011, **713**(1–2):1–7.
22. Christiani DC: **ERCC2/XPD polymorphisms and lung cancer risk.** *J Thorac Oncol* 2011, **6**(1):233. author reply 233–235.
23. Zhang J, Qiu LX, Leaw SJ, Hu XC, Chang JH: **The association between XPD Asp312Asn polymorphism and lung cancer risk: a meta-analysis including 16,949 subjects.** *Med Oncol* 2011, **28**(3):655–660.
24. Sergentanis TN, Economopoulos KP: **Cyclin D1 G870A polymorphism and breast cancer risk: a meta-analysis comprising 9,911 cases and 11,171 controls.** *Mol Biol Rep* 2011, **38**(8):4955–4963.
25. Millar EK, Dean JL, McNeil CM, O'Toole SA, Henshall SM, Tran T, Lin J, Quong A, Comstock CE, Witkiewicz A, Musgrove EA, Rui H, Lemarchand L, Setiawan VW, Haiman CA, Knudsen KE, Sutherland RL, Knudsen ES: **Cyclin D1b protein expression in breast cancer is independent of cyclin D1a and associated with poor disease outcome.** *Oncogene* 2009, **28**(15):1812–1820.
26. Miyashita H, Mori S, Tanda N, Nakayama K, Kanzaki A, Sato A, Morikawa H, Motegi K, Takebayashi Y, Fukumoto M: **Loss of heterozygosity of nucleotide excision repair factors in sporadic oral squamous cell carcinoma using microdissected tissue.** *Oncol Rep* 2001, **8**(5):1133–1138.
27. Ghosh-Choudhury N, Ghosh-Choudhury G, Celeste A, Ghosh PM, Moyer M, Abboud SL, Kreisberg J: **Bone morphogenetic protein-2 induces cyclin kinase inhibitor p21 and hypophosphorylation of retinoblastoma protein in estradiol-treated MCF-7 human breast cancer cells.** *Biochim Biophys Acta* 2000, **1497**(2):186–196.
28. Musgrove EA, Hui R, Sweeney KJ, Watts CK, Sutherland RL: **Cyclins and breast cancer.** *J Mammary Gland Biol Neoplasia* 1996, **1**(2):153–162.
29. Sutherland RL, Hamilton JA, Sweeney KJ, Watts CK, Musgrove EA: **Expression and regulation of cyclin genes in breast cancer.** *Acta Oncol* 1995, **34**(5):651–656.
30. Taneja P, Frazier DP, Kendig RD, Maglic D, Sugiyama T, Kai F, Taneja NK, Inoue K: **MMTV mouse models and the diagnostic values of MMTV-like sequences in human breast cancer.** *Expert Rev Mol Diagn* 2009, **9**(5):423–440.
31. Yang C, Ionescu-Tiba V, Burns K, Gadd M, Zukerberg L, Louis DN, Sgroi D, Schmidt EV: **The role of the cyclin D1-dependent kinases in ErbB2-mediated breast cancer.** *Am J Pathol* 2004, **164**(3):1031–1038.
32. Zhou GW, Hu J, Li Q: **CYP2E1 PstI/RsaI polymorphism and colorectal cancer risk: a meta-analysis.** *World J Gastroenterol* 2010, **16**(23):2949–2953.
33. Silva TD, Felipe AV, Pimenta CA, Barao K, Forones NM: **CYP2E1 RsaI and 96-bp insertion genetic polymorphisms associated with risk for colorectal cancer.** *Genet Mol Res* 2012, **11**(3):3138–3145.
34. Sameer AS, Nissar S, Qadri Q, Alam S, Baba SM, Siddiqi MA: **Role of CYP2E1 genotypes in susceptibility to colorectal cancer in the Kashmiri population.** *Hum Genomics* 2011, **5**(6):530–537.
35. Yang H, Zhou Y, Zhou Z, Liu J, Yuan X, Matsuo K, Takezaki T, Tajima K, Cao J: **A novel polymorphism rs1329149 of CYP2E1 and a known polymorphism rs671 of ALDH2 of alcohol metabolizing enzymes are associated with colorectal cancer in a southwestern Chinese population.** *Cancer Epidemiol Biomarkers Prev* 2009, **18**(9):2522–2527.
36. Kury S, Buecher B, Robiou-du-Pont S, Scoul C, Sebille V, Colman H, Le Houerou C, Le Neel T, Bourdon J, Faroux R, Ollivry J, Lafraise B, Chupin LD, Bézieau S: **Combinations of cytochrome P450 gene polymorphisms enhancing the risk for sporadic colorectal cancer related to red meat consumption.** *Cancer Epidemiol Biomarkers Prev* 2007, **16**(7):1460–1467.
37. Chen K, Jin MJ, Fan CH, Song L, Jiang QT, Yu WP, Ma XY, Yao KY: **A case–control study on the association between genetic polymorphisms of metabolic enzymes and the risk of colorectal cancer.** *Zhonghua Liu Xing Bing Xue Za Zhi* 2005, **26**(9):659–664.
38. van der Logt EM, Bergevoet SM, Roelofs HM, Te Morsche RH, Dijk Y, Wobbes T, Nagengast FM, Peters WH: **Role of epoxide hydrolase, NAD(P)H: quinone oxidoreductase, cytochrome P450 2E1 or alcohol dehydrogenase genotypes in susceptibility to colorectal cancer.** *Mutat Res* 2006, **593**(1–2):39–49.
39. Landi S, Gemignani F, Moreno V, Gioia-Patricola L, Chabrier A, Guino E, Navarro M, de Oca J, Capella G, Canzian F: **A comprehensive analysis of phase I and phase II metabolism gene polymorphisms and risk of colorectal cancer.** *Pharmacogenet Genomics* 2005, **15**(8):535–546.
40. Cotterchio M, Boucher BA, Manno M, Gallinger S, Okey AB, Harper PA: **Red meat intake, doneness, polymorphisms in genes that encode carcinogen-metabolizing enzymes, and colorectal cancer risk.** *Cancer Epidemiol Biomarkers Prev* 2008, **17**(11):3098–3107.
41. Chen J, Huang XF: **The signal pathways in azoxymethane-induced colon cancer and preventive implications.** *Cancer Biol Ther* 2009, **8**(14):1313–1317.

42. Tang K, Li Y, Zhang Z, Gu Y, Xiong Y, Feng G, He L, Qin S: **The PstI/RsaI and DraI polymorphisms of CYP2E1 and head and neck cancer risk: a meta-analysis based on 21 case–control studies.** *BMC Cancer* 2010, **10**:575.
43. Lu D, Yu X, Du Y: **Meta-analyses of the effect of cytochrome P450 2E1 gene polymorphism on the risk of head and neck cancer.** *Mol Biol Rep* 2011, **38**(4):2409–2416.
44. Garcia SM, Curioni OA, de Carvalho MB, Gattas GJ: **Polymorphisms in alcohol metabolizing genes and the risk of head and neck cancer in a Brazilian population.** *Alcohol Alcohol* 2010, **45**(1):6–12.
45. Economopoulos KP, Sergentanis TN: **GSTM1, GSTT1, GSTP1, GSTA1 and colorectal cancer risk: a comprehensive meta-analysis.** *Eur J Cancer* 2010, **46**(9):1617–1631.
46. Ebrahimkhani S, Asgharian AM, Nourinaier B, Ebrahimkhani K, Vali N, Abbasi F, Zali MR: **Association of GSTM1, GSTT1, GSTP1 and CYP2E1 single nucleotide polymorphisms with colorectal cancer in Iran.** *Pathol Oncol Res* 2012, **18**(3):651–656.
47. Sameer AS, Qadri Q, Siddiqi MA: **GSTP1 I105V polymorphism and susceptibility to colorectal cancer in Kashmiri population.** *DNA Cell Biol* 2012, **31**(1):74–79.
48. Wang J, Joshi AD, Corral R, Siegmund KD, Marchand LL, Martinez ME, Haile RW, Ahnen DJ, Sandler RS, Lance P, Stern MC: **Carcinogen metabolism genes, red meat and poultry intake, and colorectal cancer risk.** *Int J Cancer* 2012, **130**(8):1898–1907.
49. Sainz J, Rudolph A, Hein R, Hoffmeister M, Buch S, von Schonfels W, Hampe J, Schafmayer C, Volzke H, Frank B, Brenner H, Försti A, Hemminki K, Chang-Claude J: **Association of genetic polymorphisms in ESR2, HSD17B1, ABCB1, and SHBG genes with colorectal cancer risk.** *Endocr Relat Cancer* 2011, **18**(2):265–276.
50. Jones BA, Christensen AR, Wise JP Sr, Yu H: **Glutathione S-transferase polymorphisms and survival in African-American and white colorectal cancer patients.** *Cancer Epidemiol* 2009, **33**(3–4):249–256.
51. Skjelbred CF, Saebo M, Hjartaker A, Grotmol T, Hansteen IL, Tveit KM, Hoff G, Kure EH: **Meat, vegetables and genetic polymorphisms and the risk of colorectal carcinomas and adenomas.** *BMC Cancer* 2007, **7**:228.
52. Talseth BA, Meldrum C, Suchy J, Kurzawski G, Lubinski J, Scott RJ: **Genetic polymorphisms in xenobiotic clearance genes and their influence on disease expression in hereditary nonpolyposis colorectal cancer patients.** *Cancer Epidemiol Biomarkers Prev* 2006, **15**(11):2307–2310.
53. Romero RZ, Morales R, Garcia F, Huarriz M, Bandres E, De la Haba J, Gomez A, Aranda E, Garcia-Foncillas J: **Potential application of GSTT1-null genotype in predicting toxicity associated to 5-fluouracil irinotecan and leucovorin regimen in advanced stage colorectal cancer patients.** *Oncol Rep* 2006, **16**(3):497–503.
54. Probst-Hensch NM, Sun CL, Van Den Berg D, Ceschi M, Koh WP, Yu MC: **The effect of the cyclin D1 (CCND1) A870G polymorphism on colorectal cancer risk is modified by glutathione-S-transferase polymorphisms and isothiocyanate intake in the Singapore Chinese health study.** *Carcinogenesis* 2006, **27**(12):2475–2482.
55. Gaustadnes M, Orntoft TF, Jensen JL, Torring N: **Validation of the use of DNA pools and primer extension in association studies of sporadic colorectal cancer for selection of candidate SNPs.** *Hum Mutat* 2006, **27**(2):187–194.
56. Yu KD, Di GH, Fan L, Chen AX, Yang C, Shao ZM: **Lack of an association between a functional polymorphism in the interleukin-6 gene promoter and breast cancer risk: a meta-analysis involving 25,703 subjects.** *Breast Cancer Res Treat* 2010, **122**(2):483–488.
57. Xu B, Niu XB, Wang ZD, Cheng W, Tong N, Mi YY, Min ZC, Tao J, Li PC, Zhang W, Wu HF, Zhang ZD, Wang ZJ, Hua LX, Feng NH, Wang XR: **IL-6–174G>C polymorphism and cancer risk: a meta-analysis involving 29,377 cases and 37,739 controls.** *Mol Biol Rep* 2011, **38**(4):2589–2596.
58. Dong X, Wu J, Liang P, Li J, Yuan L, Liu X: **Methylenetetrahydrofolate reductase C677T and A1298C polymorphisms and gastric cancer: a meta-analysis.** *Arch Med Res* 2010, **41**(2):125–133.
59. Wang Z, Chen JQ, Liu JL, Qin XG, Huang Y: **Polymorphisms in ERCC1, GSTs, TS and MTHFR predict clinical outcomes of gastric cancer patients treated with platinum/5-Fu-based chemotherapy: a systematic review.** *BMC Gastroenterol* 2012, **12**:137.
60. Balassiano K, Lima S, Jenab M, Overvad K, Tjonneland A, Boutron-Ruault MC, Clavel-Chapelon F, Canzian F, Kaaks R, Boeing H, Meidtner K, Trichopoulou A, Laglou P, Vineis P, Panico S, Palli D, Grioni S, Tumino R, Lund E, Bueno-de-Mesquita HB, Numans ME, Peeters PH, Ramon Quirós J, Sánchez MJ, Navarro C, Ardanaz E, Dorronsoro M, Hallmans G, Stenling R, *et al*: **Aberrant DNA methylation of cancer-associated genes in gastric cancer in the European Prospective Investigation into Cancer and Nutrition (EPIC-EURGAST).** *Cancer Lett* 2011, **311**(1):85–95.
61. Qi X, Ma X, Yang X, Fan L, Zhang Y, Zhang F, Chen L, Zhou Y, Jiang J: **Methylenetetrahydrofolate reductase polymorphisms and breast cancer risk: a meta-analysis from 41 studies with 16,480 cases and 22,388 controls.** *Breast Cancer Res Treat* 2010, **123**(2):499–506.
62. Qiu LX, Zhang J, Li WH, Zhang QL, Yu H, Wang BY, Wang LP, Wang JL, Wang HJ, Liu XJ, Luo ZG, Wu XH: **Lack of association between methylenetetrahydrofolate reductase gene A1298C polymorphism and breast cancer susceptibility.** *Mol Biol Rep* 2011, **38**(4):2295–2299.
63. Perel'muter VM, Zav'ialova MV, Vtorushin SV, Slonimskaia EM, Kritskaia NG, Garbukov E, Litviakov NV, Stakhceva MN, Babyshkina NN, Malinovskaia EA, Denisov EV, Grigor'eva ES, Nazarenko MS, Sennikov SV, Goreva EP, Kozlov VA, Voevoda MI, Maksimov VN, Beliavskaia VA, Cherdyntseva NV: **Genetic and clinical and pathological characteristics of breast cancer in premenopausal and postmenopausal women.** *Adv Gerontol* 2008, **21**(4):643–653.
64. Stevens VL, McCullough ML, Pavluck AL, Talbot JT, Feigelson HS, Thun MJ, Calle EE: **Association of polymorphisms in one-carbon metabolism genes and postmenopausal breast cancer incidence.** *Cancer Epidemiol Biomarkers Prev* 2007, **16**(6):1140–1147.
65. Qiu LX, Mao C, Yao L, Yu KD, Zhan P, Chen B, Liu HG, Yuan H, Zhang J, Xue K, Hu XC: **XRCC3 5'-UTR and IVS5-14 polymorphisms and breast cancer susceptibility: a meta-analysis.** *Breast Cancer Res Treat* 2010, **122**(2):489–493.
66. Chen Y, Pei J: **Possible risk modifications in the association between MnSOD Ala-9Val polymorphism and breast cancer risk: subgroup analysis and evidence-based sample size calculation for a future trial.** *Breast Cancer Res Treat* 2011, **125**(2):495–504.
67. Qi X, Zhang F, Yang X, Fan L, Zhang Y, Chen L, Zhou Y, Chen X, Zhong L, Jiang J: **Transforming growth factor-beta1 polymorphisms and breast cancer risk: a meta-analysis based on 27 case–control studies.** *Breast Cancer Res Treat* 2010, **122**(1):273–279.
68. Huang Y, Hao Y, Li B, Xie J, Qian J, Chao C, Yu L: **Lack of significant association between TGF-beta1-590C/T polymorphism and breast cancer risk: a meta-analysis.** *Med Oncol* 2011, **28**(2):424–428.
69. Woo SU, Park KH, Woo OH, Yang DS, Kim AR, Lee ES, Lee JB, Kim YH, Kim JS, Seo JH: **Association of a TGF-beta1 gene −509 C/T polymorphism with breast cancer risk: a meta-analysis.** *Breast Cancer Res Treat* 2010, **124**(2):481–485.
70. Gu D, Zhuang L, Huang H, Cao P, Wang D, Tang J, Chen J: **TGFB1 T29C polymorphism and breast cancer risk: a meta-analysis based on 10,417 cases and 11,455 controls.** *Breast Cancer Res Treat* 2010, **123**(3):857–861.
71. Wei BB, Xi B, Wang R, Bai JM, Chang JK, Zhang YY, Yoneda R, Su JT, Hua LX: **TGFbeta1 T29C polymorphism and cancer risk: a meta-analysis based on 40 case–control studies.** *Cancer Genet Cytogenet* 2010, **196**(1):68–75.
72. Ma X, Chen C, Xiong H, Li Y: **Transforming growth factorbeta1 L10P variant plays an active role on the breast cancer susceptibility in Caucasian: evidence from 10,392 cases and 11,697 controls.** *Breast Cancer Res Treat* 2010, **124**(2):453–457.
73. Huang Y, Li B, Qian J, Xie J, Yu L: **TGF-beta1 29T/C polymorphism and breast cancer risk: a meta-analysis involving 25,996 subjects.** *Breast Cancer Res Treat* 2010, **123**(3):863–868.
74. Qiu LX, Yao L, Mao C, Chen B, Zhan P, Xue K, Zhang J, Yuan H, Hu XC: **TGFB1 L10P polymorphism is associated with breast cancer susceptibility: evidence from a meta-analysis involving 47,817 subjects.** *Breast Cancer Res Treat* 2010, **123**(2):563–567.
75. Radisky DC, Hartmann LC: **Mammary involution and breast cancer risk: transgenic models and clinical studies.** *J Mammary Gland Biol Neoplasia* 2009, **14**(2):181–191.
76. Stuelten CH, Busch JI, Tang B, Flanders KC, Oshima A, Sutton E, Karpova TS, Roberts AB, Wakefield LM, Niederhuber JE: **Transient tumor-fibroblast interactions increase tumor cell malignancy by a TGF-Beta mediated mechanism in a mouse xenograft model of breast cancer.** *PLoS One* 2010, **5**(3):e9832.
77. Zheng W: **Genetic polymorphisms in the transforming growth factor-beta signaling pathways and breast cancer risk and survival.** *Methods Mol Biol* 2009, **472**:265–277.

78. Hu Z, Li X, Qu X, He Y, Ring BZ, Song E, Su L: **Intron 3 16 bp duplication polymorphism of TP53 contributes to cancer susceptibility: a meta-analysis.** *Carcinogenesis* 2010, **31**(4):643–647.
79. Ma Y, Yang J, Liu Z, Zhang P, Yang Z, Wang Y, Qin H: **No significant association between the TP53 codon 72 polymorphism and breast cancer risk: a meta-analysis of 21 studies involving 24,063 subjects.** *Breast Cancer Res Treat* 2011, **125**(1):201–205.
80. Chunder N, Mandal S, Roy A, Roychoudhury S, Panda CK: **Differential association of BRCA1 and BRCA2 genes with some breast cancer-associated genes in early and late onset breast tumors.** *Ann Surg Oncol* 2004, **11**(12):1045–1055.
81. Rebbeck TR: **Inherited genetic predisposition in breast cancer. A population-based perspective.** *Cancer* 1999, **86**(11 Suppl):2493–2501.
82. Rossner P Jr, Gammon MD, Zhang YJ, Terry MB, Hibshoosh H, Memeo L, Mansukhani M, Long CM, Garbowski G, Agrawal M, Agrawal M, Kalra TS, Gaudet MM, Teitelbaum SL, Neugut AI, Santella RM: **Mutations in p53, p53 protein overexpression and breast cancer survival.** *J Cell Mol Med* 2009, **13**(9B):3847–3857.
83. Nkhata KJ, Ray A, Schuster TF, Grossmann ME, Cleary MP: **Effects of adiponectin and leptin co-treatment on human breast cancer cell growth.** *Oncol Rep* 2009, **21**(6):1611–1619.
84. Palanca Suela S, Esteban Cardenosa E, Barragan Gonzalez E, de Juan Jimenez I, Chirivella Gonzalez I, Segura Huerta A, Guillen Ponce C, Montalar Salcedo J, Martinez de Duenas E, Castel Sanchez V, Bolufer Gilabert P, Group for Assessment of Hereditary Cancer of Valencia Community: **CASP8 D302H polymorphism delays the age of onset of breast cancer in BRCA1 and BRCA2 carriers.** *Breast Cancer Res Treat* 2010, **119**(1):87–93.
85. Fanale D, Amodeo V, Corsini LR, Rizzo S, Bazan V, Russo A: **Breast cancer genome-wide association studies: there is strength in numbers.** *Oncogene* 2012, **31**(17):2121–2128.
86. Cherdyntseva NV, Denisov EV, Litviakov NV, Maksimov VN, Malinovskaya EA, Babyshkina NN, Slonimskaya EM, Voevoda MI, Choinzonov EL: **Crosstalk between the FGFR2 and TP53 genes in breast cancer: data from an association study and epistatic interaction analysis.** *DNA Cell Biol* 2012, **31**(3):306–316.
87. Lo Nigro C, Vivenza D, Monteverde M, Lattanzio L, Gojis O, Garrone O, Comino A, Merlano M, Quinlan PR, Syed N, Purdie CA, Thompson A, Palmieri C, Crook T: **High frequency of complex TP53 mutations in CNS metastases from breast cancer.** *Br J Cancer* 2012, **106**(2):397–404.
88. Mathoulin-Portier MP, Viens P, Cowen D, Bertucci F, Houvenaeghel G, Geneix J, Puig B, Bardou VJ, Jacquemier J: **Prognostic value of simultaneous expression of p21 and mdm2 in breast carcinomas treated by adjuvant chemotherapy with antracyclin.** *Oncol Rep* 2000, **7**(3):675–680.
89. Blackburn AC, Jerry DJ: **Knockout and transgenic mice of Trp53: what have we learned about p53 in breast cancer?** *Breast Cancer Res* 2002, **4**(3):101–111.
90. Bennett CN, Green JE: **Genomic analyses as a guide to target identification and preclinical testing of mouse models of breast cancer.** *Toxicol Pathol* 2010, **38**(1):88–95.
91. Girardini JE, Napoli M, Piazza S, Rustighi A, Marotta C, Radaelli E, Capaci V, Jordan L, Quinlan P, Thompson A, Mano M, Rosato A, Crook T, Scanziani E, Means AR, Lozano G, Schneider C, Del Sal G: **A Pin1/mutant p53 axis promotes aggressiveness in breast cancer.** *Cancer Cell* 2011, **20**(1):79–91.
92. Alsner J, Jensen V, Kyndi M, Offersen BV, Vu P, Borresen-Dale AL, Overgaard J: **A comparison between p53 accumulation determined by immunohistochemistry and TP53 mutations as prognostic variables in tumours from breast cancer patients.** *Acta Oncol* 2008, **47**(4):600–607.
93. Bourdon JC, Khoury MP, Diot A, Baker L, Fernandes K, Aoubala M, Quinlan P, Purdie CA, Jordan LB, Prats AC, Lane DP, Thompson AM: **p53 mutant breast cancer patients expressing p53gamma have as good a prognosis as wild-type p53 breast cancer patients.** *Breast Cancer Res* 2011, **13**(1):R7.
94. Besaratinia A, Pfeifer GP: **Applications of the human p53 knock-in (Hupki) mouse model for human carcinogen testing.** *FASEB J* 2010, **24**(8):2612–2619.
95. Jiang DK, Ren WH, Yao L, Wang WZ, Peng B, Yu L: **Meta-analysis of association between TP53 Arg72Pro polymorphism and bladder cancer risk.** *Urology* 2010, **76**(3):765–767. e761.
96. Burger M, Burger SJ, Denzinger S, Wild PJ, Wieland WF, Blaszyk H, Obermann EC, Stoehr R, Hartmann A: **Elevated microsatellite instability at selected tetranucleotide repeats does not correlate with clinicopathologic features of bladder cancer.** *Eur Urol* 2006, **50**(4):770–775. discussion 776.
97. Zuiverloon TC, Abas CS, van der Keur KA, Vermeij M, Tjin SS, van Tilborg AG, Busstra M, Zwarthoff EC: **In-depth investigation of the molecular pathogenesis of bladder cancer in a unique 26-year old patient with extensive multifocal disease: a case report.** *BMC Urol* 2010, **10**:5.
98. Kompier LC, van Tilborg AA, Zwarthoff EC: **Bladder cancer: novel molecular characteristics, diagnostic, and therapeutic implications.** *Urol Oncol* 2010, **28**(1):91–96.
99. Jarmalaite S, Andrekute R, Scesnaite A, Suziedelis K, Husgafvel-Pursiainen K, Jankevicius F: **Promoter hypermethylation in tumour suppressor genes and response to interleukin-2 treatment in bladder cancer: a pilot study.** *J Cancer Res Clin Oncol* 2010, **136**(6):847–854.
100. Lin HY, Huang CH, Yu TJ, Wu WJ, Yang MC, Lung FW: **p53 codon 72 polymorphism as a progression index for bladder cancer.** *Oncol Rep* 2012, **27**(4):1193–1199.
101. Dahabreh IJ, Linardou H, Bouzika P, Varvarigou V, Murray S: **TP53 Arg72Pro polymorphism and colorectal cancer risk: a systematic review and meta-analysis.** *Cancer Epidemiol Biomarkers Prev* 2010, **19**(7):1840–1847.
102. Economopoulos KP, Sergentanis TN, Zagouri F, Zografos GC: **Association between p53 Arg72Pro polymorphism and colorectal cancer risk: a meta-analysis.** *Onkologie* 2010, **33**(12):666–674.
103. Wang JJ, Zheng Y, Sun L, Wang L, Yu PB, Dong JH, Zhang L, Xu J, Shi W, Ren YC: **TP53 codon 72 polymorphism and colorectal cancer susceptibility: a meta-analysis.** *Mol Biol Rep* 2011, **38**(8):4847–4853.
104. Goodman JE, Mechanic LE, Luke BT, Ambs S, Chanock S, Harris CC: **Exploring SNP-SNP interactions and colon cancer risk using polymorphism interaction analysis.** *Int J Cancer* 2006, **118**(7):1790–1797.
105. Zhang Y, Liu L, Tang Y, Chen C, Wang Q, Xu J, Yang C, Miao X, Wei S, Chen J, Nie S: **Polymorphisms in TP53 and MDM2 contribute to higher risk of colorectal cancer in Chinese population: a hospital-based, case–control study.** *Mol Biol Rep* 2012, **39**(10):9661–9668.
106. Lopez I, PO L, Tucci P, Alvarez-Valin F, AC R, Marin M: **Different mutation profiles associated to P53 accumulation in colorectal cancer.** *Gene* 2012, **499**(1):81–87.
107. Kanaan Z, Rai SN, Eichenberger MR, Barnes C, Dworkin AM, Weller C, Cohen E, Roberts H, Keskey B, Petras RE, Crawford NP, Galandiuk S: **Differential microRNA expression tracks neoplastic progression in inflammatory bowel disease-associated colorectal cancer.** *Hum Mutat* 2012, **33**(3):551–560.
108. Aizat AA, Shahpudin SN, Mustapha MA, Zakaria Z, Sidek AS, Abu Hassan MR, Ankathil R: **Association of Arg72Pro of P53 polymorphism with colorectal cancer susceptibility risk in Malaysian population.** *Asian Pac J Cancer Prev* 2011, **12**(11):2909–2913.
109. Wang B, Wang D, Zhang D, Li A, Liu D, Liu H, Jin H: **Pro variant of TP53 Arg72Pro contributes to esophageal squamous cell carcinoma risk: evidence from a meta-analysis.** *Eur J Cancer Prev* 2010, **19**(4):299–307.
110. Zhao Y, Wang F, Shan S, Qiu X, Li X, Jiao F, Wang J, Du Y: **Genetic polymorphism of p53, but not GSTP1, is association with susceptibility to esophageal cancer risk - a meta-analysis.** *Int J Med Sci* 2010, **7**(5):300–308.
111. Bashash M, Yavari P, Hislop TG, Shah A, Sadjadi A, Babaei M, Le N, Brooks-Wilson A, Malekzadeh R, Bajdik C: **Comparison of two diverse populations, British Columbia, Canada, and Ardabil, Iran, indicates several variables associated with gastric and esophageal cancer survival.** *J Gastrointest Cancer* 2011, **42**(1):40–45.
112. Duenas M, Santos M, Aranda JF, Bielza C, Martinez-Cruz AB, Lorz C, Taron M, Ciruelos EM, Rodriguez-Peralto JL, Martin M, Larrañaga P, Dahabreh J, Stathopoulos GP, Rosell R, Paramio JM, García-Escudero R: **Mouse p53-deficient cancer models as platforms for obtaining genomic predictors of human cancer clinical outcomes.** *PLoS One* 2012, **7**(8):e42494.
113. Perez-Morales R, Mendez-Ramirez I, Castro-Hernandez C, Martinez-Ramirez OC, Gonsebatt ME, Rubio J: **Polymorphisms associated with the risk of lung cancer in a healthy Mexican Mestizo population: application of the additive model for cancer.** *Genet Mol Biol* 2011, **34**(4):546–552.
114. Deeb KK, Michalowska AM, Yoon CY, Krummey SM, Hoenerhoff MJ, Kavanaugh C, Li MC, Demayo FJ, Linnoila I, Deng CX, Lee EY, Medina D, Shih JH, Green JE: **Identification of an integrated SV40 T/t-antigen cancer signature in aggressive human breast, prostate, and lung carcinomas with poor prognosis.** *Cancer Res* 2007, **67**(17):8065–8080.

115. Campling BG, el-Deiry WS: **Clinical implications of p53 mutations in lung cancer.** *Methods Mol Med* 2003, **75**:53–77.
116. Meylan E, Dooley AL, Feldser DM, Shen L, Turk E, Ouyang C, Jacks T: **Requirement for NF-kappaB signalling in a mouse model of lung adenocarcinoma.** *Nature* 2009, **462**(7269):104–107.
117. Fujiwara T, Cai DW, Georges RN, Mukhopadhyay T, Grimm EA, Roth JA: **Therapeutic effect of a retroviral wild-type p53 expression vector in an orthotopic lung cancer model.** *J Natl Cancer Inst* 1994, **86**(19):1458–1462.
118. Jiang DK, Yao L, Ren WH, Wang WZ, Peng B, Yu L: **TP53 Arg72Pro polymorphism and endometrial cancer risk: a meta-analysis.** *Med Oncol* 2011, **28**(4):1129–1135.
119. Chen MB, Li C, Shen WX, Guo YJ, Shen W, Lu PH: **Association of a LSP1 gene rs3817198T>C polymorphism with breast cancer risk: evidence from 33,920 cases and 35,671 controls.** *Mol Biol Rep* 2011, **38**(7):4687–4695.
120. Bachelder RE, Crago A, Chung J, Wendt MA, Shaw LM, Robinson G, Mercurio AM: **Vascular endothelial growth factor is an autocrine survival factor for neuropilin-expressing breast carcinoma cells.** *Cancer Res* 2001, **61**(15):5736–5740.
121. Eriksson L, Ahluwalia M, Spiewak J, Lee G, Sarma DS, Roomi MJ, Farber E: **Distinctive biochemical pattern associated with resistance of hepatocytes in hepatocyte nodules during liver carcinogenesis.** *Environ Health Perspect* 1983, **49**:171–174.
122. Volm M, Koomagi R, Rittgen W: **Clinical implications of cyclins, cyclin-dependent kinases, RB and E2F1 in squamous-cell lung carcinoma.** *Int J Cancer* 1998, **79**(3):294–299.
123. Anayama T, Furihata M, Takeuchi T, Sonobe H, Sasaguri S, Matsumoto M, Ohtsuki Y: **Insufficient effect of p27(KIP1) to inhibit cyclin D1 in human esophageal cancer in vitro.** *Int J Oncol* 2001, **18**(1):151–155.
124. Buschges R, Weber RG, Actor B, Lichter P, Collins VP, Reifenberger G: **Amplification and expression of cyclin D genes (CCND1, CCND2 and CCND3) in human malignant gliomas.** *Brain Pathol* 1999, **9**(3):435–442. discussion 432–433.
125. Comstock CE, Augello MA, Benito RP, Karch J, Tran TH, Utama FE, Tindall EA, Wang Y, Burd CJ, Groh EM, Hoang HN, Giles GG, Severi G, Hayes VM, Henderson BE, Le Marchand L, Kolonel LN, Haiman CA, Baffa R, Gomella LG, Knudsen ES, Rui H, Henshall SM, Sutherland RL, Knudsen KE: **Cyclin D1 splice variants: polymorphism, risk, and isoform-specific regulation in prostate cancer.** *Clin Cancer Res* 2009, **15**(17):5338–5349.
126. Murata M, Watanabe M, Yamanaka M, Kubota Y, Ito H, Nagao M, Katoh T, Kamataki T, Kawamura J, Yatani R, Shiraishi T: **Genetic polymorphisms in cytochrome P450 (CYP) 1A1, CYP1A2, CYP2E1, glutathione S-transferase (GST) M1 and GSTT1 and susceptibility to prostate cancer in the Japanese population.** *Cancer Lett* 2001, **165**(2):171–177.
127. Uematsu F: **Genetic polymorphisms of drug-metabolizing enzymes and susceptibility to lung cancer-relevance to smoking.** *Nihon Rinsho* 1996, **54**(2):513–517.
128. Murray GI, Taylor VE, McKay JA, Weaver RJ, Ewen SW, Melvin WT, Burke MD: **Expression of xenobiotic metabolizing enzymes in tumours of the urinary bladder.** *Int J Exp Pathol* 1995, **76**(4):271–276.
129. Hu YY, Yuan H, Jiang GB, Chen N, Wen L, Leng WD, Zeng XT, Niu YM: **Associations between XPD Asp312Asn polymorphism and risk of head and neck cancer: a meta-analysis based on 7,122 subjects.** *PLoS One* 2012, **7**(4):e35220.
130. Yuan H, Niu YM, Wang RX, Li HZ, Chen N: **Association between XPD Lys751Gln polymorphism and risk of head and neck cancer: a meta-analysis.** *Genet Mol Res* 2011, **10**(4):3356–3364.
131. Kumar A, Pant MC, Singh HS, Khandelwal S: **Associated risk of XRCC1 and XPD cross talk and life style factors in progression of head and neck cancer in north Indian population.** *Mutat Res* 2012, **729**(1–2):24–34.
132. Clapper ML: **Genetic polymorphism and cancer risk.** *Curr Oncol Rep* 2000, **2**(3):251–256.
133. Likhin FA, Bartnovskii AE, Vdovichenko KK, Abramov AA, Belokhvostov AS: **Characteristics of methyl-specific PCR-test of glutathione-S-transferase P1 gene in plasm DNA and cellular urinary precipitate for differential diagnosis of prostatic adenoma and adenocarcinoma.** *Urologiia* 2005, **4**:12–15.
134. Zhang Z, Liu W, Jia X, Gao Y, Hemminki K, Lindholm B: **Use of pyrosequencing to detect clinically relevant polymorphisms of genes in basal cell carcinoma.** *Clin Chim Acta* 2004, **342**(1–2):137–143.
135. Krajinovic M, Lemieux-Blanchard E, Chiasson S, Primeau M, Costea I, Moghrabi A: **Role of polymorphisms in MTHFR and MTHFD1 genes in the outcome of childhood acute lymphoblastic leukemia.** *Pharmacogenomics J* 2004, **4**(1):66–72.
136. Petra BG, Janez J, Vita D: **Gene-gene interactions in the folate metabolic pathway influence the risk for acute lymphoblastic leukemia in children.** *Leuk Lymphoma* 2007, **48**(4):786–792.
137. Matakidou A, El Galta R, Rudd MF, Webb EL, Bridle H, Eisen T, Houlston RS: **Prognostic significance of folate metabolism polymorphisms for lung cancer.** *Br J Cancer* 2007, **97**(2):247–252.
138. Moore LE, Malats N, Rothman N, Real FX, Kogevinas M, Karami S, Garcia-Closas R, Silverman D, Chanock S, Welch R, Tardón A, Serra C, Carrato A, Dosemeci M, García-Closas M: **Polymorphisms in one-carbon metabolism and trans-sulfuration pathway genes and susceptibility to bladder cancer.** *Int J Cancer* 2007, **120**(11):2452–2458.
139. Curtin K, Slattery ML, Ulrich CM, Bigler J, Levin TR, Wolff RK, Albertsen H, Potter JD, Samowitz WS: **Genetic polymorphisms in one-carbon metabolism: associations with CpG island methylator phenotype (CIMP) in colon cancer and the modifying effects of diet.** *Carcinogenesis* 2007, **28**(8):1672–1679.
140. Weiner AS, Beresina OV, Voronina EN, Voropaeva EN, Boyarskih UA, Pospelova TI, Filipenko ML: **Polymorphisms in folate-metabolizing genes and risk of non-Hodgkin's lymphoma.** *Leuk Res* 2011, **35**(4):508–515.
141. Lee KM, Lan Q, Kricker A, Purdue MP, Grulich AE, Vajdic CM, Turner J, Whitby D, Kang D, Chanock S, Rothman N, Armstrong BK: **One-carbon metabolism gene polymorphisms and risk of non-Hodgkin lymphoma in Australia.** *Hum Genet* 2007, **122**(5):525–533.
142. Suzuki T, Matsuo K, Hasegawa Y, Hiraki A, Wakai K, Hirose K, Saito T, Sato S, Ueda R, Tajima K: **One-carbon metabolism-related gene polymorphisms and risk of head and neck squamous cell carcinoma: case–control study.** *Cancer Sci* 2007, **98**(9):1439–1446.
143. Kim SH, Lee SH, Choi YL, Wang LH, Park CK, Shin YK: **Extensive alteration in the expression profiles of TGFB pathway signaling components and TP53 is observed along the gastric dysplasia-carcinoma sequence.** *Histol Histopathol* 2008, **23**(12):1439–1452.
144. Gemma A, Uematsu K, Hagiwara K, Takenoshita S, Kudoh S: **Mechanism of resistance to growth inhibition by transforming growth factor-beta 1 (TGF-beta 1) in primary lung cancer and new molecular targets in therapy.** *Gan To Kagaku Ryoho* 2000, **27**(8):1253–1259.
145. Jonson T, Albrechtsson E, Axelson J, Heidenblad M, Gorunova L, Johansson B, Hoglund M: **Altered expression of TGFB receptors and mitogenic effects of TGFB in pancreatic carcinomas.** *Int J Oncol* 2001, **19**(1):71–81.
146. Franzen P, Ichijo H, Miyazono K: **Different signals mediate transforming growth factor-beta 1-induced growth inhibition and extracellular matrix production in prostatic carcinoma cells.** *Exp Cell Res* 1993, **207**(1):1–7.
147. Maggio-Price L, Treuting P, Bielefeldt-Ohmann H, Seamons A, Drivdahl R, Zeng W, Lai L, Huycke M, Phelps S, Brabb T, Iritani BM: **Bacterial infection of Smad3/Rag2 double-null mice with transforming growth factor-beta dysregulation as a model for studying inflammation-associated colon cancer.** *Am J Pathol* 2009, **174**(1):317–329.
148. Hirshfield KM, Rebbeck TR, Levine AJ: **Germline mutations and polymorphisms in the origins of cancers in women.** *J Oncol* 2010, **2010**:297671.
149. Volate SR, Kawasaki BT, Hurt EM, Milner JA, Kim YS, White J, Farrar WL: **Gossypol induces apoptosis by activating p53 in prostate cancer cells and prostate tumor-initiating cells.** *Mol Cancer Ther* 2010, **9**(2):461–470.
150. Bernardini MQ, Baba T, Lee PS, Barnett JC, Sfakianos GP, Secord AA, Murphy SK, Iversen E, Marks JR, Berchuck A: **Expression signatures of TP53 mutations in serous ovarian cancers.** *BMC Cancer* 2010, **10**:237.
151. Shimada S, Mimata A, Sekine M, Mogushi K, Akiyama Y, Fukamachi H, Jonkers J, Tanaka H, Eishi Y, Yuasa Y: **Synergistic tumour suppressor activity of E-cadherin and p53 in a conditional mouse model for metastatic diffuse-type gastric cancer.** *Gut* 2012, **61**(3):344–353.
152. Sano D, Xie TX, Ow TJ, Zhao M, Pickering CR, Zhou G, Sandulache VC, Wheeler DA, Gibbs RA, Caulin C, Myers JN: **Disruptive TP53 mutation is associated with aggressive disease characteristics in an orthotopic murine model of oral tongue cancer.** *Clin Cancer Res* 2011, **17**(21):6658–6670.
153. Furth PA, Cabrera MC, Diaz-Cruz ES, Millman S, Nakles RE: **Assessing estrogen signaling aberrations in breast cancer risk using genetically engineered mouse models.** *Ann N Y Acad Sci* 2011, **1229**:147–155.

154. de Jonge R, Hooijberg JH, van Zelst BD, Jansen G, van Zantwijk CH, Kaspers GJ, Peters GJ, Ravindranath Y, Pieters R, Lindemans J: **Effect of polymorphisms in folate-related genes on in vitro methotrexate sensitivity in pediatric acute lymphoblastic leukemia.** *Blood* 2005, **106**(2):717–720.
155. Durfort T, Tkach M, Meschaninova MI, Rivas MA, Elizalde PV, Venyaminova AG, Schillaci R, Francois JC: **Small interfering RNA targeted to IGF-IR delays tumor growth and induces proinflammatory cytokines in a mouse breast cancer model.** *PLoS One* 2012, **7**(1):e29213.
156. Calogero RA, Cordero F, Forni G, Cavallo F: **Inflammation and breast cancer. Inflammatory component of mammary carcinogenesis in ErbB2 transgenic mice.** *Breast Cancer Res* 2007, **9**(4):211.
157. Schiff R, Osborne CK: **Endocrinology and hormone therapy in breast cancer: new insight into estrogen receptor-alpha function and its implication for endocrine therapy resistance in breast cancer.** *Breast Cancer Res* 2005, **7**(5):205–211.
158. Lahm H, Petral-Malec D, Yilmaz-Ceyhan A, Fischer JR, Lorenzoni M, Givel JC, Odartchenko N: **Growth stimulation of a human colorectal carcinoma cell line by interleukin-1 and –6 and antagonistic effects of transforming growth factor beta 1.** *Eur J Cancer* 1992, **28A**(11):1894–1899.
159. Yu C, Yao Z, Jiang Y, Keller ET: **Prostate cancer stem cell biology.** *Minerva Urol Nefrol* 2012, **64**(1):19–33.
160. Peng B, Cao L, Ma X, Wang W, Wang D, Yu L: **Meta-analysis of association between matrix metalloproteinases 2, 7 and 9 promoter polymorphisms and cancer risk.** *Mutagenesis* 2010, **25**(4):371–379.
161. Zhang YM, Cao C, Liang K: **Genetic polymorphism of epidermal growth factor 61A>G and cancer risk: a meta-analysis.** *Cancer Epidemiol* 2010, **34**(2):150–156.
162. Willmarth NE, Ethier SP: **Amphiregulin as a novel target for breast cancer therapy.** *J Mammary Gland Biol Neoplasia* 2008, **13**(2):171–179.
163. Guise TA: **Breaking down bone: new insight into site-specific mechanisms of breast cancer osteolysis mediated by metalloproteinases.** *Genes Dev* 2009, **23**(18):2117–2123.
164. Lacroix M, Body JJ: **Regulation of c-fos and c-jun expression by calcitonin in human breast cancer cells.** *Calcif Tissue Int* 1997, **60**(6):513–519.
165. Chen MB, Wu XY, Shen W, Wei MX, Li C, Cai B, Tao GQ, Lu PH: **Association between polymorphisms of trinucleotide repeat containing 9 gene and breast cancer risk: evidence from 62,005 subjects.** *Breast Cancer Res Treat* 2011, **126**(1):177–183.
166. Gu D, Wang M: **VEGF 936C>T polymorphism and breast cancer risk: evidence from 5,729 cases and 5,868 controls.** *Breast Cancer Res Treat* 2011, **125**(2):489–493.
167. Qiu LX, Wang K, Yang S, Mao C, Zhao L, Yao L, Zhang J, Zhang QL, Sun S, Xue K: **Current evidences on vascular endothelial growth factor polymorphisms and breast cancer susceptibility.** *Mol Biol Rep* 2011, **38**(7):4491–4494.
168. Yang DS, Park KH, Woo OH, Woo SU, Kim AR, Lee ES, Lee JB, Kim YH, Kim JS, Seo JH: **Association of a vascular endothelial growth factor gene 936 C/T polymorphism with breast cancer risk: a meta-analysis.** *Breast Cancer Res Treat* 2011, **125**(3):849–853.
169. Xu B, Li JM, Tong N, Tao J, Li PC, Song NH, Zhang W, Wu HF, Feng NH, Hua LX: **VEGFA +936C>T polymorphism and cancer risk: a meta-analysis.** *Cancer Genet Cytogenet* 2010, **198**(1):7–14.
170. Liu X, Wang Z, Yu J, Lei G, Wang S: **Three polymorphisms in interleukin-1beta gene and risk for breast cancer: a meta-analysis.** *Breast Cancer Res Treat* 2010, **124**(3):821–825.
171. Oh JS, Kucab JE, Bushel PR, Martin K, Bennett L, Collins J, DiAugustine RP, Barrett JC, Afshari CA, Dunn SE: **Insulin-like growth factor-1 inscribes a gene expression profile for angiogenic factors and cancer progression in breast epithelial cells.** *Neoplasia* 2002, **4**(3):204–217.
172. Cao C, Ying T, Fang JJ, Sun SF, Lv D, Chen ZB, Ma HY, Yu YM, Ding QL, Shu LH, Deng Z-C: **Polymorphism of vascular endothelial growth factor −2578C/A with cancer risk: evidence from 11263 subjects.** *Med Oncol* 2011, **28**(4):1169–1175.
173. Xue H, Lin B, Ni P, Xu H, Huang G: **Interleukin-1B and interleukin-1 RN polymorphisms and gastric carcinoma risk: a meta-analysis.** *J Gastroenterol Hepatol* 2010, **25**(10):1604–1617.
174. Gao LB, Pan XM, Jia J, Liang WB, Rao L, Xue H, Zhu Y, Li SL, Lv ML, Deng W, Chen TY, Wei YG, Zhang L: **IL-8-251A/T polymorphism is associated with decreased cancer risk among population-based studies: evidence from a meta-analysis.** *Eur J Cancer* 2010, **46**(8):1333–1343.
175. Liu L, Zhuang W, Wang C, Chen Z, Wu XT, Zhou Y: **Interleukin-8-251 A/T gene polymorphism and gastric cancer susceptibility: a meta-analysis of epidemiological studies.** *Cytokine* 2010, **50**(3):328–334.
176. Peng B, Cao L, Wang W, Xian L, Jiang D, Zhao J, Zhang Z, Wang X, Yu L: **Polymorphisms in the promoter regions of matrix metalloproteinases 1 and 3 and cancer risk: a meta-analysis of 50 case–control studies.** *Mutagenesis* 2010, **25**(1):41–48.
177. Wysoczynski M, Ratajczak MZ: **Lung cancer secreted microvesicles: underappreciated modulators of microenvironment in expanding tumors.** *Int J Cancer* 2009, **125**(7):1595–1603.
178. Xie Y, Zhang H, Sheng W, Xiang J, Ye Z, Yang J: **Adenovirus-mediated ING4 expression suppresses lung carcinoma cell growth via induction of cell cycle alteration and apoptosis and inhibition of tumor invasion and angiogenesis.** *Cancer Lett* 2008, **271**(1):105–116.
179. Gao Y, Cao Y, Tan A, Liao C, Mo Z, Gao F: **Glutathione S-transferase M1 polymorphism and sporadic colorectal cancer risk: an updating meta-analysis and HuGE review of 36 case–control studies.** *Ann Epidemiol* 2010, **20**(2):108–121.
180. Lu S, Wang Z, Cui D, Liu H, Hao X: **Glutathione S-transferase P1 Ile105Val polymorphism and breast cancer risk: a meta-analysis involving 34,658 subjects.** *Breast Cancer Res Treat* 2011, **125**(1):253–259.
181. Qiu LX, Yuan H, Yu KD, Mao C, Chen B, Zhan P, Xue K, Zhang J, Hu XC: **Glutathione S-transferase M1 polymorphism and breast cancer susceptibility: a meta-analysis involving 46,281 subjects.** *Breast Cancer Res Treat* 2010, **121**(3):703–708.
182. Singh V, Parmar D, Singh MP: **Do single nucleotide polymorphisms in xenobiotic metabolizing genes determine breast cancer susceptibility and treatment outcomes?** *Cancer Invest* 2008, **26**(8):769–783.
183. Curran JE, Weinstein SR, Griffiths LR: **Polymorphisms of glutathione S-transferase genes (GSTM1, GSTP1 and GSTT1) and breast cancer susceptibility.** *Cancer Lett* 2000, **153**(1–2):113–120.
184. Economopoulos KP, Sergentanis TN, Vlahos NF: **Glutathione S-transferase M1, T1, and P1 polymorphisms and ovarian cancer risk: a meta-analysis.** *Int J Gynecol Cancer* 2010, **20**(5):732–737.
185. Zeng FF, Liu SY, Wei W, Yao SP, Zhu S, Li KS, Wan G, Zhang HT, Zhong M, Wang BY: **Genetic polymorphisms of glutathione S-transferase T1 and bladder cancer risk: a meta-analysis.** *Clin Exp Med* 2010, **10**(1):59–68.
186. Moore LE, Baris DR, Figueroa JD, Garcia-Closas M, Karagas MR, Schwenn MR, Johnson AT, Lubin JH, Hein DW, Dagnall CL, Colt JS, Kida M, Jones MA, Schned AR, Cherala SS, Chanock SJ, Cantor KP, Silverman DT, Rothman N: **GSTM1 null and NAT2 slow acetylation genotypes, smoking intensity and bladder cancer risk: results from the New England bladder cancer study and NAT2 meta-analysis.** *Carcinogenesis* 2011, **32**(2):182–189.
187. Tsukuda M, Nagahara T, Yago T, Matsuda H, Yanoma S: **Production of granulocyte colony-stimulating factor by head and neck carcinomas.** *Biotherapy* 1993, **6**(3):183–187.
188. Lagadec PF, Saraya KA, Balkwill FR: **Human small-cell lung-cancer cells are cytokine-resistant but NK/LAK-sensitive.** *Int J Cancer* 1991, **48**(2):311–317.
189. Enzmann V, Faude F, Kohen L, Wiedemann P: **Secretion of cytokines by human choroidal melanoma cells and skin melanoma cell lines in vitro.** *Ophthalmic Res* 1998, **30**(3):189–194.
190. Kimura F, Nakamura Y, Sato K, Wakimoto N, Kato T, Tahara T, Yamada M, Nagata N, Motoyoshi K: **Cyclic change of cytokines in a patient with cyclic thrombocytopenia.** *Br J Haematol* 1996, **94**(1):171–174.
191. Reinhold D, Bank U, Buhling F, Lendeckel U, Ulmer AJ, Flad HD, Ansorge S: **Transforming growth factor-beta 1 (TGF-beta 1) inhibits DNA synthesis of PWM-stimulated PBMC via suppression of IL-2 and IL-6 production.** *Cytokine* 1994, **6**(4):382–388.
192. Nikolova PN, Pawelec GP, Mihailova SM, Ivanova MI, Myhailova AP, Baltadjieva DN, Marinova DI, Ivanova SS, Naumova EJ: **Association of cytokine gene polymorphisms with malignant melanoma in Caucasian population.** *Cancer Immunol Immunother* 2007, **56**(3):371–379.
193. Freedman RS, Deavers M, Liu J, Wang E: **Peritoneal inflammation - a microenvironment for epithelial ovarian cancer (EOC).** *J Transl Med* 2004, **2**(1):23.
194. Jarnicki A, Putoczki T, Ernst M: **Stat3: linking inflammation to epithelial cancer - more than a "gut" feeling?** *Cell division* 2010, **5**:14.
195. Rundhaug JE, Fischer SM: **Molecular mechanisms of mouse skin tumor promotion.** *Cancers* 2010, **2**(2):436–482.
196. Mischek D, Steinborn R, Petznek H, Bichler C, Zatloukal K, Sturzl M, Gunzburg WH, Hohenadl C: **Molecularly characterised xenograft tumour**

mouse models: valuable tools for evaluation of new therapeutic strategies for secondary liver cancers. *J Biomed Biotechnol* 2009, **2009**:437284.

197. Hiss D: **Optimizing molecular-targeted therapies in ovarian cancer: the renewed surge of interest in ovarian cancer biomarkers and cell signaling pathways.** *Journal of Oncology* 2012, **2012**:737981.
198. Luo J, Solimini NL, Elledge SJ: **Principles of cancer therapy: oncogene and non-oncogene addiction.** *Cell* 2009, **136**(5):823–837.
199. Chen Z, Yan B, Van Waes C: **The role of the NF-kappaB transcriptome and proteome as biomarkers in human head and neck squamous cell carcinomas.** *Biomark Med* 2008, **2**(4):409–426.
200. Shimada Y, Imamura M: **Prognostic factors for esophageal cancer–from the viewpoint of molecular biology.** *Gan To Kagaku Ryoho* 1996, **23**(8):972–981.
201. Ziober BL, Turner MA, Palefsky JM, Banda MJ, Kramer RH: **Type I collagen degradation by invasive oral squamous cell carcinoma.** *Oral Oncol* 2000, **36**(4):365–372.
202. Nuovo GJ: **In situ detection of PCR-amplified metalloproteinase cDNAs, their inhibitors and human papillomavirus transcripts in cervical carcinoma cell lines.** *Int J Cancer* 1997, **71**(6):1056–1060.
203. Liss C, Fekete MJ, Hasina R, Lam CD, Lingen MW: **Paracrine angiogenic loop between head-and-neck squamous-cell carcinomas and macrophages.** *Int J Cancer* 2001, **93**(6):781–785.
204. Stachel D, Albert M, Meilbeck R, Kreutzer B, Haas RJ, Schmid I: **Bone marrow Th2 cytokine expression as predictor for relapse in childhood acute lymphoblastic leukemia (ALL).** *Eur J Med Res* 2006, **11**(3):102–113.
205. Melinceanu L, Sarafoleanu C, Lerescu L, Tucureanu C, Caras I, Salageanu A: **Impact of smoking on the immunological profile of patients with laryngeal carcinoma.** *J Med Life* 2009, **2**(2):211–218.
206. Lazar-Molnar E, Hegyesi H, Toth S, Falus A: **Autocrine and paracrine regulation by cytokines and growth factors in melanoma.** *Cytokine* 2000, **12**(6):547–554
207. Inoue K, Wood CG, Slaton JW, Karashima T, Sweeney P, Dinney CP: **Adenoviral-mediated gene therapy of human bladder cancer with antisense interleukin-8.** *Oncol Rep* 2001, **8**(5):955–964.
208. Snarskaia ES, Molochkov VA, Frank GA, Zavalishina LA: **Matrix metalloproteinases and their tissue inhibitors in basal cell and metatypical cancer of the skin.** *Arkhiv Patologii* 2005, **67**(3):14–16.
209. Lievre A, Milet J, Carayol J, Le Corre D, Milan C, Pariente A, Nalet B, Lafon J, Faivre J, Bonithon-Kopp C, Olschwang S, Bonaiti-Pellié C, Laurent-Puig P, Members of the ANGH group: **Genetic polymorphisms of MMP1, MMP3 and MMP7 gene promoter and risk of colorectal adenoma.** *BMC Cancer* 2006, **6**:270.
210. Ricketts C, Zeegers MP, Lubinski J, Maher ER: **Analysis of germline variants in CDH1, IGFBP3, MMP1, MMP3, STK15 and VEGF in familial and sporadic renal cell carcinoma.** *PLoS One* 2009, **4**(6):e6037.
211. Esteller M, Garcia A, Martinez-Palones JM, Xercavins J, Reventos J: **Susceptibility to endometrial cancer: influence of allelism at p53, glutathione S-transferase (GSTM1 and GSTT1) and cytochrome P-450 (CYP1A1) loci.** *Br J Cancer* 1997, **75**(9):1385–1388.
212. Kozhemiakin LA, Bulavin DV, Morozov VI, Osipov EV, Zolotarev DV: **Effectiveness of the glutathione s-transferase assay in diagnosing lung cancer.** *Vopr Onkol* 1995, **41**(1):33–38.
213. Schilthuizen C, Broyl A, van der Holt B, de Knegt Y, Lokhorst H, Sonneveld P: **Influence of genetic polymorphisms in CYP3A4, CYP3A5, GSTP1, GSTM1, GSTT1 and MDR1 genes on survival and therapy-related toxicity in multiple myeloma.** *Haematologica* 2007, **92**(2):277–278.
214. Lavender NA, Benford ML, VanCleave TT, Brock GN, Kittles RA, Moore JH, Hein DW, Kidd LC: **Examination of polymorphic glutathione S-transferase (GST) genes, tobacco smoking and prostate cancer risk among men of African descent: a case–control study.** *BMC Cancer* 2009, **9**:397.
215. Saadat I, Saadat M: **The glutathione *S*-transferase mu polymorphism and susceptibility to acute lymphocytic leukemia.** *Cancer Lett* 2000, **158**(1):43–45.
216. Ovsepian VA, Vinogradova E, Sherstneva ES: **Cytochrome P4501A1, glutathione S-transferase M1 and T1 gene polymorphisms in chronic myeloid leukemia.** *Genetika* 2010, **46**(10):1360–1362.
217. Vrana D, Pikhart H, Mohelnikova-Duchonova B, Holcatova I, Strnad R, Slamova A, Schejbalova M, Ryska M, Susova S, Soucek P: **The association between glutathione S-transferase gene polymorphisms and pancreatic cancer in a central European Slavonic population.** *Mutat Res* 2009, **680**(1–2):78–81.

3

Novel age-dependent targets in vestibular schwannomas

Amos Toren[1], Juergen K Reichardt[2], Ali Andalibi[3], Nancy Ya-Hsuan Hsu[4], Joni Doherty[5], William Slattery[6] and Ruty Mehrian-Shai[7*]

Abstract

Background: Schwannomas are the most common neurofibromatosis type 2 (NF2)-associated tumors with significant phenotypic heterogeneity in patients. The most severe subtype has an early and rapid progression and the mild type has a later onset and a less aggressive course. The aim of this study was to elucidate the underlying molecular differences between these groups. We compared the gene expression pattern between patients with early to late age of onset.

Results: A gene signature of 21 genes was constructed to differentiate between early-onset and late-onset patients. We confirmed these results by real-time PCR for SNF1LK2, NGFRAP1L1 (BEX 5), GMNN, and EPHA2.

Conclusion: Genes identified here may be additional aberrations in merlin-depleted cells that govern the disease onset. A significant number of these genes have been suggested as having a role in carcinogenesis and are used as biomarkers for prognosis in several other cancers. The role of these genes in NF2 carcinogenesis and their potential as biomarkers or drug target are worthwhile exploring.

Keywords: Neurofibromatosis, Schwannomas, Targeted therapy

Background

Neurofibromatosis type 2 (NF2) is an autosomal dominant disorder that predisposes affected individuals to several types of cerebral and spinal tumors [1]. Epidemiological studies place the incidence of NF2 at 1 in 25,000 live births [2]. The current treatment of NF2 is surgery and/or radiation therapy. However, there is no current safe therapeutic agent available at this time. Bilateral vestibular schwannomas (BVS) are the most common of NF2-associated tumors [3]. The consequences of a vestibular schwannomas (VS) are numerous, including dizziness, imbalance, tinnitus, hearing loss progressing to deafness, facial nerve paralysis, brainstem compression, and, if left untreated, death.

Mutations of the NF2 gene are thought to be the primary cause of this disease. Various types of mutations have been identified, among them single-base substitutions, insertions, and deletions [4]. The NF2 gene product, merlin, functions as a signal transduction pathway regulating cell-to-cell and cell matrix interactions. Merlin has been demonstrated to exert its antiproliferative effect by impact on several intracellular signaling pathways: inhibition of phosphatidylinositol 3-kinase (PI3-kinase), through binding to PI3-kinase enhancer, long form (PIKE-L) [5], modulation of the RAS/RAC oncogenic pathways [6], inhibition of the mitogen-activated protein kinase (MAPK) pathways [7] and repression of PAK-induced cyclin D1 expression [8]. Merlin regulates the MAPK signaling pathway by blocking the Cdc42-MLK3 interaction and MLK3 activity inhibition [9]. Furthermore, inactivation of merlin induces oncogenic gene expression, hyperproliferation, and tumorigenicity by releasing the inhibition of E3 ubiquitin ligase CRL4 (DCAF1) in the nucleus [10].

Since the disease has a variable presentation, with the severe subtype having an early and rapid progression and the milder type having a later onset and a less aggressive course, the diagnosis and management of these patients present a unique challenge [11]. Studies have indicated that a truncating NF2 mutation (nonsense and frameshift) is linked with the more severe form of NF2 [3]. The more severe form is particularly virulent, with unrelenting growth of schwannomas and meningiomas

* Correspondence: mehrian@usc.edu
[7]Institute for Genetic Medicine, University of Southern California, Keck School of Medicine, Los Angeles, CA 90089, USA
Full list of author information is available at the end of the article

from childhood, resulting in blindness, deafness, paralysis, and death by the age of 40. The mild form of NF2 is less debilitating. The schwannomas may remain the same size for years, few meningiomas will develop. The patient may not develop symptoms until later in life and will have fewer disabilities [3].

There is considerable variability in growth rates of VS in patients with NF2, but they tend to be higher in patients who are younger at onset of signs or symptoms [12]. The most important predictors of disease severity are age at diagnosis and age at onset of symptoms. The average age of onset is 18 to 24 years. Almost all affected individuals develop bilateral vestibular schwannomas by age 30 years. Vestibular schwannomas are much less common in children than adults [13]. There are age-specific risks of NF2 to an offspring of a patient. Patient presenting with BVS <20 years 29.3% and patient presenting with asymmetric disease after 40 years 5.5% [14]. Patients of ages 35 years and below show higher p53 phosphorylation compared to the tumors of older patients [15].

The development of microarray tools assists effective, current, and comprehensive understanding of complex diseases including cancer [16]. Differences in gene expression between schwannomas or between schwannoma cells from NF2 patients and normal human primary schwann cells previously examined do not confer age impact [17-19]. Here, we report whole genome gene expression variation in NF tumors differing in age of onset. Improved understanding of these molecular differences may allow elucidation of age-dependent onset etiology, novel molecular markers for prognosis, and new therapeutic targets for neurofibromatosis.

Results and discussion

We analyzed the transcriptome of VS samples from early-onset patients and late-onset patients. The results were summarized in a volcano scatter plot (Figure 1) that summarizes both fold change and t test criteria. The negative $\log_{10}$-transformed p values from the gene-specific t test was plotted against the $\log_2$ fold change between early and late onset. Genes with statistically significant differential expression according to the gene-specific t test lie above the horizontal threshold line. Genes with large fold change values lie outside the pair of vertical threshold lines. Twenty one significantly differentially expressed genes are identified by fold change >1.5 and p value <0.01: ANLN, NAV3, ZNF718, PSCD3, C180rf54, C10rf79, XPO1, GMNN, WHSC1, EPHA2, SNF1LK2, NGFRAP1L1, ELL2, SYTL3, KCNK17, IGLV1-44, PID1, RGN, PTPN1, ZNF331, and RNF19A (Table 1). Figure 2 illustrates the hierarchical expression of these genes for the two groups. The genes are clustered according to their relative expression in each group. Green color represents genes that have relatively low expression and red color represents genes that have relatively high expression. Finally, we utilized quantitative

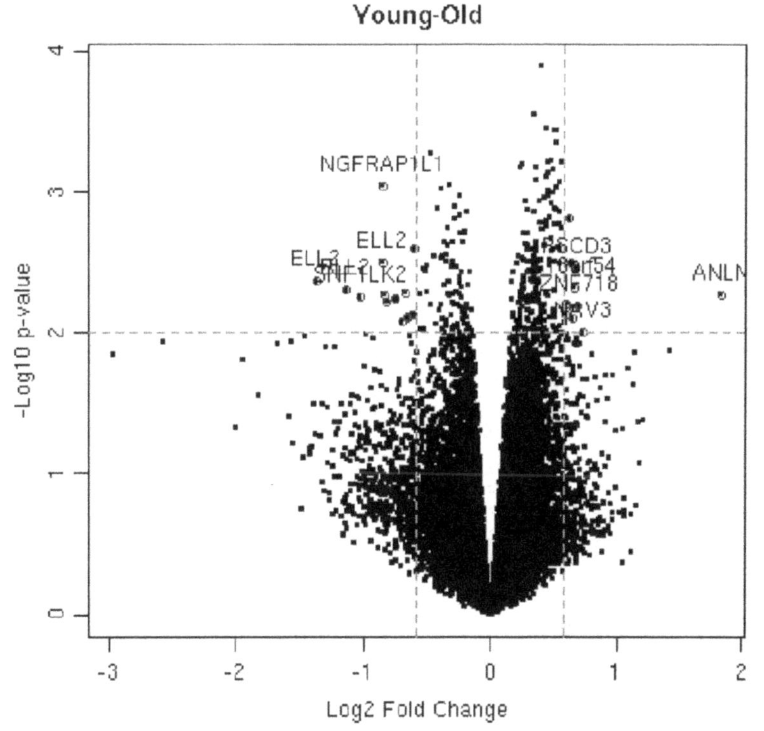

Figure 1 Volcano plot of early- and late-onset tumors.

Table 1 List of age-dependent differentially expressed genes

Gene symbol	Fold change	*p* value	Function	Activity	Role in cancer
ANLN	3.55	0.0053		Actin-binding protein	Overexpressed in pancreatic carcinoma
NAV3	1.65	0.0099	G	Neuron growth, regeneration	Neural tumorigenesis
ZNF718	1.61	0.0064		Zinc finger protein	Associated with prostate cancer
PSCD3	1.59	0.0035	T	Protein sorting and membrane trafficking	
C180rf54	1.57	0.0047			Overexpressed in multiple cancers
XPO1	1.56	0.0079	T/K	Nuclear protein transport export	
C10rf79	1.56	0.0065			
GMNN	1.55	0.0032	G	Proliferation marker	Correlated with poorer clinical outcome
WHSC1	1.51	0.006		Regulation of Wnt pathway	Expression increases with ascending glioma proliferation activity
EPHA2	1.51	0.0073	K	Tyrosine Kinase	Overexpressed in many types of cancer
SNF1LK2	−2.03	0.0055	K	Serine/Threonine kinase	Correlated with ovarian cancer poor survival
NGFRAP1L1 (BEX5)	−1.8	0.0009	G	Nerve growth factor receptor-associated	May be a tumor suppressor in VS
ELL2	−1.8	0.0031		Suppress canonical Wnt signaling	ELL translocations in malignancies.
SYTL3	−1.79	0.0053	T	Vesicular trafficking	
KCNK17	−1.76	0.006		Potassium channel	Expressed abnormally in many cancer types
IGLV1-44	−1.68	0.0057			
PID1	−1.62	0.0084		Glucose transport inhibitor	
RGN	−1.59	0.0052		Suppresses cell proliferation	Lost in breast and prostate cancer
PTPN1	−1.57	0.0076	K/G	Cell growth	
ZNF331	−1.53	0.0074	D	Induces apoptosis	
RNF19A	−1.52	0.0025	D	Neuronal cell death	

T transport, *K* kinase, *G* growth, *D* death.

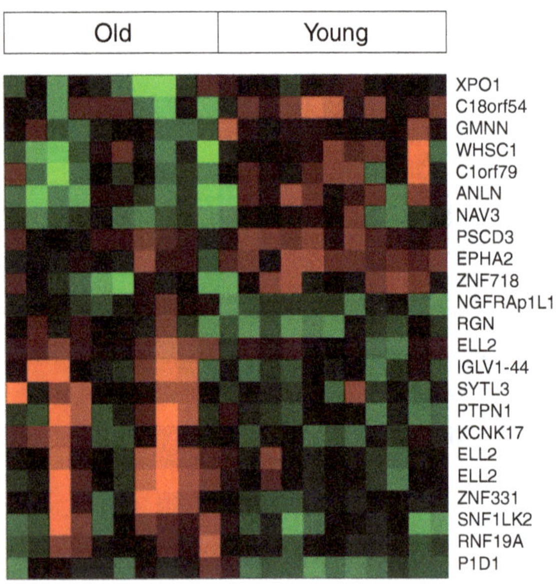

Figure 2 Heat map on age onset-dependent gene expression.

real-time RT-PCR to verify the results for four genes with the most potential future application according to the role they play in other cancers: SNF1LK2, NGFRAP1L1 (BEX 5), GMNN, and EPHA2 (Figures 3 and 4). In fact, RT-PCR confirmed the results for these genes and *t* test for all genes were significant at *p* value <0.005 (SNF1LK2 *p* value 2×10^{-7}, NGFRAP1L1 (BEX5) *p* value 0.0002, GMNN *p* value 0.0009, and EPHA2 *p* value 9×10^{-6}).

Although the NF2 locus on chromosome 22 is associated with the formation of vestibular schwannomas, it is clear that in addition to merlin gene, there are a variety of other genes whose 'dysregulation' may eventually result in tumor formation. Comparison of gene expression between early- and late-onset specimens which all are merlin depleted provides a valuable insight into the modifications of these genes. Gene expression analysis of NF2 samples resulted in 21 genes that differentiate early-onset tumors from late-onset tumors (Table 1). Some of them are widely involved in nervous system activities and have been associated with cancer as described below and summarized in Table 2.

Ten of the 21 genes we identified fall into four broad functional categories (Table 1): protein transport (genes

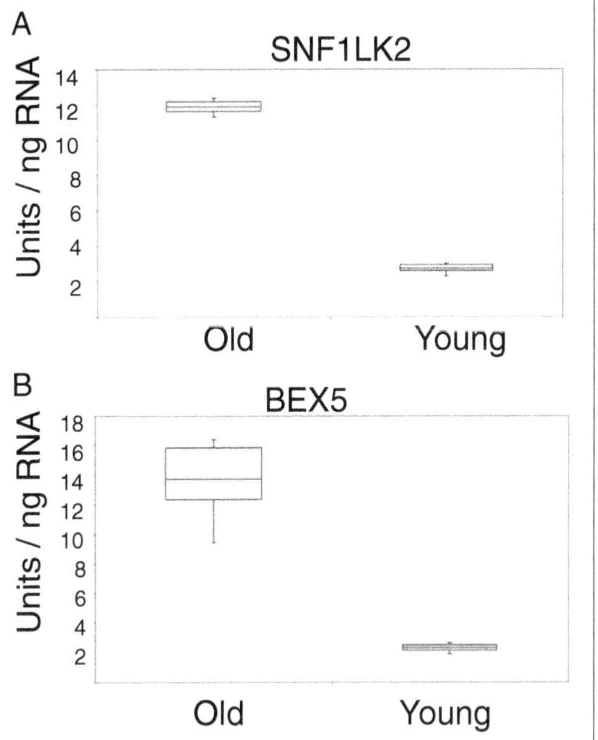

Figure 3 SNF1LK2 (A) and BEX5 (B) quantitative real-time PCR validation.

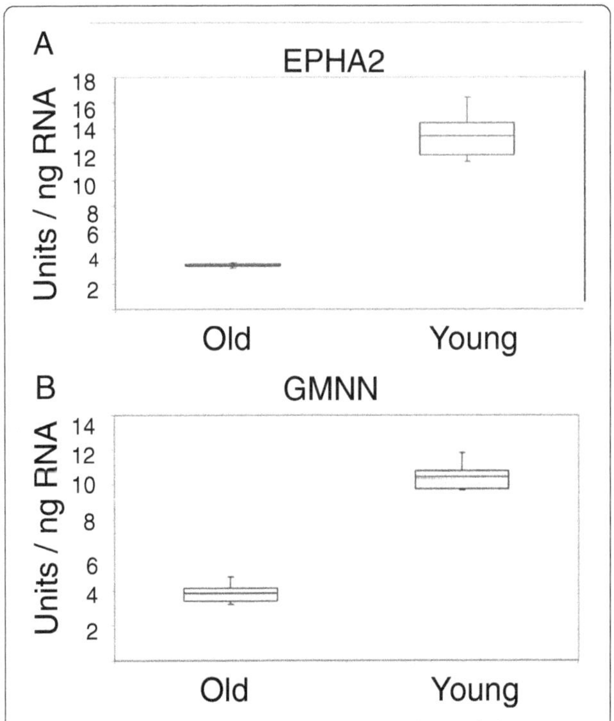

Figure 4 EPHA2 (A) and GMNN (B) quantitative real-time PCR validation.

Table 2 Proposed applicable uses of differentially expressed genes

Gene	Other cancer	Drug target	Outcome prediction	To be defined
EPHA2	Y	Y	Y	
XPO1	Y	Y	Y	
SNF1LK2	Y	Y	Y	
NAV3	Y	Y	Y	
KCNK17	Y	Y	Y	
ZNF331	Y	Y	Y	
GMNN	Y		Y	
ZNF718	Y		Y	
WHSC1	Y			
ANLN	Y			
PSCD3	Y			
RGN	Y			
ELL2	Y			
PTPN1	Y			
BEX5				Y
SYTL3				Y
RNF19A				Y
P1D1				Y

PSCD3, XPO1, and SYTL3), protein phosphorylation and dephosphorylation (XPO1, EPHA2, and SNF1LK2), cell growth (NAV3, GMNN, and NGFRAP1L1), and cell death (ZNF331 and RNF19A). The latter two are particularly relevant to cancerous growth and the first two may underpin it as well. Additional cellular functions and cancer phenotypes are also listed in Table 1. Furthermore, some, at least 14 (EPA, XPO, SNF1LK, NAV3, KCNK17, ZNF331, GNMM, ZNF718, WHSC1, ANLN, PSCD3, RGN, ELL2, and PTPN1) of the 21 genes, have been reported to be involved in cancers (Table 1).

We further grouped the 21 genes we identified into 4 subgroups according to their potential role in NF2: in carcinogenesis, as biomarker, as drug target, or potential for clinical outcome prediction. This was according to other studies findings for each gene above. Another group was constructed from genes that their role in cancer has not been indicated yet (Table 2).

In summary, we report here a gene signature comprising 21 genes that characterize the clinically important age at onset in NF2 patients. Interestingly, many of these genes have known or at least inferred functions which may lead to a more complete molecular understanding of the age-based pathogenic differences in NF2 in the future. Such data may, in turn, lead to improved pre-symptomatic diagnoses and personalized age-focused treatment.

Conclusion

There is great phenotypic difference between early and late onset in NF2. Our data indicate that these groups have distinct gene expression signatures. Most of the differentiating genes have already been shown to have important roles in other cancers. Thus, they may also have a role in VS NF2 patients. Moreover, these genes may be involved in pathogenesis, used as potential age-oriented biomarkers and treatment targets. Our gene lists will provide fertile ground for testing novel hypotheses on disease mechanism, pathogenesis, and therapeutic targets.

Methods

Thirty-seven samples from human tumor (schwannomas) tissues were obtained at the time of surgery in accordance with applicable human ethics regulations (USC IRB protocol # 97–157) and snap frozen in liquid nitrogen. Tumor specimens were divided into two groups (young and old) according to the patient's age of onset. The young-onset group included 21 specimens from patients whose age of onset was less than 16 years old (ranging from 7 to 16 years old). The old-onset group included 16 specimens from patients whose age of onset was 30 years and older (ranging from 30 to 67 years old). The average age of the young group was 12 years old. The average age of the old group was 43 years. RNA was extracted and cRNA were hybridized to Human Genome U133 Plus 2.0 Array (Affymetrix) for analysis of over 47,000 transcripts. The detailed protocol for the sample preparation and microarray processing is available from Affymetrix at www.affymetrix.com (Santa Clara, CA, USA). For real-time PCR, total RNA was extracted and RT-qPCR was performed in the DNA Engine Opticon 2 Continuous Fluorescence Detection System (Bio-Rad, Hercules, CA, USA).

Data analysis

The Bioconductor limma package [20] was used to preprocess the expression data from Human Genome U133 Plus 2.0 Affymetrix Array. To remove batch effects, the complete dataset were normalized by RMA. Before doing statistical analysis, we filter the probe sets by present/absent calls using the Wilcoxon signed rank-based algorithm. Out of 54,675 probes, 42,339 were kept and the remaining ones were removed as 'Absent' to reduce false positive rate. We identified differentially expressed gene list by fitting linear models to the normalized expression values. The empirical Bayes shrinkage was applied to t statistics using the limma package in Bioconductor. Because patient subtypes were still observed after RMA normalization, balanced samples from the same subtype were selected to identify significantly differentially expressed genes and to reduce the potential of small-sample artifacts. In general, selected genes have greater than 1.5 fold change and less than 0.01 p value.

The analysis of RT-PCR is as follows: Sample RNA was processed in triplicate with serial dilutions of Human Universal Reference RNA (Stratagene, La Jolla, CA, USA) on the same 96-well plate. Standard curves were constructed from the Universal RNA wells with arbitrary units of 1 unit equivalent to 1 pg of Universal RNA. Results were plotted as units per nanogram of RNA. Graphically, the middle line of the bar represents mean, bar size corresponds to the difference between lower quartile and upper quartile, and error bars represent the range of the raw data. t test p values were calculated for each differentiating gene.

Ethical conduct of research

The authors state that they have obtained the University of Southern California institutional review board approval and have followed the principles outlined in the Declaration of Helsinki for all human experimental investigations. In addition, informed consent has been obtained from the participants involved.

Competing interests

The authors declare that they have no competing interests.

Authors' contributions

AA and RMS developed the hypotheses underlying this study. JD, WS, and AA obtained informed consent and patient materials. AT had medical oversight of the study. RMS and NHYH performed the experimental procedures of this study. RMS, AT, and JKVR analyzed the data. RMS wrote the manuscript. AT and JKVR contributed to editing of the manuscript. All authors read and approved the final manuscript.

Author details

[1]Department of Pediatric Hemato-Oncology, The Cancer Research Center, Sheba Medical Center, 2 Sheba Road, Ramat Gan 52621, Israel. [2]School of Pharmacy and Molecular Sciences, James Cook University, Townsville QLD 4811, Australia. [3]University of Connecticut, 438 Whitney Rd. Extension, Unit 1006, Storrs, CT 06269, USA. [4]Quest Diagnostics Nichols Institute, 14225 Newbrook Drive, Chantilly, VA 20153, USA. [5]Center for Neural Tumor Research, 2100 West Third Street, Los Angeles, CA 90057, USA. [6]Department of Clinical Studies, House Ear Institute, Los Angeles, CA 90057, USA. [7]Institute for Genetic Medicine, University of Southern California, Keck School of Medicine, Los Angeles, CA 90089, USA.

References

1. Gutmann DH, Giordano MJ, Fishback AS, Guha A: **Loss of merlin expression in sporadic meningiomas, ependymomas and schwannomas.** *Neurology* 1997, **49**(1):267–270.
2. Asthagiri AR, Parry DM, Butman JA, Kim HJ, Tsilou ET, Zhuang Z, Lonser RR: **Neurofibromatosis type 2.** *Lancet* 2009, **373**(9679):1974–1986.
3. Evans DG, Trueman L, Wallace A, Collins S, Strachan T: **Genotype/phenotype correlations in type 2 neurofibromatosis (NF2): evidence for more severe disease associated with truncating mutations.** *J Med Genet* 1998, **35**(6):450–455.
4. Sughrue ME, Yeung AH, Rutkowski MJ, Cheung SW, Parsa AT: **Molecular biology of familial and sporadic vestibular schwannomas: implications for novel therapeutics.** *J Neurosurg* 2009, **114**(2):359–366.
5. Rong R, Tang X, Gutmann DH, Ye K: **Neurofibromatosis 2 (NF2) tumor suppressor merlin inhibits phosphatidylinositol 3-kinase through binding to PIKE-L.** *Proc Natl Acad Sci USA* 2004, **101**(52):18200–18205.
6. Yohay KH: **The genetic and molecular pathogenesis of NF1 and NF2.** *Semin Pediatr Neurol* 2006, **13**(1):21–26.

7. Lim JY, Kim H, Jeun SS, Kang SG, Lee KJ: **Merlin inhibits growth hormone-regulated Raf-ERKs pathways by binding to Grb2 protein.** *Biochem Biophys Res Commun* 2006, **340**(4):1151–1157.
8. Xiao GH, Gallagher R, Shetler J, Skele K, Altomare DA, Pestell RG, Jhanwar S, Testa JR: **The NF2 tumor suppressor gene product, merlin, inhibits cell proliferation and cell cycle progression by repressing cyclin D1 expression.** *Mol Cell Biol* 2005, **25**(6):2384–2394.
9. Zhan Y, Chadee DN: **Inhibition of Cdc42-mediated activation of mixed lineage kinase 3 by the tumor suppressor protein merlin.** *Small Gtpases* 2010, **1**(3):183–186.
10. Li W, Giancotti FG: **Merlin's tumor suppression linked to inhibition of the E3 ubiquitin ligase CRL4 (DCAF1).** *Cell Cycle* 2010, **9**(22):4433–4436.
11. Uppal S, Coatesworth AP: **Neurofibromatosis type 2.** *Int J Clin Pract* 2003, **57**(8):698–703.
12. Mautner VF, Baser ME, Thakkar SD, Feigen UM, Friedman JM, Kluwe L. **Vestibular schwannoma growth in patients with neurofibromatosis type 2: a longitudinal study.** *J Neurosurg* 2002, **96**(2):223–228.
13. Evans DG, Huson SM, Donnai D, Neary W, Blair V, Newton V, Harris R: **A clinical study of type 2 neurofibromatosis.** *Q J Med* 1992, **84**(304):603–618.
14. Evans DG, Wallace A: **An update on age related mosaic and offspring risk in neurofibromatosis 2 (NF2).** *J Med Genet* 2009, **46**(11):792.
15. Dayalan AH, Jothi M, Keshava R, Thomas R, Gope ML, Doddaballapur SK, Somanna S, Praharaj SS, Ashwathnarayanarao CB, Gope R: **Age dependent phosphorylation and deregulation of p53 in human vestibular schwannomas.** *Mol Carcinog* 2006, **45**(1):38–46.
16. Shai RM: **Microarray tools for deciphering complex diseases.** *Front Biosci* 2006, **11**:1414–1424.
17. Hanemann CO, Bartelt-Kirbach B, Diebold R, Kampchen K, Langmesser S, Utermark T: **Differential gene expression between human schwannoma and control Schwann cells.** *Neuropathol Appl Neurobiol* 2006, **32**(6):605–614.
18. Aarhus M, Bruland O, Saetran HA, Mork SJ, Lund-Johansen M, Knappskog PM: **Global gene expression profiling and tissue microarray reveal novel candidate genes and down-regulation of the tumor suppressor gene CAV1 in sporadic vestibular schwannomas.** *Neurosurgery* 2010, **67**(4):998–1019. discussion 1019.
19. Martinez-Glez V, Franco-Hernandez C, Alvarez L, De Campos JM, Isla A, Vaquero J, Lassaletta L, Casartelli C, Rey JA: **Meningiomas and schwannomas: molecular subgroup classification found by expression arrays.** *Int J Oncol* 2009, **34**(2):493–504.
20. Smyth GK: **Linear models and empirical Bayes methods for assessing differential expression in microarray experiments.** *Stat Appl Genet Mol Biol* 2004, **3**(1). ISSN (Online) 1544-6115, doi:10.2202/1544-6115.1027. Article3.

4

Evaluation of copy number variation and gene expression in neurofibromatosis type-1-associated malignant peripheral nerve sheath tumours

Laura E Thomas[1], Jincy Winston[1], Ellie Rad[1], Matthew Mort[1], Kayleigh M Dodd[1], Andrew R Tee[1], Fionnuala McDyer[2], Stephen Moore[2], David N Cooper[1] and Meena Upadhyaya[1*]

Abstract

Background: Neurofibromatosis type-1 (NF1) is a complex neurogenetic disorder characterised by the development of benign and malignant tumours of the peripheral nerve sheath (MPNSTs). Whilst biallelic *NF1* gene inactivation contributes to benign tumour formation, additional cellular changes in gene structure and/or expression are required to induce malignant transformation. Although few molecular profiling studies have been performed on the process of progression of pre-existing plexiform neurofibromas to MPNSTs, the integrated analysis of copy number alterations (CNAs) and gene expression is likely to be key to understanding the molecular mechanisms underlying NF1-MPNST tumorigenesis. In a pilot study, we employed this approach to identify genes differentially expressed between benign and malignant NF1 tumours.

Results: *SPP1* (osteopontin) was the most differentially expressed gene (85-fold increase in expression), compared to benign plexiform neurofibromas. Short hairpin RNA (shRNA) knockdown of *SPP1* in NF1-MPNST cells reduced tumour spheroid size, wound healing and invasion in four different MPNST cell lines. Seventy-six genes were found to exhibit concordance between CNA and gene expression level.

Conclusions: Pathway analysis of these genes suggested that glutathione metabolism and Wnt signalling may be specifically involved in NF1-MPNST development. *SPP1* is associated with malignant transformation in NF1-associated MPNSTs and could prove to be an important target for therapeutic intervention.

Keywords: NF1, MPNSTs, Copy number alterations, Gene expression profiling, *SPP1*

Background

Neurofibromatosis type 1 (NF1) (MIM# 162200), a complex autosomal dominant disorder with a highly variable clinical phenotype, affects approximately 1 in 4,000 people worldwide (Huson, 2008). Malignant complications are relatively rare manifestations of this disorder but include brain tumours, optic gliomas and malignant peripheral nerve sheath tumours (MPNSTs) [1,2]. MPNSTs can either occur sporadically or instead may develop from the malignant transformation of pre-existing NF1-associated plexiform neurofibromas (PNF) or from a focal subcutaneous neurofibroma. The lifetime risk of developing MPNSTs in NF1 patients is 10%–15% [3,4].

MPNSTs are a significant cause of morbidity and mortality in NF1. Upon first presentation, MPNSTs are often non-resectable because the tumour is already at a late stage of development; metastases may also be present, most commonly in the lung but also in the liver and brain. Consequently, the 5-year survival rate for individuals with these tumours is only 20%–50%, and the 10-year survival rate is even lower (7.5%) [5]. Currently, there are no effective treatments for MPNSTs; although complete surgical excision with clear margins is the therapy of choice, chemotherapy has sometimes also been employed despite its limited effectiveness. Several risk factors confer an increased likelihood of MPNST development, e.g. multiple internal PNFs [6], previous radiation

* Correspondence: upadhyaya@cardiff.ac.uk
[1]Institute of Medical Genetics, School of Medicine, Cardiff University, Cardiff CF14 4XN, UK

therapy, the presence of an inherited gross genomic deletion that removes the entire *NF1* gene [7], the presence of neurofibromatous neuropathy [8] or a family history of NF1-MPNSTs [9]. Since there are no reliable predictive or prognostic biomarkers for MPNSTs, the progression of a pre-existing plexiform neurofibroma to an MPNST cannot currently be predicted in advance on the basis of molecular (copy number and/or gene expression) profiling despite recent significant advances in this field. Beert et al. (2011) demonstrated recurrent homozygous loss of the *CDKN2A* locus in 15/16 atypical neurofibromas; this finding supports the notion that atypical neurofibromas constitute intermediates between benign neurofibroma and MPNSTs and further suggests that *CDKN2A* loss is an early step in the progression of neurofibroma to MPNSTs [10]. A detailed knowledge of the *NF1* somatic mutational spectrum of MPNSTs is, however, a prerequisite for the development of targeted therapies. Although somatic inactivation of the wild-type *NF1* allele is presumed to be the key step in NF1-associated tumour development, this cannot on its own explain the malignant transformation of benign plexiform neurofibromas to MPNSTs. This indicates that additional genetic (and potentially epigenetic) alterations are required to bring about malignancy.

High-throughput whole genome microarray profiling has proved to be one of the most effective methods to analyse large numbers of clinical samples across multiple tumour types. Indeed, a considerable number of studies have identified somatic copy number alterations (CNA) and concomitant gene expression changes in benign and malignant NF1-associated tumours [11-30]. However, despite the plethora of previous array-based investigations, relatively few genes have so far been identified that are consistently mutated across multiple MPNSTs. Such frequently mutated genes may harbour 'driver mutations' (as opposed to 'passenger mutations') that promote NF1 malignant transformation. MPNST development is clearly a complex multistep process in which the mutation of a large number of genes, contributing to the deregulation of multiple signalling and regulatory pathways, is to be expected. Whole genome analysis and, in particular, the focussed investigation of specific pathways are likely to be key to determining the underlying molecular mechanisms involved in MPNST tumorigenesis. Genes that could be informative in a prognostic context may be identified through the use of integrated CNA/gene expression analysis performed on the same sample sets [31,32]. To this end, the present study employed Affymetrix Human Exon 1.0 ST Arrays to screen both PNF and MPNST tumour DNAs from nine unrelated NF1 patients to generate data on differences in gene expression at the whole genome level between benign and malignant tumours with which to compare with previously generated CNA data derived from the same tumours in order to disclose novel genes and pathways that could be important in MPNST development [25].

Results

Identification of differentially expressed genes between neurofibromas and MPNSTs

For differential expression analysis, different sets of genes were identified from the various analyses (Figure 1a,b) that we performed: (1) 4 benign tumour samples vs. 5 malignant tumour samples with stringent criteria applied, (2) 4 benign tumour samples vs. 5 malignant tumour samples under less stringent criteria, (3) 3 benign tumour samples vs. 3 malignant tumour samples under stringent criteria and (4) 3 benign tumour samples vs. 3 malignant tumour samples under less stringent criteria (Additional file 1: Table S2). The genes identified employing the less stringent criteria from the 4 vs. 5 analyses were cross-compared with the corresponding list of genes identified by means of the 3 vs. 3 analysis (Figure 1a). The same process was then followed for those genes identified using the more stringent criteria (Figure 1b). Given the relatively

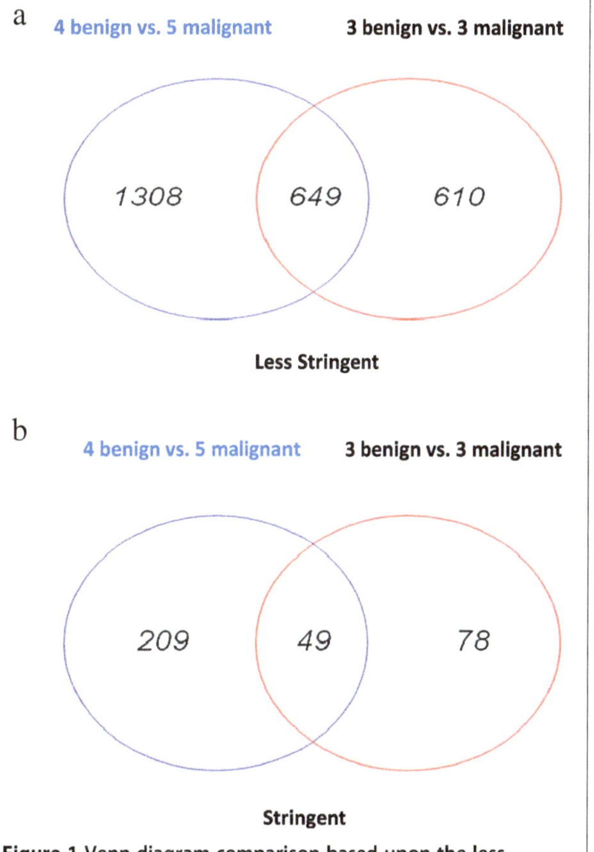

Figure 1 Venn diagram comparison based upon the less stringent and stringent gene list. a. Venn diagram based upon the less stringent gene lists from the 4 vs. 5 and 3 vs. 3 pairwise comparisons. **b.** Venn diagram based upon the stringent gene lists from the 4 vs. 5 and 3 vs. 3 pairwise comparisons.

small number of patients included in this study, the presence of outliers (patients exhibiting variable expression compared with the median) was expected to have a considerable influence on the combined results. With this in mind, the analysis as described above was performed with and without those outlier/variable samples.

The number of genes identified as being differentially expressed between benign and malignant tumours under more or less stringent criteria in the 3 vs. 3 and 4 vs. 5 analyses can be found in Table 1. Under the less stringent criteria, statistical testing employed a *P* value threshold of 0.05, which served to identify genes displaying ≥1.3-fold (absolute) differential gene expression. In the differential analysis, which considered all profiled samples (4 benign vs. 5 malignant), a total of 1,957 genes were identified as being differentially expressed between benign and malignant tumours whereas in the differential analysis which excluded the three samples at the expression range extremes (3 benign vs. 3 malignant), only 1,259 genes were identified. The two different conditions of stringency were used for the sake of comparison. However, for the final analysis, the genes identified under the more stringent criteria were used. Under the more stringent criteria, statistical testing employed a *P* value threshold of 0.005, which was deemed to be sufficient to identify genes displaying 1.5-fold or more (absolute) differential gene expression. In the 4 vs. 5 stringent gene list analysis, 258 genes were identified as being differentially expressed between benign and malignant tumours whereas in the 3 vs. 3 analyses, the number of genes identified was 127. The top 20 significantly differentially expressed genes identified using the more stringent criteria are given in Table 2.

The *SPP1* gene [NCBI: NM_001040058] (osteopontin; OPN) was found to exhibit the most significantly elevated differential mean expression level between the benign and malignant tumours. *SPP1* was therefore selected for further functional analysis to assess its possible role in malignant transformation. Exon array analysis identified a mean expression level of 12.06 (log2) for *SPP1* in malignant tumours and a mean expression level of 5.65 (log2) in benign plexiform neurofibromas. This equates to an 85-fold increase (based on anti-logged LS means) in expression in

Table 1 Definitions of stringent and less stringent analytical criteria and the numbers of genes detected by the 3 vs. 3 and 4 vs. 5 analyses under both sets of criteria

	Less stringent criteria	Stringent criteria
Statistical testing *P* value	0.05	0.005
Fold change	1.3	1.5
Number of genes 4 vs. 5	1,957	258
Number of genes 3 vs. 3	1,259	127

Definition of stringent and less stringent analytical criteria and the numbers of genes detected by the t vs. 3 and 4 vs. 5 analyses under both sets of criteria.

MPNSTs compared to benign plexiform neurofibromas ($P = 0.0002$) (Table 2). Since this was the highest fold change in expression observed between benign and malignant tumours for all the genes identified in this analysis, an association with malignant transformation was strongly suspected. Significant reductions in the expression of *ADH1B* and *GRIK2* (*P* values 0.0003 and 0.0004, respectively) in MPNSTs as compared to benign plexiform neurofibromas were however also observed (Table 2).

Quantitative real-time PCR (q-PCR)

Gene expression changes initially detected by Affymetrix Human Exon 1.0 ST Array analysis were validated by q-PCR. We aimed to determine where there was a correlation between the presence of a copy number alteration and gene expression (either a concomitant increase in copy number and gene expression or a decrease in both) as assessed by quantitative PCR. This was determined by identifying whether the same directional change as noted above was identified in the array data from the current study and CNA data from the previous analyses [25] (Additional file 2: Table S3). A correlation was noted for 11 of the 20 differentially expressed genes analysed (Additional file 3: Figure S1) (*ADH1B, FAP, FLJ42200, GRIK2, GTDC1, KIAA0746, KRTAP13-4, PEG3, NSBP1, PTGIS* and *SPP1*). For six of the genes (*CCT5, CD72, COL10A1, FAM177A1, SLC25A12* and *TDP1*), we were unable to identify a correlation (i.e. concordance) between the copy number alteration and gene expression in six of the tumour samples tested. For the remaining three genes (*CSRP1, GRIK3* and *EFHC2*), half the samples yielded findings compatible with, and anticipated from, the results of the exon array experiments; the remaining samples either demonstrated no change in gene expression or the opposite change to that anticipated on the basis of the exon array results (i.e. a decrease in gene expression identified by array, increase in gene expression identified by Q-PCR) (see Additional file 3: Figure S1).

Integration of copy number analysis with differentially expressed genes

CNA data were derived from a previously published analysis of the same tumours [25]. In total, 27 genes were common to HMM and expression analysis, whereas 120 genes were common to segmentation and expression analysis. We then selected those genes that were common to expression analysis and HMM and/or segmentation analysis (121 genes in total; see Figure 2). Of these 121 genes, gene expression and CNA data were concordant in 76 (63%) cases, with all 76 genes displaying the same directional change of both CNA and gene expression (Additional file 2: Table S3). The 76 genes that were concordant for copy number and gene expression

Table 2 The top 20 genes identified as being significantly differentially expressed between MPNSTs and PNFs in the more stringent analysis of 3 vs. 3 samples

Transcript ID	Gene symbol	Ref seq	Mean expression	Mean expression	Fold change	*P* value	Chromosome	Start	Stop
			Benign	Malignant	Benign vs. malignant	Benign vs. malignant			
2584134	*FAP*	NM_004460	4.87	8.75	14.75	0.0001	2	163027200	163101589
4013828	*NSBP1*	NM_030763	5.22	3.67	−2.92	0.0001	X	80211860	80457431
3917555	*KRTAP13n4*	NM_181600	3.77	3.13	−1.55	0.0001	21	31797943	31809269
3908934	*PTGIS*	NM_000961	4.58	6.60	4.06	0.0002	20	48120414	48185550
2764192	*KIAA0746*	NM_015187	4.33	5.82	2.80	0.0002	4	25722248	25865344
2735027	*SPP1*	NM_001040058	5.65	12.06	85.19	0.0002	4	88408243	88904561
3532353	*FAM177A1*	NM_001079519	8.01	7.11	−1.86	0.0003	14	35508201	35582327
2779231	*ADH1B*	NM_000668	6.50	3.18	−9.99	0.0003	4	100226131	100242895
2406926	*GRIK3*	NM_000831	7.20	3.85	−10.19	0.0004	1	37266614	37524753
3916290	*FLJ42200*	AK124194	3.32	4.05	1.65	0.0004	21	25353415	25920256
2970942	*COL10A1*	NM_000493	3.56	4.67	2.17	0.0004	6	116440092	116518549
2450865	*CSRP1*	NM_004078	9.09	7.28	−3.50	0.0005	1	201445919	201481500
2918982	*GRIK2*	NM_175768	7.02	3.47	−11.66	0.0005	6	101841683	102690448
3204648	*CD72*	NM_001782	4.08	5.08	1.99	0.0005	9	35609970	35646790
4006326	*EFHC2*	NM_025184	4.84	3.42	−2.67	0.0005	X	44006888	44309044
2586845	*SLC25A12*	NM_003705	5.56	6.30	1.68	0.0006	2	172639117	172750960
2579439	*GTDC1*	NM_001006636	6.95	5.92	−2.05	0.0006	2	144702190	145123135
3872053	*PEG3*	NM_006210	5.58	4.17	−2.65	0.0006	19	57285930	57352082
2801526	*CCT5*	NM_012073	8.62	9.33	1.64	0.0006	5	10250111	10266501
3548152	*TDP1*	NM_018319	4.17	5.49	2.50	0.0007	14	90421293	90511103

The top 20 genes identified as being significantly differentially expressed between MPNSTs and PNFs in the more stringent analysis of 3 vs. 3 samples.

changes were regarded as potential candidates for involvement in malignancy (Additional file 2: Table S3).

Pathway analysis

The 76 concordant genes, which were common to both the CNA and expression analyses, were interrogated using all pathways in the METACORE database. Pathways in which more than one gene was subject to concomitant alterations in both copy number and expression were then listed. The top ten pathways (by *P* value) are given in Table 3. These pathways include the glutathione metabolism, Wnt signalling, cell adhesion and alpha-6/beta 4 integrin pathways.

SPP1 knockdown in multiple MPNST cell lines impairs tumour formation, wound healing and invasion

Given that we observed significant differences in the expression level of *SPP1* in MPNSTs as compared with the benign plexiform neurofibromas and the fact that *SPP1* plays significant roles in both tumorigenesis and metastasis [33], we knocked down expression of the *SPP1* gene in four MPNST cell lines (ST8814, S462, S1844.1 and S1507.2) and examined both the ability of these cell lines to form tumours (Figure 3a) and the effect of knockdown on wound healing and invasion. Both control and *SPP1* knockdown cell lines formed tumour colonies in soft agar. However, *SPP1* knockdown caused a significant reduction in tumour spheroid size (n = 40, P = 0.0001) in all MPNST cell lines tested (Figure 3b). We next analysed the effects of *SPP1* knockdown on cell migration during wound healing (Figure 4a). In all cell lines, knockdown of *SPP1* robustly inhibited wound closure (Figure 4b) (*P* values for the ST8814, S462, S1844.1 and S1507.2 cell line were 0.03, 0.001, 0.001 and 0.003, respectively), suggesting a possible role for *SPP1* in metastasis. This role was further supported by the results of cellular invasion assays, which revealed that *SPP1* knockdown significantly reduces the cells' invasive properties (*P* values for the ST8814, S462, S1844.1 and S1507.2 cell line were 0.0001, 0.001, 0.0001 and 0.001, respectively) (Figure 4b,c). Validation of specific gene knockdown using short hairpin RNA (shRNA) clones was completed by Western blot analysis. A β-actin control blot was performed to confirm that there were no

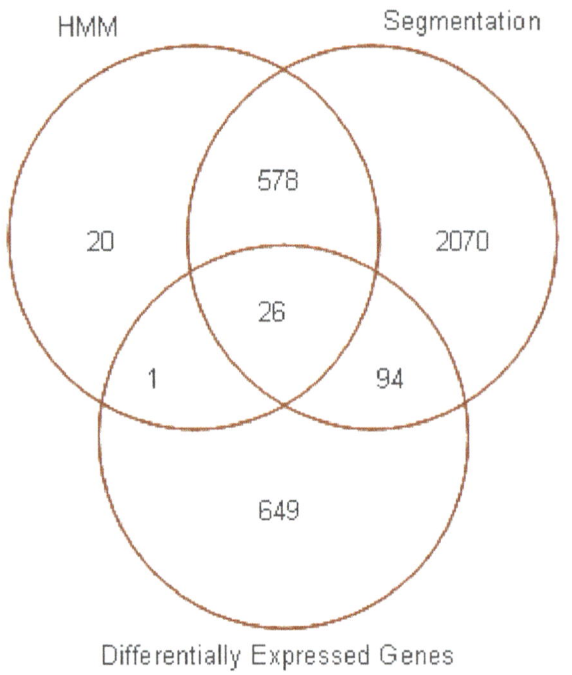

Figure 2 Venn diagram comparing the numbers of genes from the HMM and segmentation copy number analyses with the genes found to be differentially expressed.

shRNA off-target effects (Figure 5). In summary, *SPP1* knockdown with shRNA resulted in a significant reduction in both wound healing and invasiveness.

Discussion

The functional loss of neurofibromin, due to *NF1* gene inactivation, leads to increased cell growth and proliferation through constitutive Ras pathway signalling. Although this is necessary for benign neurofibroma formation, it is insufficient to explain the malignant transformation of a benign PNF to an MPNST, since additional genetic lesions (and/or epigenetic modifications) are required for this to occur [25].

Initially, this study aimed to identify genes that contribute to the malignant transformation of benign neurofibromas by establishing which genes were differentially expressed between benign and malignant tumours in NF1 patients. A previously compiled list of genes located within regions encompassed by copy number alterations (CNAs) identified in the NF1-MPNSTs which were also used in the current study [25] was then cross-compared with a list of genes differentially expressed in the same NF1-MPNST samples, which were analysed for this study through Affymetrix exon array analysis. Finally, an additional study involving pathway analysis was performed on those genes that were common to the results of the CNA and exon array analyses.

In previous studies of NF1-MPNSTs, many genetic alterations, including copy number alterations and differential gene expression, have been identified but no specific molecular signature pathognomonic of malignant transformation has so far been defined [11-30]. Identifying genes that are differentially expressed between benign and malignant tumours not only promises to improve our understanding of the process of malignant transformation but should also aid in identifying potential therapeutic targets.

This study employed the GeneChip Human Gene 1.0 ST array (Affymetrix, Santa Clara, USA). This array is a whole transcript-based array for gene expression profiling which, unlike older Affymetrix arrays, queries the entire transcript instead of just the 3′ end [34]. Additionally, this array uses a labelling protocol that generates biotinylated sense strand DNA instead of complementary RNA (cRNA), thereby yielding DNA-DNA duplexes, which are more specific than the RNA-DNA duplexes generated using standard protocols [35]. This array provides approximately 25-mer probes designed to be distributed across the transcribed regions of each gene with a median of 26 probes per gene, giving two complementary levels of expression analysis in a single experiment, both "exon-level" and "gene-level" analysis. The array interrogates 28,869 well-annotated genes with 764,885 distinct probes. The array is based on the March 2006 (UCSChg18, NCBI Build 36) human genome sequence assembly. The Affymetrix Human Exon 1.0 ST array contains 17,881 transcripts. Whole genome Affymetrix exon arrays have been employed in a number of different studies of cancer including non-small cell lung, colon, bladder and prostate cancer [36,37].

The comparative transcriptome analysis reported here identified the *SPP1* gene to be the single most differentially overexpressed gene in NF1-MPNSTs as compared to benign tumours. *SPP1* was selected for further study not only for this reason but also because of its well-documented involvement in cell signalling, tumorigenesis and metastasis [38-49]. shRNA knockdown of four different MPNST cell lines revealed a significant reduction in tumour colony size growth, wound healing and cell invasion, thereby supporting a role for the increased expression of *SPP1* in the malignant transformation and invasion of cells during NF1-MPNST development. *SPP1* is an extracellular matrix protein with cytokine properties. It is involved in extracellular matrix (ECM) and adhesion-related pathways where it performs key roles in cell-cell communication, focal adhesion, immune cell activation and immune cell migration. It plays an essential role in the pathway that leads to type I immunity, thereby enhancing the production of interferon-gamma and interleukin-12 and reducing interleukin-1 synthesis. In terms of an association with cancer, *SPP1* has been shown to

Table 3 Pathway Enrichment analysis

	Pathway name	*P* value	Genes	Fold change (3 benign vs. 3 malignant)	Fold change (4 benign vs. 5 malignant
1	Glutathione metabolism	0.00056	*GSTM1*	−3.25	−2.27
			GSTM2	−3.25	−2.27
			GSTM4	−3.25	−2.27
2	Glutathione metabolism/human version	0.00059	*GSTM1*	−3.25	−2.27
			GSTM2	−3.25	−2.27
			GSTM4	−3.25	−2.27
3	Glutathione metabolism/rodent version	0.00073	*GSTM1*	−3.25	−2.27
			GSTM2	−3.25	−2.27
			GSTM4	−3.25	−2.27
4	Development: Wnt signalling pathway. Degradation of beta-catenin in the absence Wnt signalling	0.00106	*CSNK1D*	2.42	1.99
			DAB2	3.46	2.65
5	Cell adhesion: PLAU signalling	0.00445	*HGF*	7.80	10.97
			SERPINE1	5.74	4.54
6	Role of alpha-6/beta-4 integrins in carcinoma progression	0.00589	*HGF*	7.80	10.97
			LIMK1	2.04	2.23
7	Development: TGF-beta-dependent induction of EMT via MAPK	0.00641	*DAB2*	3.46	2.65
			SERPINE1	5.74	4.54
8	Transport: macropinocytosis regulation by growth factors	0.01130	*HGF*	7.80	10.97
			LIMK1	2.04	2.23
9	Development: regulation of epithelial-to-mesenchymal transition (EMT)	0.01165	*HGF*	7.80	10.97
			SERPINE1	5.74	4.54
10	Transport: clathrin-coated vesicle cycle	0.01421	*PREB*	1.45	1.43
			DAB2	3.46	2.65

The pathways were ranked by hypergeometric *P* values, and a summary of the top ten pathways is reported. The *P* value represents the probability that a gene set of this size would co-occur by chance alone. Network objects represent the ratio of the number of genes from the list compared to the total number of genes known to be associated with the pathway.

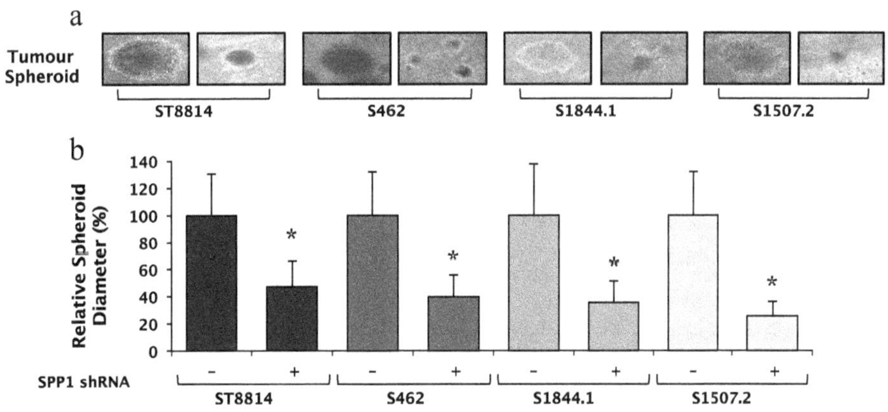

Figure 3 *SPP1* knockdown reduces tumour size in soft agar. Stable ST8814, S462, S1844.1 and S1507.2 cell lines, expressing either non-target or *SPP1* shRNA as indicated, were subjected to tumour spheroid growth assays. **a)** Photographs of 40 tumours were taken after 2 weeks of incubation. The diameter of all tumours was measured using ImageJ software; the scale bar on images represents 250 μm. **b)** The percentage of tumour size was calculated from the 40 tumours for both the control and *SPP1* shRNA. *SPP1* knockdown significantly reduced tumour size in all four MPNST cell lines, consistent with a role for *SPP1* in tumour growth ($P = 0.0001$), *$P < 0.05$ when comparing treated vs. untreated cells.

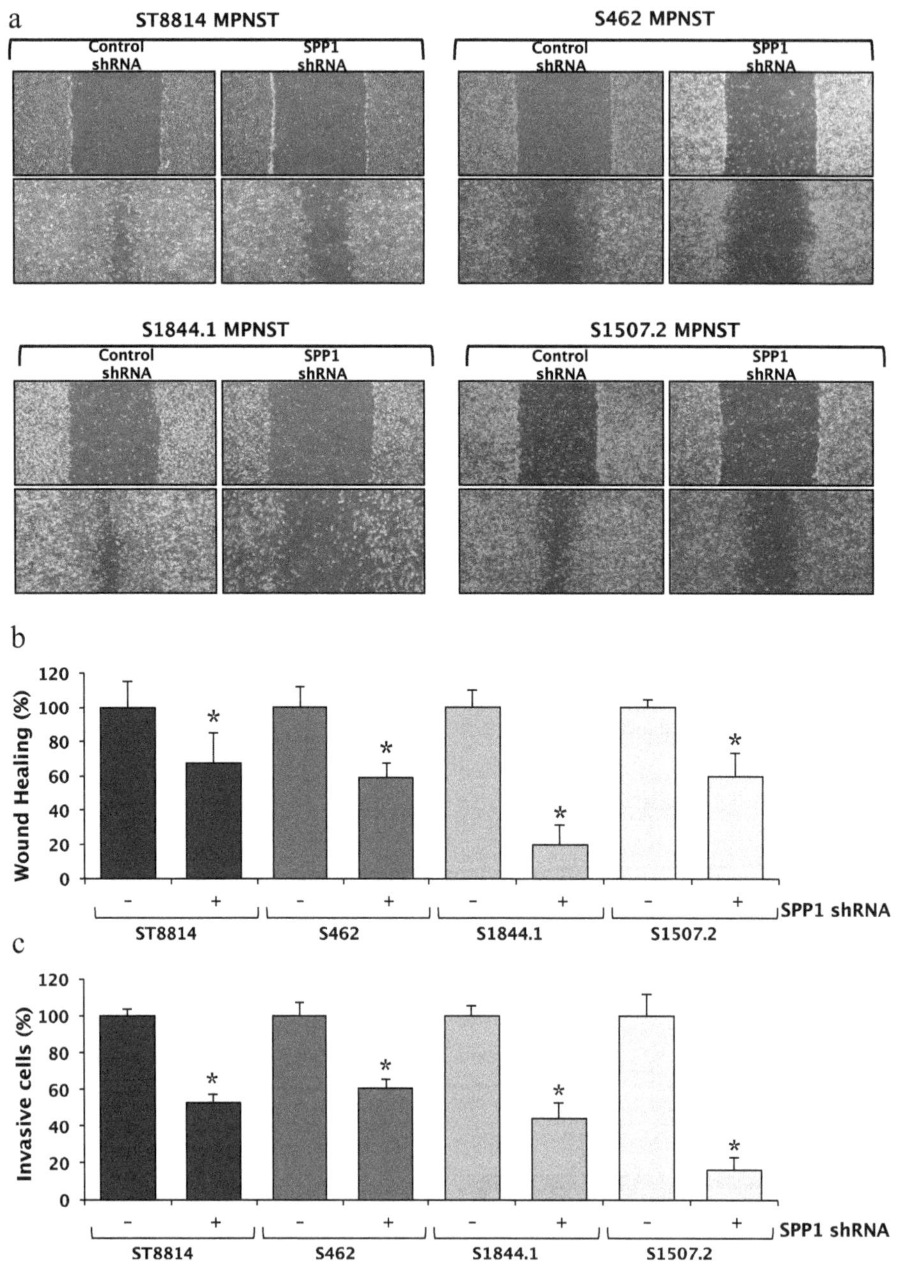

Figure 4 ***SPP1*** **knockdown impairs wound healing and cell invasion.** Stable ST8814, S462, S1844.1 and S1507.2 cell lines, expressing either non-target or *SPP1* shRNA, as indicated, were subjected to a wound healing assay. **a)** Pictures of cells were taken at 0 and 18 h after wounding. **b)** The percentage of cell migration was calculated using three individual experiments. *SPP1* knockdown significantly reduced cell migration during wound healing in all four MPNST cell lines [*P* values for the four cell lines were as follows: ST8814 (0.03), S462 (0.001), S1844.1 (0.001), S1507.2 (0.003)]. **c)** *SPP1* knockdown significantly reduced cell invasiveness; crystal violet was used to stain invasive cells. Cells were then eluted with 1% (w/v) SDS, and the absorbance was read at 550 nm on a Genova MK3 Lifescience Analyser; the number of cells was calculated by plotting the absorbance against a standard curve. The percentage of invasive cells was calculated in three individual experiments. *SPP1* knockdown significantly reduced cell invasion in all four MPNST cell lines, suggesting a potential role for *SPP1* in metastasis [*P* values for the four cell lines were as follows: ST8814 (0.0001), S462 (0.001), S1844.1 (0.0001), S1507.2 (0.001). *$P < 0.05$ when comparing treated vs. untreated cells].

promote the growth of different tumours [38-49]. Cells harbouring activated RAS have been found to exhibit a higher level of *SPP1* [50]. It could therefore be that the activation of RAS through the functional loss of neurofibromin (due to *NF1* gene inactivation) gives rise to the overexpression of *SPP1*. Furthermore, the use of *SPP1* inhibitors such as agelastatin A has successfully reduced colony formation, migration and invasion in human breast cancer cell lines [51]. Whilst *SPP1* has the highest level of differential gene expression, the remaining genes in Table 2

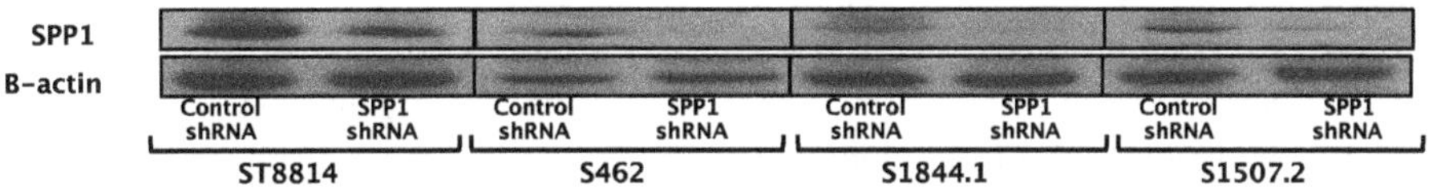

Figure 5 To confirm efficient knockdown, SPP1 protein levels were compared between control and *SPP1* knockdown cell lines by Western blot. β-actin was used as a loading control. SPP1 protein levels were significantly reduced after SPP1 knockdown in all MPNST cell lines.

would warrant further exploration in future studies. This would help to explore further the relationship with NF1 of not only SPP1 but the other identified statistically significant genes, which are differentially expressed between benign and malignant NF1 tumours.

In an attempt to explore the relationship between gene expression and copy number variation in the context of NF1 tumorigenesis, we attempted to integrate previous copy number data derived from the MPNSTs under study here [25], with the newly generated data on differentially expressed genes. The same tumour samples were utilised for both analyses. The identification of prognostic biomarkers for NF1-MPNSTs using gene expression microarrays is challenging in that there are very few candidate genes in common between the different studies so far performed [11-30]. However, over the last 5 years, studies of cancer have begun to integrate gene expression and copy number analysis in an attempt to explore underlying mechanisms of tumorigenesis and to identify potential gene and pathway biomarkers [31,32]. Such an integrative approach has led to advances in our understanding of the role of copy number alterations in tumorigenesis. Thus, for example, the Cancer Genome Atlas project [52] is generating multiple datasets using different platforms (e.g. gene expression and copy number analysis) from the same set of patients. Although the increased expression of a particular gene does not by itself constitute direct evidence for the role of that gene in tumorigenesis, concomitant copy number alterations may serve to disrupt metabolic and physiological processes, thereby contributing indirectly to tumorigenesis [31,32]. There is however compelling evidence for a *cis*-dosage effect of CNA on gene expression [53], and this relationship can facilitate the identification of novel genes involved in tumorigenesis as well as other aspects of cancer biology. In any such analysis, it is important to be aware of cellular heterogeneity within the tumour [54].

Work on different tumours, including breast, lung, prostate, hepatocellular carcinoma and melanoma, has yielded an estimate of the proportion of all differentially expressed genes whose expression is concordant with their copy number status. This has been shown to vary between 32% and 78% [31,32,55,56]. In this context, it is encouraging that in the current study, 63% of genes were found to be concordant in terms of their expression and copy number status. However, although *SPP1* was found to be the most differentially expressed gene in the initial part of this study, we failed to find any copy number changes in MPNSTs in our earlier study and thus its expression was not concordant with the copy number changes [25]. For this reason, we propose that the observed upregulation of *SPP1* gene expression may not have been modulated by a copy number alteration. This is especially in view of the fact that no copy number alterations involving *SPP1* have previously been reported in a variety of cancers and tissue types (by reference to COSMIC and CONAN) [57,58], including NF1 MPNSTs [40]. Thus, in the absence of gene duplication/amplification/deletion, it may be that there are other genetic mechanisms including DNA methylation, point mutations, up- or downregulated transcription factors, regulation of messenger RNA (mRNA) transcription or microRNAs (miRNAs) [59-61] that could influence the expression of the non-concordant genes (37%) identified in this study.

Finally, we performed pathway analysis on the 76 genes that were common to the copy number array and exon array data. Integration of clinical information with copy number and gene expression data has led to the identification of genes common to CNA regions and expression array datasets that are consistently associated with clinical outcomes including lung cancer, thereby underlining the clinical relevance and utility of such data sets [56]. The top ten statistically significant pathways were noted from those where two or more genes exhibiting alterations in copy number and/or expression belonged to the same pathway (Table 3). These pathways included glutathione metabolism, Wnt signalling, cell adhesion PLAU and intracellular signalling by alpha-6/beta-4 (a6b4) integrins. The Wnt signalling pathway, including the genes *CSNK1D* and *DAB2* in this data set (Table 3), is of particular interest. The *APC* gene belongs to the Wnt pathway and is somatically mutated in various cancers and also in familial adenomatous polyposis, which results from inherited *APC* gene mutations [62]. In human colon cancer, SPP1 is a transcriptional target of aberrant Wnt signalling, and *SPP1* expression alone predicts survival [63]. Vinas et al. (2010) demonstrated that the antiapoptotic role of Wnt was mediated by SPP1, a direct Wnt target gene, and SPP1 was reduced by Wnt antibody administration *in vivo* [64]. Using comparative transcriptome analysis, Mo et al. (2013) previously demonstrated that PI3K and β-catenin signalling are involved in the promotion of MPNST growth [26]. Furthermore, using a sleeping beauty forward genetic screen, the Wnt pathway has been found to be a driver of MPNST development [27]. Most interestingly, in a recent study, 20 Wnt genes exhibited altered expression in MPNST biopsies and cell lines in comparison to benign neurofibromas [30]. Taken together, it has become clear that progression to malignancy requires many genomic alterations acting in concert. Importantly, our results appear to concur with the findings of previous studies that the canonical Wnt signalling pathway is likely to be a key driver of MPNST development. Thus, members of the Wnt pathway may not only constitute potential biomarkers of MPNST tumorigenesis but also represent potential therapeutic targets for small molecule inhibitors [26-28].

In addition to the Wnt signalling pathway, other pathways in Table 3 are also thought to be involved in cancer progression. Specifically, although there is no clear association reported with NF1, altered glutathione (GSH) metabolism is thought to be a major mechanism of chemoresistance and GSH levels are reportedly elevated in non-small cell lung cancer [65]. In addition, genetic variations in genes involved in the glutathione and DNA repair pathways are associated with non-small cell lung cancer survival [66]. Further analysis of the pathways in Table 3 would be important to ascertain the role of the *NF1* gene in other cancers.

Conclusions

Although MPNSTs only develop in approximately 15% of NF1 patients, they represent a frequent cause of lethal progression of the NF1 phenotype. It is clear that many genetic (and potentially epigenetic) factors contribute to abnormal tumour progression in these neoplasms [67,68]. The prognosis for individuals diagnosed with an MPNST is usually very poor, especially as treatment options for MPNSTs are currently very limited and complete surgical excision with clear margins has proved to be very difficult. In knockdown experiments involving shRNA for *SPP1*, we found that cell migration was reduced in four different MPNST cell lines. This exploratory study supports the idea of a direct role for *SPP1* in MPNST development and metastasis. Although obtaining MPNST samples can be challenging, this preliminary study warrants confirmation in a larger panel of samples as the study has a limitation in that it is based on a small cohort of samples. In addition to the well-studied role of osteopontin in other cancers [38-49], the expression of *SPP1* is regulated by Wnt signalling, one of the pathways that we identified as playing a role in the progression of benign plexiform neurofibromas to MPNSTs [69]. This is most encouraging in terms of the potential for those genes and pathways newly identified in this study to help in understanding the molecular basis of tumorigenesis and malignant transformation in NF1 as well as providing targets for therapeutic intervention in NF1-MPNST development.

Methods

Patient samples and RNA preparation

DNA and RNA were isolated from the same segment of tumour. RNA was extracted from nine NF1-associated tumours with biallelic *NF1* gene mutations (comprising four benign PNFs and five high grade MPNSTs) from nine unrelated NF1 patients using the TRIZOL method (Invitrogen) as previously described [25]. The same tumour samples were utilised in the current study and the previous analyses for microarray analysis [25] to enable analysis of paired CNA and gene expression data. All total RNA samples were assessed for purity and integrity by means of an Agilent Bioanalyser. Samples were renamed and randomised in order to avoid order bias or batching effects. Analysis of gene expression by Affymetrix Human Exon 1.0 ST Array was performed by Almac Diagnostics (Craigavon, UK). The Affymetrix Human Exon 1.0 ST array contains 17,881 transcripts. Standard operating protocols, as provided by the manufacturer, were used to PCR amplify and hybridise nine NF1-associated tumour-derived cDNA samples on Affymetrix Human Exon 1.0 ST arrays.

Ethics statement

All patients provided informed consent and the study was approved by the Research Ethics Committee (REC) for Wales and appropriate institutional review boards.

Identification of differentially expressed genes between benign neurofibromas and MPNSTs

A quality control (QC) assessment of the Exon array profiles was performed to examine standard Affymetrix quality parameters, expression distribution patterns and array profile relationships. Overall, a high quality level was achieved (median percent present = 65.99%), although the average expression level of all probe sets across the array profiles was quite variable. "percent present" represents the proportion of probe sets 'present' or detected as defined by the DABG (detection above background) algorithm. The DABG algorithm yields a detection metric (*P* value) generated by comparing perfect match probes to a distribution of background probes. A probe set was considered to be 'present' if the DABG *P* value was ≤0.01. Further information is available at www.affymetrix.com. In an attempt to mitigate the variable expression profile observed, differential gene expression analysis was performed with and without those samples from either end of the observed expression range, namely S0342F0011 (malignant), S0342F0020 (malignant) and S0342F0030 (benign). The results that were common to both differential analyses were taken forward for further analysis. Probe-level data were analysed using the robust multi-array average (RMA) method to generate gene-level measurements [70].

The expression levels of all genes on the array were compared between benign PNFs and MPNSTs, at two different levels of stringency. Under the less stringent criteria, statistical testing employed a P value threshold of 0.05, which served to identify genes displaying 1.3-fold or more (absolute) differential gene expression. The two levels of stringency that were used as fold change cut-offs, in this sense, were essentially arbitrary but nevertheless provide an element of choice in terms of prioritising targets to follow up. We have filtered at 1.3, which may be interpreted as "low stringency". However, combined with a significant P value, this can often be valid in the context of those biological systems where some changes are expected to be subtle yet functionally relevant. Moreover, although the fold change estimations from microarray data compared to qPCR are frequently underestimated, it is often possible to validate findings by qPCR from the lower fold change space of microarray data. Under high stringency criteria, statistical testing employed a P value threshold of 0.005, which was deemed to be sufficient to identify genes displaying 1.5-fold or more (absolute) differential gene expression. This approach allowed us to interrogate two different sets of expression data, thereby minimising the loss of important information.

Quantitative real-time PCR (q-PCR)

All of the top 20 differentially expressed genes were independently assessed by quantitative PCR using RNA isolated from additional MPNST samples, not used in the previous or current study. Due to the small initial sample size, we felt that it was necessary to determine the validity of the top 20 genes in an independent cohort of samples. These 20 genes, plus the *B2M* [NCBI: NM_004048] endogenous control identified in our analysis were: *FAP* [NCBI: NM_004460], *NSBP1* [NCBI: NM_030763], *KRTAP13-4* [NCBI: NM_181600], *PTGIS* [NCBI: NM_000961], *KIAA0746* [NCBI: NM_015187], *SPP1* [NCBI: NM_001040058], *FAM177A1* [NCBI: NM_001079519], *ADH1B* [NCBI: NM_000668], *GRIK3* [NCBI: NM_000831], *FLJ42200* [NCBI: AK124194], *COL10A1* [NCBI: NM_000493], *CSRP1* [NCBI: NM_004078], *GRIK2* [NCBI: NM_175768], *CD72* [NCBI: NM_001782], *EFHC2* [NCBI: NM_025184], *SLC25A12* [NCBI: NM_003705], *GTDC1* [NCBI: NM_001006636], *PEG3* [NCBI: NM_006210], *CCT5* [NCBI: NM_012073] and *TDP1* [NCBI: NM_018319]. qPCR was performed as previously described [25]. Primers for all genes are listed in Additional file 4: Table S1.

Cell lines and maintenance

ST8814 MPNST-derived cell lines were purchased from ATCC (distributed by LGC Standards, Middlesex, UK). The S462, S1507.2 and S1488.1 MPNST cell lines were a kind gift from Prof. Mautner (University of Hamburg, Germany) and the late Prof. Guha (University of Toronto, Canada). After *SPP1* knockdown, cell lines were cultured and maintained in Dulbecco's Modified Eagle Medium (DMEM) supplemented with 10% (v/v) foetal bovine serum (FBS) and 1% (v/v) penicillin-streptomycin and 5 ng/ml puromycin in a humidified incubator (5% CO_2 at 37°C).

Lentivirus generation and shRNA knockdown of SPP1

Both *SPP1* shRNA (Clone ID: NM_000582.2-597s1c1) and non-target control MISSION shRNA (Clone ID: SHCO16) in pLKO.1 vector (Sigma-Aldrich Company Ltd., Dorset, UK) were packaged into lentivirus using HEK293T cells co-transfected (lipofectamine 2000, Life Technology, Paisley, UK) with pLP1, pLP2 and pLP (VSVG). Confluent MPNST cell lines were infected with shRNA-containing lentivirus (*SPP1* or non-target control) and selected over 2 weeks with 5 µg/ml puromycin (Life Technology, Paisley, UK). Puromycin-selected mixed cell populations were then used for tumour formation, wound healing and invasion assays.

Tumour spheroid assays

Two-layered soft agar assays were carried out in six-well plates. MPNST cell lines were plated in complete DMEM media in 0.3% (v/v) agar at a density of 3×10^5cells/mL over a 0.6% (v/v) agar layer. The agar was then overlaid with complete DMEM media supplemented with 0.1 µM puromycin (Life Technology, Paisley, UK). Colonies of MPNSTs were grown for 14 days at 37°C in 5% CO_2. Media were changed twice a week. Representative pictures were taken using an inverted AMG EVOS microscope equipped with an Olympus camera. The diameter of tumour spheroids was measured using ImageJ software; the chamber of a haemocytometer (250 µm) was used as a scale bar for measurement.

Wound healing

Cells were seeded in 60-mm plates and left to reach 100% confluency. Cells were then synchronised in 1% (v/v) FBS DMEM for 24 h and "wounded" with a pipette tip. Dead cells were removed with PBS wash and then replaced with DMEM (10% (v/v) FBS). Pictures were taken at 0 and 12–18 h using an inverted AMG EVOS microscope equipped with an Olympus camera.

Invasion assays

Transwell permeable supports with 6.5-mm diameter inserts, 8.0-µm pore size and a polycarbonate membrane (Corning, cat no: 3428) were used to perform the invasion assays. Cells were grown in a 75-cm^2 flask with standard medium (10% (v/v) FBS) until confluent. Cells were then harvested using Trypsin-EDTA. Cells were counted using a haemocytometer; 1 × 10^6 cells were re-suspended in DMEM containing 1% (v/v) FBS. The top chamber of the Transwell was filled with 300 μl BD Matrigel basement membrane matrix (1 mg/ml). The Matrigel was incubated at 37°C for 4 h to allow it to gel. Cells were then seeded in the upper chamber of the Transwell; the lower chamber was filled with 600 μl standard culture medium (10% (v/v) FBS) and 5 mg/mL fibronectin (R&D systems, Abingdon, UK), as an adhesive substrate. Cells were incubated at 37°C 5% CO_2 for 3 days. The proportion of adherent cells was then determined by fixing the cells with methanol and acetone (1:1) for 20 min at −20°C. Cells were then stained with crystal violet (5 mg/ml) in ethanol for 10 min, followed by a stringent wash with dH_2O until the water ran clear. Crystal violet-stained cells were eluted with 1% (w/v) SDS and the absorbance read at 550 nm on a Genova MK3 Life Science Analyser (Jenway Scientific, Staffordshire, UK). Three replicates were performed per cell line to enable statistical analysis.

Western blotting

The NuPage Novex gel system was used for electrophoresis as described in the manufacturer's protocol (Life Technology, Paisley, UK). Protein samples were resolved on 4%–12% Bis-Tris gels to identify a band size of 66 kD. Proteins were then transferred to a polyvinylidene fluoride (PDVF) membrane purchased from Millipore U.K. Ltd. (Watford, UK), blocked in 5% (w/v) dry milk powder in standard Tris-buffer saline supplemented with 0.1% (v/v) Tween [as recommended by Cell Signalling Technology Inc. (Danvers, MA, USA)] for 4 h. Membranes were incubated at 4°C overnight in primary antibody (1:200 dilutions in 2% (w/v) BSA in TBS-T) then washed twice for 4 min in TBS-T and incubated in the appropriate HRP-conjugated secondary antibody (1:10,000 dilution in 5% (w/v) Marvel in TBS-T) for a minimum of 30 min at room temperature. Membranes were washed four times for 3 min with TBS-T and then incubated in enhanced chemiluminescence (ECL) solution (GE Healthcare Life Sciences, Buckinghamshire, UK) for 1 min. Konica Medical Film was used to visualise the signal, and the exposed films were developed using a Konica Minolta SRX-101A developer.

Statistical analysis

SPSS software was used for the statistical analysis of tumour spheroid formation (n = 40) and the wound healing (n = 3) and invasion (n = 3) assays. A one-way ANOVA was performed on the data sets to obtain the requisite P values.

Additional files

Additional file 1: Table S2. The four distinct sets of genes identified from the various analyses that were performed of differentially expressed genes.

Additional file 2: Table S3. Data on copy number alterations compared with the genes found to be differentially expressed between MPNSTs and PNFs. 76/121 genes exhibited concordance between copy number changes and the level of expression.

Additional file 3: Figure S1. Results of the q-PCR analysis in relation to the top 20 genes differentially expressed between MPNSTs and PNFs.

Additional file 4: Table S1. Primers used for q-PCR analysis and results of the q-PCR analysis.

Abbreviations

CNA: copy number alteration; DABG: detection above background; HMM: hidden Markov model; MPNST: malignant peripheral nerve sheath tumour; NF1: neurofibromatosis type 1; PNF: peripheral neurofibroma; shRNA: short hairpin RNA.

Competing interests

The authors declare that they have no competing interests.

Authors' contributions

LET completed the molecular genetic studies, data analysis, coordination of the project and drafting of the manuscript. JW completed the QPCR assays. EMR carried out the cell assays. MM performed the statistical analysis. KMD completed the wWestern blot analysis. ART created the lentiviral vector and assisted with the cell assays and western blots. FM and SM completed the microarray work as part of Almac Diagnostics. DNC helped to draft the manuscript and provided guidance. MU conceived of the study, participated in its design and coordination and helped to draft the manuscript.
All authors read and approved the final manuscript.

Acknowledgements

We are grateful to Professor Victor Mautner and the late Professor Guha for providing tumour samples. We also thank Chris Lovejoy for his technical support and the Ian Owen Trust and the Wales Gene Park for their financial support. We are also grateful to Dr Ian Frayling for his encouragement.

Author details

[1]Institute of Medical Genetics, School of Medicine, Cardiff University, Cardiff CF14 4XN, UK. [2]Almac Diagnostics, 19 Seagoe Industrial Estate, Craigavon, Northern Ireland BT63 5QD, UK.

References

1. Huson S. The neurofibromatoses: classification, clinical features and genetic counselling. In: Kaufmann D, editor. Neurofibromatoses (monographs in human genetics), vol. 16. Switzerland: S Karger AG; 2008. p. 1–20.
2. Upadhyaya M. Genetic basis of tumorigenesis in NF1 malignant peripheral nerve sheath tumors. Front Biosci. 2011;16:937–51.
3. Ferner RE, Gutmann DH. International consensus statement on malignant peripheral nerve sheath tumours in neurofibromatosis 1. Cancer Res. 2002;1(62(5)):1573–7.
4. Evans DG, Baser ME, McGaughran J, Sharif S, Howard E, Moran A. Malignant peripheral nerve sheath tumours in neurofibromatosis 1. J Med Genet. 2002;9:311–4.
5. Katz D, Lazar A, Lev D. Malignant peripheral nerve sheath tumour (MPNST): the clinical implications of cellular signalling pathways. Expert Rev Mol Med. 2009;11:e30.
6. Tucker T, Wolkenstein P, Revuz J, Zeller J, Friedman J. Association between benign and malignant peripheral nerve sheath tumors in NF1. Neurology. 2005;65:205–11.
7. Mautner VF, Kluwe L, Friedrich RE, et al. Clinical characterisation of 29 neurofibromatosis type-1 patients with molecularly ascertained 1.4 Mb type-1 NF1 deletions. J Med Genet. 2010;47:623–30.

8. Ferner RE, Hughes RA, Hall SM, Upadhyaya M, Johnson MR. Neurofibromatous neuropathy in neurofibromatosis 1 (NF1). J Med Genet. 2004;41:837–41.
9. Evans DG, Huson SM, Birch JM. Malignant peripheral nerve sheath tumours in inherited disease. Clin Sarcoma Res. 2012;2:17.
10. Beert E, Brems H, Daniëls B, et al. Atypical neurofibromas in neurofibromatosis type 1 are premalignant tumors. Genes Chrom Cancer. 2011;50:1021–32.
11. Lothe RA, Karhu R, Mandahl N, et al. Gain of 17q24-qter detected by comparative genomic hybridization in malignant tumors from patients with von Recklinghausen's neurofibromatosis. Cancer Res. 1996;56:4778–81.
12. Bridge Jr RS, Bridge JA, Neff JR, Naumann S, Althof P, Bruch LA. Recurrent chromosomal imbalances and structurally abnormal breakpoints within complex karyotypes of malignant peripheral nerve sheath tumour and malignant triton tumour: a cytogenetic and molecular cytogenetic study. J Clin Pathol. 2004;57:1172–8.
13. Watson MA, Perry A, Tihan T, et al. Gene expression profiling reveals unique molecular subtypes of neurofibromatosis type I-associated and sporadic malignant peripheral nerve sheath tumors. Brain Pathol. 2004;14:297–303.
14. Storlazzi CT, Brekke HR, Mandahl N, et al. Identification of a novel amplicon at distal 17q containing the BIRC5/SURVIVIN gene in malignant peripheral nerve sheath tumours. J Pathol. 2006;209:492–500.
15. Shen MH, Mantripragada K, Dumanski JP, Frayling I, Upadhyaya M. Detection of copy number changes at the NF1 locus with improved high-resolution array CGH. Clin Genet. 2007;72:238–44.
16. Kresse SH, Skårn M, Ohnstad HO, et al. DNA copy number changes in high-grade malignant peripheral nerve sheath tumors by array CGH. Mol Cancer. 2008;7:48.
17. Mantripragada KK, Spurlock G, Kluwe L, et al. High-resolution DNA copy number profiling of malignant peripheral nerve sheath tumors using targeted microarray-based comparative genomic hybridization. Clin Cancer Res. 2008;14:1015–24.
18. Mantripragada KK, Díaz de Ståhl T, Patridge C, et al. Genome-wide high-resolution analysis of DNA copy number alterations in NF1-associated malignant peripheral nerve sheath tumors using 32 K BAC array. Genes Chrom Cancer. 2009;48:897–907.
19. Brekke HR, Kolberg M, Skotheim RI, et al. Identification of p53 as a strong predictor of survival for patients with malignant peripheral nerve sheath tumors. NeuroOncol. 2009;11:514–28.
20. Miller SJ, Jessen WJ, Mehta T, et al. Integrative genomic analyses of neurofibromatosis tumours identify *SOX9* as a biomarker and survival gene. EMBO Mol Med. 2009;1:236–48.
21. Pemov A, Park C, Reilly KM, Stewart DR. Evidence of perturbations of cell cycle and DNA repair pathways as a consequence of human and murine NF1-haploinsufficiency. BMC Genomics. 2010;11:194.
22. Brekke HR, Ribeiro FR, Kolberg M, et al. Genomic changes in chromosomes 10, 16, and X in malignant peripheral nerve sheath tumors identify a high-risk patient group. J Clin Oncol. 2010;28:1573–82.
23. Subramanian S, Thayanithy V, West RB, et al. Genome-wide transcriptome analyses reveal p53 inactivation mediated loss of miR-34a expression in malignant peripheral nerve sheath tumours. J Pathol. 2010;220:58–70.
24. Chai G, Liu N, Ma J, et al. MicroRNA-10b regulates tumorigenesis in neurofibromatosis type 1. Cancer Sci. 2010;101:1997–2004.
25. Upadhyaya M, Spurlock G, Thomas L, et al. Microarray-based copy number analysis of neurofibromatosis type-1 (NF1)-associated malignant peripheral nerve sheath tumors reveals a role for Rho-GTPase pathway genes in NF1 tumorigenesis. Hum Mutat. 2012;33:763–76.
26. Mo W, Chen J, Patel A, et al. CXCR4/CXCL12 mediate autocrine cell-cycle progression in NF1-associated malignant peripheral nerve sheath tumors. Cell. 2013;152:1077–90.
27. Rahrmann EP, Watson AL, Keng VW, et al. Forward genetic screen for malignant peripheral nerve sheath tumor formation identifies new genes and pathways driving tumorigenesis. Nat Genet. 2013;45:756–66.
28. Watson AL, Rahrmann EP, Moriarity BS, et al. Canonical Wnt/β-catenin signaling drives human Schwann cell transformation, progression, and tumor maintenance. Cancer Discov. 2013;6:674–89.
29. Largaespada D, Ratner N. Interweaving the strands: β-catenin, an HIV co-receptor, and Schwann cell tumors. Cancer Cell. 2013;23:269–71.
30. Luscan A, Shackleford G, Masliah-Planchon J, et al. The activation of the WNTWnt signalling pathway is a hallmark in Neurofibromatosis type 1 tumorigenesis. Clin Cancer Res. 2013;15(20(2)):358–71.
31. Huang N, Shah PK, Li C. Lessons from a decade of integrating cancer copy number alterations with gene expression profiles. Brief Bioinformatics. 2012;13:305–16.
32. Hassan A, Mokhtar NM, Sin K, Mohammed Rose I, Sagap I, Harun R, et al. Integrated analysis of copy number variation and genome-wide expression profiling in colorectal cancer tissues. PLoS ONE. 2014;2(9(4)):e92553.
33. Rittling SR, Chambers AF. Role of osteopontin in tumour progression. Brit J Cancer. 2004;90:1877–81.
34. Pradervand S, Paillusson A, Thomas J, et al. Affymetrix Whole-Transcript Human Gene1.0 ST array is highly concordant with standard 3′ expression arrays. Biotechniques. 2008;44:759–62.
35. Xi L, Feber A, Gupta V, et al. Whole genome exon arrays identify differential expression of alternatively spliced, cancer-related genes in lung cancer. Nucleic Acids Res. 2008;36:6535–47.
36. Thorsen K, Sørensen KD, Brems-Eskildsen AS, et al. Alternative splicing in colon, bladder, and prostate cancer identified by exon array analysis. Mol Cell Proteomics. 2008;7:1214–24.
37. Kapur K, Xing Y, Ouyang Z, Wong WH. Exon arrays provide accurate assessments of gene expression. Genome Biol. 2007;8:R82.
38. Furger KA, Menon RK, Tuck AB, Bramwell VH, Chambers AF. The functional and clinical roles of osteopontin in cancer and metastasis. Current Mol Med. 2001;1:621–32.
39. Bramwell VHC, Tuck AB, Wilson SM, et al. Expression of osteopontin and HGF/met in adult soft tissue tumors. Cancer Biol Ther. 2005;4:1336–41.
40. Hoshi N, Sugino T, Suzuki T. Regular expression of osteopontin in granular cell tumor: distinctive feature among Schwannian cell tumors. Pathol Int. 2005;55:484–90.
41. Rangaswami H, Bulbule A, Kundu G. Osteopontin: role in cell signaling and cancer progression. Trends Cell Biol. 2006;16:79–87.
42. Wai PY, Kuo PC. Osteopontin: regulation in tumor metastasis. Cancer Metastasis Rev. 2008;27:103–18.
43. Weber GF. The metastasis gene osteopontin: a candidate target for cancer therapy. Biochim Biophys Acta. 2001;1552:61–85.
44. Shevde LA, Das S, Clark DW, Samant RS. Osteopontin: an effector and an effect of tumor metastasis. Curr Mol Med. 2010;10:71–81.
45. Ahmed M, Behera R, Chakraborty G, et al. Osteopontin: a potentially important therapeutic target in cancer. Expert Opin Ther Targets. 2011;15:1113–26.
46. Luo X, Ruhland MK, Pazolli E, Lind AC, Stewart SA. Osteopontin stimulates preneoplastic cellular proliferation through activation of the MAPK pathway. Mol Cancer Res. 2011;9:1018–29.
47. Rao G, Du L, Chen Q. Osteopontin, a possible modulator of cancer stem cells and their malignant niche. Oncoimmunology. 2013;2:e24169.
48. El-Tanani MK, Campbell FC, Kurisetty V, Jin D, McCann M, Rudland PS. The regulation and role of osteopontin in malignant transformation and cancer. Cytokine Growth Factor Rev. 2006;17:463–74.
49. Tilli TM, Mello KD, Ferreira LB, et al. Both osteopontin-c and osteopontin-b splicing isoforms exert pro-tumorigenic roles in prostate cancer cells. Prostate. 2012;72:1688–99.
50. Guo X, Zhang YP, Mitchell DA, Denhardt DT, Chambers AF. Identification of a Ras-activated enhancer in the mouse osteopontin promoter and its interaction with a putative ETS-related transcription factor whose activity correlates with the metastatic potential of the cell. Mol Cell Biol. 1995;15:476–87.
51. Mason CK, McFarlane S, Johnston PG, et al. Agelastatin A: a novel inhibitor of osteopontin-mediated adhesion, invasion, and colony formation. Mol Cancer Ther. 2008;7(3):548–58.
52. The cancer genome atlas [http://cancergenome.nih.gov]
53. Gu W, Choi H, Ghosh D. Global associations between copy number and transcript mRNA microarray data: an empirical study. Cancer Inform. 2008;6:17–23.
54. Thomas L, Mautner VF, Cooper DN, Upadhyaya M. Molecular heterogeneity in malignant peripheral nerve sheath tumors associated with neurofibromatosis type 1. Hum Genomics. 2012;4(6):18.
55. Spivey TL, De Giorgi V, Zhao Y, et al. The stable traits of melanoma genetics: an alternate approach to target discovery. BMC Genomics. 2012;13:156.
56. Lu TP, Lai LC, Tsai MH, et al. Integrated analyses of copy number variations and gene expression in lung adenocarcinoma. PLoS ONE. 2011;6:e24829.
57. Conan copy number analysis [http://www.sanger.ac.uk/research/projects/cancergenome/copy_number.html]
58. COSMIC catalogue of somatic mutations in cancer [http://cancer.sanger.ac.uk/cancergenome/projects/cosmic]

59. Kleinjan DA, Lettice LA. Long-range gene control and genetic disease. Adv Genet. 2008;1:339–88.
60. Henrichsen CN, Chaignat E, Reymond A. Copy number variants, diseases and gene expression. Hum Mol Genet. 2009;18(R1):R1–8.
61. Hyman E, Kauraniemi P, Hautaniemi S, et al. Impact of DNA amplification on gene expression patterns in breast cancer. Cancer Res. 2002;62:6240–5.
62. White BD, Chien AJ, Dawson DW. Dysregulation of Wnt/β-catenin signaling in gastrointestinal cancers. Gastroenterology. 2012;142:219–32.
63. Reilly KM. Extending the convergence of canonical Wnt signaling and classic cancer pathways for treatment of malignant peripheral nerve sheath tumors. Cancer Discov. 2013;6:610–2.
64. Vinas JL, Sola A, Jung M, Mastora C, Vinuesa E, Pi F, et al. Inhibitory action of Wnt target gene osteopontin on mitochondrial cytochrome c release determines renal ischemic resistance. Am J Physiol Renal Physiol. 2010;299:F234–42.
65. Blair SL, Heerdt P, Sachar S, et al. Glutathione metabolism in patients with non-small cell lung cancers. Cancer Res. 1997;57:152–5.
66. Sun Z, Chen J, Aakre J, et al. Genetic variation in glutathione metabolism and DNA repair genes predicts survival of small-cell lung cancer patients predicts survival of small-cell lung cancer patients. Ann Oncol. 2011;21:2011–6.
67. Harder A, Titze S, Herbst L, Harder T, Guse K, Tinschert S, et al. Monozygotic twins with neurofibromatosis type 1 (NF1) display differences in methylation of NF1 gene promoter elements, 5′ untranslated region, exon and intron 1. Twin Res Hum Genet. 2010;13(6):582–94.
68. Titze S, Peters H, Währisch S, Harder T, Guse K, Buske A, et al. Differential MSH2 promoter methylation in blood cells of neurofibromatosis type 1 (NF1) patients. Eur J Hum Genet. 2010;18(1):81–7.
69. Rohde F, Rimcus C, Friederichs J, et al. Expression of osteopontin, a target gene of de-regulated Wnt signalling predicts survival of colon cancer. Int J Cancer. 2007;121:1717–23.
70. Irizarry RA, Hobbs B, Collin F, et al. Exploration, normalization, and summaries of high density oligonucleotide array probe level data. Biostatistics. 2003;4:249–64.

5

Identification of cancer predisposition variants in apparently healthy individuals using a next-generation sequencing-based family genomics approach

Ioannis Karageorgos[1†], Clint Mizzi[2,10†], Efstathia Giannopoulou[3†], Cristiana Pavlidis[1], Brock A. Peters[4,5], Zoi Zagoriti[1], Peter D. Stenson[6], Konstantinos Mitropoulos[7], Joseph Borg[8,9], Haralabos P. Kalofonos[3], Radoje Drmanac[4,5], Andrew Stubbs[10], Peter van der Spek[10], David N. Cooper[6], Theodora Katsila[1] and George P. Patrinos[1,10*]

Abstract

Cancer, like many common disorders, has a complex etiology, often with a strong genetic component and with multiple environmental factors contributing to susceptibility. A considerable number of genomic variants have been previously reported to be causative of, or associated with, an increased risk for various types of cancer. Here, we adopted a next-generation sequencing approach in 11 members of two families of Greek descent to identify all genomic variants with the potential to predispose family members to cancer. Cross-comparison with data from the Human Gene Mutation Database identified a total of 571 variants, from which 47 % were disease-associated polymorphisms, 26 % disease-associated polymorphisms with additional supporting functional evidence, 19 % functional polymorphisms with in vitro/laboratory or in vivo supporting evidence but no known disease association, 4 % putative disease-causing mutations but with some residual doubt as to their pathological significance, and 3 % disease-causing mutations. Subsequent analysis, focused on the latter variant class most likely to be involved in cancer predisposition, revealed two variants of prime interest, namely *MSH2* c.2732T>A (p.L911R) and *BRCA1* c.2955delC, the first of which is novel. *KMT2D* c.13895delC and c.1940C>A variants are additionally reported as incidental findings. The next-generation sequencing-based family genomics approach described herein has the potential to be applied to other types of complex genetic disorder in order to identify variants of potential pathological significance.

Keywords: Cancer predisposition, Family genomics, Next-generation sequencing, Genomic variants

Introduction

Cancer results from a multi-step cascade of somatic events involving the accumulation of both genetic and epigenetic changes at various genomic loci, under the influence of a variety of different environmental factors [1–5]. Single point mutations, small insertions/deletions, translocations, gene fusions, copy number changes, and loss of heterozygosity represent some of the somatic alterations frequently encountered in cancer [6] and which can lead to the increased expression of oncogenes or to the silencing of tumor suppressor genes. Genome-wide association studies (GWASs) have also identified genomic regions that appear to be associated with increased cancer risk [7–9]. It is to be expected that an improved knowledge of the genomic variants that predispose to tumor initiation, development, and progression will be advantageous in the context of informing treatment regimens. Numerous studies have been performed in an attempt to shed light on the complexity (and inter-individual variability) of the cancer genome and to examine the relationship between the possession of specific genomic variants and tumorigenesis [10, 11], often with ambiguous results.

* Correspondence: gpatrinos@upatras.gr
†Equal contributors
[1]Department of Pharmacy, University of Patras, School of Health Sciences, University Campus, Rion GR-26504, Patras, Greece
[10]Department of Bioinformatics, School of Medicine and Health Sciences, Erasmus University Medical Center, Rotterdam, The Netherlands

The advent of next-generation sequencing (NGS) has provided unprecedented opportunities to decipher the cancer genome and to dissect the molecular etiology of cancer predisposition. This has been the primary goal of the International Cancer Genome Consortium (ICGC), following the initiatives of the Human Genome Project and the HapMap Consortium [12]. The comprehensive listings of genomic abnormalities (somatic mutations, abnormal gene expression, epigenetic effects) detected in tumors from 50 cancer types and/or subtypes of clinical and societal importance are being made available to the entire research community with minimal restrictions (http://www.icgc.org/icgc). In this context, the Catalogue of Somatic Mutations in Cancer (COSMIC; http://cancer.sanger.ac.uk/cancergenome/projects/cosmic) stores and displays our current knowledge of somatic mutations detected in human cancers, including information on publications and most notably, tissue samples (i.e., benign neoplasms, in situ and invasive tumors, recurrences, metastases) and cancer cell lines. In 2004, the Cancer Gene Census (http://cancer.sanger.ac.uk/cancergenome/projects/census) indicated that mutations in more than 1 % of genes may contribute to human cancer [13]. A total of 547 entries are currently reported, of which 90 % refer to somatic mutations in cancer, 20 % correspond to germline mutations that predispose to cancer, whereas 10 % refer to both somatic and germline mutations.

Genetic susceptibility to cancer is conferred both by inherited (germline) and tumor-specific (somatic) variants and as such, it is evident in most individuals, not just in those individuals with a personal or family history of cancer. Although the deleterious alleles of cancer risk genes are generally not highly penetrant, the presence of genetic susceptibility variants at multiple loci is generally assumed to increase an individual's overall risk of cancer. It should be noted that, even in the case of highly penetrant cancer predisposition genes, such as *BRCA1* and *BRCA2*, population-based studies have revealed that about half of all heterozygous mutation carriers with incident cancers lack a family history of breast or ovarian cancer [14]. Further, individuals with no obvious indication of cancer risk from family history may nevertheless be at an increased risk of developing cancer [15]. NGS technologies have potentiated the analysis of whole genomes as a means to obtain a full picture of individual variomes [16]. Once whole genome and/or whole exome sequencing begins to take hold in routine clinical medicine, developing an understanding of the role of the detected sequence variations in guiding diagnostics and arriving at prognoses will be of paramount importance to the clinician, especially in the case of multifactorial disorders and cancer, where early detection of novel causative variants can be crucial for early disease diagnosis and health management. In the context of cancer, data interpretation will require an understanding of the heritable variation present in cancer risk-associated genes in healthy individuals. Currently, this knowledge is largely lacking.

Here, we propose a multi-step next-generation sequencing-based family genomics approach, piloted in 11 members of two families of Greek descent with no history of cancer, to identify genomic variants, particularly novel variants, that might predispose to various types of cancer. Such information could help in the assessment of personalized cancer-susceptibility risk from genome sequence data [17].

Materials and methods

Case selection, DNA isolation, and whole genome sequencing

Eleven members of two unrelated families of Greek descent were recruited for this study (Fig. 1). All individuals consented to participate. A family-based design was employed rather than a population-based design, as the former is generally considered to be robust against population admixture and stratification and may yield both within- and between-family information [18]. None of the individuals tested had a family history of cancer (germline risk variants would not be anticipated as they are quite infrequent, although they cannot altogether be excluded). We aimed to identify cancer-susceptibility variants of low penetrance in these apparently healthy individuals, information that could help in the assessment of personalized cancer-susceptibility risk from genome sequence data. It was hoped that the application of the NGS approach might lead to the identification of novel cancer-susceptibility variants. Informed consent was obtained from all individuals who took part in this study.

Genomic DNA isolation was performed from saliva samples using the Oragene collection kit (DNA Genotek, Canada). Whole genome sequencing was performed using the proprietary DNA nanoball resequencing technology of Complete Genomics [19]. DNA sequencing coverage was 110×.

Bioinformatics and in silico analyses

All variants were filtered according to the analysis required, using custom scripts and Complete Genomics Analysis Tools [CGA™ Tools]. Only high-quality call variants were included in the analysis (>93 %). Genomes were aligned with the hg19 reference genome and subsequently compared against the Human Gene Mutation Database, Professional version (HGMD v.2014.4; http://www.hgmd.org) records with respect to previously known variants in cancer predisposition genes. Subsequently, a non-redundant list of variants was generated from the 11 human genome sequences and subjected to text mining, using the following keywords: "Cancer,"

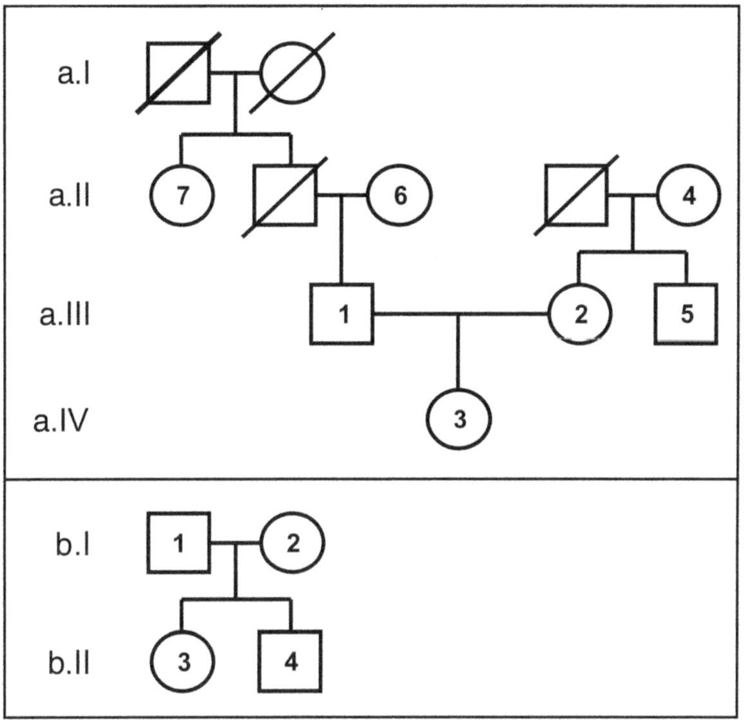

Fig. 1 Pedigrees of the two families (*a*, *b*) of Greek descent whose genomes were analyzed

"Adenoma," "Carcinoma," "Adenocarcinoma," "Melanoma," "Lymphoma," "Leukemia," "Glioma," and "Glioblastoma." Novel variants in genes that had previously been related to cancer predisposition were annotated with Annovar in Galaxy [20] and compared with NCBI dbSNP build 137 (http://www.ncbi.nlm.nih.gov/projects/SNP/snp_summary.cgi), 69 reference genomes from Complete Genomes (http://www.completegenomics.com/publicdata/69Genomes/), COSMIC v68 (http://cancer.sanger.ac.uk/cosmic/version68), and GWAS studies (http://www.genome.gov/gwastudies) to determine their novelty or otherwise.

To obtain a list of variants of potential functional significance, we employed protein variation effect analyzer (PROVEAN) v1.1.3 (PROVEAN human genome variants tool) that provides both scale-invariant feature transform (SIFT) [21] and PROVEAN [22] predictions for a given list of human genome variants as well as accessory information (dbSNP rs IDs, gene description, PFAM domain, GO terms, etc.). PROVEAN is able to make predictions for any type of protein sequence alteration, including single or multiple amino acid substitutions, deletions, and insertions [23]. In addition, we used CRAVAT (Cancer-Related Analysis of Variants Toolkit), a tool more specifically tailored to a cancer variant application, to facilitate the high-throughput assessment and prioritization of genes important for cancer tumorigenesis [24].

Downstream molecular analysis

Selected novel variants were subsequently analyzed using a polymerase chain reaction (PCR)-based conventional Sanger resequencing approach and validated in a pool of ethnically matched 60 control samples to determine whether or not they constituted frequent variants.

Results

Next-generation sequencing-based family genomics

The family genomics approach adopted herein is depicted in Fig. 2. Eleven members from two unrelated Greek families had their genomes sequenced. None of the individuals from the families selected had any history of cancer, as indicated by the participants. Our family-based approach was adopted in order to identify known cancer risk variants as well as novel variants of low penetrance—although highly penetrant genes cannot be excluded—in healthy individuals, information that could help in the assessment of personalized cancer-susceptibility risk from genome sequence data.

A list of 571 non-redundant genomic variants that might predispose family members to cancer was identified after cross-comparison with HGMD entries (Additional file 1: Table S1) and further categorized by genome/family member on the basis of the text mining terms used. To further address individual cancer risk, clinical impact data

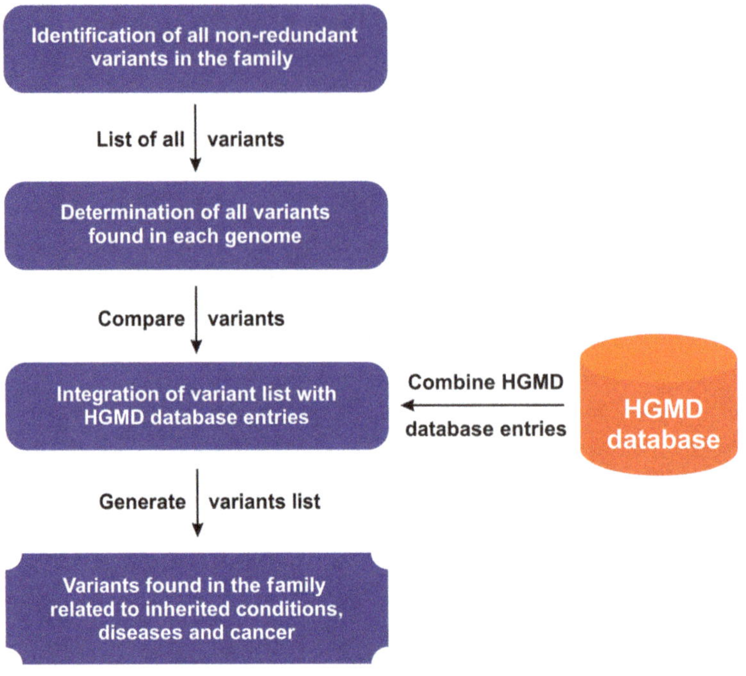

Fig. 2 Outline of the concept of the family genomics approach implemented in this study

were also incorporated accompanied by GWAS data, allele frequencies (Complete Genomics 69 diversity file), 1000 Genomes Project data as well as the input of COSMIC v68.

Analysis of 11 genomes reveals a large number of potential cancer predisposition variants

Cross-comparison with data from the Human Gene Mutation Database identified a total of 571 heritable variants that had previously been reported to be associated with cancer predisposition (Additional file 1: Table S1). Taking into account the variant classes included in the HGMD dataset, the distribution of our 571 variants was 47 % DP (disease-associated polymorphisms), 26 % DFP (disease-associated polymorphisms with additional supporting functional evidence), 19 % FP (functional polymorphisms with in vitro/laboratory or in vivo supporting evidence but no known disease association), 4 % DM? (putative disease-causing mutations but where there is some residual doubt as to pathological significance), and 3 % DM (disease-causing mutations) (Fig. 3). Subsequent analysis focused on the DMs as the variant class most likely to be involved in cancer predisposition (Table 1). Cancer predisposition to various cancer types was revealed including brain, head and neck, bladder, breast, lung, gastric, prostate, colorectal, ovarian, thyroid, oral, hereditary non-polyposis colorectal cancer (HNPCC), esophageal, upper aerodigestive tract, pancreatic, and skin cancer. The variants identified were also distributed over a broad range of tumor (tissue) types: gliomas/glioblastomas, adenomas (colorectal), lymphomas (non-Hodgkin's), adenocarcinomas (lung, gastric), melanomas, leukemias, and carcinomas (thyroid, basal cell, renal cell, esophageal, cervical, nasopharyngeal, hepatocellular). The majority of the cancer predisposition variants related to lung, colorectal, and breast cancer (Fig. 4).

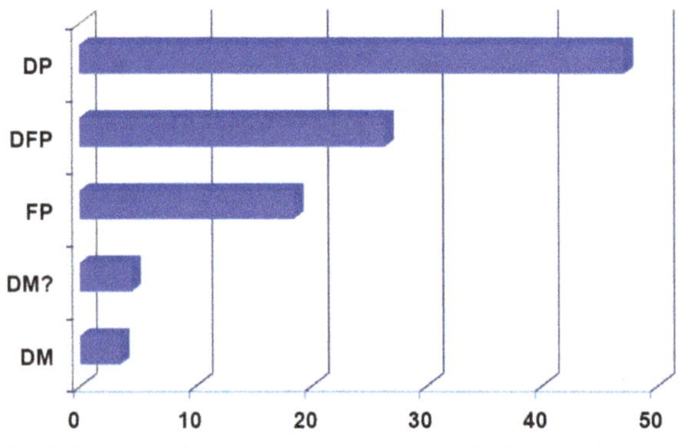

Fig. 3 Summary of the genomic variants identified, grouped per variant classes in the HGMD database. HGMD variant classes were as follows: *DP* disease-associated polymorphisms, *DFP* disease-associated polymorphisms with additional supporting functional evidence, *FP* functional polymorphisms with in vitro/laboratory or in vivo supporting evidence but no known disease association *DM* disease-causing mutations, *DM?* putative disease-causing mutations but where there is some residual doubt as to pathological significance

Table 1 The DM (disease-causing mutations) and DM? (putative disease-causing mutations but where there is some residual doubt as to pathological significance) mutations identified in each family

	Cancer type	HGMD tag
Family A, annotated variants		
dbsnp.129:rs56250729	Prostate cancer	DM?
dbsnp.125:rs28756990	Endometrial cancer	DM?
dbsnp.131:rs77067228	Cancer	DM?
dbsnp.89:rs1799966	Breast and/or ovarian cancer	DM/DM?
dbsnp.113:rs4986852	Breast cancer	DM?
COSMIC:mut:148278;dbsnp.86:rs799917	Breast and/or ovarian cancer	DM
dbsnp.89:rs1799950	Breast cancer	DM
dbsnp.98:rs2229995	Adenomatous polyposis coli	DM?
dbsnp.127:rs41545019	Colorectal cancer	DM?
dbsnp.98:rs1805324	Colorectal cancer, non-polyposis	DM?
dbsnp.129:rs61753720	Acute lymphoblastic leukemia	DM
Family B, Annotated variants		
dbsnp.126:rs33927012	Medullary thyroid carcinoma	DM?
dbsnp.98:rs2229992	Adenomatous polyposis coli	DM
dbsnp.76:rs41115	Adenomatous polyposis coli	DM
dbsnp.79:rs169547	Breast cancer	DM?
dbsnp.103:rs3092994	Breast cancer	DM?
dbsnp.89:rs1799966	Breast cancer	DM
dbsnp.86:rs1060915	Breast cancer	DM
dbsnp.125:rs28897689	Breast and/or ovarian cancer	DM
COSMIC:mut:148278;dbsnp.86:rs799917	Breast and/or ovarian cancer	DM
dbsnp.60:rs16940	Breast cancer	DM

Four variants that have not so far been annotated in either dbSNP or the 1000 Genomes Project/exome variant server data were considered to be of prime interest; *MSH2* c.2732T>A (p.Leu911Arg), *BRCA1* c.2955delC, and *KMT2D* c.13895delC and c.1940C>A variants (Additional file 1: Table S1). The *MSH2* c.2732T>A (p. Leu911Arg) variant is novel as it is not present in HGMD. The *KMT2D* c.13895delC and c.1940C>A variants are reported herein as incidental findings. All the putative cancer-associated mutations were also considered in terms of assessing personalized cancer-susceptibility risk from genome sequence data.

It became evident that, among the 571 cancer risk-associated variants identified, some were common between the two families considered, whereas others were unique (Fig. 5). In particular, 609 variants were found in both families, while 74 variants were unique to family A and 551 variants were only found in family B. Commenting on the unique variants obtained, family B comes from northern Greece, a quite distant location from Athens (300.13 km) where family A is from, implying a different genetic origin.

In silico and replication analyses

To ascertain whether the variants of interest (*MSH2* c.2732T>A (p. L911R) and *BRCA1* c.2955delC) have functional significance, in silico analysis was performed using the SIFT and PROVEAN algorithms [21, 22]. As depicted in Table 2, SIFT analysis yielded a p.L911R substitution (*MSH2* c.2732T>A) which was predicted to be "deleterious" to protein function with a score equal to or less than 0.05, implying that this could be a pathologically relevant variant. Moreover, PROVEAN's scoring scheme has been shown to perform well in separating disease-associated variants from common polymorphisms [25]. It is thought that non-synonymous SNPs exhibiting a deleterious effect on function may have become established, being potentially beneficial under some historical conditions, although today they may only be found at low frequency [26]. Using a polymerase chain reaction (PCR)-based conventional Sanger resequencing approach, *MSH2* c.2732T>A (p. L911R) was subsequently investigated in a pool of ethnically matched control samples and determined to be an infrequent variant in agreement with PROVEAN's scoring scheme.

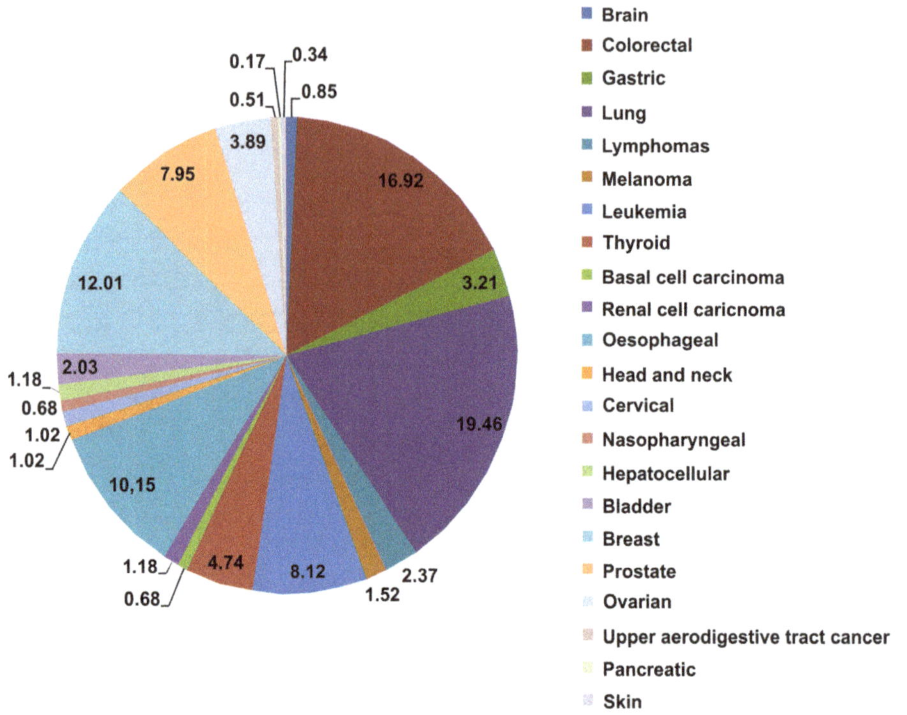

Fig. 4 Variants identified by cancer type in all 11 genomes from the two families under study

CRAVAT analysis (Table 3) was performed in two ways: firstly by querying a functional effect and then by proceeding with cancer driver analyses: a general analysis and subsequently a targeted one, choosing "colon" as the tissue type of interest, on the basis of the findings depicted in Table 1 regarding *MSH2*, as well as literature-derived evidence supporting its association with microsatellite instability and hereditary non-polyposis colorectal cancer. According to the functional analysis outcome, *MSH2* c.2732T>A (p.L911R) and *BRCA1* c.2955delC were observed in various cancer types in COSMIC (grouped by primary site). Cancer driver gene hits (tumor suppressor genes), according to Vogelstein and coworkers [27], were also obtained for *BRCA1* c.2955delC and *MSH2* c.2732T>A (p.L911R). Notably, the frameshift variant of *BRCA1* was accompanied by a TARGET (*T*umor *A*lterations *R*elevant for *GE*nomics-driven *T*herapy) drug association hit (http://www.broadinstitute.org/cancer/cga/target). TARGET

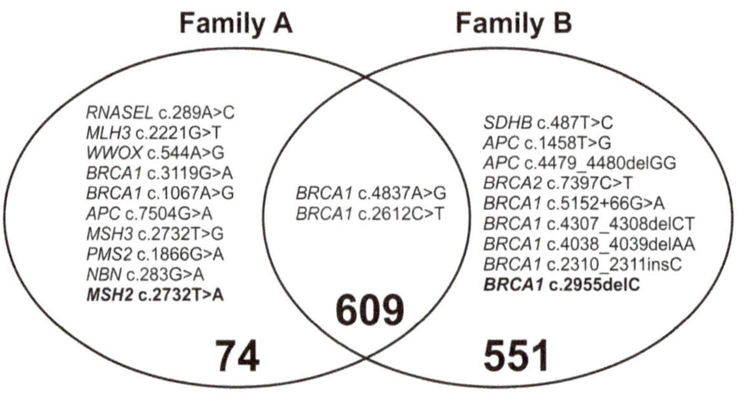

Fig. 5 Variants identified per family in all 11 genomes from the two families under study. The DM (disease-causing mutations) and DM? (putative disease-causing mutations but where there is some residual doubt as to pathological significance) mutations identified as well as our two variants of prime interest, *MSH2* c.2732T>A and *BRCA1* c.2955delC, are shown

Table 2 SIFT PROVEAN analysis outcome of the two variants of prime interest identified in the 11 family members

HUGO gene symbol	Chromosome	HGVS description of variant	HGMD tag	Aminoacid position	Reference residue	Alternative residue	Variation type	PROVEAN prediction		SIFT prediction	
								Score	Prediction	Score	Prediction
MSH2	2	c.2732T>A	NA	911	L	Q	Single AA Change	−4.14	Deleterious	0.001	Damaging
BRCA1	17	c.2955delC	DM	986			Frameshift	NA	NA	NA	NA

Source: PROVEAN v1.1.3 (PROVEAN human genome variants tool, http://provean.jcvi.org/genome_submit_2.php?species=human).PROVEAN was developed in order to predict whether a given protein sequence variation (single or multiple amino acid substitutions, micro-insertions, micro-deletions) affects protein function. To achieve this, PROVEAN introduces a delta alignment score based on the reference and variant versions of a protein query sequence with respect to sequence homologs (NCBI NR protein database through BLAST, http://www.ncbi.nlm.nih.gov/). The default score threshold was set at −2.5 for binary classification (deleterious<−2.5 vs. neutral>−2.5). Similarly (through PSI-BLAST, http://blast.ncbi.nlm.nih.gov/Blast.cgi?CMD=Web&PAGE=Proteins&PROGRAM=blastp&RUN_PSIBLAST=on), SIFT (http://sift.jcvi.org/) may be applied to naturally occurring non-synonymous polymorphisms. SIFT score ranges from 0 to 1. A SIFT score of ≤0.05 corresponds to a "damaging" prediction, whereas a SIFT score >0.05 predicts that the variant is likely to be "tolerated"

NA not available (where the precomputed score was not available in the database, the precomputed homologous protein identifiers for the query protein were retrieved in order to bypass the BLAST search and clustering, and the score was computed based on the homologs)

genes, when somatically altered in cancer, are linked to a clinical action (prediction of therapy response/ resistance, prognosis, diagnosis).

Discussion

The etiology of cancer is highly complex, being characterized by a strong genetic component (a large number of somatic as well as germline variants have been associated with different cancer types), while multiple environmental factors contribute to disease susceptibility. In 1974, Anderson stated that the two- to threefold excess observed in first-degree relatives of cancer patients is not indicative of strong genetic effects. They are more suggestive of the involvement of many genes with small effects acting in concert with environmental or nongenetic factors with larger and more important effects [28]. Although according to Peto (1980) this was a statistical fallacy [29], it seems that the overall statement is correct since current epidemiological evidence is supported by the discovery of low-penetrance genes that predispose to the majority of cancer types. Under the polygenic model, a large number of alleles each conferring a small genotypic risk (perhaps a relative risk of 1.5–2.0) combine additively or multiplicatively to confer a range of susceptibilities in the general population [30]. Hence, individuals are at elevated risk in the presence of the combined effects of several susceptibility alleles. This implies that unless a large number of the relevant alleles have been identified for a susceptible group, this group cannot be targeted for early screening or prophylactic therapy. Reduced (or incomplete) penetrance may be also of importance, in an attempt to understand why healthy individuals can harbor several potentially disadvantageous variants in their genomes without suffering any obvious ill effects. Next-generation sequencing of entire exomes or genomes of apparently normal healthy individuals from the general population supports the view that reduced penetrance is actually a widespread phenomenon in human genetics [31]. We believe that large-scale sequencing and genotyping studies of apparently healthy individuals could provide a powerful new approach to understanding the penetrance of pathological mutations/genotypes.

The advent of next-generation sequencing has provided unprecedented opportunities to decipher the cancer genome and to delineate the molecular etiology

Table 3 CRAVAT functional analysis outcome of the two variants of prime interest identified in the 11 family members

HUGO gene symbol	HGVS description of variant	HGMD tag	Sequence ontology	Driver genes	Target	Occurrences in COSMIC by primary sites (gene mutated)
MSH2	c.2732T>A	NA	Missense variant	TSG	NA	Cervix(1), large intestine (106), autonomic ganglia (2), central nervous system (2), liver(1), small intestine (1), haematopoietic and lymphoid tissue (7), endometrium (18), urinary tract (1), lung (14), breast (7), skin (4), stomach (1), esophagus (1), ovary (4), NS (2), prostate (2), kidney (6), pancreas (1)
BRCA1	c.2955delC	DM	Frameshift deletion	TSG	PARP inhibitor	Cervix (1), large intestine (66), stomach (8), central nervous system (2), pancreas (1), meninges (1), haematopoietic and lymphoid tissue (3), endometrium (23), urinary tract (5), lung (42), liver (5), skin (6), oesophagus (4), ovary (39), NS (2); prostate (2), kidney (5), breast (33)

Source: CRAVAT tool. In the case of *MSH2*, cancer driver analyses were also performed, selecting "colon" as the tissue type of interest. A driver score of 0.27 was obtained (a driver score close to zero means an increased probability of the mutation being a cancer driver)

TSG tumor suppressor gene, *NA* not available

underlying cancer predisposition, similar to the numerous applications of next-generation sequencing in the elucidation of the molecular basis of rare diseases [23] and pharmacogenomics [32]. Herein, we pursued a next-generation sequencing-based family genomics approach in 11 members of two families of Greek descent in order to identify genomic variants that might predispose family members to cancer. None of the individuals tested had a family history of cancer (germline genomic variants would not be anticipated), and hence, we aimed to identify genomic variants, particularly novel variants, that might predispose currently asymptomatic individuals to various types of cancer.

A total of 571 variants previously shown to be associated with cancer predisposition were identified. We assessed both non-synonymous and synonymous variations, since the latter can impact the mRNA phenotype (whether via transcription, splicing, mRNA transport or translation) thereby rendering the synonymous mutation non-silent [33]. In a recent study that focused on germline mutations in cancer-susceptibility genes, the authors identified non-synonymous genomic variations in 158 genes causally implicated in carcinogenesis, using high-quality whole genome sequences from an ancestrally diverse cohort of 681 healthy individuals, none of whom were first-degree relatives [34]. As in our study, all individuals were found to carry multiple variants with the potential to impact cancer-susceptibility. Bodian and coworkers, however, focused on the detailed analysis of a selected subset of five clinically important cancer genes (*BRCA1*, *BRCA2*, *KRAS*, *TP53*, and *PTEN*), highlighting differences between germline variants and reported somatic mutations, reporting on their allele frequencies by ancestry. Differences between ancestry groups (African, African-European, Central Asian, East Asian, European, Hispanic, others) were also reflected in the number of cancer-gene variants as well as the number of deleterious variants per individual. In the case of *TP53* c.215C>G (p.P72R), *BRCA1* c.2612C>T (p.P871L), *ERBB2* c.3508C>G (p. P1170A), and *FLT3* c.680C>T (p.T227M), the minor allele in one population was shown to be the major allele in another.

Our study revealed four variants—namely, *BRCA1* c.2955delC, *MSH2* c.2732T>A (p.L911R), and *KMT2D* c.13895delC and c.1940C>A—that have not been annotated in either dbSNP or the 1000 Genomes Project/exome variant server data. It should be noted that there is no HGMD entry for *MSH2* c.2732T>A (p.L911R), and hence, it may be considered to be novel. Inherited mutations in *BRCA1* are well known to confer an increased lifetime risk of developing breast or ovarian cancer. *BRCA1* is a tumor suppressor gene that is involved in the maintenance of genome stability (homologous recombination pathway for double-strand DNA repair) and hence is of paramount importance in hereditary breast and ovarian cancers. However, the identification of an evidently detrimental *BRCA1* variant in a healthy individual is not unlikely [35]. This may raise awareness regarding the use of next-generation sequencing in oncology.

MSH2 c.2732T>A (p.L911R) was predicted by PROVEAN to be "deleterious" to protein function, implying that this is a case of a disease-associated variant (amino acid variant that deviates from the frequently occurring residue) and was assigned a driver mutation score close to zero (a driver score close to zero implies increased likelihood of the mutation being a cancer driver) for colon cancer (by CRAVAT). Using a PCR-based conventional Sanger resequencing approach, this variant was verified as a non-frequent one in agreement with PROVEAN's scoring scheme, separating disease-associated variants from common polymorphisms [25]. The DNA mismatch repair protein Msh2 (also known as MutS protein homolog 2, MSH2) is encoded by the *MSH2* gene (tumor suppressor gene), which is located on chromosome 2. Mutations in the *MSH2* gene are associated with microsatellite instability and cancer (hereditary non-polyposis colorectal cancer (HNPCC)). MSH2, as a heterodimer with MSH6, forms the human MutSα mismatch repair complex. MSH3 is also a dimerization partner of MSH2 towards the formation of the MutSβ DNA repair complex. MSH2 participates in several DNA repair processes, such as transcription-coupled repair [36], homologous recombination [37] as well as base excision repair [38]. The amino acid change consequent to the identified missense variant is located within the protein domain that serves to allow MSH2 to interact with MSH6/MSH3 [38]. Although the crystal structure of an MSH2/MSH6 heterodimer in complex with a DNA fragment has been solved [39, 40], the region containing the p.L911 residue was not resolvable. For this reason, we were unable to visualize the effect that the p.L911R might have on the protein.

KMT2D c.13895delC is a mutation, which has previously been associated with Kabuki (Niikawa-Kuroki) syndrome (autosomal dominant) with a particularly severe congenital phenotype: left-sided cardiac abnormalities, facial dysmorphisms, skeletal, renal and anorectal malformations, and hypertricosis [41, 42]. Interestingly, this syndrome has also been associated with cancer predisposition in children. The KMT2D protein encoded by this gene is a histone methyltransferase that methylates the Lys-4 position of histone H3 [43]. This notwithstanding, both *KMT2D* variants obtained herein (c.13895delC and c.1940C>A) are reported as incidental findings. There is currently an ongoing debate about reporting incidental findings in the context of genomic testing. American College of Medical Genetics and Genomics (ACMG) recommendations have been established and approximately 1 %

of genome sequencing reports are expected to include an incidental variant that falls within the ACMG recommendations [44]. Although the aforementioned *KMT2D* variants were not given in the ACMG list, we chose to report and note them as incidental findings that could require further evaluation.

Our study has a number of limitations. Firstly, functional analysis of the *BRCA1* c.2955delC and *MSH2* c.2732T>A (p.L911R) variants was not performed. Secondly, although the SIFT-based in silico analysis provides an assessment of the likely pathogenicity of these novel variants, it cannot fully replace functional assays. Furthermore, our study considered only those genomic variants previously associated with cancer predisposition and that had been logged in HGMD Professional at the time of our analysis. Since this resource is frequently updated, the bioinformatics analysis of these genomes should be replicated periodically to exploit any new variants reported therein. Looking to the future, whole genome sequencing should ideally be performed once, e.g., at birth, with data analysis being frequently replicated thereafter in order to exploit the wealth of genomic knowledge that is continually becoming available. Lastly, family history is of central importance in medical/clinical practice, since it reflects both genetic and environmental exposures within families. Herein, none of the individuals reported had a family history of cancer (germline genomic variants would not be anticipated), rendering it highly questionable as to whether they would meet the normal criteria for genetic counseling. Incidental findings and reduced (incomplete) penetrance in cancer complicate decision-making even further. Nowadays, genomic data are hardly integrated in medical decision-making in cancer, given its complexity and as educational initiatives and support from specialists are also lacking [45]. In this context, a community knowledge base has been proposed by Good and coworkers (2014) to facilitate collaborative contributions and open discussions on genomic events [46].

In relation to the diagnosis and prognosis of cancer patients, data interpretation requires an understanding of the variation in cancer risk-associated genes in healthy individuals. This knowledge is still largely lacking. Herein, we followed a family-based genomics approach in healthy individuals to assess cancer risk via the identification of genomic variants, particularly novel ones that might predispose to various types of cancer. A crude assessment of the potential extent of the genome-wide cancer-susceptibility burden in normal healthy individuals was also an objective of this study, taking into account all the (putative) risk-associated mutations obtained. As whole genome and/or whole exome sequencing approaches begin to be recruited into clinical care, our understanding of detected sequence variations on diagnosis (and prognosis) needs to become more readily accessible to the clinician. This is not a trivial undertaking, especially as the polygenic model proposes that an individual's cancer risk is the net outcome of the presence of multiple variants and environmental factors [47]. The use of next-generation sequencing is expected to play a crucial role in delineating an individual's variome as well as providing the means to identify novel variants to improve therapeutic modalities. Signature-based drug-repositioning methods are also known to make use of gene signatures to uncover unknown mechanisms of action of molecules and drugs by coupling the significantly changed genes to computational approaches [48]. As whole genome sequencing services become more accurate in delivering clinical-grade genome sequences and whole genome sequencing costs continue to decline, it is expected that this approach will gradually assume an integral role in genomic medicine. The next-generation sequencing-based family genomics approach employed here could be readily replicated for other types of disorders to identify causative variants and/or in the context of signature-based drug-repositioning methods.

Competing interests

The authors declare the following competing interests: BP and RD are employees of the Complete Genomics Inc. (Mountain View, CA, USA). DNC and PDS are in receipt of financial support from BIOBASE GmbH/Qiagen Inc through a license agreement with Cardiff University.

Authors' contributions

KM and GPP conceived and designed the study. IK, EG, and ZZ carried out the PCR-based conventional Sanger resequencing approach. IK, CM, EG, and CP carried out text mining. BAP and RD supervised the next-generation sequencing analyses. CM, PvS, AS, and TK carried out the bioinformatics and in silico analyses. IK, CM, DNC, KM, JB, HPK, RD, PvS, TK, and GPP drafted the manuscript. All authors read and approved the final manuscript.

Acknowledgements

This study was funded by the European Commission (RD-CONNECT; FP7-304555) research grant to GPP and endorsed by the Genomic Medicine Alliance Cancer Genomics Working Group.

Author details

[1]Department of Pharmacy, University of Patras, School of Health Sciences, University Campus, Rion GR-26504, Patras, Greece. [2]Department of Physiology and Biochemistry, Faculty of Health Sciences, University of Malta, Msida, Malta. [3]Clinical Oncology Laboratory, Division of Oncology, Department of Medicine, University of Patras, Patras, Greece. [4]Complete Genomics Inc., Mountain View, CA, USA. [5]BGI-Shenzhen, Shenzhen 51803, China. [6]Institute of Medical Genetics, School of Medicine, Cardiff University, Cardiff, UK. [7]The Golden Helix Foundation, London, UK. [8]Department of Applied Biomedical Science, Faculty of Health Sciences, University of Malta, Msida, Malta. [9]Department of Cell Biology and Genetics, School of Medicine

and Health Sciences, Erasmus University Medical Center, Rotterdam, The Netherlands. [10]Department of Bioinformatics, School of Medicine and Health Sciences, Erasmus University Medical Center, Rotterdam, The Netherlands.

References

1. Lea IA, Jackson MA, Li X, Bailey S, Peddada SD, Dunnick JK. Genetic pathways and mutation profiles of human cancers: site- and exposure-specific patterns. Carcinogenesis. 2007;28:1851–8.
2. You JS, Jones PA. Cancer genetics and epigenetics: two sides of the same coin? Cancer Cell. 2012;22:9–20.
3. Hanahan D, Weinberg RA. Hallmarks of cancer: the next generation. Cell. 2011;144:646–74.
4. Witte T, Plass C, Gerhauser C. Pan-cancer patterns of DNA methylation. Genome Med. 2014;6:66.
5. Barrow TM, Michels KB. Epigenetic epidemiology of cancer. Biochem Biophys Res Commun. 2014;455:70–83.
6. Dutt A, Beroukhim R. Single nucleotide polymorphism array analysis of cancer. Curr Opin Oncol. 2007;19:43–9.
7. Chung CC, Chanock SJ. Current status of genome-wide association studies in cancer. Hum Genet. 2011;130:59–78.
8. Rae JM, Skaar TC, Hilsenbeck SG, Oesterreich S. The role of single nucleotide polymorphisms in breast cancer metastasis. Breast Cancer Res. 2008;10:301.
9. Teraoka SN, Bernstein JL, Reiner AS, Haile RW, Bernstein L, Lynch CF, et al. Single nucleotide polymorphisms associated with risk for contralateral breast cancer in the Women's Environment, Cancer, and Radiation Epidemiology (WECARE) study. Breast Cancer Res. 2011;13:R114.
10. Inaki K, Liu ET. Structural mutations in cancer: mechanistic and functional insights. Trends Genet. 2012;28:550–9.
11. Lopez-Lazaro M. A new view of carcinogenesis and an alternative approach to cancer therapy. Mol Med. 2010;16:144–53.
12. Stratton MR, Campbell PJ, Futreal PA. The cancer genome. Nature. 2009;458:719–24.
13. Futreal PA, Coin L, Marshall M, Down T, Hubbard T, Wooster R, et al. A census of human cancer genes. Nat Rev Cancer. 2004;4:177–83.
14. Rubinstein WS, Jiang H, Dellefave L, Rademaker AW. Cost-effectiveness of population-based *BRCA1/2* testing and ovarian cancer prevention for Ashkenazi Jews: a call for dialogue. Genet Med. 2009;11:629–39.
15. Johnston JJ, Rubinstein WS, Facio FM, Ng D, Singh LN, Teer JK, et al. Secondary variants in individuals undergoing exome sequencing: screening of 572 individuals identifies high-penetrance mutations in cancer-susceptibility genes. Am J Hum Genet. 2012;91:97–108.
16. Nekrutenko A, Taylor J. Next-generation sequencing data interpretation: enhancing reproducibility and accessibility. Nat Rev Genet. 2012;13:667–72.
17. Kilpivaara O, Aaltonen LA. Diagnostic cancer genome sequencing and the contribution of germline variants. Science. 2013;339:559–1562.
18. Laird NM, Lange C. Family-based designs in the age of large-scale gene-association studies. Nat Rev Genet. 2006;7:385–94.
19. Drmanac R, Sparks AB, Callow MJ, et al. Human genome sequencing using unchained base reads on self-assembling DNA nanoarrays. Science. 2010;327:78–81.
20. Hiltemann S, Mei H, de Hollander M, Palli I, van der Spek P, Jenster G, et al. CGtag: complete genomics toolkit and annotation in a cloud-based galaxy. Gigascience. 2014;3(1):1.
21. SIFT tool—http://sift.jcvi.org.
22. PROVEAN tool webpage—http://provean.jcvi.org/about.php#about_3.
23. Boycott KM, Vanstone MR, Bulman DE, MacKenzie AE. Rare-disease genetics in the era of next-generation sequencing: discovery to translation. Nat Rev Genet. 2013;14:681–91.
24. Douville C, Carter H, Kim R, Niknafs N, Diekhans M, Stenson PD, et al. CRAVAT: cancer-related analysis of variants toolkit. Bioinformatics. 2013;29:647–8.
25. Choi Y, Sims GE, Murphy S, Miller JR, Chan AP. Predicting the functional effect of amino acid substitutions and indels. PLoS One. 2012;7, e46688.
26. Marcel Dekker. In: Chasman DI, editor. Protein structure. Determination, analysis, and applications for drug discovery. New York-Basel: Marcel Dekker; 2003. p. 606.
27. Vogelstein B, Papadopoulos N, Velculescu VE, Zhou S, Diaz LA, Kinzler KW. Cancer genome landscapes. Science. 2013;339:1546–58.
28. Anderson DE. Genetic study of breast cancer: identification of a high-risk group. Cancer. 1974;34:1090–7.
29. Peto J. In: Cairns J, Lyon JL, Skolnick MH, editors. Banbury report 4: cancer incidence in defined populations. Cold Spring Harbor, New York: Cold Spring Harbor Laboratories; 1980. p. 203–13.
30. Houlston RS, Peto J. The search for low-penetrance cancer susceptibility alleles. Oncogene. 2004;23:6471–6.
31. Cooper DN, Krawczak M, Polychronakos C, Tyler-Smith C, Kehrer-Sawatzki H. Where genotype is not predictive of phenotype: towards an understanding of the molecular basis of reduced penetrance in human inherited disease. Hum Genet. 2013;132:1077–130.
32. Mizzi C, Peters B, Mitropoulou C, Mitropoulos K, Katsila T, Agarwal MR, et al. Personalized pharmacogenomics profiling using whole-genome sequencing. Pharmacogenomics. 2014;15:1223–34.
33. Goymer P. Synonymous mutations break their silence. Nat Rev Genet. 2007;8:92.
34. Bodian DL, McCutcheon JN, Kothiyal P, Huddleston KC, Iyer RK, Vockley JG, et al. Germline variation in cancer-susceptibility genes in a healthy, ancestrally diverse cohort: implications for individual genome sequencing. PLoS One. 2014;9, e94554.
35. Fletcher O, Houlston RS. Architecture of inherited susceptibility to common cancer. Nat Rev Cancer. 2010;10:353–61.
36. Mellon I, Rajpal DK, Koi M, Boland CR, Champe GN. Transcription-coupled repair deficiency and mutations in human mismatch repair genes. Science. 1996;272:557–60.
37. de Wind N, Dekker M, Berns A, Radman M, te Riele H. Inactivation of the mouse *Msh2* gene results in mismatch repair deficiency, methylation tolerance, hyperrecombination, and predisposition to cancer. Cell. 1995;82:321–30.
38. Pitsikas P, Lee D, Rainbow AJ. Reduced host cell reactivation of oxidative DNA damage in human cells deficient in the mismatch repair gene hMSH2. Mutagenesis. 2007;22:235–43.
39. Lützen A, de Wind N, Georgijevic D, Nielsen FC, Rasmussen LJ. Functional analysis of HNPCC-related missense mutations in *MSH2*. Mutat Res. 2008;645:44–55.
40. Warren JJ, Pohlhaus TJ, Changela A, Iyer RR, Modrich PL, Beese LS. Structure of the human MutSα DNA lesion recognition complex. Mol Cell. 2007;26:579–92.
41. Van Laarhoven PM, Neitzel LR, Quintana AM, Geiger EA, Zackai EH, Clouthier DE, et al. Kabuki syndrome genes KMT2D and KDM6A: functional analyses demonstrate critical roles in craniofacial, heart, and brain development. Hum Mol Genet 2015;ddv180. [Epub ahead of print].
42. Hannibal MC, Buckingham KJ, Ng SB, Ming JE, Beck AE, McMillin MJ, et al. Spectrum of MLL2 (ALR) mutations in 110 cases of Kabuki syndrome. Am J Med Genet A. 2011;155A:1511–6.
43. Casanova M, Selicorni A, Ferrari A. Cancer predisposition in children with Kabuki syndrome. Am J Med Genet A. 2011;155A:1504.
44. Green RC, Berg JS, Grody WW, Kalia SS, Korf BR, Martin CL, et al. ACMG recommendations for reporting of incidental findings in clinical exome and genome sequencing. Genet Med. 2013;15:565–74.
45. Vassy JL, Korf BR, Green RC. How to know when physicians are ready for genomic medicine. Sci Transl Med. 2015;7:287fs19.
46. Good BM, Ainscough BJ, McMichael JF, Su AI, Griffith OL. Organizing knowledge to enable personalization of medicine in cancer. Genome Biol. 2014;15:438.
47. Xue Y, Chen Y, Ayub Q, Huang N, Ball EV, Mort M, et al. Deleterious- and disease-allele prevalence in healthy individuals: insights from current predictions, mutation databases, and population-scale resequencing. Am J Hum Genet. 2012;91:1022–32.
48. Jin G, Wong ST. Toward better drug repositioning: prioritizing and integrating existing methods into efficient pipelines. Drug Discov Today. 2014;19:637–44.

6

Copy number alterations detected by whole-exome and whole-genome sequencing of esophageal adenocarcinoma

Xiaoyu Wang[1*], Xiaohong Li[2,3], Yichen Cheng[3], Xin Sun[4], Xibin Sun[5], Steve Self[1], Charles Kooperberg[3] and James Y. Dai[1,3]

Abstract

Background: Esophageal adenocarcinoma (EA) is among the leading causes of cancer mortality, especially in developed countries. A high level of somatic copy number alterations (CNAs) accumulates over the decades in the progression from Barrett's esophagus, the precursor lesion, to EA. Accurate identification of somatic CNAs is essential to understand cancer development. Many studies have been conducted for the detection of CNA in EA using microarrays. Next-generation sequencing (NGS) technologies are believed to have advantages in sensitivity and accuracy to detect CNA, yet no NGS-based CNA detection in EA has been reported.

Results: In this study, we analyzed whole-exome (WES) and whole-genome sequencing (WGS) data for detecting CNA from a published large-scale genomic study of EA. Two specific comparisons were conducted. First, the recurrent CNAs based on WGS and WES data from 145 EA samples were compared to those found in five previous microarray-based studies. We found that the majority of the previously identified regions were also detected in this study. Interestingly, some novel amplifications and deletions were discovered using the NGS data. In particular, *SKI* and *PRKCZ* detected in a deletion region are involved in transforming growth factor-β pathway, suggesting the potential utility of novel biomarkers for EA. Second, we compared CNAs detected in WGS and WES data from the same 15 EA samples. No large-scale CNA was identified statistically more frequently by WES or WGS, while more focal-scale CNAs were detected by WGS than by WES.

Conclusions: Our results suggest that NGS can replace microarrays to detect CNA in EA. WGS is superior to WES in that it can offer finer resolution for the detection, though if the interest is on recurrent CNAs, WES can be preferable to WGS for its cost-effectiveness.

Background

Cancer arises from gradual accumulation of somatic genomic instability and alterations, which eventually lead to carcinogenesis and cancer progression [1, 2]. Copy number alterations (CNAs), one form of somatic genome alterations, refer to somatic changes in chromosome structure that result in gains or losses of copies of DNA segments. Detection of CNA is important to understand cancer development and identify key driver events [3, 4]. Microarray technologies have been widely used in CNA detection [5–7], including array comparative genomic hybridization (array CGH) and single nucleotide polymorphisms (SNP) microarrays. In array CGH, reference and test DNAs are fluorescence-labeled and hybridized to arrays, which are composed of bacterial artificial chromosome (BAC) clones, cDNA clones, or oligonucleotides. The signal ratio is used as an estimate of the copy number ratio. SNP microarrays are also based on hybridization, but a single sample is processed on each microarray and intensity ratios are formed by comparing the intensity of the sample under investigation to a collection of reference samples, or all other samples that are studied. Compared to array CGH, SNP arrays can have better resolution and produce B allele frequency so that loss of heterozygosity (LOH) can be detected [7]. Resolution of these arrays is typically greater than 1 kb,

* Correspondence: xwang234@fredhutch.org
[1]Vaccine and Infectious Disease Division, Fred Hutchinson Cancer Research Center, Seattle, WA, USA

depending on the density, distribution, and response characteristics of their probes. More recently, next-generation sequencing (NGS) technologies offer single-nucleotide resolution and absolute counts of read numbers and therefore can provide more sensitive and accurate CNA results. Moreover, direct sequencing enables substantial increases in discoveries of smaller structural variation events [8, 9]. It is believed that, with its ever-decreasing cost, NGS will ultimately replace microarrays in copy number analyses [10].

In this paper, we conduct CNA analyses using published NGS data from [11], which contains 145 esophageal adenocarcinoma (EA) samples, as no CNA analyses were reported in the paper. The incidence of EA has strikingly increased over the past 30–40 years, and it is the seventh leading cause of cancer death among men in the USA [12]. Many studies of CNA detection in EA have been carried out using microarrays. Paulson et al. detected 19 most frequent CNAs in 15 EA patients using BAC array data [13]. Beroukhim et al. created the Tumorscape Copy Number Portal, where they collected more than 3000 copy number profiles from 26 cancer types using Affymetrix 250K StyI (Affymetrix, Santa Clara, CA) arrays [3]. They identified 33 recurrent CNAs (RCNAs), which appear in 44 EA samples more frequently than expected by chance. Dulak et al. detected 46 regions of significant recurrent events of gain and loss in 186 EA samples using 250K StyI arrays and SNP Array 6.0 arrays (Affymetrix) [14]. Zack et al. created the TCGA Copy Number Portal and identified RCNAs across multiple cancer types; they detected 88 RCNAS across 184 EA samples using Affymetrix SNP6 arrays [4, 15]. Frankel et al. detected 52 RCNAs in 54 EA samples using Illumina CytoSNP-12 arrays [16]. However, there has not been any published CNA detection study using NGS technologies. In this study, we plan to fill the gap by analyzing the NGS data from [11] and compare the result to the findings of the aforementioned papers.

Indeed, microarray-based CNA analyses are still a common approach to detect CNAs, possibly due to the following reasons: microarray technologies have been developed for a longer time and corresponding CNA detection methods were well established and accurate detection of CNA in NGS can be a challenging task due to the complexities of sequencing data processing [17]. To the best of our knowledge, only a few CNA studies have been conducted to compare the performance of microarrays and NGS side-by-side. Koboldt et al. detected CNAs on coding regions of five ovarian tumors using both a SNP array and two NGS platforms—whole-genome (WGS) and whole-exome sequencing (WES) [18]. They found the majority of CNA events were consistently detected by the three platforms. More CNAs were detected by the WGS platform than those by the array. In another study, the authors detected germline copy number variations (CNVs) in 16 breast cancer cell lines using both

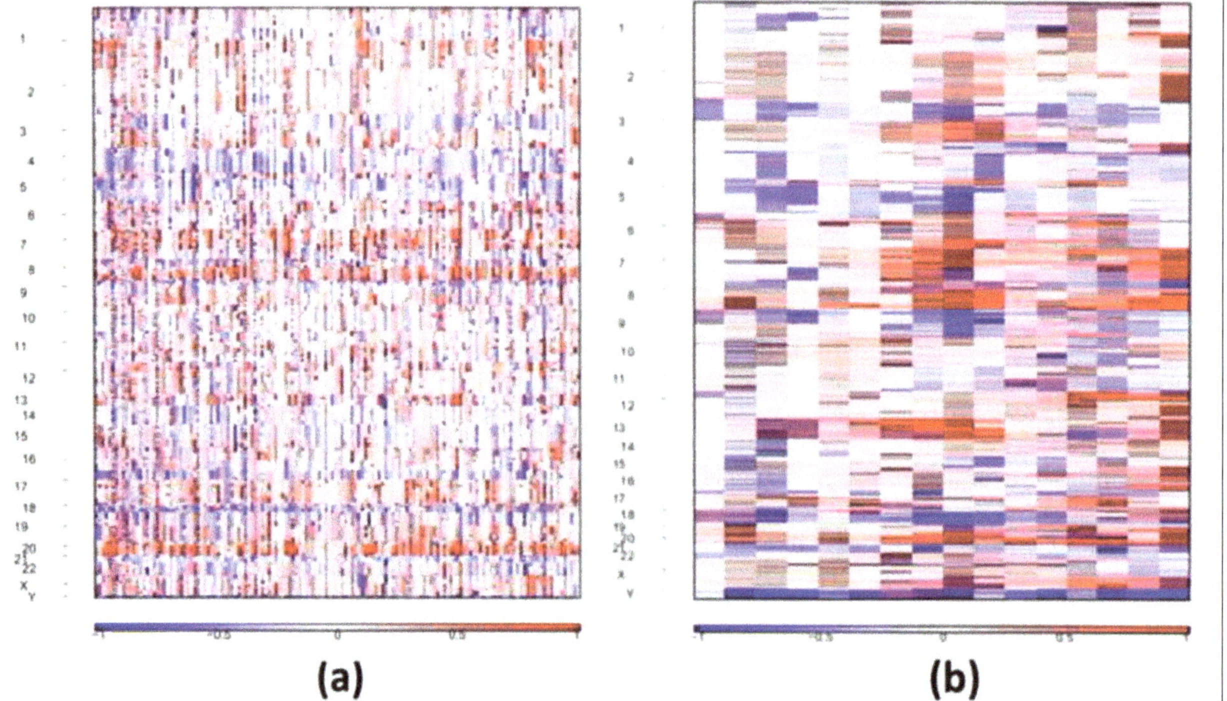

Fig. 1 Segmented copy number ratio profiles in WES and WGS. The *x*-axis represents the samples. The *y*-axis represents the chromosomes. **a** WES data. **b** WGS data

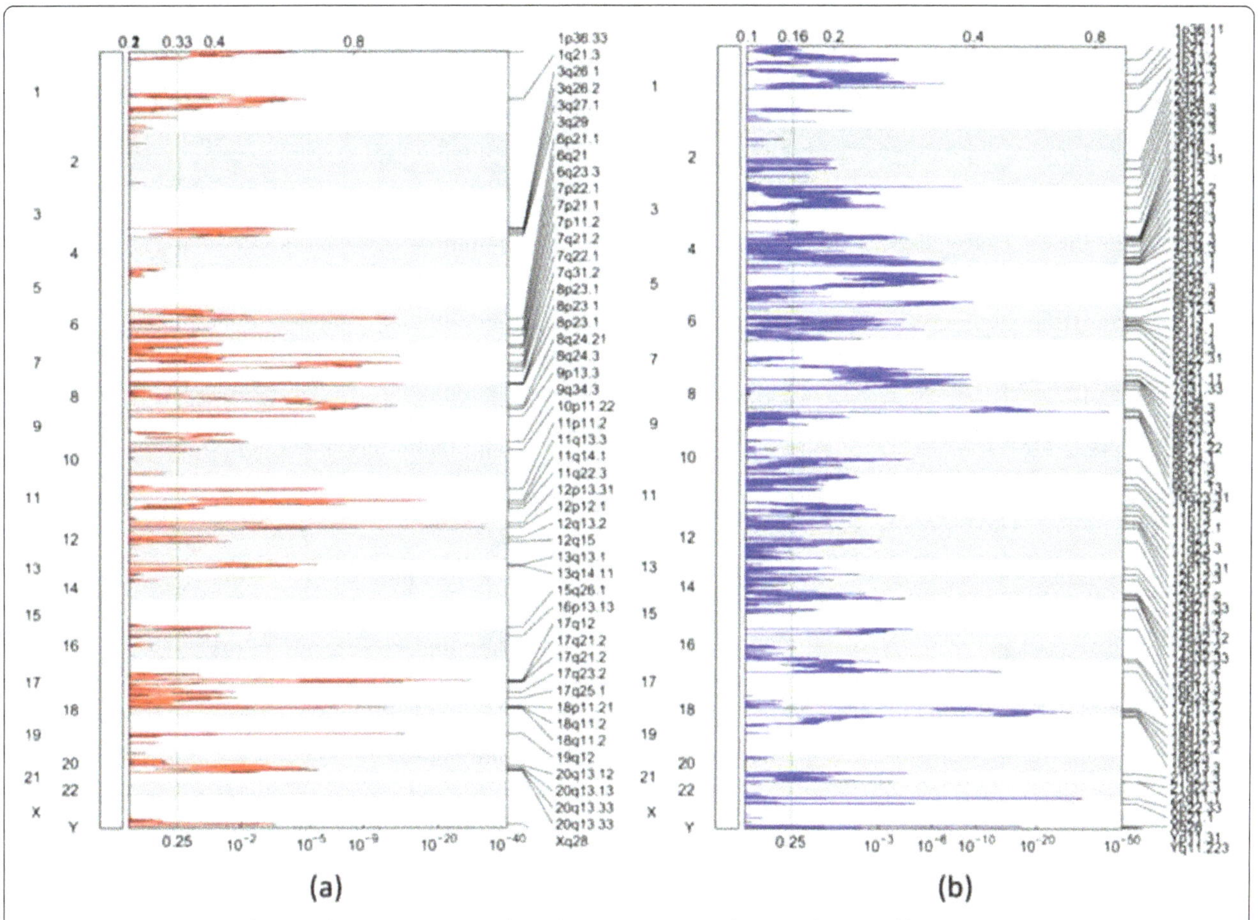

Fig. 2 Genomic positions of RCNAs detected in 145 WES data. The *x*-axis represents the normalized amplification signals (*top*) and significance by *q* value (*bottom*). The *green line* indicates the significance cutoff at $q = 0.25$. **a** Amplification regions. **b** Deletion regions

array CGH and WES [19]. Four WES-based CNV detection methods were compared, and the regions detected by the array were used to form the gold standard. They detected a greater number of focal-scale CNVs using the array. These studies were conducted on the individual sample level. In this study, we are interested to detect and compare regions frequently appearing among multiple samples between NGS data and previous findings derived from microarrays-based studies. The detected recurrent regions may contain real driver events that contribute to the cancer development.

Furthermore, there were 15 samples (patients) subjected to both WGS and WES in [11], providing a great opportunity to compare CNA detection by WES and WGS. Not much work has been conducted to address this question. Koboldt et al. found that a significant portion (79.53 %) of focal-scale CNAs detected by WES were also supported by WGS, and they recommended the use of WES-based approach, by which it is likely to detect more platform-specific focal copy number changes missed by WGS and microarray [18]. WES is an increasingly popular platform for studying tumor genomics because of itscost-effectiveness and the immediate interpretation of mutations in coding regions. It has been shown that WES data can be used to study CNA [19]. However, the uniformity of WES coverage is worse than that of WGS mostly due to exome capturing, and exons are not evenly placed within the genome so that it is difficult to detect CNAs over a long intergenic region using WES. On the other hand, if the interest is long CNA segments spanning over genes, it is not clear whether CNAs inferred by WES will lose a substantial amount of information when compared to WGS. It is quite possible that this comparison may depend on cancer site and the length of CNAs, since longer segment should be reliably detected by exome sequencing.

A number of bioinformatics and statistical methods have been developed for CNA detection using NGS data [17, 20–22]. These methods can be classified in several ways. Most methods were developed to detect CNAs on the individual sample level, and they usually detect CNAs based on read count ratios between a tumor sample and its matched normal sample. These methods can be further categorized according to the study design.

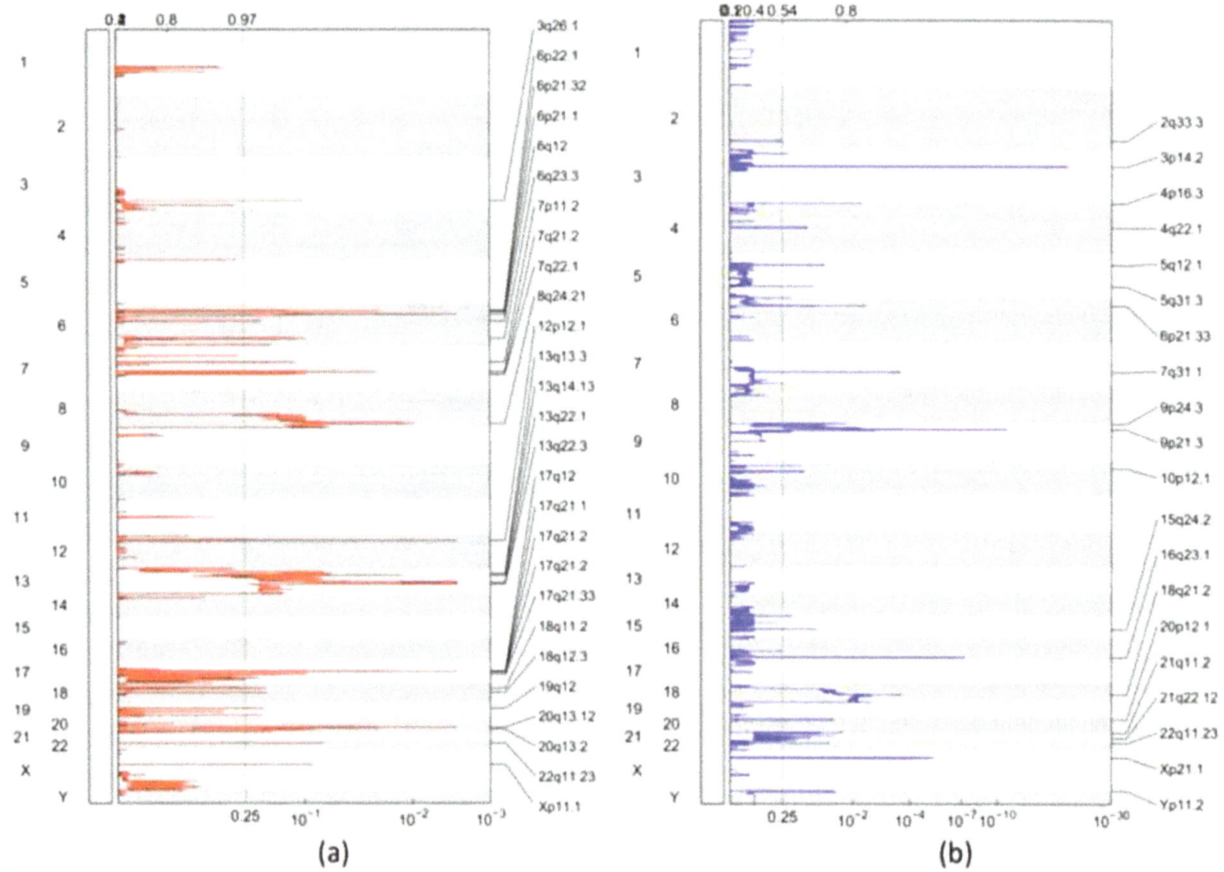

Fig. 3 Genomic positions of RCNAs detected in 15 WGS data. The *x*-axis represents the normalized amplification signals (*top*) and significance by *q* value (*bottom*). The green line indicates the significance cutoff at $q = 0.25$. **a** Amplification regions. **b** Deletion regions

Some commonly used ones are as follows. (a) CNVnator [23], RDXplorer [24], and ReadDepth [25] detect CNAs on a single tumor sample. (b) CNAseg [26], Segseq [27], ExomeCNV [28], HMMcopy [29], and VarScan2 [18] identify CNAs on matched tumor-normal samples. Control-FREEC [30, 31] can be categorized both into classes (a) and (b), as it can either work with tumor-normal pairs or with tumor-only samples. Depending on the NGS platforms, CNVnator, Segseq, RDXplorer, ReadDepth, and HMMcopy work for WGS data; ExomeCNV and VarScan work for WES data; and Control-FREEC can work for both types of the sequencing data. In addition to the above methods detecting CNA in individual samples, other methods have been developed to detect RCNAs from multiple samples. These methods take segments from all the individual samples as input and identify the (merged) segments which appear more frequently across the population than expected by chance. Only a few RCNA methods have been developed for NGS data, including JointSLM [32] and cn.MOPS [33]. They conduct copy number analyses based on read counts of segments of multiple tumor samples and usually are applied for CNV detection. On the other hand, many RCNA detection methods that were originally developed for microarray platforms [34] can also be adapted to work on NGS data. These methods include STAC [35], CMDS [36], and GISTIC2.0 [37].

In this study, Control-FREEC is selected to detect CNAs on the individual sample level using WGS and WES data from [11], and the results are compared between the two sequencing platforms. Control-FREEC is a flexible and powerful tool in that it performs multiple types of bias corrections considering GC-content, mappability, and matched normal sample, and it is among the most sensitive tools on both WGS and WES platforms [22]. GISTIC2.0, likely the most popular RCNA detection method, is chosen to detect RCNAs using both WGS and WES data. The identified RCNAs are then compared with those reported previously using microarrays. We compare our results with those from five previous studies, and four of which (all except [13]) used GISTIC2.0. By choosing GISTIC2.0, we hope to alleviate the concern that potential differences generated in the NGS data are due to different software and analytical methods being applied.

Table 1 Amplification RCNAs detected by 145 WES data and 15 WGS data

Cytoband	Peak boundary (Mb)	Width (Mb)	Platform	Residual q value	D	F	P	B	Z
1p36.33	chr1:0.99-3.16	2.174	WES	1.16E−04					
1q21.3	chr1:149.94-156.69	6.751	WES	2.14E−05	Y				
3q26.1	chr3:164.71-164.76	0.047	WES and WGS	9.75E−02					
3q26.2	chr3:169.43-170.59	1.158	WES	4.18E−02	Y	Y			Y
6p21.32	chr6:32.56-32.58	0.016	WGS	2.35E−02					
6p21.1	chr6:42.79-43.97	1.178	WES and WGS	2.00E−13	Y	Y			Y
6q23.3	chr6:135.29-135.71	0.421	WES and WGS	4.98E−04	Y				Y
7p22.1	chr7:4.29-6.89	2.609	WES	6.42E−02			Y		
7p11.2	chr7:55.00-55.46	0.455	WES	5.48E−14	Y	Y	Y	Y	Y
7q21.2	chr7:91.98-92.76	0.779	WES and WGS	5.07E−12	Y	Y	Y		Y
7q22.1	chr7:98.46-100.674	2.217	WES	7.81E−07	Y		Y	Y	
7q31.2	chr7:115.61-117.83	2.211	WES	1.71E−02	Y				
8p23.1	chr8:6.97-7.16	0.182	WES	5.08E−02	Y	Y			Y
8p23.1	chr8:7.37-7.63	0.263	WES	1.79E−03	Y	Y			Y
8p23.1	chr8:11.28-11.68	0.402	WES	4.25E−13	Y	Y			Y
8q24.21	chr8:126.45-129.02	2.572	WES and WGS	1.79E−10	Y	Y	Y	Y	Y
8q24.3	chr8:141.9-146.36	4.464	WES and WGS	1.19E−03					
9p13.3	chr9:35.4-35.97	0.571	WES	5.60E−06	Y				Y
9q33.3	chr9:124.98-141.21	16.234	WES	6.22E−03					Y
10p11.22	chr10:31.61-33.62	2.015	WES	9.75E−02					
11p11.2	chr11:46.1-47.18	1.076	WES	1.30E−06					Y
11q13.3	chr11:68.86-69.63	0.775	WES	5.25E−16	Y	Y		Y	Y
11q14.1	chr11:77.73-77.88	0.157	WES	8.70E−05					Y
12p13.31	chr12:9.63-9.72	0.082	WES	7.09E−03					
12p12.1	chr12:25.34-25.67	0.328	WES and WGS	2.63E−32	Y	Y		Y	Y
12q13.3	chr12:56.14-57.32	1.181	WES	8.56E−02					
12q15	chr12:67.07-70.19	3.116	WES	3.88E−02	Y	Y		Y	Y
13q13.2	chr13:33.28-35.25	1.972	WES	8.76E−04	Y				
13q14.11	chr13:39.36-43.16	3.798	WES	1.99E−02	Y				
13q14.13	chr13:44.73-46.64	1.906	WGS	7.11E−02					
13q22.1	chr13:72.13-78.67	6.54	WGS	5.39E−02		Y		Y	Y
15q26.1	chr15:90.03-91.79	1.765	WES	4.45E−03			Y		Y
16p13.13	chr16:11.37-12.01	0.64	WES	3.88E−02					
17q12	chr17:37.83-37.9	0.072	WES	1.04E−24	Y	Y	Y	Y	Y
17q21.2	chr17:38.82-39.02	0.2	WES and WGS	4.35E−02	Y				
17q21.2	chr17:39.85-39.99	0.146	WES and WGS	1.90E−08	Y				
17q21.33	chr17:48.68-49.12	0.442	WGS	9.71E−02					
17q25.3	chr17:68.13-81.20	13.067	WES	5.04E−02					
18p11.21	chr18:12.25-13.44	1.184	WES	9.23E−03					
18q11.2	chr18:19.75-20.52	0.766	WES	5.94E−11	Y	Y	Y		Y
19q12	chr19:30.19-30.48	0.282	WES	6.69E−15	Y	Y	Y	Y	Y
20q13.12	chr20:42.98-43.56	0.584	WES and WGS	8.36E−02			Y		
20q13.2	chr20:47.90-52.77	4.877	WES	1.00E−02		Y	Y		
20q13.33	chr20:58.42-58.51	0.099	WES	1.75E−03			Y		

Table 1 Amplification RCNAs detected by 145 WES data and 15 WGS data *(Continued)*

22q11.23	chr22:24.39-24.41	0.016	WGS	7.11E−02		
Xp11.1	chrX:58.52-58.53	0.014	WGS	8.53E−02	Y	
Xq28	chrX:152.11-153.91	1.793	WES	5.53E−04		Y

A region may span multiple cytobands, in which case the longest one was listed. The regions were verified by checking if they were identified in any of the five previous microarray-based studies

D Dulak et al. 2012 [14], *F* Frankel et al. 2014 [16], *P* Paulson et al. 2009 [13], *B* Beroukhim et al. 2010 [3], *Z* Zack et al. 2013 [4], *Y* indicates a region was identified in a study

Results

RCNA analysis

The estimated copy ratios of segments among 145 WES and 15 WGS data are shown in Fig. 1. We used GISTIC2.0 on the copy ratio profiles to perform a permutation-based significance analysis and identify significantly amplified/deleted regions. The recurrent amplification/deletion regions for WES data are shown in Fig. 2. The results of WGS data are shown in Fig. 3 accordingly. The threshold for the residual q value was set as 0.1, resulting in 41/16 amplifications and 67/19 deletions in WES/WGS data, respectively. We further combined the results from WES and WGS, and resulted in 47 amplification and 74 deletion events.

These newly identified genomic regions were verified with all the five microarray-based studies (Tables 1 and 2). It was found that the majority of the regions (68 % of deletions and 74 % of amplifications) detected in our study were also identified in those previous studies. Known cancer genes within these regions were identified according to the Cancer Gene Census [38], and the results are shown in the supplementary document (Additional file 1: Tables S1 and S2). Among all these detected regions, 13 amplification events were not reported in any of the previous studies; four of them (1p36.33, 12p13.31, 18p11.21, 8q24.3) had a residual q value less than 0.01. Twenty-nine deletion events were not identified previously, and ten of them (Xp22.33, 3p26.3, 6q22.31, 14q32.2, 1p21.1, 3p12.3, 6q12, Yq12, 6p12.3, 14p11.2) had a residual q value less than 0.01. We also examined the regions identified from the five previous studies to see whether they were also identified using the NGS data. We extracted the amplification regions (from Additional file 1: Table S2-C) and deletion regions (from Additional file 1: Table S4-B) in [14], for example. We checked if these regions were detected using the sequencing data and listed the q value for each region in Table 3. The genomic location for each region was converted from hg18 to hg19 using the University of California, Santa Cruz (UCSC) liftOver tool. The majority of those regions overlapped with our results, except for four amplifications and four deletions. The comparisons with other four studies are listed in the supplementary document (Additional file 1: Tables S3–S6), from which it can be seen that 58 % of regions in [16], 95 % of regions in [13], 64 % of regions in [3], and 57 % of regions in [4] were detected in our study. From these comparisons, we observed that the majority of regions in previous microarray studies were detected using NGS data.

To generate a consensus list of regions, we investigated all the genomic regions in terms of cytobands across all the results from the six studies including ours and listed the regions appearing in at least three of them. The results are shown in Tables 4 and 5. Only two amplifications and six deletions were not found in our study, and our result is the one that is most consistent with the consensus regions, which suggests that NGS may be a more powerful approach for detecting RCNAs.

Comparison of CNAs on WGS and WES

We detected CNAs in 15 normal-tumor sample pairs based on both WGS data and WES data using Control-FREEC and compared the results from the two platforms. The comparisons were made on different lengths of segments, including large-scale and focal-scale, where large-scale CNAs refer to those spanning more than 25 % of a chromosome arm and focal-scale CNAs refer to those shorter than 25 % of a chromosome arm. The size span of large-scale CNAs is [18.32 161.22] Mb, with a standard deviation of 37.39 Mb. The size span of small-scale CNAs is [0.001 50.65] Mb, with a standard deviation of 2.50 Mb. More than 83 % of focal-scale CNAs are shorter than 1 Mb. For each detected CNA, we used Kolmogorov-Smirnov (KS) test to assess the possibility that it was generated just by chance; furthermore, we searched the WGS and WES data of each sample to see if it contained an event that overlapped the detected CNA with at least 10 % of bases, i.e., we counted how many times it appeared in WGS data and WES data. We then applied Fisher's exact test to compare the detection frequency of each CNA by the two platforms.

The results of large-scale CNAs are shown in Table 6. Totally, 19 regions were detected from the 15 EA samples. We then counted how many times these CNAs were detected by WGS and WES and found none of them was more frequently detected by one platform than the other. In addition, we used KS test and found

Table 2 Deletion RCNAs detected by 145 WES data and 15 WGS data

Cytoband	Boundary (Mb)	Width (Mb)	Platform	Residual *q* value	D	F	P	B	Z
1p36.11	chr1:19.53-31.73	12.21	WES	9.12E−04	Y			Y	Y
1p31.1	chr1:45.53-100.32	54.79	WES	5.89E−02					
1p21.1	chr1:104.12-107.60	3.48	WES	2.86E−04					
1p13.2	chr1:115.32-115.58	0.26	WES	5.65E−04					Y
1q31.3	chr1:186.41-200.18	13.77	WES	1.16E−02					
2q22.1	chr2:136.87-149.40	12.53	WES	8.62E−02				Y	Y
2q32.1	chr2:179.23-190.43	11.20	WES	6.27E−02					
3p26.3	chr3:0.00-2.61	2.61	WES	3.97E−08					
3p24.3	chr3:12.79-69.03	56.24	WES and WGS	3.19E−02	Y	Y		Y	Y
3p12.3	chr3:75.71-88.10	12.39	WES	2.29E−03					
4p16.1	chr4:0.00-15.97	15.97	WES and WGS	2.81E−02					
4p15.31	chr4:17.84-24.53	6.69	WES	9.06E−03					Y
4p12	chr4:42.15-47.45	5.30	WES	5.30E−02					
4q13.2	chr4:69.34-71.25	1.91	WES	2.49E−02					
4q22.1	chr4:90.88-93.23	2.35	WGS	9.73E−02	Y	Y			Y
4q28.3	chr4:129.78-139.98	10.20	WES	3.52E−02					
4q32.1	chr4:154.56-159.59	5.03	WES	9.27E−02		Y			
4q32.3	chr4:164.44-165.88	1.44	WES	1.84E−02					
4q34.3	chr4:174.30-191.15	16.86	WES	2.50E−03	Y			Y	Y
5q12.1	chr5:58.15-59.79	1.64	WGS	4.42E−02	Y	Y	Y	Y	Y
5q13.1	chr5:66.46-68.46	2.00	WES	3.52E−06			Y		
5q14.3	chr5:79.47-130.52	51.04	WES	1.41E−03			Y		
6p25.3	chr6:0.00-2.62	2.62	WES	3.97E−07	Y	Y			Y
6p12.3	chr6:49.82-50.79	0.97	WES	8.30E−03					
6p22.2	chr6:24.98-25.73	0.75	WES	1.97E−02					
6p21.33	chr6:31.17-31.32	0.15	WGS	3.97E−03					
6q12	chr6:64.42-71.14	6.72	WES	3.62E−03					
6q16.1	chr6:90.58-97.25	6.67	WES	2.08E−02					Y
6q16.3	chr6:100.06-105.41	5.35	WES	4.82E−02					Y
6q22.31	chr6:123.37-124.60	1.23	WES	1.21E−04					
6q27	chr6:151.79-171.12	19.33	WES	2.27E−02	Y			Y	Y
7q31.1	chr7:105.14-128.47	23.33	WES and WGS	8.30E−03	Y			Y	Y
7q34	chr7:141.64-141.95	0.31	WES	2.45E−06	Y			Y	
8p23.2	chr8:0.00-6.26	6.27	WES	9.89E−05	Y		Y	Y	Y
8p23.1	chr8:7.83-10.39	2.55	WES	2.59E−02					
8p21.2	chr8:23.42-24.77	1.35	WES	1.73E−05			Y		
8p11.22	chr8:38.85-39.78	0.92	WES	5.30E−02				Y	
9p23	chr9:6.64-15.17	8.53	WES	1.10E−06	Y	Y	Y		Y
9p21.3	chr9:21.86-23.69	1.83	WES and WGS	1.35E−34	Y	Y	Y	Y	Y
9q12	chr9:43.13-66.51	23.38	WES	3.52E−02					
9q31.1	chr9:70.49-123.15	52.66	WES	2.49E−02					
10q23.31	chr10:89.55-94.21	4.67	WES	2.63E−05					Y
11p15.4	chr11:0.00-8.94	8.94	WES	1.05E−02					Y
11p11.12	chr11:49.00-57.07	8.07	WES	8.36E−02					

Table 2 Deletion RCNAs detected by 145 WES data and 15 WGS data *(Continued)*

11q14.1	chr11:77.96-111.96	33.99	WES	6.27E−02	Y				
11q25	chr11:126.13-135.01	8.88	WES	4.23E−03	Y			Y	Y
12p13.31	chr12:9.47-9.75	0.29	WES	4.82E−02					
12q12	chr12:33.56-48.13	14.57	WES	5.89E−02					
12q21.31	chr12:70.76-93.77	23.01	WES	4.23E−03		Y			
13q31.1	chr13:61.10-95.23	34.12	WES	2.38E−02					
14p11.2	chr14:0.00-20.48	20.48	WES	8.69E−03					
14q13.3	chr14:36.79-37.64	0.86	WES	5.30E−02					Y
14q32.13	chr14:94.16-96.85	2.69	WES	1.39E−02					
14q32.2	chr14:97.03-107.35	10.32	WES	2.37E−04					
15q11.2	chr15:20.78-22.69	1.91	WES	2.59E−02		Y	Y		Y
15q24.2	chr15:74.01-77.71	3.71	WGS	6.84E−02					
16p13.3	chr16:0.00-4.90	4.90	WES	2.10E−05					Y
16q21	chr16:29.48-90.35	60.88	WES and WGS	7.29E−02	Y	Y	Y		Y
17p12	chr17:0.00-18.02	18.02	WES	3.43E−03			Y		
17p11.2	chr17:18.42-18.54	0.12	WES	2.20E−13			Y		Y
18q12.1	chr18:24.60-28.65	4.04	WES and WGS	6.80E−03			Y		Y
18q12.3	chr18:35.15-42.28	7.14	WES and WGS	5.53E−07			Y		Y
18q21.2	chr18:48.59-50.28	1.69	WES and WGS	2.87E−13	Y	Y	Y		Y
18q23	chr18:67.87-78.08	10.21	WES and WGS	8.67E−05			Y	Y	Y
19p13.3	chr19:0.00-10.66	10.65	WES	6.47E−04					Y
20p12.1	chr20:13.97-16.04	2.06	WGS	2.93E−02	Y	Y			Y
21p11.2	chr21:0.00-15.32	15.32	WGS	1.77E−02	Y				
21q21.1	chr21:19.63-27.01	7.38	WES	4.49E−05			Y		Y
21q22.3	chr21:47.86-48.13	0.27	WES and WGS	2.64E−04			Y		
22q11.23	chr22:24.33-24.37	0.05	WGS	3.83E−02			Y		
Xp22.33	chrX:0.00-2.67	2.67	WES	8.13E−33					
Xp21.1	chrX:30.87-32.66	1.79	WES and WGS	2.99E−04		Y			Y
Xq28	chrX:154.75-155.27	0.52	WES	2.55E−17		Y			
Yq12	chrY:20.89-59.22	38.33	WES and WGS	4.08E−03					

A region may span multiple cytobands, in which case the longest one was listed. The regions were verified by checking if they were identified in any of the five previous microarray-based studies

D Dulak et al. 2012 [14], *F* Frankel et al. 2014 [16], *P* Paulson et al. 2009 [13], *B* Beroukhim et al. 2010 [3], *Z* Zack et al. 2013 [4], *O* our study, *Y* indicates a region was identified in a study

the false-positive detection rate of each identified CNA was 0.

The results of focal-scale CNAs are shown in Table 7. WGS identified 21,197 focal-scale CNAs from the 15 samples; among them, 3675 were statistically more frequently detected by WGS than by WES. WES identified 4371 focal-scale CNAs, and 144 of them were identified more frequently by the platform. We checked the false-positive detection rates of the detected CNAs using the KS test and found 19,694/3655 CNAs on WGS/WES with p values < 0.05; these CNAs are less likely to be spurious discoveries, and we only worked on these CNAs afterwards. Among them, about 18 % of CNAs detected by WGS were statistically more frequently identified by WGS than by WES, while only about 3 % of CNAs detected by WES were more frequently identified on the platform. We further investigated if the false-positive detection rates of small CNAs (<200 k) detected on the two platforms were different using one-tailed t test, which resulted in a p value of 2.2E−16 (with means 0.004 vs. 0.009), and it indicates that the false-positive detection rate of those small CNAs is significantly smaller using WGS. One possible explanation is that WGS does not contain the exome-capturing process as in WES, and the local variation/bias of sequence read coverage is smaller [39]. Compared to WGS, WES does not cover intron regions, and it only covers 2.76 % of the whole genome. So finally, we investigated the effect

Table 3 Comparison of results of Dulak et al. [14] to our results

Cytoband	Boundary (Mb)	Width (Mb)	Our study	Residual q value	Type
12p12.1	chr12:25.34-25.45	0.11	Y	2.63E−32	amp
18q11.2	chr18:19.70-19.91	0.21	Y	5.94E−11	amp
8p23.1	chr8:11.37-11.67	0.30	Y	4.25E−13	amp
19q12	chr19:30.25-30.41	0.16	Y	6.69E−15	amp
7q21.2	chr7:92.48-92.66	0.18	Y	5.07E−12	amp
11q13.3	chr11:69.26-69.81	0.55	Y	5.25E−16	amp
17q12	chr17:37.72-38.02	0.30	Y	1.04E−24	amp
17q21.2	chr17:39.77-39.96	0.19	Y	1.90E−08	amp
7p11.2	chr7:54.95-55.43	0.48	Y	5.48E−14	amp
8q24.21	chr8:128.40-128.84	0.44	Y	1.79E−10	amp
6p21.1	chr6:43.21-43.35	0.14	Y	2.00E−13	amp
9p13.3	chr9:35.48-35.94	0.46	Y	5.60E−06	amp
13q13.1	chr13:33.38-34.43	1.05	Y	8.76E−04	amp
7q22.1	chr7:99.29-100.00	0.71	Y	7.81E−07	amp
7q31.2	chr7:116.13-116.63	0.50	Y	1.71E−02	amp
12q15	chr12:67.27-70.21	2.94	Y	3.88E−02	amp
6q23.3	chr6:135.28-135.83	0.55	Y	4.98E−04	amp
10q22.2	chr10:75.33-76.13	0.80			amp
1q21.3	chr1:147.76-154.10	6.34	Y	2.14E−05	amp
10q26.13	chr10:122.76-123.92	1.16			amp
3q26.2	chr3:168.72-172.28	3.56	Y	4.18E−02	amp
18q11.2	chr18:23.45-24.21	0.76	Y	5.94E−11	amp
13q14.11	chr13:41.37-41.93	0.56	Y	1.99E−02	amp
11p14.1	chr11:27.08-27.61	0.53			amp
7q34[a]	chr7:141.92-142.26	0.34			amp
3p14.2	chr3:58.98-61.54	2.56	Y	3.19E−02	del
16q23.1	chr16:78.13-79.65	1.52	Y	7.29E−02	del
9p21.3	chr9:21.86-22.02	0.16	Y	1.35E−34	del
5q12.1	chr5:58.26-59.79	1.53	Y	4.42E−02	del
6p25.3	chr6:1.60-2.63	1.03	Y	3.97E−07	del
20p12.1	chr20:14.26-16.04	1.78	Y	2.93E−02	del
4q22.1	chr4:91.15-93.27	2.12	Y	9.73E−02	del
18q21.2	chr18:48.52-48.72	0.20	Y	2.87E−13	del
21q22.12	chr21:36.11-36.43	0.32			del
9p23	chr9:7.79-12.72	4.93	Y	1.10E−06	del
6q26	chr6:161.69-163.21	1.52	Y	2.27E−02	del
2q33.3	chr2:204.82-206.56	1.74			del
1q44	chr1:245.85-246.71	0.86			del
8p23.3	chr8:1.01-1.46	0.45	Y	9.89E−05	del
7q33	chr7:123.66-142.53	18.87	Y	8.30E−03	del
7q36.1	chr7:148.11-159.13	11.02			del
1p36.11	chr1:25.77-31.25	5.48	Y	9.12E−04	del
4q34.3	chr4:178.82-185.31	6.49	Y	2.50E−03	del

Table 3 Comparison of results of Dulak et al. [14] to our results *(Continued)*

11q22.3	chr11:105.95-112.83	6.88	Y	6.27E−02	del
11q25	chr11:121.03-134.94	13.91	Y	4.23E−03	del
21p11.2[a]	chr21:1.00-16.26	15.26	Y	1.77E−02	del

Regions detected in Dulak et al., 2012 [14] were verified in our study
[a]In cytoband indicates that the coordinate is based on hg18

of non-coverage to CNA detection and dealt with small CNAs that only reside in intron regions. As the result, no CNAs detected by WES spanned only on introns, and more than 7000 of such CNAs were identified by WGS, but only 22 % of these intron CNAs were statistically more frequently detected by WGS.

Discussion

In this study, we detected RCNAs using NGS data from 145 EA samples and compared them with those from the five microarray studies. We found that the majority of the regions detected by microarrays overlapped the regions identified by NGS and vise versa. Furthermore, based on all these six studies, we identified 22/51 consensus amplification/deletion regions, and our result was found to be the one that is most concordant with the consensus events. From the above observations, we suggest that NGS can replace microarrays to detect RCNAs in EA.

Table 4 Consensus amplification RCNAs in 6 studies

Cytoband	Boundary (Mb)	D	F	P	B	Z	O
3q26.2	chr3:167.60-170.90	Y	Y			Y	Y
6p21.1	chr6:40.50-46.20	Y	Y			Y	Y
6q23.3	chr6:135.20-139.00	Y				Y	Y
7p11.2	chr7:54.00-58.00	Y	Y	Y	Y	Y	Y
7q21.2	chr7:91.10-92.80	Y	Y	Y		Y	Y
7q21.3	chr7:92.80-98.00		Y	Y	Y		
7q22.1	chr7:98.00-103.80	Y		Y	Y		Y
8p23.1	chr8:6.20-12.70	Y	Y			Y	Y
8q24.13	chr8:122.50-127.30			Y	Y		Y
8q24.21	chr8:127.30-131.50	Y	Y	Y	Y	Y	Y
9p13.3	chr9:33.20-36.30	Y				Y	Y
11q13.3	chr11:68.40-70.40	Y	Y		Y	Y	Y
12p12.1	chr12:21.30-26.50	Y	Y		Y	Y	Y
12q14.3	chr12:65.10-67.70	Y			Y		Y
12q15	chr12:67.70-71.50	Y	Y		Y	Y	Y
13q22.1	chr13:73.30-75.40		Y		Y	Y	Y
15q26.1	chr15:89.10-94.30			Y		Y	Y
15q26.2	chr15:94.30-98.50		Y	Y		Y	
17q12	chr17:31.80-38.10	Y	Y	Y	Y	Y	Y
18q 11.2	chr18:19.00-25.00	Y	Y	Y		Y	Y
19q12	chr19:28.60-32.40	Y	Y	Y	Y	Y	Y
20q13.2	chr20:49.80-55.00		Y	Y			Y

These regions are those that appear in at least three studies
D Dulak et al. 2012 [14], *F* Frankel et al. 2014 [16], *P* Paulson et al. 2009 [13], *B* Beroukhim et al. 2010 [3], *Z* Zack et al. 2013 [4], *O* our study, *Y* indicates a region was identified in a study

However, discrepancy generally exists when comparing each specific region from all the studies. Even for the largest detected events, they are not consistent across the platforms and across the different microarray studies. The largest recurrent deletions detected by microarrays are not consistent. Two of them [3, 14] identified the largest recurrent deletions on chr7:123.66-142.52 (Mb), which corresponds to chr7:105.14-128.47 (Mb) detected both by WGS and WES in our study. The largest deletion detected by WGS and WES is on Chr16:29.48-90.35 (Mb), while only part of the region—chr16:78.13–79.65 (Mb) (in [4, 14, 16]) and chr16:31.93–33.39 (Mb) (in [16])—were detected in the microarray studies. Part of these discrepancies may just be caused by different technologies used in these platforms, such as different hybridization and scanning methods applied in these microarray studies, target-enrichment strategies applied in WES, and bias due to the effect of GC-content and uneven mappability across genome in NGS. Although our study indicates a significant overlap between RCNAs detected using microarray data and NGS data, it is still a challenge to rigorously compare these RCNA calling methods. To further compare these approaches, a well-controlled study design such as a spike-in experiment should be applied in the future.

GISTIC analysis is often used to identify driver genes that contribute to cancer development. In this study, we found several potential driver genes in the detected regions that were reported in previous studies, and the results are listed in Table 8. We detected oncogenes such as *EGFR*, *ERBB2*, *GATA6*, *KRAS*, *MYC*, and tumor suppressor genes such as *APC*, *ARID1A*, *ATM*, *CDKN2A*, *CDKN2B*, *CDK6*, *MCL1*, *MET*, *MYB*, *PDE4D*, *PRCKI*, and *PTPRD*. Those were also identified in the various previous microarray studies. In another study [11], the authors identified 26 significantly mutated genes based on the 145 WES data used in our study. Among them, ten genes such as *TP53*, *CDKN2A*, *EYS*, *ARID1A*, *TLR4*, *ARID2*, *SYNE1*, *C6orf118*, *ACTL7B*, and *SCN10A* were also identified in our study, and three of the rest (*SMAD4*, *TLL1*, and *SMARCA4*) are located within

Table 5 Consensus deletion RCNAs in six studies

Cytoband	Boundary (Mb)	D	F	P	B	Z	O
1p36.11	chr1:23.90-28.00	Y			Y	Y	Y
1p35.3	chr1:28.00-30.20	Y			Y		Y
1p35.2	chr1:30.20-32.40	Y			Y		Y
1q44	chr1:243.70-249.25	Y	Y			Y	
2q22.1	chr2:136.80-142.20				Y	Y	Y
2q22.2	chr2:142.20-144.10				Y	Y	Y
2q33.3	chr2:204.90-209.00	Y			Y	Y	
3p14.2	chr3:58.60-63.70	Y	Y		Y	Y	Y
4q22.1	chr4:88.00-93.70	Y	Y			Y	Y
4q34.1	chr4:171.90-176.30				Y	Y	Y
4q34.2	chr4:176.30-177.50				Y	Y	Y
4q34.3	chr4:177.50-183.20	Y			Y	Y	Y
4q35.1	chr4:183.20-187.10	Y			Y	Y	Y
5q11.2	chr5:50.70-58.90	Y	Y	Y	Y	Y	Y
5q12.1	chr5:58.90-62.90	Y	Y	Y	Y	Y	Y
6p25.3	chr6:0.00-2.30	Y	Y			Y	Y
6p25.2	chr6:2.30-4.20	Y	Y				Y
6q26	chr6:161.00-164.50	Y			Y	Y	Y
7q31.1	chr7:107.40-114.60				Y	Y	Y
7q31.32	chr7:121.10-123.80	Y			Y		Y
7q31.33	chr7:123.80-127.10	Y			Y		Y
7q32.1	chr7:127.10-129.20	Y			Y		Y
7q34	chr7:138.20-143.10	Y			Y		Y
7q36.3	chr7:155.10-159.14	Y			Y	Y	
8p23.3	chr8:0.00-2.20	Y		Y	Y	Y	Y
8p23.2	chr8:2.20-6.20				Y	Y	Y
8p23.1	chr8:6.20-12.70				Y	Y	Y
9p24.1	chr9:4.60-9.00	Y	Y	Y		Y	Y
9p23	chr9:9.00-14.20	Y	Y	Y		Y	Y
9p21.3	chr9:19.90-25.60	Y	Y	Y	Y	Y	Y
11q24.2	chr11:123.90-127.80	Y			Y		Y
11q24.3	chr11:127.80-130.80	Y			Y	Y	Y
11q25	chr11:130.80-135.01	Y			Y	Y	Y
16q23.1	chr16:74.10-79.20	Y	Y	Y		Y	Y
16q23.2	chr16:79.20-81.70	Y	Y			Y	Y
17p11.2	chr17:16.00-22.20			Y		Y	Y
18q12.2	chr18:32.70-37.20			Y		Y	Y
18q12.3	chr18:37.20-43.50			Y		Y	Y
18q21.2	chr18:48.20-53.80	Y	Y	Y		Y	Y
18q21.33	chr18:59.00-61.60			Y	Y	Y	
18q22.1	chr18:61.60-66.80			Y	Y	Y	
18q22.2	chr18:66.80-68.70			Y	Y	Y	Y
18q22.3	chr18:68.70-73.10			Y	Y	Y	Y
18q23	chr18:73.10-78.077			Y	Y	Y	Y
20p12.1	chr20:12.10-17.90	Y	Y			Y	Y
21q11.2	chr21:14.30-16.40	Y		Y		Y	Y
21q21.1	chr21:16.40-24.00			Y		Y	Y
21q21.2	chr21:24.00-26.80			Y		Y	Y
21q22.12	chr21:35.80-37.80	Y	Y	Y		Y	
Xp21.2	chrX:29.30-31.50		Y			Y	Y
Xp21.1	chrX:31.50-37.60		Y			Y	Y

These regions are those that appear in at least three studies

1 Mb of the detected regions of this study. It is worth to point out that some of the potential driver genes such as *ERBB2* and *TP53* were reported as implicated in the progression of esophageal Barrett to EA [13]. However, CNA regions are usually large and contain many genes. It is difficult to distinguish driver genes from passengers by just studying copy numbers [40]. Although more common driver genes were detected in this study than those found in [16], the discrepancy still implies the need of an integrated approach to identify driver genes of EA, which can consider CNA, mutation, gene expression, and methylation altogether.

In addition to the common regions, we found some novel ones, including four amplification regions and ten deletion regions with statistically high frequency of appearance in the population. These regions may provide

Table 6 Large-scale CNAs detected in WGS and WES

Boundary (Mb)	Width (Mb)	Type	WGS count	WES count	*p* value
chrX: 2.70-44.00	41	Gain	0	1	1.00
chr12:58.34-110.00	52.05	Gain	1	3	0.60
chr8:87.08-126.00	39.3	Gain	0	1	1.00
chr14:37.15-65.00	27.5	Gain	0	1	1.00
chr20:36.79-55.00	18.32	Gain	0	1	1.00
chr4:20.88-69.00	48.46	Gain	0	1	1.00
chrX:46.95-139.00	91.93	Loss	1	4	0.33
chr8:0.12-86.00	86.27	Loss	1	2	1.00
chr13:35.76-115.00	79.35	Loss	2	5	0.39
chr4:75.26-178.00	103.1	Loss	1	3	0.60
chr5:19.47-181.00	161.22	Loss	2	4	0.65
chrY:10.01-29.00	18.71	Loss	0	5	0.04
chr17:0.00-21.00	21.19	Loss	2	1	1.00
chr18:19.84-78.00	58.18	Loss	5	4	1.00
chr15:32.02-60.00	28.39	Loss	1	0	1.00
chr19:0.25-25.00	24.26	Loss	3	0	0.22
chr19:36.81-55.00	18.42	Loss	1	0	1.00
chr7:93.74-152.00	58.36	Loss	2	1	1.00
chr21:15.00-45.00	29.63	Loss	1	1	1.00

p value is used to assess if the detected CNA is more frequently identified by WGS or WES

Table 7 Focal-scale CNAs detected in WGS and WES

	WGS	WES
All CNAs	21,197/3675	4371/144
Filtered CNAs	19,694/3456	3655/121
Small CNAs (<200 k)	11,480/2175	1201/36
Small and intron CNAs	7452/1603	0/0

A number before/indicates how many CNAs detected in the specific platform; a number after/indicates how many CNAs are more frequently detected in the platform. Filtered CNAs represent detected CNAs with p-value < 0.05. Small and Intron CNAs are CNAs with width < 200 k and only cover introns

more clues to understand the cancer genomics of EA. In particular, *SKI* and *PRKCZ* in 1p36.33 have been reported to contribute to the loss function of *TGFBR2* and *SMAD4* in cancer [41]. *TGFBR2* and *SMAD4* are involved in the transforming growth factor (TGF)-β pathway and were identified as driver genes in gastric cancer [42] and colorectal cancer [43]. The novel deletion event identified on Yq12 in our study, along with previously found deletion events on X chromosome (e.g., Xp21.1 and Xp21.2) may help to understand the greater incidence of EA in males over the past three decades. For example, the *DMD* gene in Xp21.1 was identified as a driver gene in gastric cancer [42], and our result suggests that it may also contribute to EA development.

The recurrently detected regions are likely to harbor "common mutations" that are of great interest in cancer studies. However, each tumor sample can contain private driver mutations for that individual patient's tumor. To verify it, we compared the CNAs detected at individual sample level (Tables 6 and 7) with the recurrent events (Tables 1 and 2). We found only about 25.2 % of individual deletions overlapped identified deletion RCNAs. More extremely, only 10.2 % of amplifications detected at individual sample level overlapped those amplification RCNAs. Even for large-scale events, we found 88.0 % of individual deletions overlapped the recurrent deletion events, and only 35 % of individual amplifications overlapped the recurrent amplification events. The above observation implies that a considerable amount of driver mutations in a specific tumor sample is not located in the recurrent regions and personalized studies are required to identify these rare events.

In our study, the medians of spans of recurrent amplification/deletion events are 1.0/6.6 Mb for WES (and possibly WGS) and 0.2/2.1 Mb for those identified only from WGS (Tables 1 and 2). Also, we detected more individual small CNAs by WGS (Table 7). Compared to WES, WGS appears more powerful to detect small events, especially for those that mostly reside in non-coding regions. The limitation of this comparison is that only 15 WGS/WES samples were available. For future studies, a larger sample size should provide more precision to calibrate the performance of WES relative to WGS.

Conclusions

In this study, we detected RCNAs in EA using the NGS data from [11] and compared the results with those from the previous microarray studies. The majority of the events detected in our study also were detected in those previous studies. Furthermore, novel regions and genes were found using NGS technologies. We also compared carefully WGS and WES in detecting CNA on an individual level. We found large-scale segments can be more consistently detected by both platforms, whereas WGS does detect more focal events. Importantly, the recurrent events on the population level appear to be successfully identified by WES. Given that the cost of WES is much less than that of WGS, and the mutations in WES is much more interpretable, our study suggests that WES may be the viable platform to detect recurrent copy number events in EA research.

Table 8 Potential driver genes reported in previous studies and corresponding RCNAs detected in this study

Genes	Cytoband	Boundary (Mb)
ARID1A	1p36.11	chr1:19.53-31.73
SKI.PRKCZ	1p36.33	chr1:0.99-3.16
MCL1	1q21.3	chr1:149.94-156.69
SCN10A	3p24.3	chr3:12.79-69.03
PRCKI	3q26.2	chr3:169.43-170.59
PDE4D	5q12.1	chr5:58.15-59.79
APC	5q14.3	chr5:79.47-130.52
EYS	6q12	chr6:64.42-71.14
MYB	6q23.3	chr6:135.29-135.71
C6orf118, SYNE1	6q27	chr6:151.79-171.12
EGFR	7p11.2	chr7:55.00-55.46
CDK6	7q21.2	chr7:91.98-92.76
MET	7q31.2	chr7:115.61-117.83
MYC	8q24.21	chr8:126.45-129.02
CDKN2A, CDKN2B	9p21.3	chr9:21.86-23.69
PTPRD	9p23	chr9:6.64-15.17
TLR4	9q31.1	chr9:70.49-123.15
ATM	11q14.1	chr11:77.96-111.96
KRAS	12p12.1	chr12:25.34-25.67
ARID2	12q12	chr12:33.56-48.13
GATA6	18q11.2	chr18:19.75-20.52
DMD	Xp21.1	chrX:30.87-32.66

Methods

Esophageal adenocarcinoma cancer data

The NGS data, including both WGS and WES data, were generated in [11] and stored in the database of Genotypes and Phenotypes (dbGaP) (study accession: phs000598.v1.p1). The dataset is comprised of 145 matched tumor-normal samples. Among them, 15 samples both have WGS and WES data, and the rest 130 samples have only WES data. The EA samples include those from the gastric-esophageal junction, not treated with chemotherapy or radiation before surgery. The tumor samples were examined by a board-certified pathologist and ensured that their carcinoma content >70 %. The samples were sequenced on multiple Illumina HiSeq flow cells to have the average target exome coverage of ~80× in WES data, and sequenced on the Illumina Genome Analyzer Iix or the Illumina HiSeq sequencer with an average of ~30× coverage depth in WGS data. The details of the sample collection, DNA extraction, and sequencing procedures can be found in [11].

The raw sequence data were extracted from dbGaP using the NCBI SRA Toolkit; the sequences were aligned to the NCBI build 37 (hg19) reference using BWA [44] and processed following GATK best practices. The base score re-calibrated bam files were used for CNA detection.

CNA detection methods

Control-FREEC was applied in this study on both WGS and WES data. It divided the genome into small contiguous regions using sliding windows. The read count profiles in each region for normal and tumor samples were computed and normalized accounting for GC-content and mappability. The read count ratios of tumors to matched normal samples were calculated and used as the proxy of the copy number ratios. A LASSO-based algorithm was used to segment the data. LASSO is a widely used generalized linear regression method that involves penalizing the absolute size of its regression coefficients [45]. Using LASSO, a piecewise constant smoothed step profile was used to model the copy number ratios, and the positions with nonzero coefficients were considered as change points. For WES data, the window size was set to 500, and the step size was set to 250, which were recommended by the authors. For WGS data, those parameters were set as 2000 and 1000, respectively. Control-FREEC estimates the normal cell contamination in tumor samples by comparing the observed and predicted copy numbers. It uses the Kolmogorov-Smirnov test to assess the false-positive rate of each detected CNA. Control-FREEC can predict absolute copy numbers if the ploidy information is provided. We used ABSOLUTE [46] to estimate the ploidy of the 15 EA samples using WES data, and the results are listed in the supplement. In this study we classified the identified CNAs based on their status (amplification or deletion) instead of their absolute copy numbers. Control-FREEC ignored genomic regions with mappability less than 0.85 by default, and hence, we did not consider the effect of unmappable regions in this study.

GISTIC2.0 was used to identify regions with a statistically high frequency of copy number aberrations over background aberrations. It evaluated both the frequency and the significance to identify regions of interest. The G score measured both the frequency of aberrations, and the magnitude of the copy number changes (log ratio intensity) in each sample. Each location was scored separately for gains and losses. Then locations in each sample were permuted to simulate random aberrations. This random distribution was compared to the observed statistic to identify scores that are statistically significant. A false discovery rate (FDR) multiple testing correction was applied to calculate a q-bound significance score. Within each statistically significant region, a peak region was identified so that the region with a maximal G score and a minimal q value is most likely to contain affected genes. In addition to the q value, it also computed the residual q value, which measured the q value of a peak region after removing events that overlap with other more significant peak regions in the same chromosome. The 145 WES data were segmented using circular binary segmentation (CBS) algorithm [47] and combined to form the segmentation file, while the 15 WGS data were segmented using Control-FREEC as described above. The parameter settings were as follows: amplification threshold = 0.1, deletion threshold = 0.1, broad length cutoff = 0.98, remove X-chromosome = 0, and confidence level = 0.95.

Whenever possible, default parameters and recommended settings were used in the implementation of these tools.

Competing interests

The authors declare that they have no competing interests.

Authors' contributions

JD, XL, XW, and YC conceived of the ideas in this manuscript. XW wrote the code and ran the analysis. CK, JD, SS, XBS, XL, XS, XW, and YC wrote the manuscript. All authors read and approved the final manuscript.

Acknowledgements

This work was directly supported by the National Institutes of Health (R01HL114901 to J.Y.D. and X.W., P01CA53996 to J.Y.D.)

Author details
[1]Vaccine and Infectious Disease Division, Fred Hutchinson Cancer Research Center, Seattle, WA, USA. [2]Human Biology, Fred Hutchinson Cancer Research Center, Seattle, WA, USA. [3]Public Health Science Division, Fred Hutchinson Cancer Research Center, Seattle, WA, USA. [4]Institute of Occupational Health and Poison Control, Chinese Center for Disease Control and Prevention, Beijing, China. [5]Henan Office for Cancer Research and Control, Henan Cancer Hospital, Zhengzhou, Henan, China.

References

1. Nowell P. The clonal evolution of tumor cell populations. Science. 1976;194(4260):23–8.
2. Greaves M, Maley CC. Clonal evolution in cancer. Nature. 2012;481(7381):306–13.
3. Beroukhim R, Mermel CH, Porter D, Wei G, Raychaudhuri S, Donovan J, et al. The landscape of somatic copy-number alteration across human cancers. Nature. 2010;463(7283):899–905.
4. Zack TI, Schumacher SE, Carter SL, Cherniack AD, Saksena G, Tabak B, et al. Pan-cancer patterns of somatic copy number alteration. Nat Genet. 2013;45(10):1134–40.
5. Greshock J, Feng B, Nogueira C, Ivanova E, Perna I, Nathanson K, et al. A comparison of DNA copy number profiling platforms. Cancer Res. 2007;67(21):10173–180.
6. Carter NP. Methods and strategies for analyzing copy number variation using DNA microarrays. Nat Genet. 2007;39:S16–21.
7. Alkan C, Coe BP, Eichler EE. Genome structural variation discovery and genotyping. Nat Rev Genet. 2011;12(5):363–76.
8. Korbel JO, Urban AE, Affourtit JP, Godwin B, Grubert F, Simons JF, et al. Paired-end mapping reveals extensive structural variation in the human genome. Science. 2007;318(5849):420–26.
9. Hurd PJ, Nelson CJ. Advantages of next-generation sequencing versus the microarray in epigenetic research. Brief Funct Genomic Proteomic. 2009;8(3):174–83.
10. Chin L, Hahn WC, Getz G, Meyerson M. Making sense of cancer genomic data. Genes Dev. 2011;25(6):534–55.
11. Dulak AM, Stojanov P, Peng S, Lawrence MS, Fox C, Stewart C, et al. Exome and whole genome sequencing of esophageal adenocarcinoma identifies recurrent driver events and mutational complexity. Nat Genet. 2013;45(5):478–86.
12. Stewart BW, Wild CP. World cancer report 2014. Lyon, France: IARC Nonserial Publication; 2014.
13. Paulson TG, Maley CC, Li X, Li H, Sanchez CA, Chao DL, et al. Chromosomal instability and copy number alterations in Barrett's esophagus and esophageal adenocarcinoma. Clin Cancer Res. 2009;15(10):3305–14.
14. Dulak AM, Schumacher S, van Lieshout J, Imamura Y, Fox C, Shim B, et al. Gastrointestinal adenocarcinomas of the esophagus, stomach and colon exhibit distinct patterns of genome instability and oncogenesis. Cancer Res. 2012;72(17):4383–93.
15. TCGA Genome Data Analysis Center. SNP6 copy number analysis (GISTIC2). TCGA Genome Data Analysis Center. 2014. https://www.broadinstitute.org/tcga/gistic/browseGisticByTissue?gisticAnalysisId=21. Accessed 15 Aug 2015.
16. Frankel A, Armour N, Nancarrow D, Krause L, Hayward N, Lampe G, et al. Genome-wide analysis of esophageal adenocarcinoma yields specific copy number aberrations that correlate with prognosis. Genes Chromosom Cancer. 2014;53(4):324–38.
17. Liu B, Morrison CD, Johnson CS, Trump DL, Qin M, Conroy JC, et al. Computational methods for detecting copy number variations in cancer genome using next generation sequencing: principles and challenges. Oncotarget. 2013;4(11):1868–81.
18. Koboldt DC, Zhang Q, Larson DE, Shen D, McLellan MD, Lin L, et al. VarScan 2: somatic mutation and copy number alteration discovery in cancer by exome sequencing. Genome Res. 2012;22(3):568–76.
19. Guo Y, Sheng Q, Samuels DC, Lehmann B, Bauer JA, Pietenpol J, et al. Comparative study of exome copy number variation estimation tools using array comparative genomic hybridization as control. Biomed Res Int. 2013;2013:915636.
20. Pabinger S, Dander A, Fischer M, Snajder R, Sperk M, Efremova M, et al. A survey of tools for variant analysis of next-generation genome sequencing data. Brief Bioinform. 2014;15(2):256–78.
21. Zhao M, Wang Q, Wang Q, Jia P, Zhao Z. Computational tools for copy number variation (CNV) detection using next-generation sequencing data: features and perspectives. BMC Bioinformatics. 2013;14(11):S1.
22. Alkodsi A, Louhimo R, Hautaniemi S. Comparative analysis of methods for identifying somatic copy number alterations from deep sequencing data. Brief Bioinform. 2015;16(2):242–54.
23. Abyzov A, Urban AE, Snyder M, Gerstein M. CNVnator: an approach to discover, genotype, and characterize typical and atypical CNVs from family and population genome sequencing. Genome Res. 2011;21(6):974–84.
24. Yoon S, Xuan Z, Makarov V, Ye K, Sebat J. Sensitive and accurate detection of copy number variants using read depth of coverage. Genome Res. 2009;19(9):1586–92.
25. Miller CA, Hampton O, Coarfa C, Milosavljevic A. ReadDepth: a parallel R package for detecting copy number alterations from short sequencing reads. PLoS ONE. 2011;6(1):16327.
26. Ivakhno S, Royce T, Cox AJ, Evers DJ, Cheetham RK, Tavaré S. CNAseg-a novel framework for identification of copy number changes in cancer from second-generation sequencing data. Bioinformatics. 2010;26(24):3051–58.
27. Chiang DY, Getz G, Jaffe DB, O'Kelly MJT, Zhao X, Carter SL, et al. High-resolution mapping of copy-number alterations with massively parallel sequencing. Nat Meth. 2009;6(1):99–103.
28. Sathirapongsasuti JF, Lee H, Horst BAJ, Brunner G, Cochran AJ, Binder S, et al. Exome sequencing-based copy-number variation and loss of heterozygosity detection: ExomeCNV. Bioinformatics. 2011;27(19):2648–54.
29. Ha G, Roth A, Lai D, Bashashati A, Ding J, Goya R, et al. Integrative analysis of genome-wide loss of heterozygosity and monoallelic expression at nucleotide resolution reveals disrupted pathways in triple-negative breast cancer. Genome Research. 2012;22(10):1995-2007.
30. Boeva V, Zinovyev A, Bleakley K, Vert JP, Janoueix-Lerosey I, Delattre O, et al. Control-free calling of copy number alterations in deep-sequencing data using GC-content normalization. Bioinformatics. 2011;27(2):268–69.
31. Boeva V, Popova T, Bleakley K, Chiche P, Cappo J, Schleiermacher G, et al. Control-FREEC: a tool for assessing copy number and allelic content using next-generation sequencing data. Bioinformatics. 2012;28(3):423–25.
32. Magi A, Benelli M, Yoon S, Roviello F, Torricelli F. Detecting common copy number variants in high-throughput sequencing data by using JointSLM algorithm. Nucleic Acids Res. 2011;39(10):65.
33. Klambauer G, Schwarzbauer K, Mayr A, Clevert DA, Mitterecker A, Bodenhofer U, et al. cn.MOPS: mixture of Poissons for discovering copy number variations in next-generation sequencing data with a low false discovery rate. Nucleic Acids Res. 2012;40(9):69.
34. Yuan X, Zhang J, Zhang S, Yu G, Wang Y. Comparative analysis of methods for identifying recurrent copy number alterations in cancer. PLoS ONE. 2012;7(12):52516.
35. Diskin SJ, Eck T, Greshock J, Mosse YP, Naylor T, Stoeckert CJ, et al. STAC: a method for testing the significance of DNA copy number aberrations across multiple array-CGH experiments. Genome Res. 2006;16(9):1149–58.
36. Zhang Q, Ding L, Larson DE, Koboldt DC, McLellan MD, Chen K, et al. CMDS: a population-based method for identifying recurrent DNA copy number aberrations in cancer from high-resolution data. Bioinformatics. 2010;26(4):464–69.
37. Mermel CH, Schumacher SE, Hill B, Meyerson ML, Beroukhim R, Getz G. Gistic2.0 facilitates sensitive and confident localization of the targets of focal somatic copy-number alteration in human cancers. Genome Biol. 2011;12(4):41.
38. Futreal PA, Coin L, Marshall M, Down T, Hubbard T, Wooster R, et al. A census of human cancer genes. Nat Rev Cancer. 2004;4(3):177–83.
39. Meynert AM, Ansari M, FitzPatrick DR, Taylor MS. Variant detection sensitivity and biases in whole genome and exome sequencing. BMC Bioinformatics. 2014;15(1):247.
40. Akavia UD, Litvin O, Kim J, Sanchez-Garcia F, Kotliar D, Causton HC, et al. An integrated approach to uncover drivers of cancer. Cell. 2010;143(6):1005–17.
41. Milacic M, Haw R, Rothfels K, Wu G, Croft D, Hermjakob H, et al. Annotating cancer variants and anti-cancer therapeutics in reactome. Cancers. 2012;4(4):1180–211.
42. Wang K, Yuen ST, Xu J, Lee SP, Yan HH, Shi ST, et al. Whole-genome sequencing and comprehensive molecular profiling identify new driver mutations in gastric cancer. Nat Genet. 2014;46(6):573–82.
43. Fleming NI, Jorissen RN, Mouradov D, Christie M, Sakthianandeswaren A, Palmieri M, et al. SMAD2, SMAD3 and SMAD4 mutations in colorectal cancer. Cancer Res. 2012;73(2):725–35.
44. Li H, Durbin R. Fast and accurate short read alignment with burrows-wheeler transform. Bioinformatics. 2009;25(14):1754–60.

7

Cancer classification in the genomic era: five contemporary problems

Qingxuan Song[1], Sofia D. Merajver[2] and Jun Z. Li[1*]

Abstract

Classification is an everyday instinct as well as a full-fledged scientific discipline. Throughout the history of medicine, disease classification is central to how we develop knowledge, make diagnosis, and assign treatment. Here, we discuss the classification of cancer and the process of categorizing cancer subtypes based on their observed clinical and biological features. Traditionally, cancer nomenclature is primarily based on organ location, e.g., "lung cancer" designates a tumor originating in lung structures. Within each organ-specific major type, finer subgroups can be defined based on patient age, cell type, histological grades, and sometimes molecular markers, e.g., hormonal receptor status in breast cancer or microsatellite instability in colorectal cancer. In the past 15+ years, high-throughput technologies have generated rich new data regarding somatic variations in DNA, RNA, protein, or epigenomic features for many cancers. These data, collected for increasingly large tumor cohorts, have provided not only new insights into the biological diversity of human cancers but also exciting opportunities to discover previously unrecognized cancer subtypes. Meanwhile, the unprecedented volume and complexity of these data pose significant challenges for biostatisticians, cancer biologists, and clinicians alike. Here, we review five related issues that represent contemporary problems in cancer taxonomy and interpretation. (1) How many cancer subtypes are there? (2) How can we evaluate the robustness of a new classification system? (3) How are classification systems affected by intratumor heterogeneity and tumor evolution? (4) How should we interpret cancer subtypes? (5) Can multiple classification systems co-exist? While related issues have existed for a long time, we will focus on those aspects that have been magnified by the recent influx of complex multi-omics data. Exploration of these problems is essential for data-driven refinement of cancer classification and the successful application of these concepts in precision medicine.

Keywords: Cancer, Classification, Genomics, Integration, Evolution, Uncertainty, Precision

Introduction

Classification and labeling represent the most intuitive forms of learning. According to Confucius, "If the name is not right then speech will not be in order, and if speech is not in order then nothing will be accomplished." Instances of classification can be found in every aspect of life: the Linnaean system in biology is a seven-level framework for cataloging living organisms; E-commerce companies must organize their holdings in an easy-to-search system. Whether the goal is to recommend movies, screen job candidates, or rank colleges, a system of summarizing and dividing is involved, and uncertainties inherent to this task are common. In a quote attributed to Albert Einstein [1], classification is "an attempt to make the chaotic diversity of our sense experience correspond to a logically uniform system of thought." The tension between "chaotic diversity" on one hand and a "logically uniform system" on the other makes classification a long-standing subject in scientific research. In practice, it was regarded more often as an art than a science, as there is no axiomatic classification theory that applies to all problems. This review will discuss the topic of cancer classification. Instead of offering a systematic review of specific cancers, we will focus on the implicit assumptions and common caveats of classification, especially how it has been confronted with new challenges in the genomic era. We organize the many strands of this topic under the heading of five contemporary problems, although in many ways they are new, more acute forms of old problems. A recurring theme of our discussion is that the merit of a classification system

* Correspondence: junzli@med.umich.edu
[1]Department of Human Genetics, University of Michigan, Ann Arbor, MI, USA

depends on what it will be used for. Often, a new map is drawn, but its intended application is unclear. Only by spelling out the purpose of a proposed system can we evaluate its merit according to what it aims to achieve. The potential measures of merit for classification systems include statistical robustness, connections with existing standards, prognostic value [2], insights into biological mechanisms, and predictive power of treatment outcomes [3]. As we discuss below, sometimes these merits cannot be achieved all at once, and multiple classification systems can be simultaneously "correct" depending on which purpose they are designed to serve.

A few notes of terminology before we begin. In the field of statistical learning, the term "classification" refers to *supervised sample assignment*, using features identified in a training set containing samples with known class labels. Here, we adopt its other, more commonly understood meaning, referring to ab initio pattern recognition, also known as *unsupervised class discovery*. We will use the terms (sub)class and (sub)type interchangeably and will only discuss sample classification, not gene clustering. We sometimes use "genomics" to refer to all high-throughput -omics data. We will focus on subtype discovery within a major organ-specific cancer type, not between the major types.

How many cancer types are there?

The short answer is about 200: the National Cancer Institute keeps an A–Z list of nearly 200 cancer types (http://www.cancer.gov/types/by-body-location), organized by organ location, although with some exceptions, such as "HIV-related" or "unknown primary." This organ-centric system is further stratified, most often by the known cell type of origin within the organ, e.g., "astrocytomas," as a subtype of brain tumors [4], or by patient age, e.g., "childhood leukemia." If each of these major types has four subtypes, there will be 800 subtypes of cancer. As stated above, we will focus on how to identify subtypes within a broadly recognized organ-specific entity.

"Endless forms most beautiful"

While the organ-derived naming system has been used for over a century by doctors, patients, and cancer registries, there has always been the drive to recognize finer subtypes, and this trend has accelerated dramatically with genomic data. For example, in the clinic, primary breast cancers have traditionally been classified by their expression status of hormone receptors into three subtypes: estrogen receptor (ER) positive or progesterone receptor (PR) positive, human epidermal growth factor receptor 2 (HER2) positive, and triple negative [5]. The result of the immunohistochemical (IHC) assays of these receptors can thus guide the selection of patients for different hormonal therapies or targeted therapies [6, 7]. The arrival of microarray-based gene expression data led to the division of breast cancers into five intrinsic molecular subtypes: luminal A, luminal B, HER2 overexpression, normal like, and basal like, and they showed notable differences in clinical outcome [8, 9]. More recently, analyses of copy number and gene expression data for several thousand malignant breast tumor samples revealed 10 molecular subtypes [10, 11]. Meanwhile, the triple-negative subtype was further divided [12, 13], and with a sample size of >10,000 and additional basal markers, Blow et al. [14] identified six IHC subtypes for breast cancer by splitting the basal group.

At least three factors contribute to the continued fracturing of cancer subtypes. First, increasingly larger sample cohorts are being used—they contain not only more phenotypic heterogeneity but also greater power to define and replicate rare subtypes. Second, simultaneous collection of diverse -omics data types, for aberrations in DNA, gene expression, epigenetic features, etc., tends to recognize additional "structures" in a given tumor series [15–17]. Third, intrinsic gene-gene correlations in the data, often unrelated to the disease itself, may create illusions of stable clusters with the use of some methods [18] even in cases where the structure is weak.

An ever finer classification system has many potential benefits. It is needed to capture the full spectrum of biological diversity—the "endless forms" that Darwin spoke of. It could lead to a better recognition of patient-specific disease mechanisms and, importantly, could suggest treatment options that are more accurately matched to the patient's tumor [2, 3]. Precision medicine, at its very foundation, relies on valid and constantly optimized disease classification that reflects the underlying mechanisms. However, a fine-grained classification system also has many potential drawbacks. The newly proposed splits may not be technically robust (see "Is the classification system robust?"). Even when the finer categories are robustly supported by statistical significance and by replication, they may still lack a clear biological meaning, or have little impact on treatment options ("Can classification capture intratumor heterogeneity and evolutionary progression?" and "Caveats in interpreting cancer subtypes" below) if it turns out that some subtypes share the same clinical endpoint, or if treatment options are limited.

Is the classification system robust?

Here, we delve into the issue of robustness: how can we tell if a classification scheme is more reliable than alternative systems? The value of any classification depends critically on its robustness. Without evaluating robustness, we face profound problems in downstream analyses, including integration across studies and clinical translation. For example, the reported number of subtypes for a certain cancer could differ between two studies, simply because one or neither study had strong evidence to formally distinguish K clusters from $(K - 1)$ or $(K + 1)$. Similarly, if the reported optimal K varies among DNA, mRNA, and methylation data, the discrepancy could either reflect a real biological distinction or be explained by trivial methodological differences or by the mere absence of a strong cluster signal.

Is there a p value?

In epidemiological or genetic association studies, evidence of credible association is measured by effect size and statistical significance, the latter being expressed by a p value and a hypothesis-testing procedure used to calculate it. For example, a DNA variant's additive effect on a continuous trait can be evaluated by linear regression. However, the task of classification cannot be easily cast into a hypothesis-testing framework: when declaring K clusters for a sample, is the null hypothesis "no cluster" or "$K - 1$ and $K + 1$ clusters"? While the confidence of *class assignment* can be assessed by cross-validation in test samples for which the class labels are already known, there is no well-established statistics to compare the performance of *class discovery*. In theory, one can quantify the degree of clustering by indices such as compactness, connectedness, separation [19], or silhouette width [20]; however, there is no universally accepted quantitative measure—a p value-like index—to report how likely the observed clusters could arise merely due to naturally occurring data "structure." Two types of structure are frequently encountered in high-dimensional molecular profiling data: that due to separations between groups, i.e., stratification, and that due to locally tight clusters, i.e., cryptic relatedness. These terms are borrowed from human population genetics studies, where both types of structure ultimately came from shared ancestry of sampled individuals at different time depths. Their impact on association tests can be monitored and corrected by well-established procedures [21, 22]. However, for gene expression or other functional genomics data (such as proteomic, metabolomic, epigenomic data), the information used in classification is sample-sample similarity in high-dimensional feature space, and the basis of co-ancestry is lacking, at least not self-evident. Indeed, how to evaluate competing algorithms or alternative results is an active topic of research [23]. Many groups have studied the issue of cluster validation and have proposed the use of either internal or external standards [24–26]. More often, however, there is no real dataset that can serve as a reliable external standard. Our recent analyses have shown that even the datasets that are said to contain well-separated clusters can have an uncertain number of clusters (i.e., the true K), thus making it difficult to use them as benchmarks for comparing class discovery methods [18]. As sample size increases, the number of clusters will increase and exhibit increasing apparent stability [18, 27]. Given this, we recommend the use of simulations to create fully transparent standard data, in which the number of clusters (K) and the degree of separation are known, and the gene-gene correlations can be introduced based on empirical data. Using such simulated data as a benchmark, we can systematically compare different clustering methods for their performance, especially their rate of over- and under-calling K over data that span a wide range of known K values and pre-specified degrees of cluster separation.

Quantitative reporting of the robustness of clustering results is often lacking in publications that propose new classification systems. Sometimes the data structure was *illustrated* by pre-selecting the best discriminating genes and showing how they could visually separate the reported clusters crisply. Although this form of presentation is well suited for annotation—showing which genes appeared in which group—it is not appropriate as a demonstration of cluster strength, because with many more genes than samples (i.e., the $p >> n$ situation), seemingly informative discriminators can always be found for any random partition, even for samples without clear groupings. When classification strength is not properly assessed, visual display of clusters using the best genes can inadvertently turn into an exaggerated inference, even if subsequent interpretations seem appealing [18].

Can classification capture intratumor heterogeneity and evolutionary progression?

Every living cancer inevitably changes its character in time and every solid tumor is spatially heterogeneous, yet most samples used in research so far are bulk tissue blocks collected as a single time point. Thus, most of today's cancer genomics data, by the very nature of sampling, provide a one-time view of a mixed pool of changeable cells. Standard cancer classifications are aimed at capturing *inter*tumor heterogeneity, while treating each tumor as homogeneous and unvarying. For a given cohort of patients, classifying their bulk tumor data is an attempt to find natural groupings among many mixed cell populations, while ignoring the within-population diversity and its variation in space and time. Not surprisingly, the cancer subtypes reported are often driven by, and therefore reflect, *intra*tumor heterogeneity and tumor evolution.

Spatial heterogeneity

With bulk tissue data, spatial heterogeneity is an unobserved property. If the sample consists of a limited number of clonal populations, the number and molecular features of these component populations can be potentially "deconvolved" computationally. As sequencing costs drop, spatial heterogeneity can be analyzed with increasing resolution: first by multi-region analysis of smaller sectors of the same tumor [28–30], ultimately by DNA or RNA sequencing of single cells [31, 32]. In multi-region analyses, a typical assumption is that individual regions are clonally "pure," and the results can be presented as such. However, it remains the rule rather than the exception that each region still contains a mixture of many cell types, albeit with presumed lower heterogeneity compared to the entire tumor [33]. Single-cell analysis provides the ultimate solution, as it describes the smallest unit of cancer heterogeneity and provides truly clonal data for use in classification. Single-cell studies have identified many more cell types than previously seen with bulk tissue analysis. For example, a single-cell RNAseq study of cortical tissues [34] has found nine major classes and 47 "molecularly distinct" subclasses of brain cells, significantly expanding the known cellular repertoire of the mammalian cortex. Due to the higher cost of single-cell analysis, bulk tissue samples will remain the predominant source of cancer genomics data for the foreseeable future, both in basic research and in real-time clinical testing. By sampling smaller and smaller "core" regions, the spatial heterogeneity can be reduced, but it cannot be fully removed. In this regard, the traditional, *hard* classification into disjoint categories is a poor fit for admixed samples, as they contain cancer cells carrying somatic mutations or aneuploid segments as well as surrounding normal-like cells that are euploid and carrying only germline mutations. Partial membership modeling has been proposed to address this scenario [35, 36], reminiscent of similar methods for ancestry inference using genotype data for individuals with mixed ancestry [37, 38]. Alternatively, phylogeny-based methods can be applied to explicitly account for the polyclonal nature of each regional sample in a multi-region dataset [39, 40].

Cancer life history and impact on classification

Classification of cancers can also be viewed as a task of cataloging evolutionary trajectories of complex genomes [41, 42]. Each cancer genome carries many variations, with a distribution of fitness effects as defined in a specific but changeable environment. Each tumor thus undergoes its own Darwinian evolution, with many intricate details that make it distinct from all other tumors [43]. However, our effort to classify them is predicated on the notion that convergent evolution does happen, such that a limited number of evolutionary paths are traveled repeatedly by tumors from different patients, leading to recognizable major hallmarks recurring in different tumors. The discovery of N subtypes of breast cancer, for example, detects N destinations of convergent evolution in this cancer type. But N needs not be a fixed parameter. For example, if the tissue has K cell types that could eventually turn to cancer cells, the precancerous cells have K starting points from which to explore the initial evolutionary paths, and multiple paths may merge or split during the life history of a cancer before congregating to one of N major types at the time of sampling. Metastasis and treatment response would further extend, diversify, or reshuffle the evolutionary trajectories [44, 45].

Current cancer classification systems can only reflect, but not accurately portray, this complex succession of events, as different tumors may be sampled at different stages along their own life histories. In a typical lifespan of a malignant tumor, some cells start acquiring oncogenic potential, showing increased proliferation, escaping apoptosis and immunosuppression, competing successfully for resources with other cells in the tissue niche, and harnessing the right combination of driver mutations with enough fitness gain to overcome the fitness burden incurred by the larger number of passenger mutations (for reviews of common hallmarks and pathways for cancer, see [46–48]). To become more "successful," the cancer needs to grow sufficiently large and clonally diverse before tissue turnover and, sometimes, to acquire migration and invasion properties that are essential for metastasis. It may also carry treatment-resistant subclones that can thrive after therapy. Viewed in this light, cancers are chronic diseases with changeable character, punctuated by rare episodes of acceleration, essentially slow-evolving populations that occasionally rush to a new, more successful endpoint. A given sample collection may have captured the tumors at different "stations" of their life history. For example, the mesenchymal subtype of glioblastoma multiforme (GBM) possesses the signature of macrophages/microglial infiltration [49, 50] and has a greater degree of mixing of aneuploid and euploid cells. More recently, Ozawa et al. reported that most non-GCIMP mesenchymal GBMs may evolve from another known subtype, a proneural-like precursor of GBM [51].

Caveats in interpreting cancer subtypes

In most cases, the task after class discovery is to explain the meaning of the found classes. Typical actions include the following: describe the involvement of known cancer-related genes as a way to report specific signaling pathways active in different subtypes; map the new class nomenclature to those of the previously established systems; assess differences in clinical outcome, e.g., survival time or treatment responsiveness; and dissect tissue-specific signatures or enrichment of previously curated gene clusters. In the following sections, we discuss three caveats in such interpretations. Both marker selection and analysis method have a strong impact on classification results and how the resulting classes can be explained. Further, the third factor affecting interpretation is the strength of clustering inherent in the dataset, which is not known until a specific collection of tumors has been assembled and analyzed.

Feature selection bias

We illustrate the importance of feature selection by first drawing analogies with population genetics studies, where DNA variation data can be used to (1) infer historical demography or (2) detect natural selection. These two tasks are related, but are also inherently different, even conflicting with each other, and relying on different features. Demographic inference tries to describe historical changes of population size and distribution, including migration, self-isolation, expansion, and admixture. The best genetic features for this task are "neutral" variations, those not under natural selection, or more accurately, those not likely to affect the Darwinian fitness of the individuals. Typical examples of such neutral markers are those found in intergenic regions of the genome. In contrast, the second task, inference of natural selection, relies on markers with a fitness effect, and they can be detected after specifying a null model of genetic drift, because demographic forces could have generated DNA variation patterns similar to those due to natural selection.

In cancer evolution, the concept of *driver* and *passenger* mutations are almost exact parallels of the *adaptive* (*positively selected*) and *neutral* variants recognized in population genetics [48, 52]. However, we rarely ask whether the emphasis of cancer classification is for understanding the tumors' past demography or their future evolution. The story of the cancer's past is shaped by the drivers but may be best recorded by the passengers, and the drivers in the past may not experience the forces of selection acting in the future. The type of features selected for use in classification will therefore directly affect the downstream interpretation. For example, if the analysis of gene expression data pre-selects transcripts that correlate with survival time, these markers, by being most informative for future outcome, are likely to reveal tumor subtypes that differ in outcome, and this in turn will lead to the interpretation that the subtypes thus discovered have a stronger prognostic/predictive value than classes discovered using other features. Alternatively, if the selected transcripts correspond to cell type or pathway-specific genes, the resulting classes will likely exhibit differential loading of pathway or source cell signals and make it easy to map the discovered classes to biological mechanisms. Even the presumably "unbiased" choice of selecting the most variable genes may have inadvertently loaded the interpretation towards the most dynamic or most strongly co-expressed pathways, such as those for stress response or immune cell infiltration.

Hidden assumptions in choosing a clustering method

Unsupervised clustering is the basic tool for ab initio class discovery. The term "unsupervised" refers to statistical inference of data structure without relying on existing knowledge of sample labels. However, "unsupervised" does not mean assumption-free. Some important assumptions have always been made, sometimes unknowingly, in marker selection, data processing (such as how to treat outliers and how to deal with batch effects), and the choice of the clustering method. This methodological choice is already based on an implied data-generating model, i.e., what type of biological heterogeneity could have produced the observed data structure. If we assume that the objects—different tumor samples—arise from distinct, non-overlapping causes, methods for finding disjoint taxonomy, such as *k*-means clustering, are appropriate. If, alternatively, we see each tumor sample as a mixed population of cells comprising a small number of canonical clones, a mixed membership model is more powerful [35, 36, 53], as has been routinely applied in studies of human population diversity involving individuals of mixed ancestry [37]. The number of co-existing clones and the rate of clonal replacement depend on population size, mutation rate, and the distribution of fitness effects of the new mutations. If the task is to classify cells in a single evolving population with major branches, it would be best to capture the lineage relationship by using hierarchical clustering—akin to the coalescence analysis in classic population genetics [54]—aiming to identify hierarchical classes to reflect their shared ancestry as the historical truth. When using simulated data to compare methods such as *k*-means clustering or hierarchical clustering, the data-generating model will usually dictate the winner: the method that matches the model will fit the simulated data best.

Inherent intensity of data structure

Perhaps it is worth reiterating that when the clustering signal is strong, most methods will perform well and they will be in good agreement. Conversely, when the data structure is subtle, slight differences in sampling, data processing, feature selection, or the choice of method will yield highly discordant results, and it is difficult to tell which method is better. A recent example of a strong clustering signal is from a joint analysis of 3527 specimens of 12 cancer types by the Cancer Genome Atlas (TCGA) Research Network [16]. Most identified classes follow the cancer's known organ of origin, undoubtedly due to the distinct cell types found in different tissues. This result is as expected, because it affirms the earliest insight that cancer cells are transformed normal cells rather than entirely "foreign" cells (as is the case in bacterial infection). As cells are "canalized" during differentiation, a tumor occurs in one of

Waddington's valleys and bears its local hallmark. Speaking in more modern terms, the malignant transformation, although a radical step in the adaptive evolution of the cancer cells, usually could not have erased their tissue-of-origin signature inherited from prior differentiation. This identity, perhaps coded in the epigenomes of the fate-committed cells, remains the most noticeable molecular character in matured organs despite subsequent oncogenesis. Meanwhile, this study also revealed remarkable examples of cross-tissue subtypes [16], e.g., squamous-like lung, head and neck, and bladder cancers that are more similar to each other than other cancers from the same organ, and they appear to have overcome the ontological divergence of the source tissues. Is this because convergent evolution—newly acquired oncogenic characters overwriting history, or shared lineage—the same group of differentiated cells "seeded" into two different body sites? Either scenario would be immensely interesting. In principle, it is entirely possible that the same pathways are activated in different cell types as the oncogenic driver and manifest as the same subtype. Such cross-tissue classification is at the forefront of pan-cancer analysis today, made possible by the availability of multi-cancer datasets collected under uniform technical conditions. With such data, we are entering the best time to study population genetics of somatic cells. This discipline will stimulate new theoretic work on the evolution of non-recombining populations, will produce patterns that can be contrasted with experimental evolution of microbial systems, and will provide increasingly strong knowledge support for the practice of precision oncology.

Can multiple classification schemes co-exist?

Traditional classification methods rely on organ type, appearance, and histological markers. Multiple systems, such as tumor grade and stage, have co-existed for decades. In recent years, the arrival of high-throughput molecular studies has rapidly increased the number of competing systems. For example, the analyses of human breast tumors by the TCGA [55] produced multiple answers to the "how many subtypes" question for the same sample series. It found that breast tumors' gene expression data supported 13 classes with the use of a consensus cluster-based method, 12 classes with a second method, and five classes with the semi-supervised PAM50 method [56]. The concordance rate among the three results was modest, as the best-matched classes between any two methods only account for 50–60 % of the samples (our unpublished observation). Further, the study found seven breast tumor subtypes from microRNA data, five subtypes from methylation data, and five subtypes from copy number alterations, again with poor to modest agreement (per our analysis). While the classification solutions were described as "correlated" across data types, their differences impacted a large fraction of the samples, making it difficult to find a straight answer to the simple question: how many subtypes are there for breast cancer? To integrate such complex data requires a quantitative assessment of clustering strength within each data type and a system to truly integrate the solutions rather than recounting them side-by-side. Multiple methods have been developed to meet this growing need [57–60].

When the same data type lead to two or more different classifications by the use of different methods, it becomes a methodological imperative to arrive at a consensus: there is no sound reason for multiple "truths" within the same raw data. However, across different genomic data types, it is less clear that there must be a single unifying classification. In the example of TCGA breast tumor study mentioned above, it may not be possible, or necessary, to forge a single classification by reconciling the observed groupings across all omics layers. If we assume that biological information flows from DNA to epigenetic marks, then RNA, and then to proteins, if the cells commit to its differentiated fate primarily using epigenetic codes yet react to short-term needs by gene expression adaptation, further, if the cells interact with their microenvironment chiefly through variations of metabolites, it is conceivable that different levels of biology coalesce to different grouping patterns, and the same sample could truly belong to different groups depending on the level of inquiry. We think it remains an open question whether different layers of genomic data signify different archetypes of cellular states and could lead to different but equally valid classification systems. To test such a multi-layered classification would require very large datasets that can validate the class-to-class mapping across layers.

Conclusions

Cancer classification is both a scientific technique and a living art, to be performed for each dataset with individualized care. Classification results are widely used and form the foundational knowledge for both basic and translational oncology. In this review, we outlined five contemporary challenges at the interface of computational data mining, biological understanding, and clinical utility. To classify late-stage tumors is to engage in probabilistic cataloging and reverse storytelling, not unlike other observational sciences such as archeology or anthropology. The arrival of genomic data has dramatically increased the power to peer into the past, but even now, in the midst of the excitement of many new opportunities, it is useful to keep in mind that sometimes the sample series at hand may not be sufficient to support the full ambition of fine-grained classification or to trace the entire evolutionary trajectories. Whether intratumor heterogeneity is so strong as to destabilize intertumor classification, and whether a newly observed cluster represents a robust, recurrent, and meaningful subtype, ultimately need to be settled by empirical data for each major tumor type. The usefulness of classification ultimately rests on increased prognostic power or more precisely targeted therapies. Assessing and communicating the strength of data, in quantitative terms whenever possible, is essential for the long-term management of predictive uncertainty and for the successful application of genomics in patient care.

Competing interests

The authors declare that they have no competing interests.

Authors' contributions

QS and JZL conceived the article and took the lead in writing the initial draft. All authors contributed to the research discussed in the article. All authors have read and approved the manuscript.

Acknowledgements

QS is supported by funding from the Joint Institute for Translational and Clinical Research of the University of Michigan Health System and Peking University Health Sciences Center. SDM is supported by the Breast Cancer Research Foundation and the Metavivor Foundation. JZL is supported by general funds of the Department of Human Genetics and the Department of Computational Medicine and Bioinformatics of the University of Michigan. We thank two anonymous reviewers for their insightful comments.

Author details

[1]Department of Human Genetics, University of Michigan, Ann Arbor, MI, USA. [2]Department of Internal Medicine and Epidemiology, University of Michigan, 5789A Medical Science II, Box 5618, Ann Arbor, MI 48109-5618, USA.

References

1. McKusick VA. On lumpers and splitters, or the nosology of genetic disease. Perspect Biol Med. 1969;12(2):298–312.
2. Weitzel JN, Blazer KR, MacDonald DJ, Culver JO, Offit K. Genetics, genomics, and cancer risk assessment: state of the art and future directions in the era of personalized medicine. CA Cancer J Clin. 2011;61(5):327–59.
3. Levy MA, Lovly CM, Pao W. Translating genomic information into clinical medicine: lung cancer as a paradigm. Genome Res. 2012;22(11):2101–8.
4. Louis DN, Ohgaki H, Wiestler OD, Cavenee WK, Burger PC, Jouvet A, et al. The 2007 WHO classification of tumours of the central nervous system. Acta Neuropathol. 2007;114(2):97–109.
5. Prat A, Perou CM. Deconstructing the molecular portraits of breast cancer. Mol Oncol. 2011;5(1):5–23.
6. Morrison DH, Rahardja D, King E, Peng Y, Sarode VR. Tumour biomarker expression relative to age and molecular subtypes of invasive breast cancer. Br J Cancer. 2012;107(2):382–7.
7. Caudle AS, Yu TK, Tucker SL, Bedrosian I, Litton JK, Gonzalez-Angulo AM, et al. Local-regional control according to surrogate markers of breast cancer subtypes and response to neoadjuvant chemotherapy in breast cancer patients undergoing breast conserving therapy. Breast Cancer Res. 2012;14(3):R83.
8. Perou CM, Sorlie T, Eisen MB, van de Rijn M, Jeffrey SS, Rees CA, et al. Molecular portraits of human breast tumours. Nature. 2000;406(6797):747–52.
9. Sorlie T, Tibshirani R, Parker J, Hastie T, Marron JS, Nobel A, et al. Repeated observation of breast tumor subtypes in independent gene expression data sets. Proc Natl Acad Sci U S A. 2003;100(14):8418–23.
10. Need AC, McEvoy JP, Gennarelli M, Heinzen EL, Ge D, Maia JM, et al. Exome sequencing followed by large-scale genotyping suggests a limited role for moderately rare risk factors of strong effect in schizophrenia. Am J Hum Genet. 2012;91(2):303–12.
11. Ali HR, Rueda OM, Chin SF, Curtis C, Dunning MJ, Aparicio SA, et al. Genome-driven integrated classification of breast cancer validated in over 7,500 samples. Genome Biol. 2014;15(8):431.
12. Prat A, Parker J, Karginova O, Fan C, Livasy C, Herschkowitz J, et al. Phenotypic and molecular characterization of the claudin-low intrinsic subtype of breast cancer. Breast Cancer Res. 2010;12(5):R68.
13. Lehmann BD, Bauer JA, Chen X, Sanders ME, Chakravarthy AB, Shyr Y, et al. Identification of human triple-negative breast cancer subtypes and preclinical models for selection of targeted therapies. J Clin Invest. 2011;121(7):2750–67.
14. Blows FM, Driver KE, Schmidt MK, Broeks A, van Leeuwen FE, Wesseling J, et al. Subtyping of breast cancer by immunohistochemistry to investigate a relationship between subtype and short and long term survival: a collaborative analysis of data for 10,159 cases from 12 studies. PLoS Med. 2010,7(5).e1000279.
15. Heim D, Budczies J, Stenzinger A, Treue D, Hufnagl P, Denkert C, et al. Cancer beyond organ and tissue specificity: next-generation-sequencing gene mutation data reveal complex genetic similarities across major cancers. Int J Cancer. 2014;135(10):2362–9.
16. Hoadley KA, Yau C, Wolf DM, Cherniack AD, Tamborero D, Ng S, et al. Multiplatform analysis of 12 cancer types reveals molecular classification within and across tissues of origin. Cell. 2014;158(4):929–44.
17. Russnes HG, Vollan HK, Lingjaerde OC, Krasnitz A, Lundin P, Naume B, et al. Genomic architecture characterizes tumor progression paths and fate in breast cancer patients. Sci Transl Med. 2010;2(38):38ra47.
18. Şenbabaoğlu Y, Michailidis G, Li JZ. Critical limitations of consensus clustering in class discovery. Sci Rep. 2014;4:6207.
19. Handl J, Knowles J, Kell DB. Computational cluster validation in post-genomic data analysis. Bioinformatics. 2005;21(15):3201–12.
20. Rousseeuw PJ. Silhouettes—a graphical aid to the interpretation and validation of cluster-analysis. J Comput Appl Math. 1987;20:53–65.
21. Price AL, Patterson NJ, Plenge RM, Weinblatt ME, Shadick NA, Reich D. Principal components analysis corrects for stratification in genome-wide association studies. Nat Genet. 2006;38(8):904–9.
22. Kang HM, Sul JH, Service SK, Zaitlen NA, Kong SY, Freimer NB, et al. Variance component model to account for sample structure in genome-wide association studies. Nat Genet. 2010;42(4):348–54.
23. Hand DJ. Classifier technology and the illusion of progress. Stat Sci. 2006;21(1):1–15.
24. Kleinberg J. An impossibility theorem for clustering. Adv Neural Inf Process Syst. 2002. http://papers.nips.cc/paper/2340-an-impossibility-theorem-forclustering. Accessed on 08 July 2014.
25. Lange T, Roth V, Braun ML, Buhmann JM. Stability-based validation of clustering solutions. Neural Comput. 2004;16(6):1299–323.
26. de Souto MC, Costa IG, de Araujo DS, Ludermir TB, Schliep A. Clustering cancer gene expression data: a comparative study. BMC Bioinformatics. 2008;9:497.
27. Ben-David S, von Luxburg U, Pal D. A sober look at clustering stability. In: Learning theory: lecture notes in computer science, vol. 4005. Berlin: Springer; 2006. p. 5–19.
28. de Bruin EC, McGranahan N, Mitter R, Salm M, Wedge DC, Yates L, et al. Spatial and temporal diversity in genomic instability processes defines lung cancer evolution. Science. 2014;346(6206):251–6.
29. Gerlinger M, Horswell S, Larkin J, Rowan AJ, Salm MP, Varela I, et al. Genomic architecture and evolution of clear cell renal cell carcinomas defined by multiregion sequencing. Nat Genet. 2014;46(3):225–33.
30. Zhang J, Fujimoto J, Zhang J, Wedge DC, Song X, Zhang J, et al. Intratumor heterogeneity in localized lung adenocarcinomas delineated by multiregion sequencing. Science. 2014;346(6206):256–9.
31. Wang Y, Waters J, Leung ML, Unruh A, Roh W, Shi X, et al. Clonal evolution in breast cancer revealed by single nucleus genome sequencing. Nature. 2014;512(7513):155–60.
32. Ting DT, Wittner BS, Ligorio M, Vincent Jordan N, Shah AM, Miyamoto DT, et al. Single-cell RNA sequencing identifies extracellular matrix gene expression by pancreatic circulating tumor cells. Cell reports. 2014;8(6):1905–18.
33. Polyak K. Heterogeneity in breast cancer. J Clin Invest. 2011;121(10):3786–8.
34. Zeisel A, Munoz-Manchado AB, Codeluppi S, Lonnerberg P, La Manno G, Jureus A, et al. Brain structure. Cell types in the mouse cortex and hippocampus revealed by single-cell RNA-seq. Science. 2015;347(6226):1138–42.
35. Oesper L, Mahmoody A, Raphael BJ. THetA: inferring intra-tumor heterogeneity from high-throughput DNA sequencing data. Genome Biol. 2013;14(7):R80.

36. Roth A, Khattra J, Yap D, Wan A, Laks E, Biele J, et al. PyClone: statistical inference of clonal population structure in cancer. Nat Methods. 2014;11(4):396–8.
37. Pritchard JK, Stephens M, Donnelly P. Inference of population structure using multilocus genotype data. Genetics. 2000;155(2):945–59.
38. Bryc K, Auton A, Nelson MR, Oksenberg JR, Hauser SL, Williams S, et al. Genome-wide patterns of population structure and admixture in West Africans and African Americans. Proc Natl Acad Sci U S A. 2010;107(2):786–91.
39. Hong WS, Shpak M, Townsend JP. Inferring the origin of metastases from cancer phylogenies. Cancer Res. 2015;75:4021–5.
40. Niknafs N, Beleva-Guthrie V, Naiman DQ, Karchin R. Subclonal hierarchy inference from somatic mutations: automatic reconstruction of cancer evolutionary trees from multi-region next generation sequencing. PLoS computational biology 2015;11(10):e1004416.
41. Greaves M, Maley CC. Clonal evolution in cancer. Nature. 2012;481(7381):306–13.
42. Burrell RA, McGranahan N, Bartek J, Swanton C. The causes and consequences of genetic heterogeneity in cancer evolution. Nature. 2013;501(7467):338–45.
43. Ogino S, Fuchs CS, Giovannucci E. How many molecular subtypes? Implications of the unique tumor principle in personalized medicine. Expert Rev Mol Diagn. 2012;12(6):621–8.
44. Ding L, Ellis MJ, Li S, Larson DE, Chen K, Wallis JW, et al. Genome remodelling in a basal-like breast cancer metastasis and xenograft. Nature. 2010;464(7291):999–1005.
45. Ding L, Ley TJ, Larson DE, Miller CA, Koboldt DC, Welch JS, et al. Clonal evolution in relapsed acute myeloid leukaemia revealed by whole-genome sequencing. Nature. 2012;481(7382):506–10.
46. Hanahan D, Weinberg RA. Hallmarks of cancer: the next generation. Cell. 2011;144(5):646–74.
47. Greaves M. Evolutionary determinants of cancer. Cancer Discov. 2015;5(8):806–20.
48. Vogelstein B, Papadopoulos N, Velculescu VE, Zhou S, Diaz Jr LA, Kinzler KW. Cancer genome landscapes. Science. 2013;339(6127):1546–58.
49. Li B, Senbabaoglu Y, Peng W, Yang M-I, Xu J, Li JZ. Genomic estimates of aneuploid content in glioblastoma multiforme and improved classification. Clin Cancer Res. 2012;18(20):5595–605.
50. Bhat KP, Balasubramaniyan V, Vaillant B, Ezhilarasan R, Hummelink K, Hollingsworth F, et al. Mesenchymal differentiation mediated by NF-kappaB promotes radiation resistance in glioblastoma. Cancer Cell. 2013;24(3):331–46.
51. Ozawa T, Riester M, Cheng YK, Huse JT, Squatrito M, Helmy K, et al. Most human non-GCIMP glioblastoma subtypes evolve from a common proneural-like precursor glioma. Cancer Cell. 2014;26(2):288–300.
52. Holderegger R, Kamm U, Gugerli F. Adaptive vs. neutral genetic diversity: implications for landscape genetics. Landscape Ecol. 2006;21(6):797–807.
53. Miller CA, White BS, Dees ND, Griffith M, Welch JS, Griffith OL, et al. SciClone: inferring clonal architecture and tracking the spatial and temporal patterns of tumor evolution. PLoS Comput Biol. 2014;10(8):e1003665.
54. Bouaziz M, Paccard C, Guedj M, Ambroise C. SHIPS: spectral hierarchical clustering for the inference of population structure in genetic studies. PLoS One. 2012;7(10):e45685.
55. TCGA. Comprehensive molecular portraits of human breast tumours. Nature. 2012;490(7418):61–70.
56. Parker JS, Mullins M, Cheang MCU, Leung S, Voduc D, Vickery T, et al. Supervised risk predictor of breast cancer based on intrinsic subtypes. J Clin Oncol. 2009;27(8):1160–7.
57. Kirk P, Griffin JE, Savage RS, Ghahramani Z, Wild DL. Bayesian correlated clustering to integrate multiple datasets. Bioinformatics. 2012;28(24):3290–7.
58. Lock EF, Hoadley KA, Marron JS, Nobel AB. Joint and individual variation explained (JIVE) for integrated analysis of multiple data types. Ann Appl Stat. 2013;7(1):523–42.
59. Shen R, Wang S, Mo Q. Sparse integrative clustering of multiple omics data sets. Ann Appl Stat. 2013;7(1):269–94.
60. Wang B, Mezlini AM, Demir F, Fiume M, Tu Z, Brudno M, et al. Similarity network fusion for aggregating data types on a genomic scale. Nat Methods. 2014;11(3):333–7.

8

Integrative genomic analysis reveals functional diversification of APOBEC gene family in breast cancer

Yanfeng Zhang[1,2], Ryan Delahanty[1], Xingyi Guo[1], Wei Zheng[1] and Jirong Long[1*]

Abstract

Background: The human APOBEC protein family plays critical but distinct roles in host defense. Recent studies revealed that APOBECs mediate C-to-T mutagenesis in multiple cancers, including breast cancer. It is still unclear whether APOBEC gene family shows functional diversification involved in cancer mutagenesis.

Results: We performed an integrated analysis to characterize the functional diversification of APOBEC gene family associated with breast cancer mutagenesis relative to estrogen receptor (ER) status. Among the APOBEC family, we found that both *APOBEC3B* and *APOBEC3C* mRNA levels were significantly higher in estrogen receptor negative (ER–) subtype compared with estrogen receptor positive (ER+) subtype ($P < 2.2 \times 10^{-16}$ and $P < 3.1 \times 10^{-5}$, respectively). Epigenomic data further reflected the distinct chromatin states of *APOBEC3B* and *APOBEC3C* relative to ER status. Notably, we observed the significantly positive correlation between the APOBEC3B-mediated mutagenesis and *APOBEC3B* expression levels in ER+ cancers but not in ER– cancers. In contrast, we discovered the negative correlation of *APOBEC3C* mRNA levels with base-substitution mutations in ER– tumors. Meanwhile, we observed that breast cancers in carriers of germline deletion of *APOBEC3B* gene harbor similar mutation patterns, but higher mutation rates in the TCW motif (W corresponds to A or T) than cancers in non-carriers, indicating additional factors may also induce carcinogenic mutagenesis.

Conclusions: These results suggest that functional potential of APOBEC3B and APOBEC3C involved in cancer mutagenesis is associated with ER status.

Keywords: APOBEC family, Estrogen receptor, Breast cancer, Methylation, Mutagenesis, Chromatin state

Background

In the human genome, APOBEC family comprises of a total of 11 genes. They have been known to encode Zn^{2+}-dependent DNA cytosine deaminases. Of these 11 members, seven apolipoprotein B mRNA editing enzyme, catalytic polypeptide-like 3 genes (*APOBEC3A, APOBEC3B, APOBEC3C, APOBEC3D, APOBEC3F, APOB EC3G*, and *APOBEC3H*) are tandemly distributed on chromosome 22 [1]. The other four members are located on other chromosomes, including *APOBEC1*, *APOBEC2*, *APOBEC4*, and activation-induced cytidine deaminase (*AICDA*). The APOBEC family proteins show different classes of DNA cytosine deaminase domains and distinct tissue expression profiles [2–5], indicating they may have diverse biological functions. For example, the APOBEC proteins exhibit different activities in restricting virus replication and inhibiting LINE-1 retrotransposition [6–8].

Recent studies showed the elevated expression of *APOBEC3B* in multiple tumors [9–12]. Meanwhile, the strong correlation of somatic base-substitution mutation with *APOBEC3B* mRNA levels in cancer samples has implicated APOBEC3B as an enzymatic source inducing the C-to-T somatic mutations [9, 10, 13, 14]. However, in breast cancer subtypes, the distinct mutational patterns and genomic changes have also been reported [15–18], meaning that the APOBEC-mediated mutagenesis and APOBEC family expression may be variable in cancer subtypes [14].

Thanks to two projects, The Cancer Genome Atlas (TCGA) [17] and the Encyclopedia of DNA Elements

* Correspondence: jirong.long@vanderbilt.edu
[1]Division of Epidemiology, Department of Medicine, Vanderbilt University Medical Center, Nashville 37203, USA
Full list of author information is available at the end of the article

(ENCODE) project [19], leveraging these diverse types of data to interpret functional features of genes or gene families in particular cancer types is possible. Here, we performed integrated analysis on diverse high-throughput sequencing data involved in somatic mutation, gene expression, and epigenetic profiles. The aim of this study is to investigate the functional diversification of the APOBEC family genes in breast cancer, in cancer subtypes with a focus on estrogen receptor (ER) status.

Results

Data summary

For breast cell lines, a total of 42 high-throughput sequencing data, including 10 RNA sequencing (RNA-seq) data from two data sets [20, 21], 18 ChIP sequencing (ChIP-seq) data, 4 corresponding input DNA (control) from five data sets, and 10 bisulfite sequencing (BS-seq) data from two data sets [19–22], were collected in this study (Additional file 1: Table S1). Among ten RNA-seq data, eight are from breast cancer cell lines and two are from normal breast cell lines.

Of the 18 ChIP-seq datasets, six histone modifications, including histone H3 lysine 4 methylations (H3K4me1, H3K4me3), lysine 9 trimethylation (H3K9me3), lysine 27 trimethylation (H3K27me3), lysine 36 trimethylation (H3K36me3), and histone H3 lysine 27 acetylations (H3K27ac), were conducted in each of the HCC1954 cell line, an estrogen receptor negative (ER−) breast cancer cell line, MCF-7 cell line, an estrogen receptor positive (ER+) breast cancer cell line, and human mammary epithelial cells (HMEC), a normal breast cell line.

For the ten bisulfite-seq datasets, two included whole-genome BS-seq at the single nucleotide resolution in the ER− breast cancer cell line HCC1954 and the normal cell line HMEC [20]. Eight were generated by reduced representation bisulfite sequencing (RRBS) in low depth [21]. As no or low sequencing coverage in the proximal promoters of APOBECs in the initial analysis, we discarded these eight RRBS data for further analyses.

RNA-seq data was available for 1000 breast tissue specimens from TCGA database, including 915 breast carcinoma samples and 85 adjacent normal breast tissues (Table 1). Among 915 breast tumor samples, 664, 196, and 55 are from breast tumor patients with ER+, ER−, and unknown ER status, respectively.

Expression profiling of APOBECs in breast cancer

We quantified mRNA levels for each of the 11 APOBEC family members in ten breast cell lines including cancer and normal cell types (Additional file 1: Table S2). Consistent with the previous findings [9], only *APOBEC3B* shows the over-expression in the range of two- to four-fold changes in breast cancer cells relative to normal cells. Other APOBEC family members have no or very low expression levels in normal or cancer cells with an exception of *APOBEC3C*, whose expression levels are highest in normal cells and decline slightly in the ER− cancer cell lines, but drop sharply in the ER+ cancer cell lines (Fig. 1a). Relative to ER− cancer cell lines, these results show the down-regulation of both the *APOBEC3B* and *APOBEC3C* genes in ER+ cancer cells.

We then expanded this analysis to include a total of 1000 RNA-seq data from TCGA project. In agreement with observation in cancer cell lines, both the *APOBEC3B* and *APOBEC3C* genes show higher expression levels in ER− cancers ($P < 2.2 \times 10^{-16}$ and $P < 3.1 \times 10^{-5}$, respectively, two-sided Wilcoxon rank sum test) relative to ER+ cancers (Fig. 1b). For other APOBEC family members (Additional file 2: Figure S1), they show either extremely low (median log2-transformed RPKM < 0)

Table 1 Summary of breast cell lines and tissue specimens in the study

	Breast non-tumor cell lines	Breast cancer cell lines	Breast tumor tissues	Adjacent normal breast tissues
No. of samples	2	8	915	85
ER status				
ER+	0	4 (50 %)	664 (72.6 %)	67 (78.9 %)
ER−	2 (100 %)	4 (50 %)	196 (21.4 %)	15 (17.6 %)
Unknown	0	0	55 (6.0 %)	3 (3.5 %)
CNV				
CN0	na	na	28 (3.1 %)	2 (2.4 %)
CN1	na	na	162 (17.7 %)	17 (20 %)
CN2	na	na	597 (65.2 %)	66 (77.6 %)
Unknown	na	na	128 (14.0 %)	0
Availablity of exome-seq data				
Yes	na	na	750 (82.0 %)	na
No	na	na	165 (18.0 %)	na

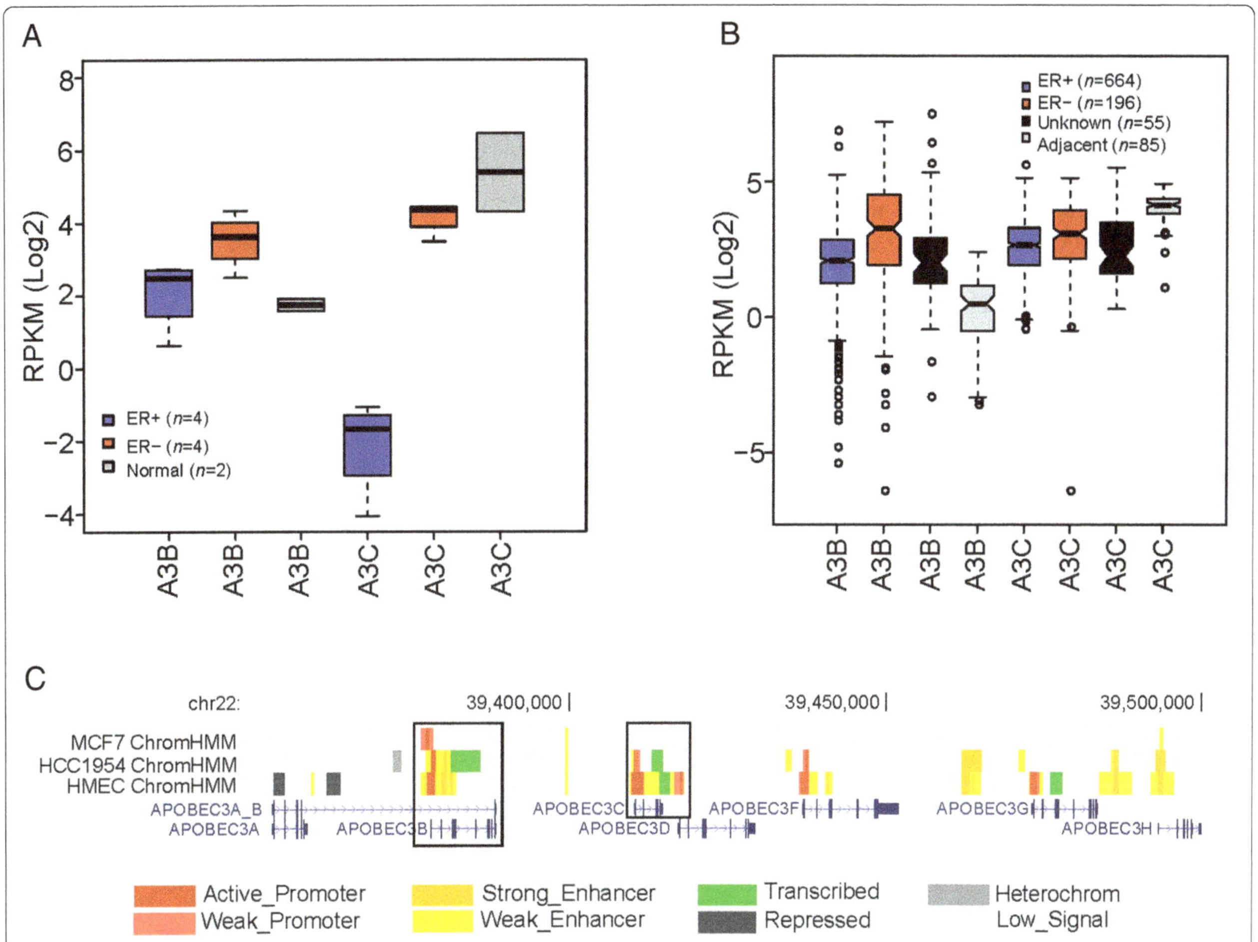

Fig. 1 Expression of *APOBEC3B* and *APOBEC3C* genes in breast cancer cell lines and tissues in relation to ER status. **a** mRNA levels of *APOBEC3B* and *APOBEC3C* in breast cancer cell lines with ER subtypes and normal cell lines. **b** mRNA levels of *APOBEC3B* and *APOBEC3C* in breast tumor tissues with ER subtypes and adjacent normal tissues. **c** Comparison of chromatin states in APOBEC3 family genes in ER+ (MCF-7), ER− (HCC1954) breast cancer cells, and normal cells (HMEC). The highlight with rectangle is on *APOBEC3B* and *APOBEC3C* genes. Chromatin states characterized by the ChromHMM algorithm are represented by different colors shown in the *bottom*

mRNA levels (including *APOBEC3A*, *APOBEC3H*, *APOBEC1*, *APOBEC2*, *APOBEC4*, and *AICDA*), or no obvious expression differences between ER+ and ER− breast cancers (including *APOBEC3D*, *APOBEC3F*, and *APOBEC3G*). Additionally, the expression levels of APOBEC family genes in 55 breast cancer tissues with unknown ER status are similar with those samples of ER+ subtypes, indicating many of these 55 patients probably belong to ER+ subtype. These results together indicate that the expression patterns of *APOBEC3B* and *APOBEC3C* genes may be associated with ER status.

Chromatin states of APOBEC gene family in breast cancer cells

To investigate whether the different expression profiles of APOBEC family members could show different chromatin states in relation to ER status, we integrated ChIP-seq data for six histone modifications, including H3K4me3 and H3K36me3 (two epigenetic markers connected with gene activity) [23, 24], H3K27ac and H3K4me1 (two enhancer-associated hallmarks) [25, 26], and H3K9me3 and H3K27me3 (two typical epigenetic markers indicative of transcriptional repression and heterochromatin formation) [23, 27], across three breast tissue relevant cell types: ER+ (MCF-7), ER− (HCC1954) breast cancer cells, and normal mammary epithelial cells (HMEC). Notably, in the ER− cell line HCC1954, we observed active promoter and clustered enhancers surrounding both the *APOBEC3B* and *APOBEC3C* loci (Fig. 1c). Meanwhile, these two genes show strong transcription signal. In addition, parts of active promoters or enhancers at the *APOBEC3F* and *APOBEC3G* genes were also found. For the other APOBEC family genes, we did not observe active promoter or enhancers (Additional file 2: Figure S2).

In contrast, in the ER+ cancer cell line MCF-7, we only observed promoter (Fig. 1c) activity at the *APOBEC3B*, but not at the *APOBEC3C* and the other APOBEC family genes (Additional file 2: Figure S2). Furthermore, compared with the normal HMECs, the loss of promoter activity at the *APOBEC3C*, *APOBEC3F*, and *APOBEC3G* genes was specifically detected in the ER+ cancer cell (Fig. 1c). The observed chromatin state profiles of the APOBEC family genes are quite concordant with the gene expression patterns, further suggesting that the functional divergence of the *APOBEC3B* and *APOBEC3C* genes may be related to the ER status.

In addition, with respect to several APOBEC family members (including *APOBEC3A*, *APOBEC3H*, *APOBEC1*, *APOBEC2*, *APOBEC4*, and *AICDA*) showing no or extremely low expression levels in both ER+ and ER− breast cancers, we did not find any enrichment of repressive chromatin modifications (H3K9me3 and H3K27me3) in these genes (Fig. 1c and Additional file 2: Figure S2), suggesting some additional molecular mechanisms probably participate in the regulation of these genes.

DNA methylation of APOBECs in breast cancer cells

DNA methylation at the proximal promoter of genes is well-characterized as an epigenetically repressive marker [28, 29]. We further analyzed the DNA methylation profiles of APOBECs using BS-seq data to detect methylation signatures. Due to unavailability of whole-genome BS-seq data for ER+ cancer cells, we could not conduct the comparative DNA methylation analysis between ER+ and ER− cancer cells. Here, we only compared the DNA methylation levels of APOBECs between the ER− breast cancer cells and normal cells (Fig. 2a, b). As expected, highly expressed genes possess low DNA methylation levels in their proximal transcription start site (TSS) regions (defined as ± 0.5 kb of TSS). For example, *APOBEC3B* and *APOBEC3C* show low DNA methylation levels (median methylation ratio ≤20 %) in both HMEC and ER− breast cancer cells, although a slight increase in ER− cancer cells (Fig. 2c). While for other APOBEC members, including *APOBEC3D*, *APOBEC3F*, and *APOBEC3G*, they show DNA hyper-methylation in ER− breast cancer cells when compared to HMEC ($P < 0.01$, Wilcoxon signed rank test). In addition, except the *APOBEC3H* gene, we found high DNA methylation levels of the remaining APOBEC members, including *APOBEC1*, *APOBEC2*, *APOBEC3A*, *APOBEC4*, and *AICDA*, in both HMEC and ER− breast cancer cells (Fig. 2c). Together, these findings are in agreement with the observation from the gene expression data.

Clinical outcome with mRNA levels of APOBECs

We then assessed whether the mRNA levels of both *APOBEC3B* and *APOBEC3C* genes were associated with clinical outcome. Compared to patients who are deceased, surviving patients show lower expression levels of *APOBEC3B* and higher expression levels of *APOBEC3C* (Fig. 3a). Meanwhile, a similar trend was observed for TNM stage, with higher *APOBEC3B* (Fig. 3b) and lower *APOBEC3C* (Fig. 3c) mRNA level associated with advanced breast cancer stage. However, no association was observed between the *APOBEC3B* and *APOBEC3C* mRNA levels with survival times (Additional file 2: Figure S3).

APOBEC-mediated mutagenesis in relation to ER status

We examined whether the correlation between APOBEC-mediated mutagenesis and expression levels of APOBEC family genes would be associated with ER status. A total of 46,096 somatic single nucleotide variants (SNVs) (57.9 ± 50.9, mean ± SD, Additional file 2: Figure S4A) from 750 exome-sequencing (exome-seq) data and matched RNA-seq data were combined to conduct such test. Among these somatic SNVs, 21,339 are C>T/G>A mutations (27.1 ± 24.8, mean ± SD, Additional file 2: Figure S4B). Interestingly, the significantly positive correlation between the number of C>T/G>A mutations per tumor exome and *APOBEC3B* mRNA levels is observed in ER+ cancers ($\rho = 0.32$, $P = 7.09 \times 10^{-15}$), but not in ER− cancers ($\rho = 0.04$, $P = 0.60$, Fig. 4a). Locally weighted polynomial regression also shows a similar trend. Conversely, we found a significantly negative correlation between the total number of C>T/G>A mutations per tumor exome and *APOBEC3C* mRNA levels in ER− cancers ($\rho = -0.26$, $P = 0.001$), which is also supported by the locally weighted regression (Fig. 4b). However, the negative correlation for *APOBEC3C* is not obvious in ER+ cancers. Similar observations exist for both *APOBEC3B* and *APOBEC3C* when including all somatic mutations (Additional file 2: Figure S5).

APOBEC-mediated mutagenesis in relation to germline deletion of *APOBEC3B*

In the analysis of the CNV status of *APOBEC3B* [30] in 787 breast tumor samples, we detected 190 breast cancer samples in carriers of germline deletion of *APOBEC3B* gene. Among them, 28 (75 % being ER+) and 162 (80 % being ER+) samples bear homozygous (zero copy, CN0) and heterozygous (one copy, CN1) deletions, respectively. Among the CN2 group (wild-type), 74 % of them are ER+. Figure 5a shows that the group with CN0 (homozygous deletion) effectively eliminates the transcription of *APOBEC3B*, and the CN1 group reduced mRNA level of *APOBEC3B*, compared to the CN2 group, indicating the high confidence of

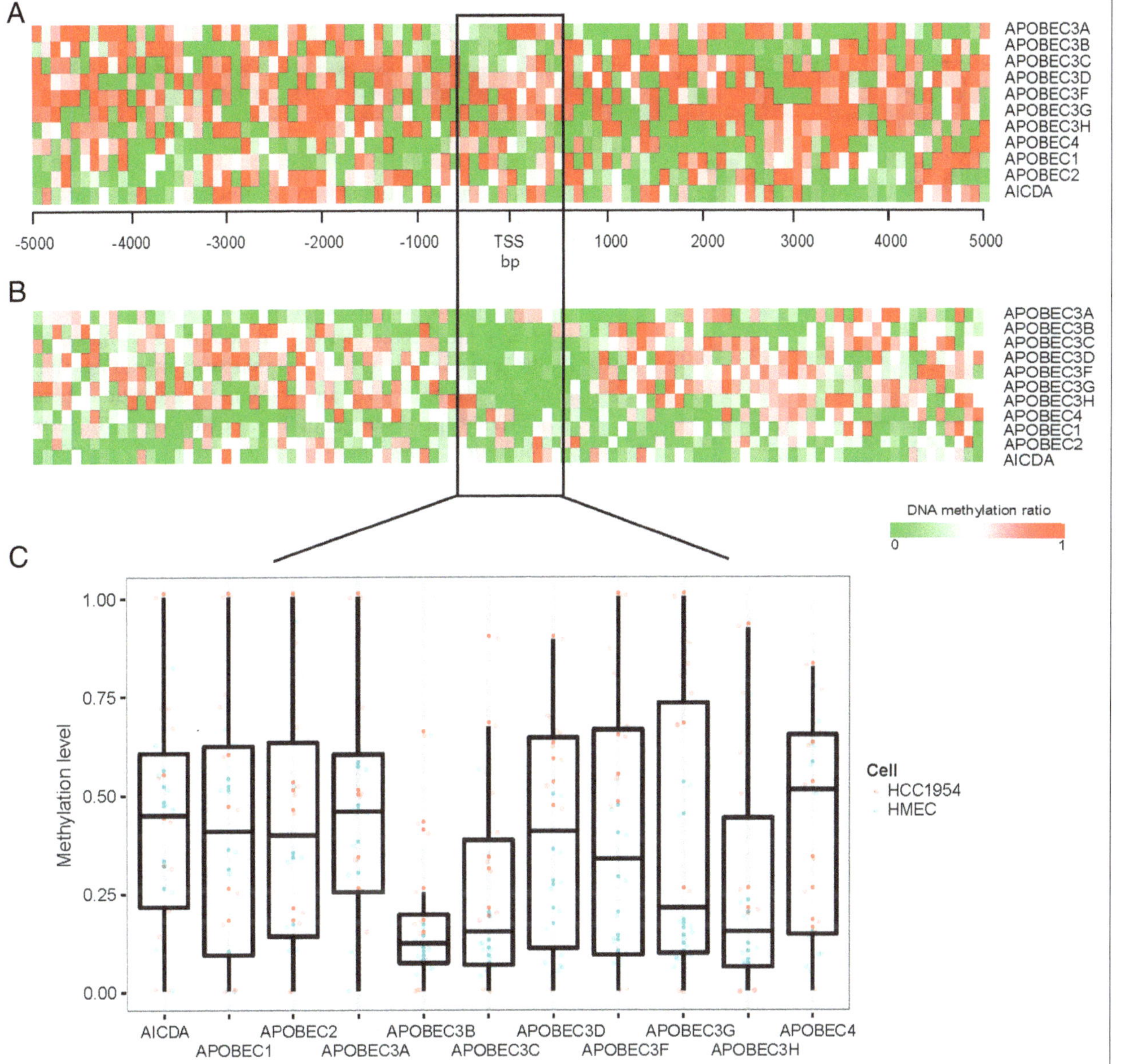

Fig. 2 DNA methylation of APOBECs in breast cancer cells. Heatmap of DNA methylation levels per 100 bp bin within ±5 kb regions of APOBEC gene family transcription start sites (TSS) in HCC1954 ER– breast cancer cells (**a**) and HMEC normal breast cells (**b**). The *color bar* shown represents the DNA methylation ratio from the lowest (*green*) to the highest (*red*). **c** Boxplot of DNA methylation levels of APOBECs in breast cancer and normal cells in the proximal regions (defined as ±0.5 kb of TSS)

CNV calling in this study. We then examined the possibility of functional interaction between *APOBEC3B* and other APOBEC family members. In cancer samples with the depletion of *APOBEC3B*, although the expression level of the *APOBEC3A* is decreased, such change is likely a false positive as reported by Leonard et al. [13]. The mRNA levels for other APOBEC family members do not exhibit the remarkable alteration (Additional file 2: Figure S6), including the *APOBEC3C* gene (Fig. 5a), further raising the possibility that there are less functionally direct interactions between APOBEC family members, at least between *APOBEC3B* and other members.

To address whether the APOBEC-mediated mutagenesis in breast tumors is directly induced by the *APOBEC3B* protein, stratified by CNV of *APOBEC3B* locus, we further compared the number of mutations per tumor exome in breast cancer tissues. The results show the remarkably positive correlation ($r = 0.33$, $P = 8.9 \times 10^{-16}$) between the number of SNVs per exome and *APOBEC3B* expression levels for *APOBEC3B* with CN2, but not for CN1 and CN0 types (Fig. 5b). Similar

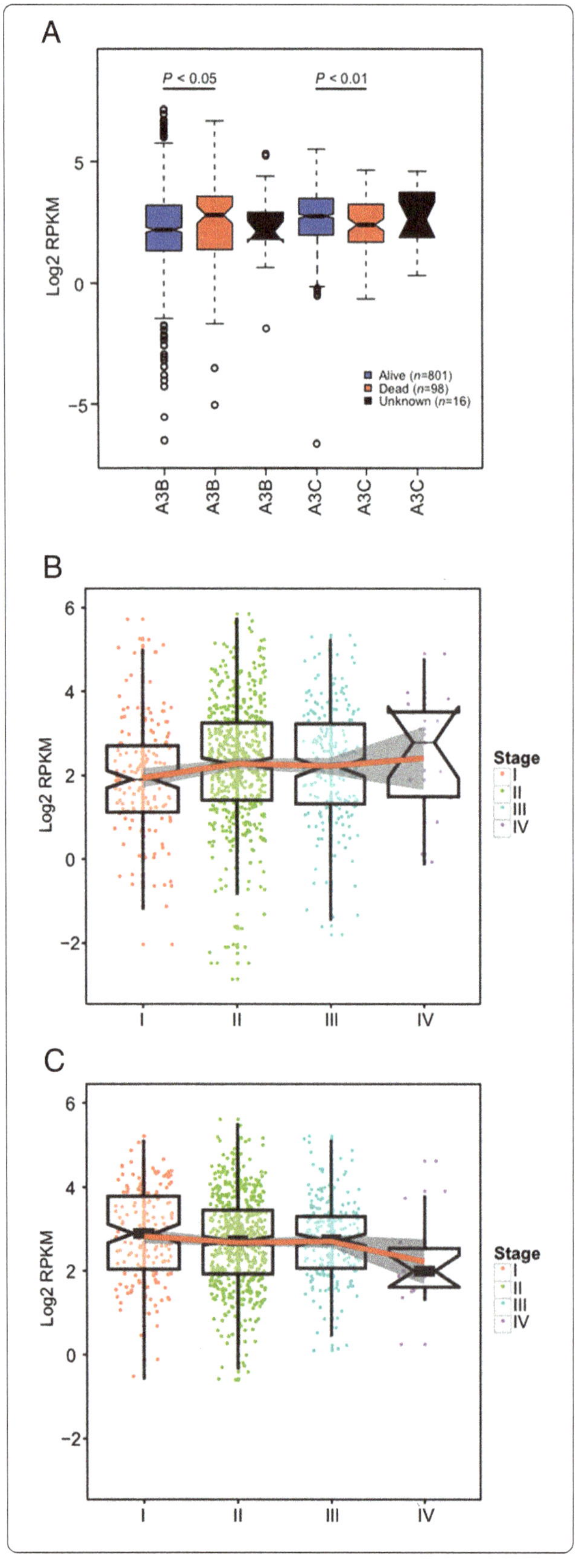

Fig. 3 Association of clinical outcome with expression levels of *APOBEC3B* and *APOBEC3C*. **a** Expression levels of *APOBEC3B* and *APOBEC3C* in breast cancer patients who are alive or not. **b** and **c** Association of mRNA levels of *APOBEC3B* and *APOBEC3C* with breast tumor stages ranging from I to IV

but negative correlation of mutations per exome with *APOBEC3C* expression levels is observed. Meanwhile, the comparative results show that the number of somatic SNVs in the absence of *APOBEC3B* (CN0) is not significantly different with the other two genotypes (CN1 and CN2, Fig. 5c), although some biases could be introduced in the comparison, including the unequal sample size and regional (not whole-genome) variants for three genotypes. Furthermore, in terms of mutation types, the mutation patterns are quite similar with predominance of C-T transition for all three *APOBEC3B* genotypes (Fig. 5d). Compared with samples with CN1 and CN2 of *APOBEC3B*, we observed elevated frequency of C-G mutation in samples containing the CN0 of *APOBEC3B* (Fig. 5d). The excessive analysis of trinucleotide motifs with centered C>A, C>G, and C>T mutation types shows a significantly increased TCW motif occurrence in CN0 group (where W corresponds to A or T, Fig. 5e) compared with CN1 ($P = 2.4 \times 10^{-4}$) and CN2 groups ($P < 2.2 \times 10^{-16}$) based on Fisher's exact test.

Discussion

In this study, we investigated the genomic, transcriptomic, and epigenetic regulation of APOBEC gene family in breast cancers by integrating diverse high-throughput sequencing data. The transcriptome data from both breast cancer cell lines and tumor specimens reveal that the *APOBEC3B* and *APOBEC3C* genes show significant differences at the transcription levels between ER+ and ER− breast tumors. On the one hand, we recapitulated previous findings that the up-regulation of *APOBEC3B* gene represents a growing enzyme-catalyzed cytosine-to-uracil deamination activity in carcinogenesis [9, 10]. On the other hand, the substantial up-regulation of *APOBEC3B* gene and absence of down-regulation of *APOBEC3C* gene in ER− subtypes suggest that the cytosine deaminase activity for APOBECs may be distinct in cancer subtypes. Furthermore, our study also suggests that the APOBEC-induced cancer mutagenesis is distinct regarding ER status, in agreement with the phenomena of different mutational spectrum observed between ER+ and ER− breast cancers [15].

Our results provide an additional support of the functional significance of *APOBEC3B* and probably *APOBEC3C* in breast carcinogenesis [12]. Based on the overall similar mutation patterns between breast cancers

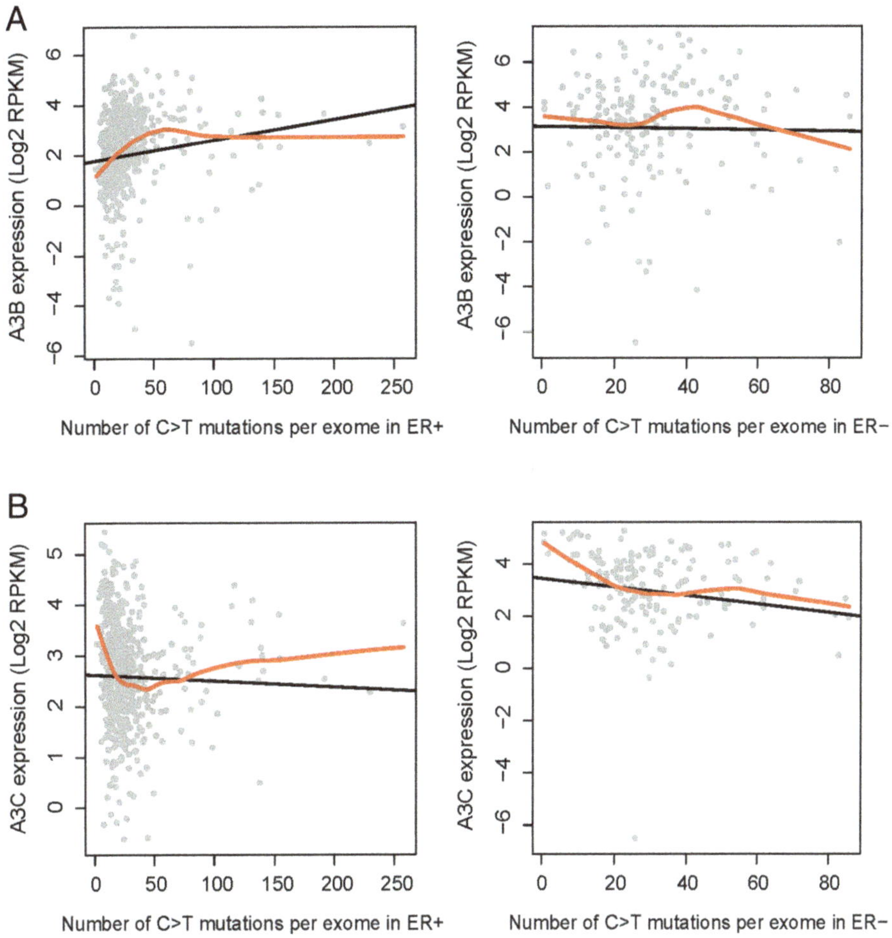

Fig. 4 Relationship between mRNA levels of *APOBEC3B* (**a**) and *APOBEC3C* (**b**) and number of C>T/G>A per tumor exome stratified by the ER status. The *black lines* and *red curves* are drawn from the linear regression model and local regression smoothing, respectively

in carriers of germline deletion of *APOBEC3B* genes and non-carriers, and a higher occurrence of somatic mutations on the TCW motif in *APOBEC3B* deletion samples, we speculate that germline deletion of *APOBEC3B*, expression of *APOBEC3B* and *APOBEC3C*, and somatic mutation may interact in contributing to breast cancer.

Integrated analysis of functional genomic data is a powerful approach with broad applications in many areas, including prediction of gene activity [31] and annotation of non-coding RNAs [32]. Using a similar approach, our integrated analyses illuminate the difference of chromatin states among APOBECs in breast cancer subtypes, which is highly consistent with the gene expression data. For instance, the active promoter and enhancer states at the *APOBEC3B* gene are concordant with the over-expression of *APOBEC3B*, particularly in ER− subtype. Meanwhile, the loss of active promoter and enhancer signals at the *APOBEC3C* gene in the ER+ cancer cell reflects the down-regulation of this gene observed in the ER+ subtype. In addition, the DNA hypermethylation may explain no or low expression profiles of other APOBECs. These results are concordant with Isobe's report [33, 34] in blood cells. Meanwhile, Pauklin et al. [35] have reported the estrogen induced increase of *APOBEC3B* gene expression by nearly 1.5-fold in a dose-dependent manner, but not *APOBEC3C* gene and other members in human MCF-7 cells, suggesting the possibility that ER may directly (or indirectly) regulate APOBECs in breast cancer cells through recruiting chromatin modifiers [36].

Compared with *APOBEC3B*, the *APOBEC3C* gene may play a different role in the cancer genome mutagenesis. For example, we observed that the elevated expression levels of *APOBEC3C* but lowered expression levels of *APOBEC3B* in breast cancer patients have better clinical outcomes. The opposite correlation of *APOBEC3B* and *APOBEC3C* genes' expression with clinical outcomes further provides a possibility of using both two genes as potential biomarkers in prognosis. Although no functional assays are performed in this study, several lines of

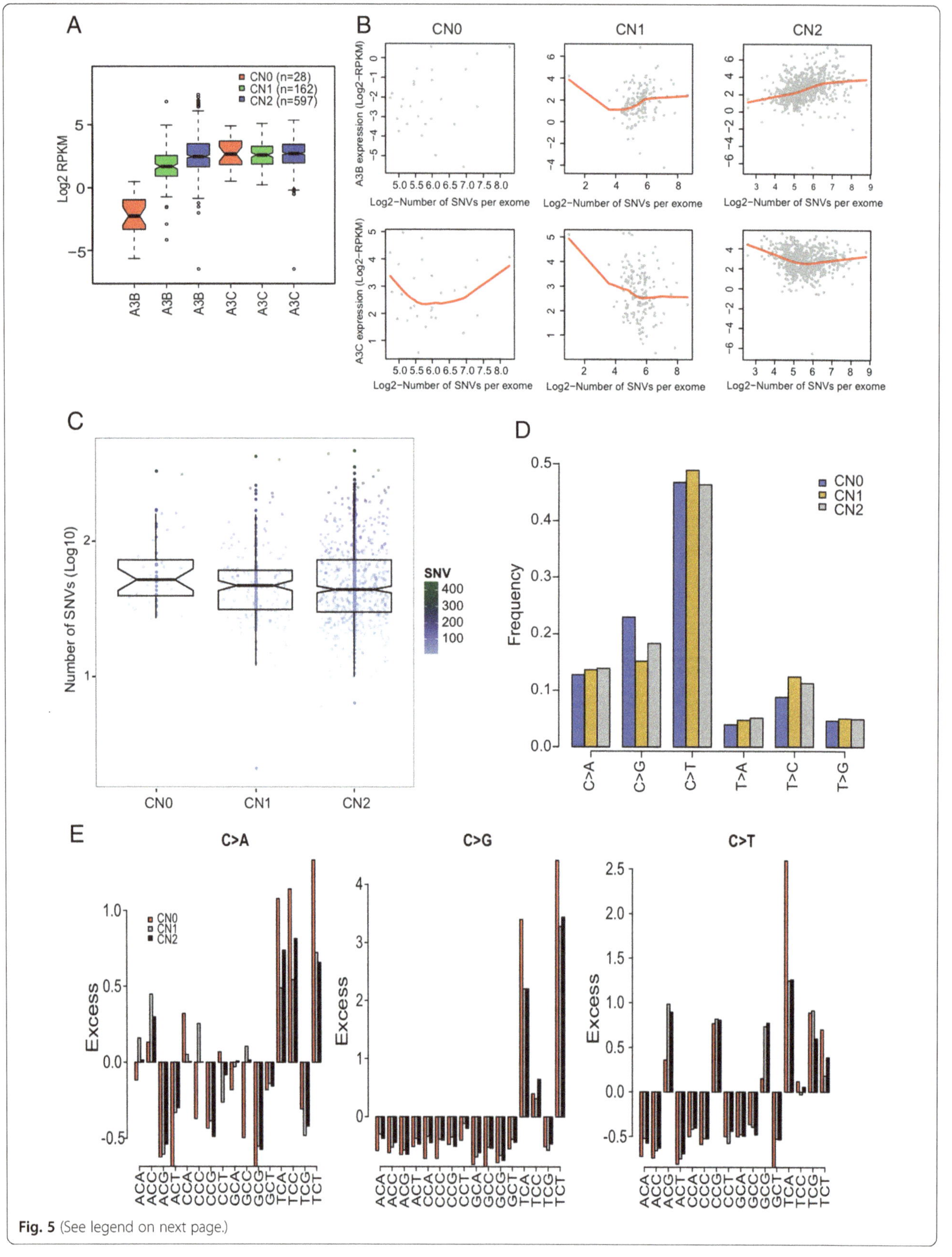

Fig. 5 (See legend on next page.)

(See figure on previous page.)
Fig. 5 Gene expression and somatic mutation signatures in breast tumors stratified by copy numbers of *APOBEC3B* gene. **a** Boxplot of mRNA levels of *APOBEC3B* and *APOBEC3C* in totally 787 breast tumors. **b** Relationship between *APOBEC3B* (*upper panel*) and *APOBEC3C* (*lower panel*) expression levels and number of somatic SNVs per tumor exome. The *red curves* are drawn from the local regression smoothing. **c** Boxplot of the total number of somatic mutations per tumor exome (*y*-axis, log10 scaled). The *color bars* shown in the *right* are the original number of somatic SNVs per exome. **d** Frequency of each of six somatic mutation types. **e** Excess rate of trinucleotide motifs with centered C>A, C>G, and C>T mutations shown from *left* to *right panels*. The excess rate is calculated by (observed occurrence – mean occurrence) / mean occurrence. CN0, CN1, and CN2 present the zero, one, and two copies of *APOBEC3B* gene, respectively

evidence support the possible functionality of the APOBEC3C protein in breast cancer.

First, *APOBEC3C* is localized in both the cytoplasmic and nuclear compartments, which is not only observed in human cells [37–39], but also observed in the rhesus counterparts [7], suggesting functionally constrained localization of *APOBEC3C*. However, for other APOBECs, they show either tissue-restricted expression patterns (*APOBEC3A*, *APOBEC1*, *APOBEC2*, *APOBEC4*, and *AICDA*) or cytoplasmic localization (*APOBEC3D*, *APOBEC3F*, *APOBEC3G*, and *APOBEC3H*) in human cells [3, 4, 6, 7, 10, 39, 40]. Along with high expression levels of *APOBEC3C* gene in ER− breast cancer cells, it is possible that both *APOBEC3B* and *APOBEC3C* retain DNA cytosine deaminase activity in breast cancer. Meanwhile, Lackey et al. reported that throughout mitosis in HEK293T and HeLa cells, *APOBEC3C* has access to genomic DNA during interphase and telophase, while *APOBEC3B* is excluded from the genomic DNA during mitosis [37]. Such phenomena are consistent with our findings that there is less functional interaction between *APOBEC3C* and *APOBEC3B* proteins, suggesting they may perform different roles in cancer cells.

Second, given that the *APOBEC3C* possesses a single active Z2-cytosine deaminase domain, while the *APOBEC3B* has double Z-coordinating (Z1 and Z2) deaminase domains [8, 41], the crystal structure determinants and functional comparison have revealed the distinct substrate preferences for binding HIV-1 DNA between the single- and double-domained *APOBEC3* enzymes [42–44], raising the possibility that these two enzymes have differential DNA binding specificity which might help explain the relative differences in their observed mutagenesis in breast cancer cells, especially in the ER− cancers.

Third, besides the deaminase activity for APOBECs, the *APOBEC3* family proteins also contribute to inhibit the L1 retrotransposition in a deaminase independent manner [6, 38, 45]. For instance, depletion of *APOBEC3C* significantly increases the L1 retrotransposition activity by ~80 % in HeLa cells [39]. Meanwhile, many studies have strongly indicated the enhanced activity of LINE-1 retrotransposons in human cancers induces genome instability, DNA damage, and genetic variation [46–51], further implying the potentially functional roles of *APOBEC3C* in breast cancer.

Conclusions

In conclusion, our integrated analyses suggested that *APOBEC3B* and *APOBEC3C* expression patterns were correlated with ER status and clinical outcome, providing an additional implication that these two genes may contribute to mutation profile and clinical outcome in breast cancer subtypes.

Methods

Data collection

We collected functional genomics data from experiments including the following: (1) RNA-seq, (2) chromatin immunoprecipitation followed by high-throughput DNA sequencing (ChIP-seq), and (3) bisulfite sequencing (BS-seq) data, for breast cell lines (including both normal and cancer) from the Gene Expression Omnibus (GEO) database [52] and ENCODE project. We initially searched the GEO database using the following terms: breast [AND] sequencing. After manual curation to rule out data where cell lines were treated by additional chemicals or siRNAs in experiments, all relevant data with no redundancy were retained for further analyses. We retrieved the ChIP-seq data released by the ENCODE project for well-characterized chromatin modifications in two breast cell lines: one normal cell line, called human mammary epithelial cells (HMEC), and the other ER+ breast cancer cell line (MCF-7). We also downloaded a total of 1000 RNA-seq data with approval (BAM files, Level 1) and corresponding clinical data (Biotab format) for breast tissue specimens (including 915 cancer and 85 adjacent normal tissue specimens) from TCGA (https://tcga-data.nci.nih.gov/tcga/). In addition, we downloaded 840 CEL files (Affymetrix SNP 6.0 array, level 1) and processed somatic mutation data (level 2) from 776 whole exome-sequencing (exome-seq) for the breast cancer from TCGA data portal, where 787 and 750 have matched RNA-seq data, respectively.

Data processing and statistics

All raw sequencing data (FASTQ format) were initially mapped to the human reference genome (hg19) using Bowtie2 program [53] with the default setting. Aligned data in SAM format were processed and converted into BAM files using SAMtools program [54]. As each type of sequencing data conveys specifically biological purpose, we used the following methods to process the corresponding sequencing data. Except relevant programs described, all other bioinformatics analyses were implemented using Perl and R programming.

For RNA-seq data, we used similar methods described elsewhere [55]. In brief, to characterize the quantitative expression of each RefSeq gene, the reads per kilobase and million mapped reads (RPKM) was calculated as the number of mapped reads with the mapping quality (MAQ) $\geq$30 aligning to each transcript multiplied by 1 million and divided by the length of the transcript times the total number of aligned reads. Then the RPKM values for APOBEC family members were extracted to quantify their expression levels. The same method was also utilized to process BAM files for TCGA RNA-seq data.

To uniformly analyze and visualize ChIP-seq data, we used the MACS14 (version 1.4.2) algorithm [56] to call peaks of ChIP-seq data for histone modifications against the corresponding control data in 20 bp resolution (−−space = 20) at $P < 1 \times 10^{-5}$. The resulting peak files (.bed) were then implemented into the ChromHMM algorithm [57] at a 200-bp resolution for chromatin state characterization. We ran ChromHMM with a range of possible states and settled on a 9 state model as it accurately captured biologically meaningful patterns in a reproducible way. The resulting genome segmentation files were uploaded to the UCSC Genome Browser as a custom track to visualize the chromatin sates and comparison among APOBEC family members.

For BS-seq data, we employed the BSMAP (version 2.74) program [58] to analyze DNA methylation ratios on each CpG site. Each CpG site supported by $\geq$4 reads was considered. To compare the DNA methylation ratios among APOBECs, we calculated mean DNA methylation levels within each 100-bp sliding window across ±5 kb regions of transcription start site (TSS) for each of APOBEC family members.

Level 1 CEL files for the breast cancer were used for copy number variation (CNV) calling. CNVs were detected based on the signal intensities of over 1.8 million SNP or copy number probes on the Affymetrix SNP 6.0 array. The Affymetrix Power Tools (APT-1.14.3) package was used to normalize for samples run on the same plate according to file handles and the chemistry file available. CNVs were called using Birdsuite (version 1.4) [59], which calls both common and rare CNVs. The *APOBEC3B* deletion is named as CNP2576 (hg19, chr22: 39363620–39375307) in Canary and was determined by 24 probes. In the present study, we only focus on this *APOBEC3B* deletion and copy number states of 0, 1, and 2 (CN0, CN1, and CN2) were used. Genotypes were checked against sample barcodes and participant IDs to identify possible duplicate samples.

For somatic mutation data, both somatic single nucleotide variants (SNVs) and C>T/G>A mutations per tumor were first summed. The correlation between the number of C>T/G>A mutations (or somatic SNVs) and expression levels of APOBECs was calculated using nonparametric Spearman's Rank correlation statistics. The same analysis was employed stratifying for *APOBEC3B* germline deletion states. Six types of somatic SNVs (C>A/G>T, C>G/G>C, C>T/G>A, T>A/A>T, T>C/A>G, T>G/A>C) were counted and their relative frequencies were then calculated and compared. Following the method reported in the previous study [10], we compared the trinucleotides motif patterns with the background distribution normalized among breast cancer samples in different copies of *APOBEC3B* gene.

Additional files

Additional file 1: Tables S1 and S2. Table S1. Data characteristics in this study. Table S2. Expression levels of APOBEC family genes across ten breast cell lines.

Additional file 2: Figures S1–S6. Figure S1. Expression profiles of APOBEC family genes in breast tumor tissues and adjacent normal tissues in relation to ER status. Figure S2. Comparison of chromatin states in *APOBEC1* (A), *APOBEC2* (B), *APOBEC4* (C), and *AICDA* (D) genes in ER+ (MCF-7), ER− (HCC1954) breast cancer cells, and normal cells (HMEC). Chromatin states characterized by the ChromHMM algorithm are represented by different colors shown in the bottom. Figure S3. Kaplan-Meier curve for overall survival of four patient groups with higher (top 50 %) or lower (bottom 50 %) expression of *APOBEC3B* and *APOBEC3C* genes in breast cancer. Figure S4. Distribution of the number of somatic mutations (A) and C>T/G>A mutations (B) per tumor exome. The red curve is a kernel density estimate. Figure S5. Relationship between mRNA levels of *APOBEC3B* (upper panel) and *APOBEC3C* (lower panel) and number of somatic SNVs per tumor exome stratified by the ER status. The black lines and red curves are drawn from the linear regression model and local regression smoothing, respectively. Figure S6. Expression profiles of APOBEC family genes in breast tumor tissues in relation with copy numbers of *APOBEC3B*

Competing interests
The authors declare that they have no competing interests.

Authors' contributions
YZ, WZ, and JL conceived and designed the study. YZ, RD, and XG analyzed the sequencing data and performed the statistical tests. WZ and JL supervised the study. YZ, RD, and JL wrote the manuscript. All authors participated in the elaboration of the manuscript. All authors read and approved the final manuscript.

Acknowledgements
We thank Jing He and Yan Guo for data processing and analyses and Samantha Stansel for clerical support in the preparation of this manuscript. The content is solely the responsibility of the authors and does not necessarily represent the official views of the funding agents. This work was supported in part by US National Institutes of Health grants R01CA137013.

Author details
[1]Division of Epidemiology, Department of Medicine, Vanderbilt University Medical Center, Nashville 37203, USA. [2]Present address: HudsonAlpha Institute for Biotechnology, Huntsville 35806, USA.

References

1. Jarmuz A, Chester A, Bayliss J, Gisbourne J, Dunham I, Scott J, et al. An anthropoid-specific locus of orphan C to U RNA-editing enzymes on chromosome 22. Genomics. 2002;79(3):285–96.
2. Rogozin IB, Basu MK, Jordan IK, Pavlov YI, Koonin EV. APOBEC4, a new member of the AID/APOBEC family of polynucleotide (deoxy)cytidine deaminases predicted by computational analysis. Cell Cycle. 2005;4(9):1281–5.
3. Sato Y, Probst HC, Tatsumi R, Ikeuchi Y, Neuberger MS, Rada C. Deficiency in APOBEC2 leads to a shift in muscle fiber type, diminished body mass, and myopathy. J Biol Chem. 2010;285(10):7111–8.
4. Muramatsu M, Sankaranand VS, Anant S, Sugai M, Kinoshita K, Davidson NO, et al. Specific expression of activation-induced cytidine deaminase (AID), a novel member of the RNA-editing deaminase family in germinal center B cells. J Biol Chem. 1999;274(26):18470–6.
5. Daniel J, Nussenzweig A. The AID-induced DNA damage response in chromatin. Mol Cell. 2013;50(3):309–21.
6. Kinomoto M, Kanno T, Shimura M, Ishizaka Y, Kojima A, Kurata T, et al. All APOBEC3 family proteins differentially inhibit LINE-1 retrotransposition. Nucleic Acids Res. 2007;35(9):2955–64.
7. Hultquist JF, Lengyel JA, Refsland EW, LaRue RS, Lackey L, Brown WL, et al. Human and rhesus APOBEC3D, APOBEC3F, APOBEC3G, and APOBEC3H demonstrate a conserved capacity to restrict vif-deficient HIV-1. J Virol. 2011; 85(21):11220–34.
8. Langlois MA, Beale RCL, Conticello SG, Neuberger MS. Mutational comparison of the single-domained APOBEC3C and double-domained APOBEC3F/G anti-retroviral cytidine deaminases provides insight into their DNA target site specificities. Nucleic Acids Res. 2005;33(6):1913–23.
9. Burns MB, Lackey L, Carpenter MA, Rathore A, Land AM, Leonard B, et al. APOBEC3B is an enzymatic source of mutation in breast cancer. Nature. 2013;494(7437):366–70.
10. Burns MB, Temiz NA, Harris RS. Evidence for APOBEC3B mutagenesis in multiple human cancers. Nat Genet. 2013;45(9):977–83.
11. Tsuboi M, Yamane A, Horiguchi J, Yokobori T, Kawabata-Iwakawa R, Yoshiyama S, et al. APOBEC3B high expression status is associated with aggressive phenotype in Japanese breast cancers. Breast Cancer. 2015:1–9. doi:10.1007/s12282-015-0641-8
12. Cescon DW, Haibe-Kains B, Mak TW. APOBEC3B expression in breast cancer reflects cellular proliferation, while a deletion polymorphism is associated with immune activation. Proc Natl Acad Sci. 2015;112(9):2841–6.
13. Leonard B, Hart SN, Burns MB, Carpenter MA, Temiz NA, Rathore A, et al. APOBEC3B upregulation and genomic mutation patterns in serous ovarian carcinoma. Cancer Res. 2013;73(24):7222–31.
14. Roberts SA, Lawrence MS, Klimczak LJ, Grimm SA, Fargo D, Stojanov P, et al. An APOBEC cytidine deaminase mutagenesis pattern is widespread in human cancers. Nat Genet. 2013;45(9):970–6.
15. Nik-Zainal S, Alexandrov LB, Wedge DC, Van Loo P, Greenman CD, Raine K, et al. Mutational processes molding the genomes of 21 breast cancers. Cell. 2012; 149(5):979–93.
16. Kan Z, Jaiswal BS, Stinson J, Janakiraman V, Bhatt D, Stern HM, et al. Diverse somatic mutation patterns and pathway alterations in human cancers. Nature. 2010;466(7308):869–73.
17. Network TCGA. Comprehensive molecular portraits of human breast tumours. Nature. 2012;490(7418):61–70.
18. Stephens PJ, McBride DJ, Lin ML, Varela I, Pleasance ED, Simpson JT, et al. Complex landscapes of somatic rearrangement in human breast cancer genomes. Nature. 2009;462(7276):1005–10.
19. Consortium TEP. An integrated encyclopedia of DNA elements in the human genome. Nature. 2012;489(7414):57–74.
20. Hon GC, Hawkins RD, Caballero OL, Lo C, Lister R, Pelizzola M, et al. Global DNA hypomethylation coupled to repressive chromatin domain formation and gene silencing in breast cancer. Genome Res. 2012;22(2):246–58.
21. Sun Z, Asmann YW, Kalari KR, Bot B, Eckel-Passow JE, Baker TR, et al. Integrated analysis of gene expression, CpG island methylation, and gene copy number in breast cancer cells by deep sequencing. PLoS ONE. 2011;6(2):e17490.
22. Frietze S, Wang R, Yao L, Tak Y, Ye Z, Gaddis M, et al. Cell type-specific binding patterns reveal that TCF7L2 can be tethered to the genome by association with GATA3. Genome Biol. 2012;13(9):R52.
23. Kouzarides T. Chromatin modifications and their function. Cell. 2007;128(4): 693–705.
24. Mikkelsen TS, Ku M, Jaffe DB, Issac B, Lieberman E, Giannoukos G, et al. Genome-wide maps of chromatin state in pluripotent and lineage-committed cells. Nature. 2007;448(7153):553–60.
25. Wang Z, Zang C, Rosenfeld JA, Schones DE, Barski A, Cuddapah S, et al. Combinatorial patterns of histone acetylations and methylations in the human genome. Nat Genet. 2008;40(7):897–903.
26. Heintzman ND, Stuart RK, Hon G, Fu Y, Ching CW, Hawkins RD, et al. Distinct and predictive chromatin signatures of transcriptional promoters and enhancers in the human genome. Nat Genet. 2007;39(3):311–8.
27. Zhao XD, Han X, Chew JL, Liu J, Chiu KP, Choo A, et al. Whole-genome mapping of histone H3 Lys4 and 27 trimethylations reveals distinct genomic compartments in human embryonic stem cells. Cell Stem Cell. 2007;1(3):286–98.
28. Jones PA. Functions of DNA methylation: islands, start sites, gene bodies and beyond. Nat Rev Genet. 2012;13(7):484–92.
29. Weisenberger DJ. Characterizing DNA, methylation alterations from The Cancer Genome Atlas. J Clin Invest. 2014;124(1):17–23.
30. Kidd JM, Newman TL, Tuzun E, Kaul R, Eichler EE. Population stratification of a common APOBEC gene deletion polymorphism. PLoS Genet. 2007;3(4):e63.
31. Creyghton MP, Cheng AW, Welstead GG, Kooistra T, Carey BW, Steine EJ, et al. Histone H3K27ac separates active from poised enhancers and predicts developmental state. Proc Natl Acad Sci. 2010;107(50):21931–6.
32. Guttman M, Amit I, Garber M, French C, Lin MF, Feldser D, et al. Chromatin signature reveals over a thousand highly conserved large non-coding RNAs in mammals. Nature. 2009;458(7235):223–7.
33. Fujimura S, Matsui T, Kuwahara K, Maeda K, Sakaguchi N. Germinal center B-cell-associated DNA hypomethylation at transcriptional regions of the AID gene. Mol Immunol. 2008;45(6):1712–9.
34. Isobe T, Song SN, Tiwari P, Ito H, Yamaguchi Y, Yoshizaki K. Activation-induced cytidine deaminase auto-activates and triggers aberrant gene expression. FEBS Lett. 2013;587(16):2487–92.
35. Pauklin S, Sernandez IV, Bachmann G, Ramiro AR, Petersen-Mahrt SK. Estrogen directly activates AID transcription and function. J Exp Med. 2009;206(1):99–111.
36. Gaughan L, Stockley J, Coffey K, ONeill D, Jones DL, Wade M, et al. KDM4B is a master regulator of the estrogen receptor signalling cascade. Nucleic Acids Res. 2013;41(14):6892–904.
37. Lackey L, Law EK, Brown WL, Harris RS. Subcellular localization of the APOBEC3 proteins during mitosis and implications for genomic DNA deamination. Cell Cycle. 2013;12(5):762–72.
38. Niewiadomska AM, Tian C, Tan L, Wang T, Sarkis PTN, Yu XF. Differential inhibition of long interspersed element 1 by APOBEC3 does not correlate with high-molecular-mass-complex formation or P-body association. J Virol. 2007;81(17):9577–83.
39. Muckenfuss H, Hamdorf M, Held U, Perkovic M, Lower J, Cichutek K, et al. APOBEC3 proteins inhibit human LINE-1 retrotransposition. J Biol Chem. 2006;281(31):22161–72.
40. Fujino T, Navaratnam N, Scott J. Human apolipoprotein B RNA editing deaminase gene (APOBEC1). Genomics. 1998;47(2):266–75.
41. LaRue RS, Andresdottir V, Blanchard Y, Conticello SG, Derse D, Emerman M, et al. Guidelines for naming nonprimate APOBEC3 genes and proteins. J Virol. 2009; 83(2):494–7.
42. Kitamura S, Ode H, Nakashima M, Imahashi M, Naganawa Y, Kurosawa T, et al. The APOBEC3C crystal structure and the interface for HIV-1 Vif binding. Nat Struct Mol Biol. 2012;19(10):1005–10.
43. Siu KK, Sultana A, Azimi FC, Lee JE. Structural determinants of HIV-1 Vif susceptibility and DNA binding in APOBEC3F. Nat Commun. 2013;4–2593.
44. Mitra M, Hercik K, Byeon IJ, Ahn J, Hill S, Hinchee-Rodriguez K, et al. Structural determinants of human APOBEC3A enzymatic and nucleic acid binding properties. Nucleic Acids Research. 2014;42(2):1095-110.
45. Horn AV, Klawitter S, Held U, Berger A, Jaguva Vasudevan AA, Bock A, et al. Human LINE-1 restriction by APOBEC3C is deaminase independent and mediated by an ORF1p interaction that affects LINE reverse transcriptase activity. Nucleic Acids Res. 2014;42(1):396–416.
46. Gary LB, Robert DCR, Thomas GF. Expression of LINE-1 retrotransposons in human breast cancer. Cancer. 1994;73(9):2333–6.
47. Belgnaoui SM, Gosden R, Semmes OJ, Haoudi A. Human LINE-1 retrotransposon induces DNA damage and apoptosis in cancer cells. Cancer Cell Int. 2006;6(1):13.
48. Gasior SL, Wakeman TP, Xu B, Deininger PL. The human LINE-1 retrotransposon creates DNA double-strand breaks. J Mol Biol. 2006; 357(5):1383–93.
49. Daskalos A, Nikolaidis G, Xinarianos G, Savvari P, Cassidy A, Zakopoulou R, et al. Hypomethylation of retrotransposable elements correlates with genomic instability in non-small cell lung cancer. Int J Cancer. 2009;124(1):81–7.

50. Hancks DC, Kazazian J. Active human retrotransposons: variation and disease. Curr Opin Genet Dev. 6/20122012. 2012;22(3):191–203.
51. Symer DE, Connelly C, Szak ST, Caputo EM, Cost GJ, Parmigiani G, et al. Human L1 retrotransposition is associated with genetic instability in vivo. Cell. 2002;110(3):327–38.
52. Barrett T, Troup DB, Wilhite SE, Ledoux P, Evangelista C, Kim IF, et al. NCBI GEO: archive for functional genomics data sets—10 years on. Nucleic Acids Res. 2011;39 suppl 1:D1005–D10.
53. Langmead B, Salzberg SL. Fast gapped-read alignment with Bowtie 2. Nat Meth. 2012;9(4):357–9.
54. Li H, Handsaker B, Wysoker A, Fennell T, Ruan J, Homer N, et al. The Sequence Alignment/Map (SAM) Format and SAMtools. Bioinformatics. 2009.
55. Yan G, Zhang G, Fang X, Zhang Y, Li C, Ling F, et al. Genome sequencing and comparison of two nonhuman primate animal models, the cynomolgus and Chinese rhesus macaques. Nat Biotech. 2011;29(11):1019–23.
56. Zhang Y, Liu T, Meyer C, Eeckhoute J, Johnson D, Bernstein B, et al. Model-based Analysis of ChIP-Seq (MACS). Genome Biol. 2008;9(9):R137.
57. Ernst J, Kellis M. ChromHMM: automating chromatin-state discovery and characterization. Nat Meth. 2012;9(3):215–6.
58. Xi Y, Li W. BSMAP: whole genome bisulfite sequence MAPping program. BMC Bioinformatics. 2009;10(1):232.
59. Korn JM, Kuruvilla FG, McCarroll SA, Wysoker A, Nemesh J, Cawley S, et al. Integrated genotype calling and association analysis of SNPs, common copy number polymorphisms and rare CNVs. Nat Genet. 2008;40(10):1253–60.

The clinical significance of snail protein expression in gastric cancer

Xiaoya Chen[1], Jinjun Li[1*], Ling Hu[2], William Yang[3], Lili Lu[1], Hongyan Jin[4], Zexiong Wei[4], Jack Y. Yang[5], Hamid R. Arabnia[7], Jun S. Liu[6], Mary Qu Yang[5] and Youping Deng[1,8*]

Abstract

Background: Snail is a typical transcription factor that could induce epithelial-mesenchymal transition (EMT) and cancer progression. There are some related reports about the clinical significance of snail protein expression in gastric cancer. However, the published results were not completely consistent. This study was aimed to investigate snail expression and clinical significance in gastric cancer.

Results: A systematic review of PubMed, CNKI, Weipu, and Wanfang database before March 2015 was conducted. We established an inclusion criterion according to subjects, method of detection, and results evaluation of snail protein. Meta-analysis was conducted using RevMan4.2 software. And merged odds ratio (OR) and 95 % CI (95 % confidence interval) were calculated. Also, forest plots and funnel plot were used to assess the potential of publication bias.

A total of 10 studies were recruited. The meta-analysis was conducted to evaluate the positive rate of snail protein expression. OR and 95 % CI for different groups were listed below: (1) gastric cancer and para-carcinoma tissue [OR = 6.15, 95 % CI (4.70, 8.05)]; (2) gastric cancer and normal gastric tissue [OR = 17.00, 95 % CI (10.08, 28.67)]; (3) non-lymph node metastasis and lymph node metastasis [OR = 0.40, 95 % CI (0.18, 0.93)]; (4) poor differentiated cancer, highly differentiated cancer, and moderate cancer [OR = 3.34, 95 % CI (2.22, 5.03)]; (5) clinical stage TI + TII and stage TIII + TIV [OR = 0.38, 95 % CI (0.23, 0.60)]; (6) superficial muscularis and deep muscularis [OR = 0.18, 95 % CI (0.11, 0.31)].

Conclusions: Our results indicated that the increase of snail protein expression may play an important role in the carcinogenesis, progression, and metastasis of gastric cancer. And this result might provide instruction for the diagnosis, therapy, and prognosis of gastric cancer.

Keywords: Gastric cancer, Snail, Meta-analysis

Background

Epithelial-mesenchymal transition (EMT), a developmental process whereby epithelial cells reduce intercellular adhesion and acquire myofibroblastic features, is critical to tumor progression [1–3]. Meanwhile, the dissolution of intercellular adhesions and the acquisition of a more motile mesenchymal phenotype as part of epithelial-to-mesenchymal transition (EMT) are crucial capacities of invading cancer cells [4]. Snail can induce EMT partly by suppressing the expression of E-cadherin. Reduced expression of E-cadherin may lead to the loss of cell-cell adhesion and cancer progression [5]. In recent years, snail was found to be highly expressed in several carcinomas, including non-small cell lung carcinomas, ovarian carcinomas, urothelial carcinomas, breast cancer, and hepatocellular carcinoma [6–10]. Studies of immunohistochemical analyses suggest that snail is highly expressed in gastric cancer and significantly associated with tumor progression and metastasis [11–13].

* Correspondence: entry2003@126.com; Youpingd@gmail.com
[1]Medical College, Wuhan University of Science and Technology, Wuhan 430065, China
[8]Department of Internal Medicine and Rush University Cancer Center, Rush University Medical Center, Chicago, IL 60612, USA

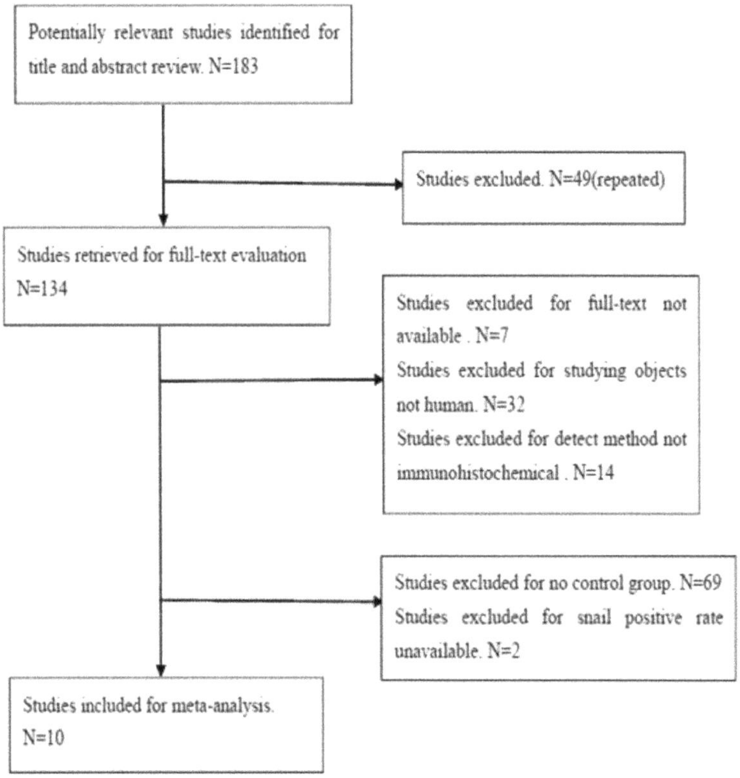

Fig. 1 Studies identified with criteria for inclusion and exclusion. After reviewing the abstracts and titles of 183 studies, 173 of them were excluded. In detail, 49 studies were excluded due to repetition; 32 studies were due to non-human subjects; 7 studies were due to non-full-text; 14 studies were due to non-IHC study; 69 studies were due to missing control group; 2 studies were due to missing the snail positive rate. Eventually, 10 articles were collected

Methods

Study search protocol

A total of 10 studies were identified by primary search strategies using the keywords "snail" combined with "gastric cancer" and synonyms in PubMed, CNKI, Weipu, and Wanfang database.

Inclusion criteria and exclusion criteria

Studies that were included in this meta-analysis met the following criteria: (1) the official published literature or master's and doctoral dissertation in both Chinese and English before March 2015; (2) the detection method used immunohistochemical and the results experienced

Table 1 Main characteristics of the studies included in this meta-analysis

First author	Year	Positive rate											Quality
		Cancer tissue	Adjacent tissue	Normal tissue	Low differentiation	Highly + moderate	TI + TII	TIII + TIV	Superficial	Deep	No metastasis	Metastasis	
Yingfeng Zhu	2007	80/96	33/80	–	56/62	24/34	21/29	59/67	10/16	70/80	23/32	57/64	D
Zhifeng Tang	2010	159/189	26/54	6/32	82/100	61/89	29/46	114/143	–	–	49/73	94/116	D
Yaqin Hao	2011	41/54	22/54	9/30	20/22	21/32	–	–	4/9	17/19	5/11	16/17	D
Shengxi Wang	2011	92/112	28/79	–	66/75	26/37	–	–	15/23	77/89	29/42	63/70	E
Li Jin	2011	78/87	–	7/24	–	–	–	–	–	–	–	–	E
Lina Wang	2011	32/60	16/60	3/20	26/42	6/18	–	–	2/9	30/51	4/7	28/53	D
Wude Zhang	2012	41/48	15/48	–	32/34	9/14	23/27	18/21	22/29	19/19	24/30	7/18	E
Xiaoli Cao	2013	32/45	5/20	–	24/27	8/18	11/20	21/25	9/19	23/26	10/20	22/25	E
Qianjun Li	2013	38/65	–	0/65	–	–	–	–	–	–	–	–	D
Limin Liu	2014	57/80	24/80	–	–	–	6/14	51/66	6/15	51/65	11/24	46/56	C

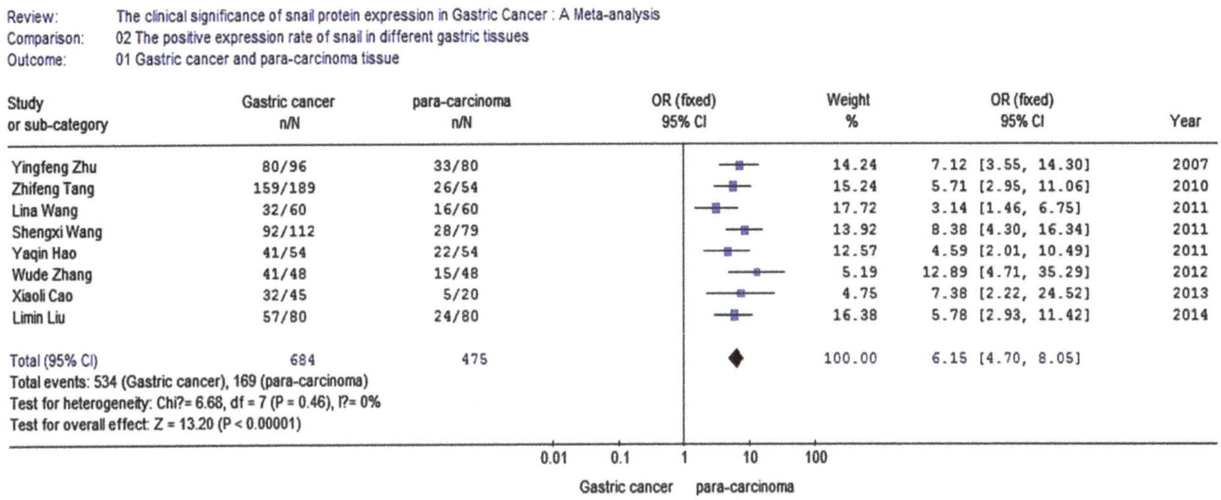

Fig. 2 Meta-analysis for the expression of snail protein in gastric cancer and para-carcinoma. Eight of the ten studies compared the expression of snail protein in gastric cancer tissues and the adjacent tissues, including 684 gastric cancer samples and 475 para-carcinoma samples. The I2 value was 0 % and less than 50 %; thus, we chose fixed-effect Mantel-Haenszel model for further analysis. The overall effect was $Z = 13.20$. The odds ratio (OR) was 6.15 with 95 % CI = (4.70, 8.05), and $P < 0.001$

quantitative analysis; (3) when duplicate articles were published, we included the newest or the most informative single study; (5) the snail positive rate was given or could be calculated based on the information from tables or figures.

Exclusion criteria included (1) repetitive studies; (2) research on animal and cellular level; (3) studies without reviews, letters, abstracts and editorials; and (4) the studies without control group.

Data extraction and quality assessment

Two reviewers screened the titles and abstracts according to the inclusion and exclusion criteria listed above independently. Then, they cross-checked the articles and removed disagreements. Information extracted from the eligible articles included first author, publication year, detection method, the number of cases and controls, the clinical pathology states of cases and controls, and the location of snail protein expression. The quality of these studies is assessed by the following: (1) whether the gold standard method is set up; (2) whether the gold standard test stayed is independent of the evaluation test; (3) whether the blind method is used; (4) whether quantitative data is given or is able to be calculated; (5) whether the definition and diagnosis of the case are correct, independent, and standard; (6) whether the diagnostic steps are detailed; (7) whether the case has a good representation; (8) whether cases and controls are selected and

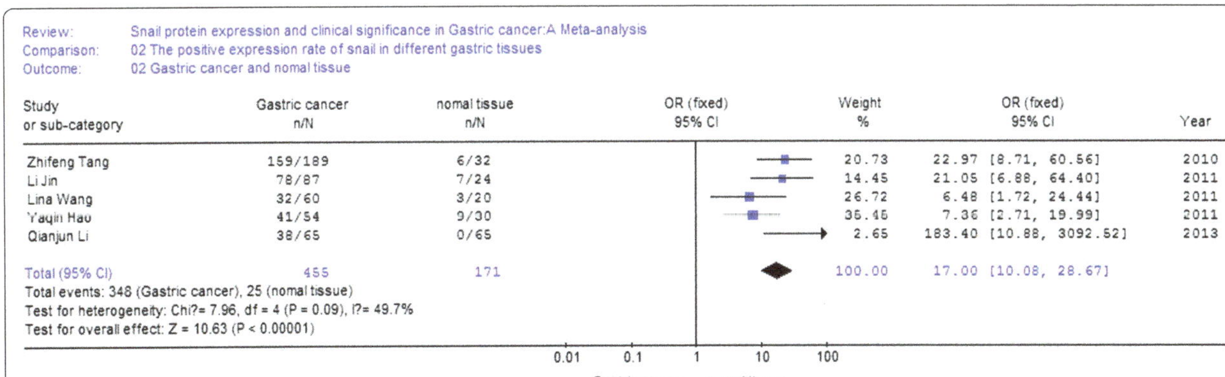

Fig. 3 Meta-analysis for the expression of snail protein in gastric cancer and normal tissue. Five of the ten studies compared the positive expression of snail protein in gastric cancer tissues with that in normal tissues, including 455 gastric cancer tissue samples and 171 normal samples. The I2 value was 49.7 % and less than 50 %; thus, we chose fixed-effect Mantel-Haenszel model for further analysis. The overall effect was $Z = 10.63$, OR = 17, 95 % CI = (10.08, 28.67), and $P < 0.001$

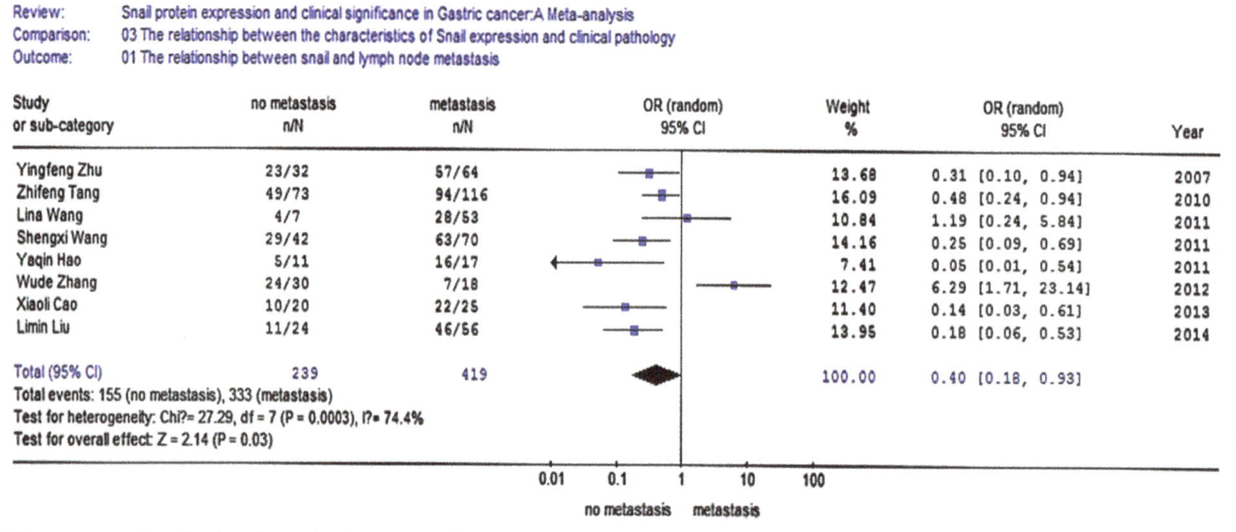

Fig. 4 Meta-analysis for the relationship between snail expression and lymph node metastasis. Eight studies analyzed the relationship between snail expression and lymph node metastasis. The results indicated that the I2 value was 74.4 % and greater than 50 %; thus, we chose random-effect model for further analysis. The overall effect was $Z = 2.14$, $OR = 0.40$, 95 % $CI = (0.18, 0.93)$, and $P < 0.001$

analyzed based on the most important factor. Based on the above standards, we classified the qualities of the research into five grades: (A) meets all 8 quality standards; (B) meets 7 standards; (C) meets 6 standards; (D) meets 5 standards; (E) meets 4 standards.

Statistical analysis

Meta-analysis was conducted with RevMan4.2 software. Odds ratio (OR) with 95 % confidence interval was calculated. Heterogeneity between studies was examined using the I2 statistic [14, 15]. When I2 value was greater than 50 %, we considered that heterogeneity was significant. Fixed-effect Mantel-Haenszel model was chosen as the main analysis method when the heterogeneities were not confirmed statistically significant. Otherwise, random-effect model was adopted. Funnel plots were used to check for the potential of publication bias. All the P values were two-sided, and statistically significant difference was defined as $P < 0.05$.

Results

Literature search and study characteristics

After reviewing the abstracts and titles of 183 studies, 173 of them were excluded. In detail, 49 studies were excluded due to repetition; 32 studies were due to non-human subjects; 7 studies were due to non-full-

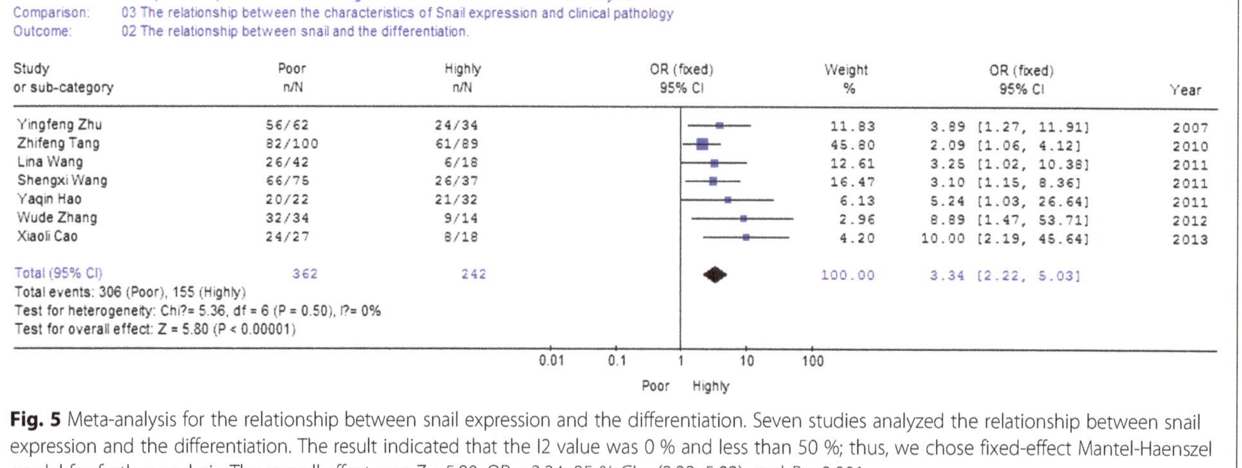

Fig. 5 Meta-analysis for the relationship between snail expression and the differentiation. Seven studies analyzed the relationship between snail expression and the differentiation. The result indicated that the I2 value was 0 % and less than 50 %; thus, we chose fixed-effect Mantel-Haenszel model for further analysis. The overall effect was $Z = 5.80$, $OR = 3.34$, 95 % $CI = (2.22, 5.03)$, and $P < 0.001$

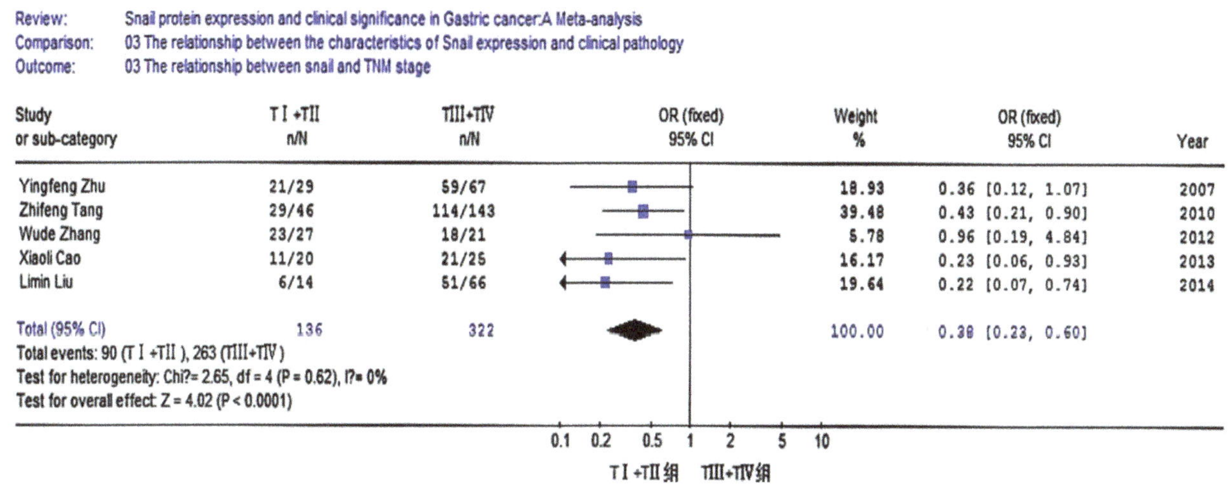

Fig. 6 Meta-analysis for the relationship between snail expression and TNM stage. Five studies analyzed the relationship between snail expression and the TNM stage. The result showed that the I2 value was 0 % and less than 50 %, thus we chose fixed-effect Mantel-Haenszel model for further analysis. The overall effect was $Z = 4.02$, OR = 0.38, 95 % CI = (0.23, 0.60), and $P < 0.001$

text; 14 studies were due to non-IHC study; 69 studies were due to missing control group; 2 studies were due to missing the snail positive rate. Eventually, 10 articles were collected [16–25] (Fig. 1). Detailed characteristics of these 10 eligible studies are summarized in Table 1. A total of 756 gastric cancer tissue samples, 346 para-carcinoma tissue samples, and 171 normal tissue samples were used in these 10 studies. Eight of them reported the relationship between the snail expression and clinical pathology, enrolled the degree of differentiation, the lymph node metastasis, TNM stage, and invasion depth.

Stratification analysis

Eight of the ten studies compared the expression of snail protein in gastric cancer tissues and the adjacent tissues, including 684 gastric cancer samples and 475 para-carcinoma samples. The I2 value was 0 % and less than 50 %; thus, we chose fixed-effect Mantel-Haenszel model for further analysis. The overall effect was $Z = 13.20$. The odds ratio (OR) was 6.15 with 95 % CI = (4.70, 8.05), and $P < 0.001$ (Fig. 2).

Five of the ten studies compared the positive expression of snail protein in gastric cancer tissues with that in normal tissues, including 455 gastric cancer tissue samples and 171 normal samples. The I2 value was 49.7 % and less than 50 %; thus, we chose fixed-effect Mantel-Haenszel model for further analysis. The overall effect was $Z = 10.63$. The odds ratio was 17 with 95 % CI = (10.08, 28.67), and $P < 0.001$ (Fig. 3).

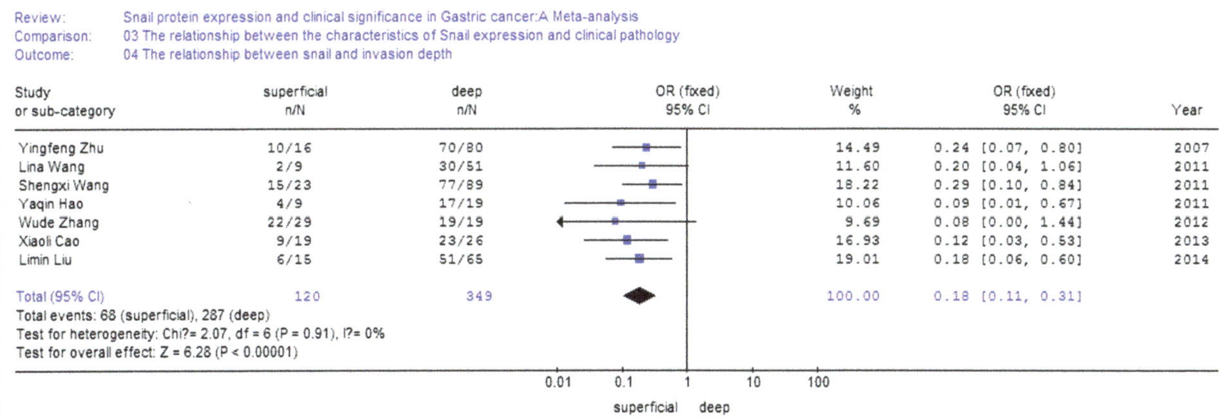

Fig. 7 Meta-analysis for the relationship between snail expression and invasion depth. Seven studies analyzed the relationship between snail expression and invasion depth. The result showed that I2 value was 0 % and less than 50 %; thus, we chose fixed-effect Mantel-Haenszel model for further analysis. The overall effect was $Z = 6.28$, OR = 0.18, 95 % CI = (0.11, 0.31), and $P < 0.001$

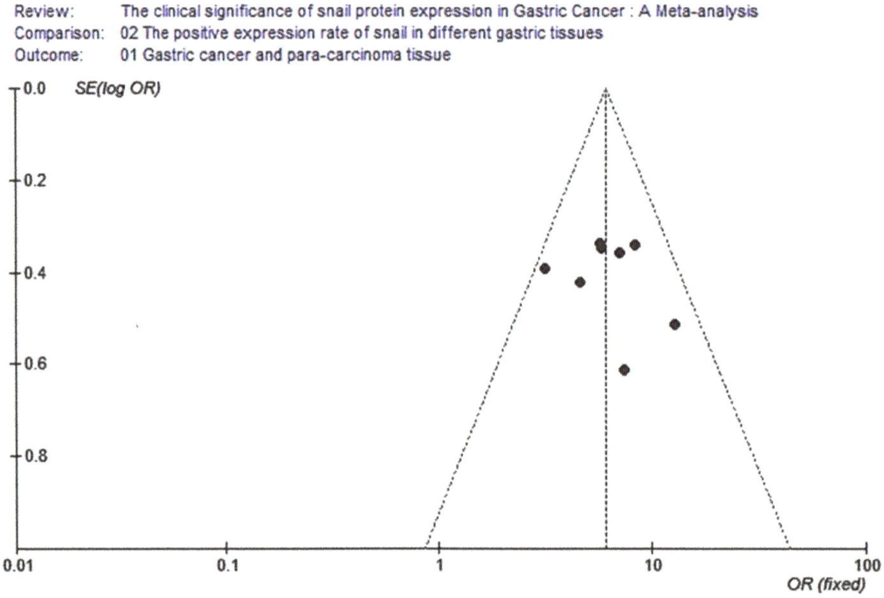

Fig. 8 Funnel plot analysis for the expression of snail protein in gastric cancer and para-carcinoma. Funnel plot analysis for publication bias indicated a low likelihood of publication bias

The relationship between the expression of snail protein and the characteristics of clinical pathology

Eight studies analyzed the relationship between snail expression and lymph node metastasis. The results indicated that the I2 value was 74.4 % and greater than 50 %; thus, we chose random-effect model for further analysis. The overall effect was $Z = 2.14$, OR = 0.40, 95 % CI = (0.18, 0.93), and $P < 0.001$ (Fig. 4). Seven studies analyzed the relationship between snail expression and the differentiation. The result indicated that the I2 value was 0 % and less than 50 %; thus, we chose fixed-effect Mantel-Haenszel model for further analysis. The overall effect was $Z = 5.80$, OR = 3.34, 95 % CI = (2.22, 5.03), and $P < 0.001$ (Fig. 5). Five studies analyzed the relationship between snail expression and the TNM stage. The result showed that the I2 value was 0 % and less than 50 %;

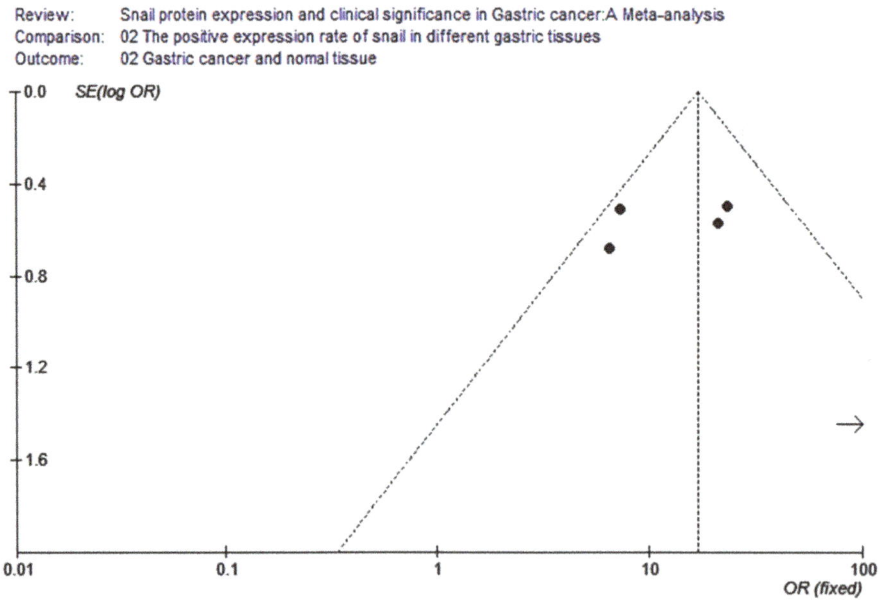

Fig. 9 Funnel plot analysis for the expression of snail protein in gastric cancer and normal tissue. Funnel plot analysis for publication bias indicated a low likelihood of publication bias

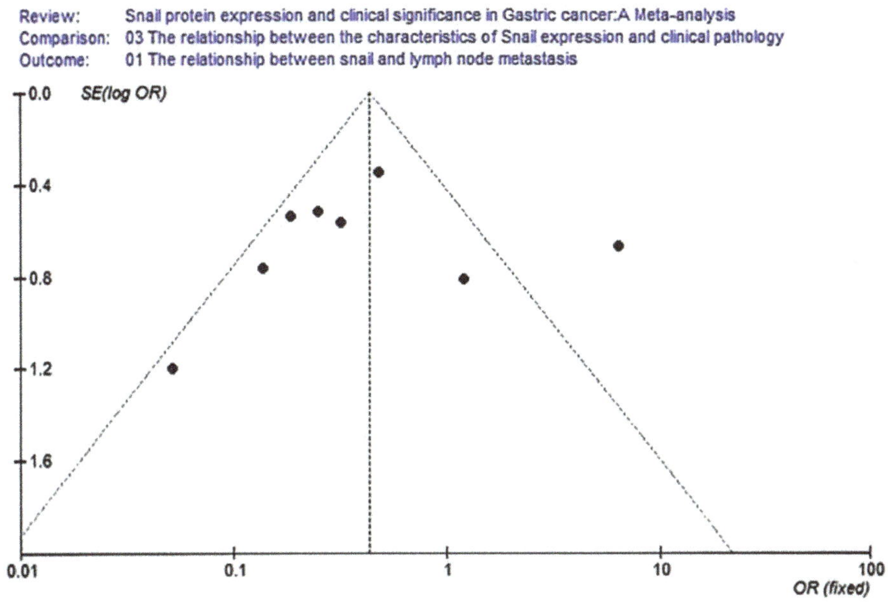

Fig. 10 Funnel plot analysis for the relationship between snail expression and lymph node metastasis. Funnel plot analysis for publication bias indicated a low likelihood of publication bias

thus, we chose fixed-effect Mantel-Haenszel model for further analysis. The overall effect was $Z = 4.02$, OR = 0.38, 95 % CI = (0.23, 0.60), and $P < 0.001$ (Fig. 6). Seven studies analyzed the relationship between snail expression and invasion depth. The result showed that I2 value was 0 % and less than 50 %; thus, we chose fixed-effect Mantel-Haenszel model for further analysis. The overall effect was $Z = 6.28$, OR = 0.18, 95 % CI = (0.11, 0.31), and $P < 0.001$ (Fig. 7).

Publication bias analysis

Funnel plot analysis for publication bias of these analytical studies (as shown in Figs. 8, 9, 10, 11, 12, and 13) indicated a low likelihood of publication bias.

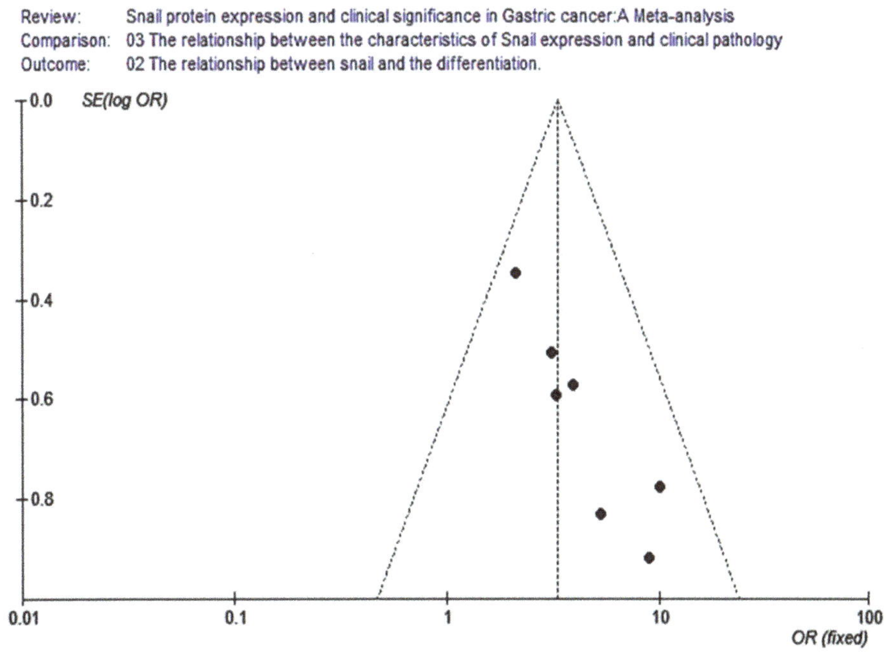

Fig. 11 Funnel plot analysis for the relationship between snail expression and the differentiation. Funnel plot analysis for publication bias indicated a low likelihood of publication bias

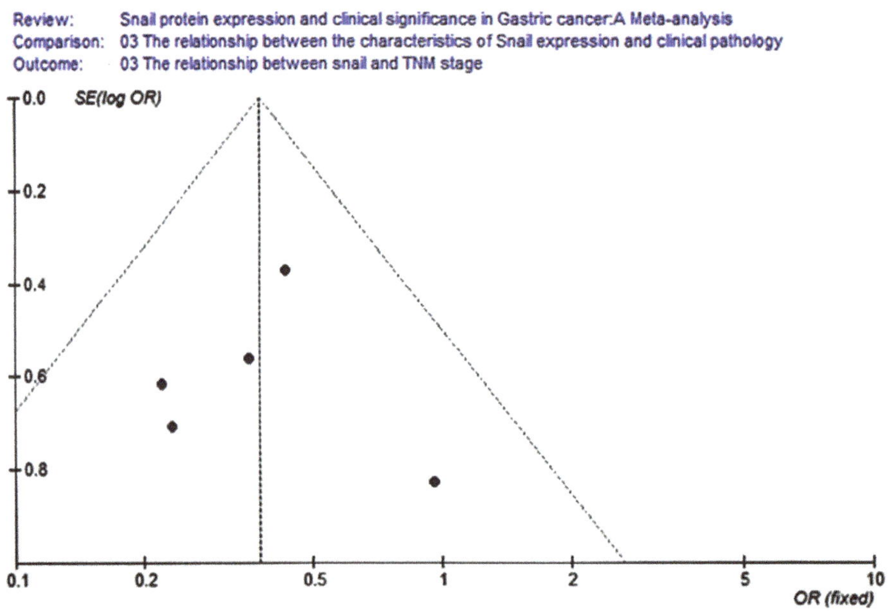

Fig. 12 Funnel plot analysis for the relationship between snail expression and the TNM stage. Funnel plot analysis for publication bias indicated a low likelihood of publication bias

Discussion and conclusions

The emerging roles of some key, EMT-related proteins in cancer progression and their close relationship with clinical pathology parameters make them attractive for developing diagnostic biomarkers and therapies [26]. The transcriptional repression of E-cadherin is mediated mainly by zinc finger transcription factors related to the snail family (SNAIL1), zinc finger E-box binding homeobox-2 (ZEB2), and basic helix-loop-helix family (TWIST) [27, 28]. Network analysis (Fig. 14) revealed that snail expression was significantly correlated with the expression of ZEB2, TWIST (Twist1 and Twist2), and N-cadherin (CDH2). These gene expressions may be regulated by snail at transcriptional level, and they also interact with each other. N-cadherin, encoded by the CDH2 gene, mediates cell-cell adhesion and renders

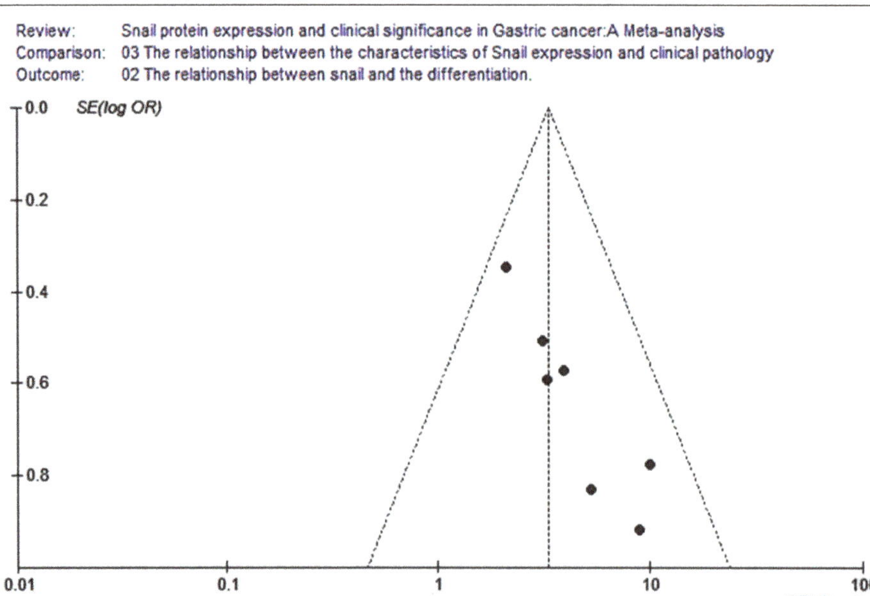

Fig. 13 Funnel plot analysis for the relationship between snail expression and the invasion depth. Funnel plot analysis for publication bias indicated a low likelihood of publication bias

tumor cell migration and invasion [29]. N-cadherin was reported to be a prognostic marker [30], and the up-regulation correlated with advanced TNM stage and poor survival [31]. In addition, TWIST can modulate N-cadherin expression through directly interacting with an E-box, a regulatory element within intron 1 of CDH2 [32], and expression of TWIST appears to be indispensable for the entry of tumor cells into the bloodstream, a significant early step towards metastasis [33]. ZEB2 is also known as SIP1, which interacts through its COOH-terminal region with E-box element of E-cadherin gene promoter and mediates its transcriptional repression by recruiting corepressor complexes [34, 35]. These transcription factors form signaling networks that could initiate and sustain the mesenchymal phenotypes of tumor cells; therefore, the expression of these proteins could define EMT occurrence in a tumor setting. For example, a study in primary human gastric cancers revealed elevated snail and twist expressions in diffuse-type gastric cancer, whereas ZEB2/SIP1 was primarily expressed in the intestinal type [36] (Fig. 14).

This meta-analysis was aimed to examine the expression of transcription factor snail in different tissue samples and the relationship between increased snail expression and clinicopathological features of gastric cancer. This study combined 756 gastric cancer tissue samples, 346 para-carcinoma samples, and 171 normal tissue samples from 10 individual studies. The results indicated that snail expression is higher in gastric cancer tissues than that in para-carcinoma tissues and normal tissues, respectively (OR = 6.15, 95 % CI = 4.70, 8.05; OR = 17, 95 % CI = 10.08, 28.67). Furthermore, closed correlations were observed between snail expression and clinicopathological characteristics that included the lymph node metastasis, the degree of differentiation, TNM stage, and invasion depth. The positive expression rate of snail was higher in gastric cancer tissues with lymphatic metastasis, OR = 0.40, 95 % CI = (0.18, 0.93). The higher positive rate of snail is

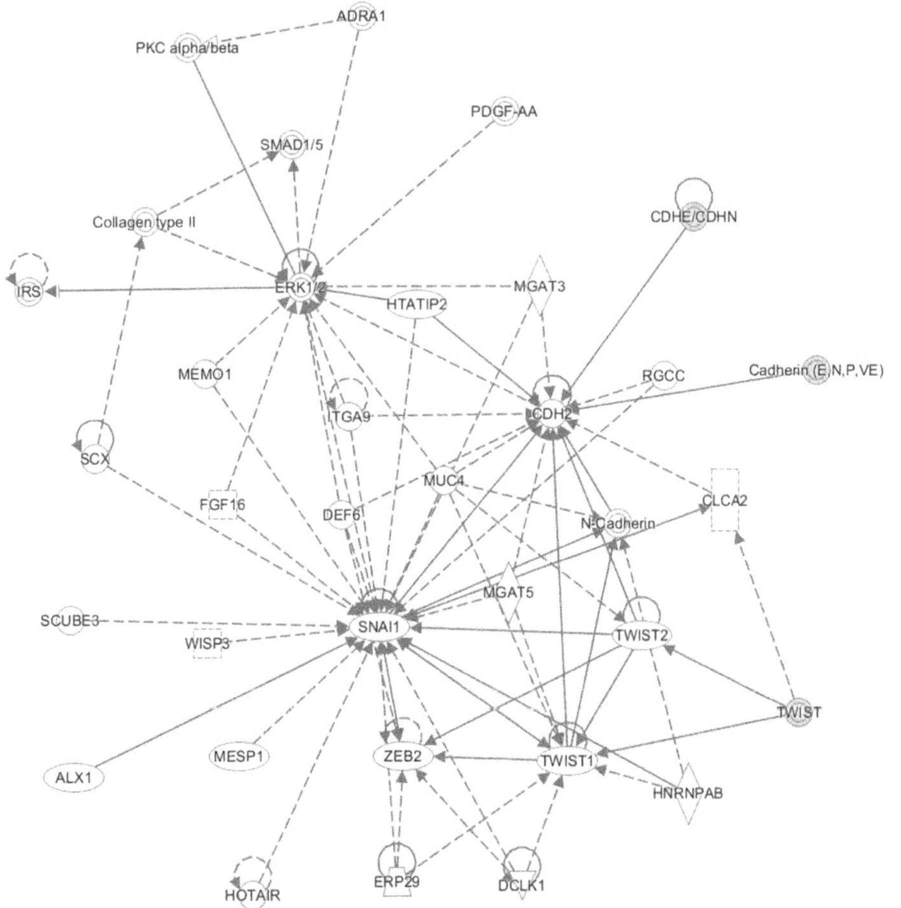

Fig. 14 Gene network analysis. The target genes of cancer-induced differentially expressed protein were used to run the IPA tool for gene network analysis. These genes around *triangles* highlighted genes that are involved in immunity system development function. The network score described in the "Methods" section for the network is 39. The *solid lines* connecting the molecules here represent a direct relation and *dotted lines* an indirect relation

connected with the lower differentiation degree, OR = 3.34, 95 % CI = (2.22, 5.03). The positive expression of snail was higher at late clinical stage, OR = 0.38, 95 % CI = (0.23, 0.60). Moreover, it appeared that the deeper the infiltration was, the higher the expression of snail was, OR = 0.18, 95 % CI = (0.11, 0.31).

The result of funnel plot indicated an imminent possibility of publication bias. Two potential biases might be introduced. First, the languages in collected papers were used in both Chinese and English, which may lead to a language bias. Second, the majority of collected studies did not use blind method, which might result in a measurement bias. Hence, the large-scale samples and double blind statistical tests will be investigated in the future study. Additionally, our review only collected the publications that have full text, since data that can be used for the methodology assessment and meta-analysis were only available in these publications with full text.

Our meta-analysis indicated that snail was highly expressed in gastric cancer. In addition, the overexpression of snail is significantly associated with tumor progression and metastasis.

Competing interests

The authors declare that they have no competing interests.

Authors' contributions

YC, YD, and JL envisioned the project. YC and LL designed the work. YC and LH constructed and validated the pathway models and performed the data analysis, with assistance from WY. YC, ZW, and HJ screened the data. YC, MY, WG, and HRA wrote the manuscript. YL polished the English. All authors read and approved the final manuscript.

Declarations

The research and publication of the research were supported by the Natural Science Foundation Hubei Province of China (2011CDB236 and 2012FFB04903). This article has been published as part of *Human Genomics* Volume 10 Supplement 2, 2016: From genes to systems genomics: human genomics. The full contents of the supplement are available online at http://humgenomics.biomedcentral.com/articles/supplements/volume-10-supplement-2.

Author details

[1]Medical College, Wuhan University of Science and Technology, Wuhan 430065, China. [2]Department of Anesthesiology, Tianyou Hospital, Wuhan University of Science and Technology, Wuhan 430064, China. [3]Texas Advanced Computing Center, University of Texas at Austin, 10100 Burnet Road, Austin, TX 78758, USA. [4]Puren Hospital, Wuhan University of Science and Technology, Wuhan 430081, China. [5]MidSouth Bioinformatics Center, Department of Information Science, George Washington Donaghey College of Engineering and Information Technology and Joint Bioinformatics Graduate Program, University of Arkansas at Little Rock and University of Arkansas for Medical Sciences, 2801 S. University Avenue, Little Rock, AR 72204, USA. [6]Department of Statistics and Harvard School of Public Health, Harvard University, One Oxford St., Cambridge 02138 Massachusetts, USA. [7]Department of Computer Science, University of Georgia, Athens, GA 30602, USA. [8]Department of Internal Medicine and Rush University Cancer Center, Rush University Medical Center, Chicago, IL 60612, USA.

References

1. Polyak K, Weinberg RA. Transitions between epithelial and mesenchymal states: acquisition of malignant and stem cell traits. Nat Rev Cancer. 2009;9:265–73.
2. Thompson EW, Newgreen DF, Tarin D. Carcinoma invasion and metastasis: a role for epithelial-mesenchymal transition. Cancer Res. 2005;65:5991–5.
3. Thiery JP, Sleeman JP. Complex networks orchestrate epithelial-mesenchymal transitions. Nat Rev Mol Cell Biol. 2006;7:131–42.
4. Sanchez-Tillo E, Liu Y, de Barrios O, Siles L, Fanlo L, Cuatrecasas M, et al. EMT-activating transcription factors in cancer: beyond EMT and tumor invasiveness. Cell Mol Life Sci. 2012;69:3429–56.
5. Iwatsuki M, Mimori K, Yokobori T, Ishi H, Beppu T, Nakamori S, et al. Epithelial-mesenchymal transition in cancer development and its clinical significance. Cancer Sci. 2010;101:293–9.
6. Jin H, Yu Y, Zhang T, Zhou X, Zhou J, Jia L, Wu Y, Zhou BP, Feng Y. Snail is critical for tumor growth and metastasis of ovarian carcinoma. Int J Cancer. 2010;126:2102–11.
7. Yanagawa J, Walser TC, Zhu LX, Hong L, Fishbein MC, Mah V, Chia D, Goodglick L, Elashoff DA, Luo J, Magyar CE, Dohadwala M, Lee JM, St John MA, Strieter RM, Sharma S, Dubinett SM. Snail promotes CXCR2 ligand dependent tumor progression in non-small cell lung carcinoma. Clin Cancer Res. 2009;15:6820–9.
8. Kosaka T, Kikuchi E, Mikami S, Miyajima A, Shirotake S, Ishida M, Okada Y, Oya M. Expression of snail in upper urinary tract urothelial carcinoma: prognostic significance and implications for tumor invasion. Clin Cancer Res. 2010;16:5814–23.
9. Muenst S, Daester S, Obermann EC, Droeser RA, Weber WP, von Holzen U, et al. Nuclear expression of snail is an independent negative prognostic factor in human breast cancer. Dis Markers. 2013;35:337–4.
10. Yang MH, Chen CL, Chau GY, Chiou SH, Su CW, Chou TY, Peng WL, Wu JC. Comprehensive analysis of the independent effect of twist and snail in promoting metastasis of hepatocellular carcinoma. Hepatology. 2009;50: 1464–74.
11. Kim MA, Lee HS, Lee HE, Kim JH, Yang HK, Kim WH. Prognostic importance of epithelial-mesenchymal transition-related protein expression in gastric carcinoma. Histopathology. 2009;54:442–51.
12. Ryu HS, do Park J, Kim HH, Kim WH, Lee HS. Combination of epithelial-mesenchymal transition and cancer stem cell-like phenotypes has independent prognostic value in gastric cancer. Hum Pathol. 2012;43:520–8.
13. Shin NR, Jeong EH, Choi CI, Moon HJ, Kwon CH, Chu IS, et al. Overexpression of snail is associated with lymph node metastasis and poor prognosis in patients with gastric cancer. BMC Cancer. 2012;12:521.
14. Higgins JPT, Thompson SG, Deeks JJ, Altman DG. Measuring inconsistency in meta-analyses. Br Med J. 2003;327(7414):557–60.
15. Ioannidis JPA, Patsopoulos NA, Evangelou E. Uncertainty in heterogeneity estimates in meta-analyses. Br Med J. 2007;335(7626):914–6.
16. Zhu Y, Wu J, et al. Expression of TGF-β1, snail, E-cadherin and N-cadherin in gastric cancer and its significance. Chin J Clin Oncol. 2007;4(6):384–9.
17. Tang Z, Zhou Y, et al. Expression and clinical significance of transcriptional factor Snail and adhesion factor E-cadherin in gastric cancer. China J Emerg Resuscitat Disaster Med. 2010;5(8):696–9.
18. Hao Y, Ouyang X, et al. Combined detection of Shh, Glil, snail and E-cadherin expression in gastric cancer and its significance. Chin J Clin Oncol. 2011;38(7):382–5.
19. Wang S, Jiang R, Song W. The expression and significance of snail, E-cadherin protein in gastric carcinoma. Shandong Med. 2011;51(38):48–50.
20. Wang L et al. Expression and significance of Cox-2, snail and E-cadherin in gastric cancer. Lanzhou: Master degree thesis of Lanzhou university; 2011. p. 69.
21. Jin L et al. Expression of Snail, CK18 and Fn in gastric carcinoma and their relations with epithelial-mesenchymal transformation. J Hebei Med Univ. 2011;32(3):313–6.
22. Wu D et al. Expression and clinical significance of snail in gastric cancer. Henan. J Surg. 2012;18(4):26–7.
23. Cao X et al. Expression and significance of snail and E-cadherin in gastric cancer. Acta Acad Med Weifang. 2013;35(1):45–8.
24. Li Q et al. Snail, a zinc-finger transcriptional factor, induces gastric carcinoma invasion and metastasis via suppression of E-cadherin expression. Chin J Biomed Eng. 2013;19(6):433–7.
25. Liu L, Li J. Expression and clinical significance of E-cadherin, snail and twist in gastric cancer tissue and lymph node metastases. J Clin Med Pract. 2014;18(21):71–4.

26. Peinado H, Olmeda D, Cano A. Snail, ZEB and bHLH factors in tumor progression: an alliance against the epithelial phenotype. Nat Rev Cancer. 2007;7(6):415–28.
27. Drasin DJ, Robin TP, Ford HL. Breast cancer epithelial-to-mesenchymal transition: examining the functional consequences of plasticity. Breast Cancer Res. 2011;13:226.
28. Peng Z, Wang CX, Fang EH, Wang GB, Tong Q. Role of epithelial-mesenchymal transition in gastric cancer initiation and progression. World J Gastroenterol. 2014;20:5403–10.
29. Shirakihara T, Saitoh M, Miyazono K. Differential regulation of epithelial and mesenchymal markers by deltaEF1 proteins in epithelial mesenchymal transition induced by TGF-beta. Mol Biol Cell. 2007;18:3533–44.
30. Lascombe I, Clairotte A, Fauconnet S, Bernardini S, Wallerand H, Kantelip B, et al. N-cadherin as a novel prognostic marker of progression in superficial urothelial tumors. Clin Cancer Res. 2006;12:2780–7.
31. Hui L, Zhang S, Dong X, Tian D, Cui Z, Qiu X. Prognostic significance of twist and N-cadherin expression in NSCLC. PLoS One. 2013;8:e62171.
32. Alexander NR, Tran NL, Rekapally H, Summers CE, Glackin C, Heimark RL. N-cadherin gene expression in prostate carcinoma is modulated by integrin-dependent nuclear translocation of Twist1. Cancer Res. 2006;66:3365–9.
33. Yang J, Mani SA, Donaher JL, Ramaswamy S, Itzykson RA, Come C, Savagner P, Gitelman I,Richardson A, Weinberg RA. Twist, a master regulator of morphogenesis, plays an essential role in tumor metastasis. Cell. 2004;117: 927–39.
34. Fabregat I, Malfettone A, Soukupova J. New Insights into the Crossroads between EMT and Stemness in the Context of Cancer. Edel MJ, ed. J Clin Med. 2016;5(3):37.
35. Vandewalle C, Van Roy F, Berx G. The role of the ZEB family of transcription factors in development and disease. Cell Mol Life Sci. 2009;66:773–87.
36. Rosivatz E, Becker I, Specht K, Fricke E, Luber B, Busch R, Hofler H, Becker KF. Differential expression of the epithelial-mesenchymal transition regulators snail, SIP1, and twist in gastric cancer. Am J Pathol. 2002;161:1881–91.

10

Hypomethylation coordinates antagonistically with hypermethylation in cancer development

Garima Kushwaha[1,2], Mikhail Dozmorov[3], Jonathan D. Wren[4], Jing Qiu[5], Huidong Shi[6,7*] and Dong Xu[1,2,8*]

Abstract

Background: Methylation changes are frequent in cancers, but understanding how hyper- and hypomethylated region changes coordinate, associate with genomic features, and affect gene expression is needed to better understand their biological significance. The functional significance of hypermethylation is well studied, but that of hypomethylation remains limited. Here, with paired expression and methylation samples gathered from a patient/control cohort, we attempt to better characterize the gene expression and methylation changes that take place in cancer from B cell chronic lymphocyte leukemia (B-CLL) samples.

Results: Across the dataset, we found that consistent differentially hypomethylated regions (C-DMRs) across samples were relatively few compared to the many poorly consistent hypo- and highly conserved hyper-DMRs. However, genes in the hypo-C-DMRs tended to be associated with functions antagonistic to those in the hyper-C-DMRs, like differentiation, cell-cycle regulation and proliferation, suggesting coordinated regulation of methylation changes. Hypo-C-DMRs in B-CLL were found enriched in key signaling pathways like B cell receptor and p53 pathways and genes/motifs essential for B lymphopoiesis. Hypo-C-DMRs tended to be proximal to genes with elevated expression in contrast to the transcription silencing-mechanism imposed by hypermethylation. Hypo-C-DMRs tended to be enriched in the regions of activating H4K4me1/2/3, H3K79me2, and H3K27ac histone modifications. In comparison, the polycomb repressive complex 2 (PRC2) signature, marked by *EZH2*, *SUZ12*, *CTCF* binding-sites, repressive H3K27me3 marks, and "repressed/poised promoter" states were associated with hyper-C-DMRs. Most hypo-C-DMRs were found in introns (36 %), 3′ untranslated regions (29 %), and intergenic regions (24 %). Many of these genic regions also overlapped with enhancers. The methylation of CpGs from 3′UTR exons was found to have weak but positive correlation with gene expression. In contrast, methylation in the 5′UTR was negatively correlated with expression. To better characterize the overlap between methylation and expression changes, we identified correlation modules that associate with "apoptosis" and "leukocyte activation".

Conclusions: Despite clinical heterogeneity in disease presentation, a number of methylation changes, both hypo and hyper, appear to be common in B-CLL. Hypomethylation appears to play an active, targeted, and complementary role in cancer progression, and it interplays with hypermethylation in a coordinated fashion in the cancer process.

Keywords: Epigenetic regulation, DNA methylation, Hypomethylation, CLL, Cancer, Signaling pathway, 3′UTR, Enhancer

* Correspondence: hshi@gru.edu; xudong@missouri.edu
[6]GRU Cancer Center, Georgia Regents University, Augusta, GA 30912, USA
[1]Christopher S. Bond Life Sciences Center, University of Missouri, Columbia, MO 65211, USA
Full list of author information is available at the end of the article

Background

Loss of DNA methylation, also known as hypomethylation, in cancer cells relative to normal cells was one of the first-described epigenetic changes in human cancers. Hypomethylation has been detected at both a global level and on a local scale [1] in cancer genomes. Many cancer types have been reported to have global loss of methylation like glioblastoma [2], ovarian epithelial carcinoma [3], prostate metastatic tumors [4], B cell chronic lymphocytic leukemia [5, 6], hepatocellular carcinoma [7], cervical cancer [8], colon adenocarcinoma [9], and Wilms' tumor [10]. However, the biological significance of DNA hypomethylation remains understudied owning to its unclear role in carcinogenesis, in contrast to hypermethylation, which is commonly viewed as a transcription silencing mechanism [11, 12]. Yet, hypomethylation of DNA, despite its unclear role, has been linked to tumor progression [8, 13] in different tumor types and in individual specimens [3, 14]. Also, some experiments have indicated the importance of induced DNA hypomethylation in oncogenesis by using DNA methylation inhibitors in vivo and in vitro [15, 16]. However, the role of hypomethylation is not clearly understood. Hence, it is critical to analyze hypomethylation data in depth to achieve a better understanding of its biological roles in carcinogenesis.

DNA hypomethylation in cancer is often seen in satellite DNAs, Arthrobacter luteus (ALU) repeats, and long interspersed nuclear elements (LINEs) [17, 18], etc. These DNA repeats comprise approximately half of the genome. Hence, DNA hypomethylation is generally considered a global phenomenon not suitable for use as a biomarker. One advantage of the global hypomethylation phenomenon (as it pertains to its genome composition) is that it is often considered a technique to balance focal and conserved hypermethylation in the promoter regions of key genes. Also, it is believed that these hypomethylated genomic regions are randomly spread over the genome, mostly in repetitive regions whose functions, if any, are unclear. Again, this reported disadvantage might actually be an advantage due to recent findings indicating that ALU elements can act as enhancers [19], which further emphasizes the need for defining the role of hypomethylation in cancers.

As part of our study of hypomethylation patterns, we used B cell chronic lymphocytic leukemia (B-CLL) as an example case. This B-CLL cancer type has a predominant global hypomethylation as its characteristic feature [5, 6], and it is the most common form of blood cancer. It is a clinically heterogeneous disease, with some patients experiencing rapid disease progression and others living for decades without requiring treatment [20]. Although a number of cellular and molecular prognostic markers, i.e., surface markers *ZAP70* and *CD38*, cytogenetic abnormalities, and IGHV mutational status [21–23], have been identified to help classify CLL into molecular and clinical subgroups and to predict their course of progression, they do not provide clear insight into the underlying biology necessary to develop better targeted and more effective treatments.

In addition to various molecular and genetic changes, several genome-wide DNA methylation studies have identified many aberrantly methylated genes in CLL samples [24]. Initially, DNA hypermethylation in CLL patients was found to affect 4.8 % of CpG islands on average [25]. Furthermore, hypermethylation in the promoters of tumor suppressor genes such as *DAPK1* [26], *SFRP1* [27], and *ID4* [28] genes involved in apoptosis, cell cycle regulators *p16* and *p15* [29], and prognostic markers *ZAP70* [21] and *TWIST2* [30] were identified. DNA methylation changes were also found to be associated with disease progression in the E_{μ}-TCL1 transgenic mouse model of CLL [28]. In addition to hypermethylation, hypomethylation of proto-oncogenes has also been observed particularly in liver tumors and leukemia such as the *c-fos*, *c-myc*, *ras*, *Erb-A1* [31], and the *bcl-2* gene [32]. Along with this, many studies have indicated widespread hypomethylation compared to instances of hypermethylation, particularly in the CLL cancer type. However, a detailed account on the genome-wide hypomethylation pattern and its contributing role towards cancer development has not been conducted for CLL. Hence, it is clear that an in-depth methylation analysis focusing more on hypomethylation can be very helpful to unveil the underlying mechanism regulating the disease.

Here, we studied the genome-wide DNA methylation pattern in CLL and investigated whether hypomethylation is also consistent at some locations like hypermethylation across multiple CLL patients. We also investigated the biological role of consistent hypomethylation towards tumor initiation and progression; and finally, we compared instances of consistent hypomethylation to that of consistent hypermethylation. We characterized the epigenetic context of hyper- and hypomethylated regions in CLL and further investigated association of hypomethylation with change in expression of the neighborhood genes along with their potential mechanism of influence.

Results

Methylation data analysis

In order to study genome-wide methylation changes in the CLL genome, we computed differentially methylated regions (DMRs) from genome-wide methylation data of 30 samples from publically available CLL samples in GEO (http://www.ncbi.nlm.nih.gov/geo/). DMRs of size 1000 bp were obtained by comparing each patient sample against each control normal sample individually using Fisher's exact test. False discovery rate (FDR) was used to correct for multiple testing errors with a q value threshold of 0.01. Hence, three sets of DMRs were obtained by comparing all 30 CLL samples against each of the three control samples.

Entropy and permutation analysis

Having obtained a list of all hypo- and hyper-DMRs for each CLL against each control sample, we first plotted the distribution of the number of samples in which each DMR (hypo and hyper) existed. Figure 1a shows that the majority of hypo-DMRs are present in less than 50 % of samples. Out of the DMRs present in 20 or more samples, hyper-DMRs outnumbered hypo-DMRs. This showed that overall hypomethylated regions are less conserved than hypermethylated regions across samples.

Next, in order to check randomness in contrast to conservation of methylation change in each 1000 bp region across all CLL samples, methylation entropies were calculated using a probability distribution of methylation changes for each region. Figure 1b shows this opposite pattern of entropy and average methylation change. This plot shows that a high percentage methylation of specific regions is more consistent across all patients; however, as the average methylation goes down, their conservation tends to fluctuate, thereby leading to an increase in entropy (Fig. 1b). After comparing these methylation entropies for each region against the average methylation change across 30 CLL samples, we observed a negative correlation (Pearson correlation = −0.22, p value <0.05) in each of the 3-control sample tests.

Identification of consistent differentially methylated regions (C-DMRs)

In order to obtain consistent DMRs, a binomial test was used to check the significance of each DMR with the probability of being hypo/hypermethylated in 25 or more CLL samples (q value <0.01). Hence, three lists of significant DMRs were obtained for each control sample. Next, 658 hypo- and 982 hypermethylated regions that were found common in all three lists and referred to as C-DMRs (see Tables S1–S4 in Additional file 1 and Additional file 2 for lists and details).

To further check the statistical significance of our lists of hypo- and hyper-C-DMRs, we performed two permutation tests, one by permuting samples and the other by permuting methylation values for 1000 bp regions (see Methods in Additional file 1 for more details). The sample permutation test helped in detecting whether we observed hyper/hypo-C-DMR patterns by chance if there was no difference among cancer vs. normal samples. On the other hand, the methylated region permutation test detected whether hyper/hypo-C-DMR pattern can occur by chance if there is no difference between regions. In both permutation tests, all of our obtained C-DMRs had q values <0.05, showing the statistical significance of hyper- and hypo-C-DMRs in cancer samples against normal and non-DMRs.

Differences in positional genomic location analysis of hyper- and hypo-C-DMRs

By checking the genomic-location distribution of C-DMRs, we found that a higher number of hyper-C-DMRs mapped to promoters (64 %) and 5′UTRs (43 %) as compared to hypo-C-DMRs (14 % for promoters and 12 % for 5′UTR) and genomic background regions (30 % for promoters and 29 % for 5′UTRs). A higher percentage of promoter and 5′UTR hypermethylation confirmed their role in interfering with transcription factor binding (Fig. 2a, b). However, hypo-C-DMRs outnumbered both hyper-C-DMRs and background genomic regions for 3′UTRs (29 % in hypo-C-DMRs, 8 % in hyper-C-DMRs, and 7 % in background) and introns (36 % in hypo-C-DMRs, 4 % in hyper-C-DMRs, and 15 % in background). There were also more hypo-C-DMRs (24 %) in the intergenic regions than hyper-C-DMRs (18 %), but comparable with genomic background regions (26 %). CpG sites from hypo- and hyper-C-DMRs were also checked against "weak/strong enhancer regions" chromatin states as defined by chromHMM [33] and were found coming mostly from intronic and intergenic regions on a genome. (Figure S6 in Additional file 1). Strong enhancers were overlapped more by hypo-C-DMRs in comparison to hyper-C-DMRs. Genes overlapping with hypomethylated strong enhancers were *ELN, GTF2I, KLC1, MIF4GD, MIR6821, MOB2, PTBP1, RGS3, SH3BGRL3, TBC1D14, TCIRG1*, and *VASH2*.

Across each sample data, we found 25–30 % of all DMRs as hypomethylated, and only 10–15 % hypermethylated, as shown in Figure S1 in Additional file 1. However, they were not targeted for any specific chromosomal region (Figure S2 in Additional file 1). Also, only 100 hypo-C-DMRs (15.2 %) co-localized with CpG islands, while 955 out of 982 hyper-C-DMRs (97.2 %) co-localized with CpG islands. Hypo-C-DMRs were mostly present in regions outside CpG islands and shores (Fig. 2c). Next, Fig. 2d shows that almost half of hypo-C-DMRs (46 %) were present on non-repeat regions along with ones mapped on the repeat regions. Overall, hypo-C-DMRs were found more in 3′UTR, intronic, and intergenic regions, mostly outside CpG islands and overlapping both repeat and non-repeat regions over enhancers. Additional file 3 lists the genes with genic-regions overlapped by these C-DMRs.

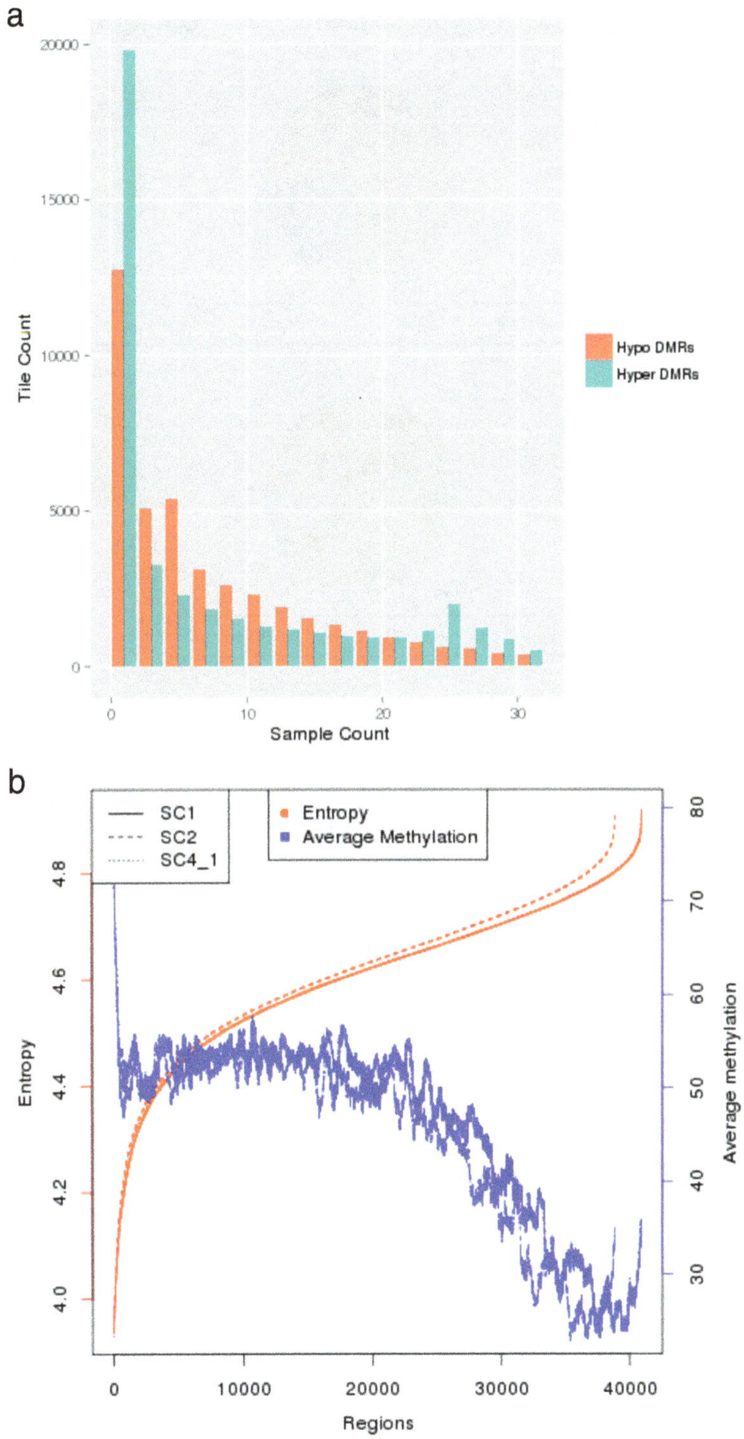

Fig. 1 Overall representation of methylation. **a** Distribution of hyper/hypo-DMRs (tiles) over number of samples. This illustration shows that a higher proportion of hypo-DMRs (compared to hyper-DMRs) are consistent in small subsets of samples. It also shows the presence of few hypo-DMRs present in all 30 samples. **b** Relationship between average methylation difference across all CLL patients against control samples (SC1, SC2, and SC4_1) and methylation entropy per 1000 bp region

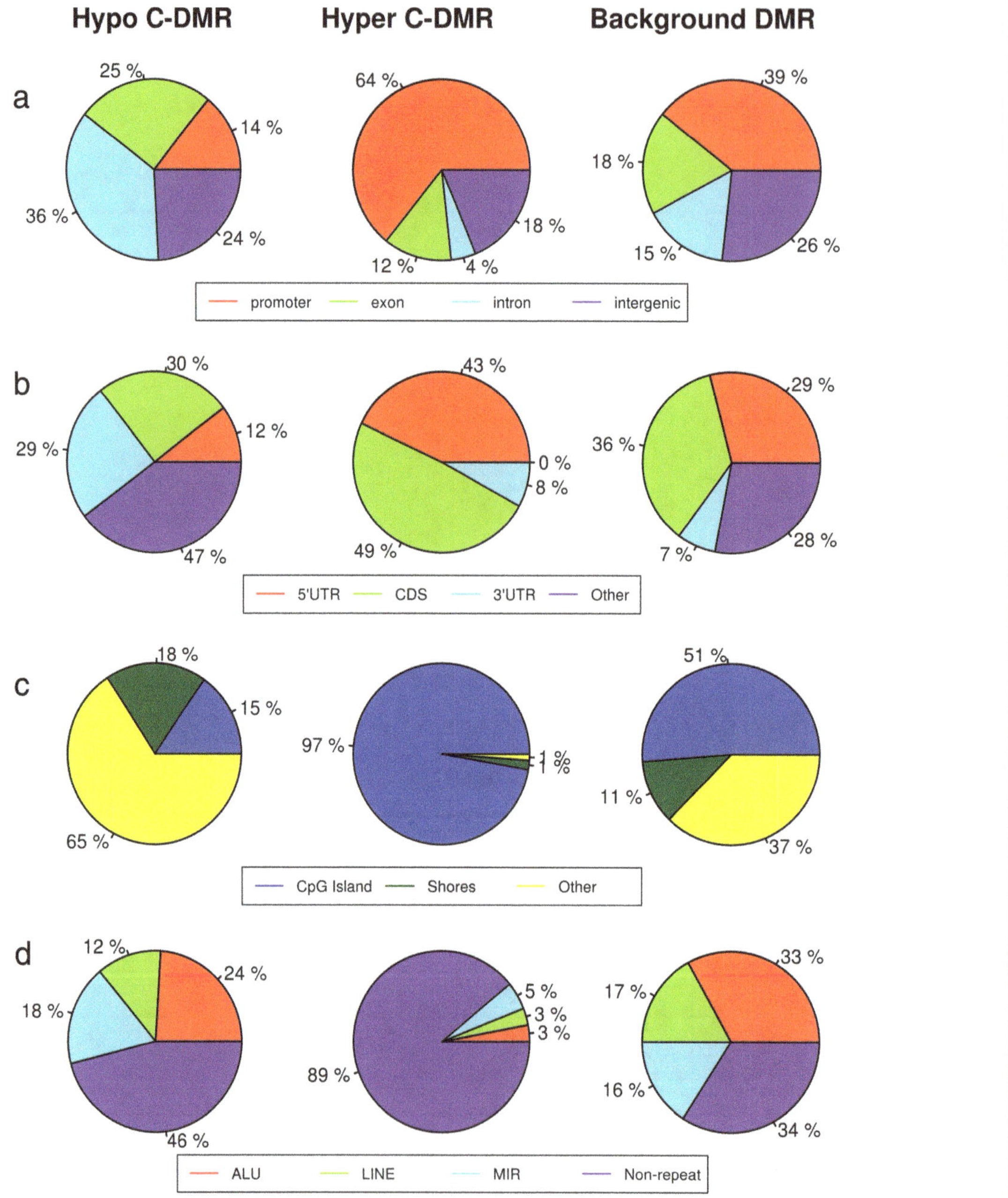

Fig. 2 Distributions of C-DMRs. **a**, **b** Over different genic parts. **c** Over CpG islands. **d** Over genomic repeats and non-repeat regions

Enrichment of KEGG pathways, GO annotations and phenotypes

For our obtained lists of hypo- and hyper-C-DMRs, we performed enrichment analysis of genes overlapped by C-DMRs (Additional file 3) for gene ontology (GO) [34] categories and KEGG [35] pathways. The most significantly enriched KEGG pathways in hypo-C-DMRs were "B cell receptor (BCR) signaling pathway" (adjusted p value (p.adj) = 2.21E-02), "*p53* signaling pathway" (p.adj = 3.69E-02), and "pathways in cancer" (p.adj = 3.69E-02), along with a few other signaling pathways and pathways involved in cancer. In contrast, hyper-C-DMRs were not enriched for any leukemia-related pathway such as *BCR* signaling. Hyper-C-DMRs were enriched for "neuroactive ligand-receptor interaction" (p.adj = 7.29E-05) and for the "calcium-signaling pathway" (p.adj = 9.86E-03) (Fig. 3). See Additional file 4 for complete enrichment results.

Among the GO annotations, the most important and significantly enriched biological processes for hypo-C-DMRs were "negative regulation of transcription" (p.adj = 4.28E-02), "chromatin modification" (p.adj = 3.92E-02),

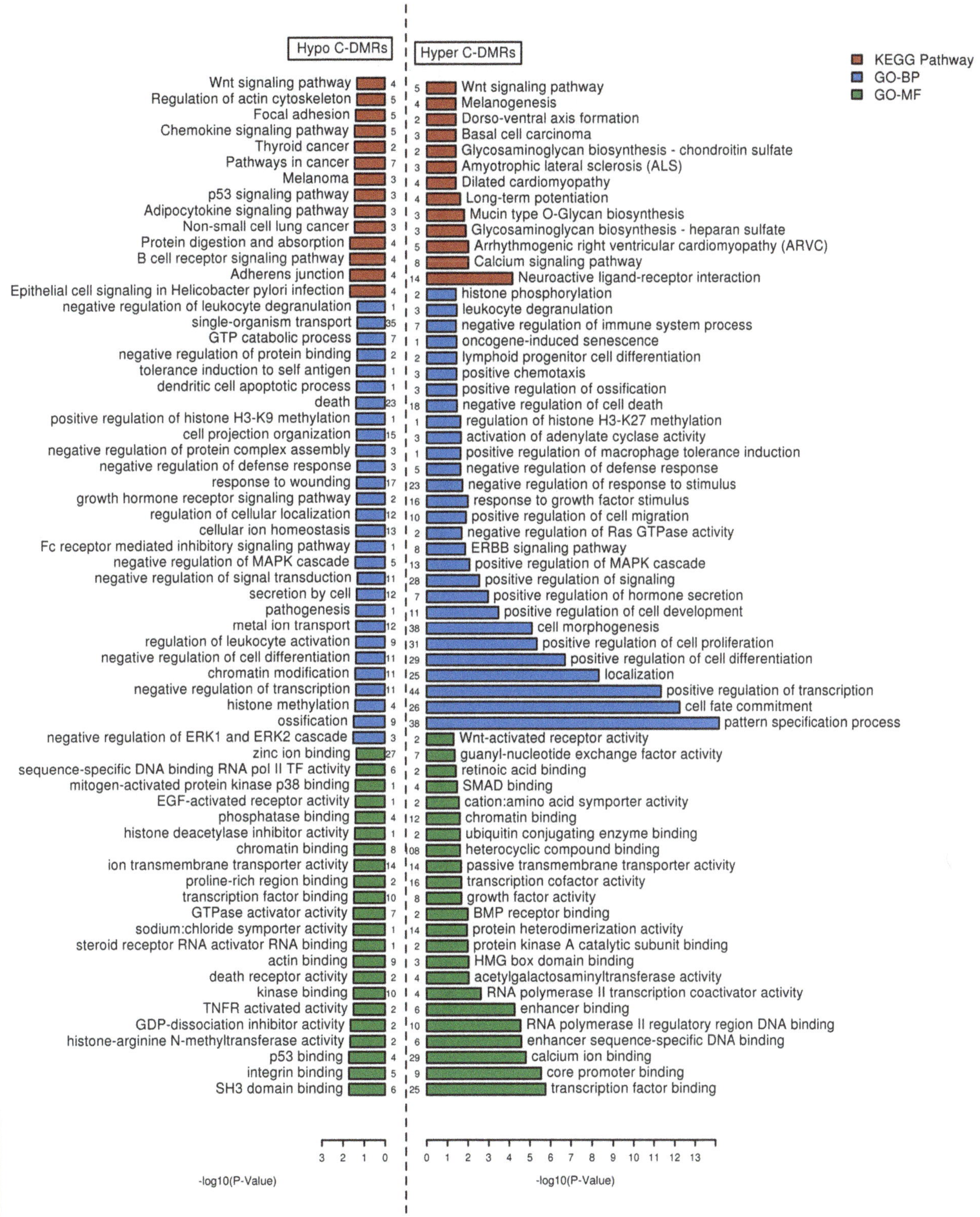

Fig. 3 GO annotation and KEGG pathway enrichment for C-DMRs

"regulation of signaling" (p.adj = 3.92E-02), "histone methylation" (p.adj = 3.92E-02); "positive regulation of histone H3-K9 methylation" (p.adj = 4.29E-02), "protein alkylation" (p.adj = 4.28E-02), "programmed cell death" (p.adj = 4.30E-02), "negative regulation of cell proliferation" (p.adj = 4.40E-02), and "negative regulation of leukocyte differentiation" (p.adj = 3.04E-02), "leukocyte activation" (p.adj = 4.28E-02), and "cell morphogenesis involved in differentiation" (p.adj = 4.29E-02). On the other hand, hyper-C-DMRs were enriched for processes which are antagonistic to the processes enriched in hypo-C-DMRs. Hyper-C-DMRs were enriched for processes like "positive regulation of transcription" (p.adj = 4.81E-12) and "positive regulation of cell differentiation" (p.adj = 1.99E-07), "positive regulation cell proliferation" (p.adj = 4.75E-06), "regulation of signaling" (p.adj = 3.53E-05) with more processes related to "cell-fate commitment" (p.adj = 6.09E-13), "cell morphogenesis involved in differentiation" (p.adj = 7.69E-08), and similar processes like "protein and cell localization" (p.adj = 4.77E-06). Also, hypo-C-DMRs were enriched for "H3K9 methylation" but hyper for "H3-K27 methylation."

Molecular functions (Fig. 3) showed a strong enrichment for binding functions like "protein binding" (like integrin, p.adj = 1.92E-02), "SH3 domain binding" (p.adj = 1.92E-02), "p53 binding" (p.adj = 1.92E-02), "histone-arginine *N*-methyltransferase activity" (p.adj = 2.20E-02), "tumor necrosis factor-activated receptor activity" (p.adj = 3.20E-02), GTPase regulator activity (p.adj = 3.20E-02), and "transcription factor binding" (p.adj = 3.40E-02) in hypo-C-DMRs. In comparison, hyper-C-DMRs were specifically highly enriched for "sequence-specific DNA binding" (p.adj = 5.49E-32), transcription factor (or regulator, p.adj = 3.86E-25), and transmembrane transporter activity (p.adj = 6.58E-03), along with also metal/ion (calcium, p.adj = 6.72E-07) and "enhancer binding" (p.adj = 5.47E-05). In summary, both C-DMR types (hypo and hyper) affected similar processes but in different directions, with hypomethylation focusing on transcription and leukocyte activation and hypermethylation focusing on transcription suppression through transcription factors and cell-fate commitment.

We did not observe any differences in enriched phenotypes between hypo- and hyper-C-DMRs. Specific associations with the hematopoietic system, homeostasis/metabolism, mortality/aging, immune system, and growth/size phenotype were enriched in both types of C-DMRs, except embryogenesis (or related terms like differentiation), which was specific to hypermethylation. Genes falling under each enriched top attribute are listed in Additional file 5. These results suggest the importance of both hypo- and hyper-C-DMRs in CLL, and emphasize the functional significance of hypo-C-DMRs.

Enrichment of TFBS, histone modifications, and chromatin states

Next, in order to identify epigenomic signatures associated with both C-DMRs, we systematically tested for enrichment in transcription factor binding sites (TFBSs), histone modification marks, and chromatin states provided by ENCODE project [36].

TFBS enrichment analysis identified EZH2 as strongly associated with hyper-C-DMRs (p.adj = 1.70E-23), in contrast to hypo-C-DMRs (p.adj = 4.27E-05, Fig. 4a). On the contrary, *EBF1, POL2, CHD2, WHIP,* and *TBLR1* were strongly associated with hypo-C-DMRs (p.adj = 2.53E-37, 1.06E-30, 2.17E-22, 6.024E-22, and 5.78E-19, respectively), in contrast to hyper-C-DMRs (p.adj = 1.65E-09 and 3.50E-07) (Fig. 4). Other than these, the HAIB dataset in ENCODE showed additional B lymphopoiesis-related enriched TFBS like *RUNX3* (p.adj = 3.58E-31), *TCF3* (p.adj = 4.04E-14), *PU.1* (p.adj = 7.42E-11), and *PAX5* (p.adj = 7.43E-11). Both hyper- and hypo-C-DMRs were enriched in *ZNF143, CTCF, MAZ,* and *MXI1* TFBSs (Fig. 4a). These findings were confirmed by using TFBS data from all cell lines provided by the ENCODE project (Figure S3 (a), S4 in Additional file 1 and Additional file 6).

Among histone modification marks, we found H3K27me3 to be highly enriched in hyper-C-DMRs (Fig. 4b, p.adj = 2.31E-40). On the contrary, hypo-C-DMRs were strongly enriched in H3K4me1 (p.adj = 1.11E-54), H3K27ac (p.adj = 1.22E-38), and H3K79me2 (p.adj = 1.44E-34) histone modification marks (Fig. 4b). Both C-DMRs were enriched in H3K4me2, H3K4me3, and H2AZ histone modification marks (Fig. 4a). The specificity of the H3K27me3 mark for hyper-C-DMRs was confirmed by using histone modification data from all cell lines provided by the ENCODE project (Figure S3 (b) in Additional file 1 and Additional file 6).

Furthermore, hyper-C-DMRs were significantly enriched for homeobox, *E2F* and TATAbox/promoter motifs, and hypo-C-DMRS for *ETS, IRF4, EGR, ZFX, RUNX1, PU.1, Pax5, BATF, Erra,* and *bZIP* motifs (Table S5 in Additional file 1). All motifs enriched for hypo-C-DMR have been shown to contribute to cell proliferation, B cell development and pathogenesis of lymphomas [37–39].

Using chromatin state annotations from multiple cell lines (Figure S3 (c) in Additional file 1 and Additional file 6), we found hyper-C-DMRs to be enriched in "repressed" (p.adj = 5.63E-182) and "poised promoters" (p.adj = 1.24E-69) chromatin states (Fig. 4c). In contrast, hypo-C-DMRs were consistently enriched in both "strong/weak enhancers" (p.adj = 6.73E-36 for both) and "weak transcription" (p.adj = 2.73E-24). Both C-DMRs were similarly enriched in "weak promoters" (p.adj = 1.70E-19 and 2.93E-15 for hyper- and hypo-C-DMRs, respectively). These results suggest that distant enhancer regions tend to be hypomethylated in cancer whereas regions associated with repressed or poised transcription are hypermethylated.

Also, 17,811 hyper- and 15,599 hypo-differentially methylated regions (DMRs) were obtained from pooled CLL and control sample comparison (Table S2 in Additional file 1). Each of these region lists exhaustively included all hyper- and hypo-C-DMRs, respectively. KEGG and GO annotation enrichment analysis of

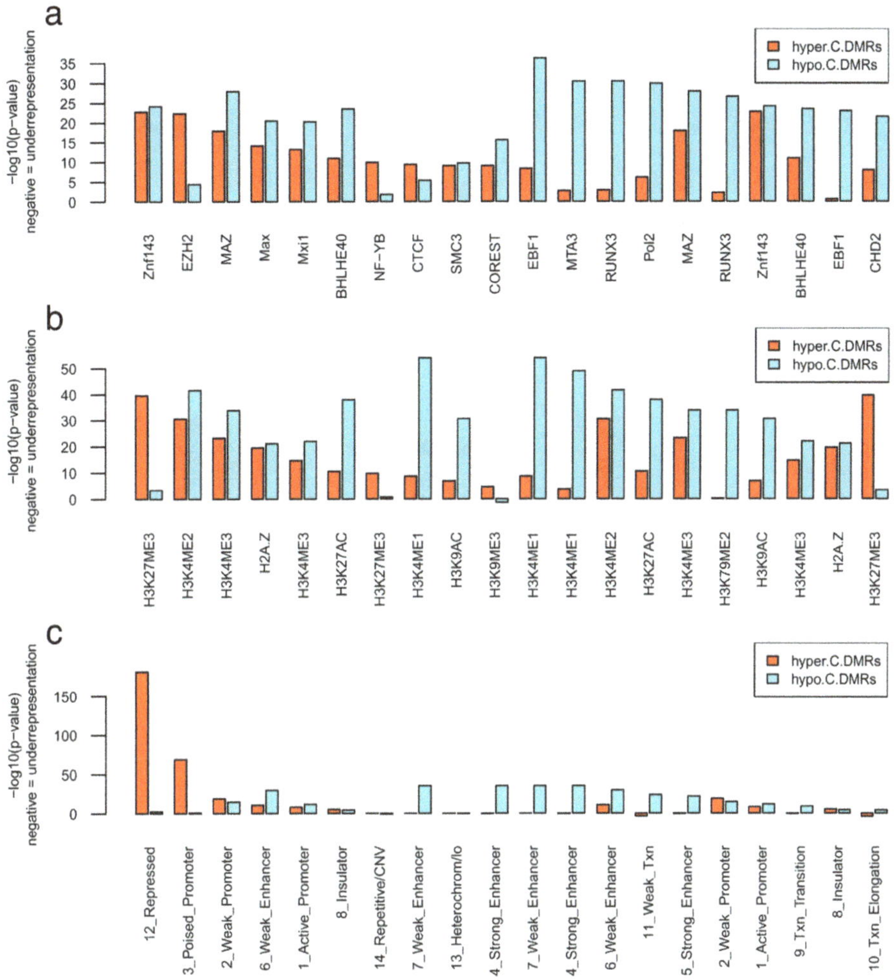

Fig. 4 Enrichment of C-DMRs in the regulatory regions. The ENCODE genome annotation datasets for Gm12878 lymphoblastoid cell line from Broad and Stanford/Yale/USC/Harvard were used for transcription factor and Histone enrichment analyses (**a**, **b**). Broad datasets were used for chromatin states enrichment (**c**). See Figures S3, S4 in Additional file 1 for the results for all cell lines. The vertical axis shows −log10-transformed enrichment *p* values, FDR corrected. Left/right parts of the *bar-plots* show top 10 most significant enrichments for hyper/hypo-C-DMRs, respectively. **a** Transcription factor binding sites enrichment. **b** Histone modification sites enrichment. **c** Chromatin states enrichment

pooled sample DMRs also showed a strong enrichment of similar terms (Additional files 1 and 4). Results from pooled sample analysis show that C-DMRs are more specific and significant subset of DMRs that are consistently present in all samples.

Expression data analysis

Expression profiles in relation with methylation

Next, we looked at the association between gene expression changes and methylation differences. For this, expression values of all transcripts from 19 matching CLL samples were divided into four expression quartiles and referred to as lowest to highest expression groups. Methylation profiles for genes in each of these quartiles were then extracted for comparison. Figure 5a shows a significant reduction of methylation at gene boundaries for all expression quartile groups. At the peripheral region, methylation in the highest expression genes is reduced the most. Towards the center, methylation of CpGs and expression has an inverse relationship, with the lowest expression genes having the lowest percent methylation. Overall, average methylation for whole gene regions for all genes had a negative correlation (Pearson correlation = −0.07; *p* value = 3.1E-09) with expression.

Next, we looked for expression (transcript FPKM values) and methylation (for overlapped CpG sites) relationship in exons and introns individually (Fig. 5d, e). We observed that among exons (Fig. 5d), transcripts in the lowest expression quartile had the highest and most distinct methylation pattern. Overall, all exons combined from transcripts in all expression quartiles had a negative correlation (corr = −0.13; *p* value <2.2E-16). For introns (Fig. 5e), this relationship appeared to be opposite with the highest expression quartile transcripts showing the highest methylation but almost no correlation

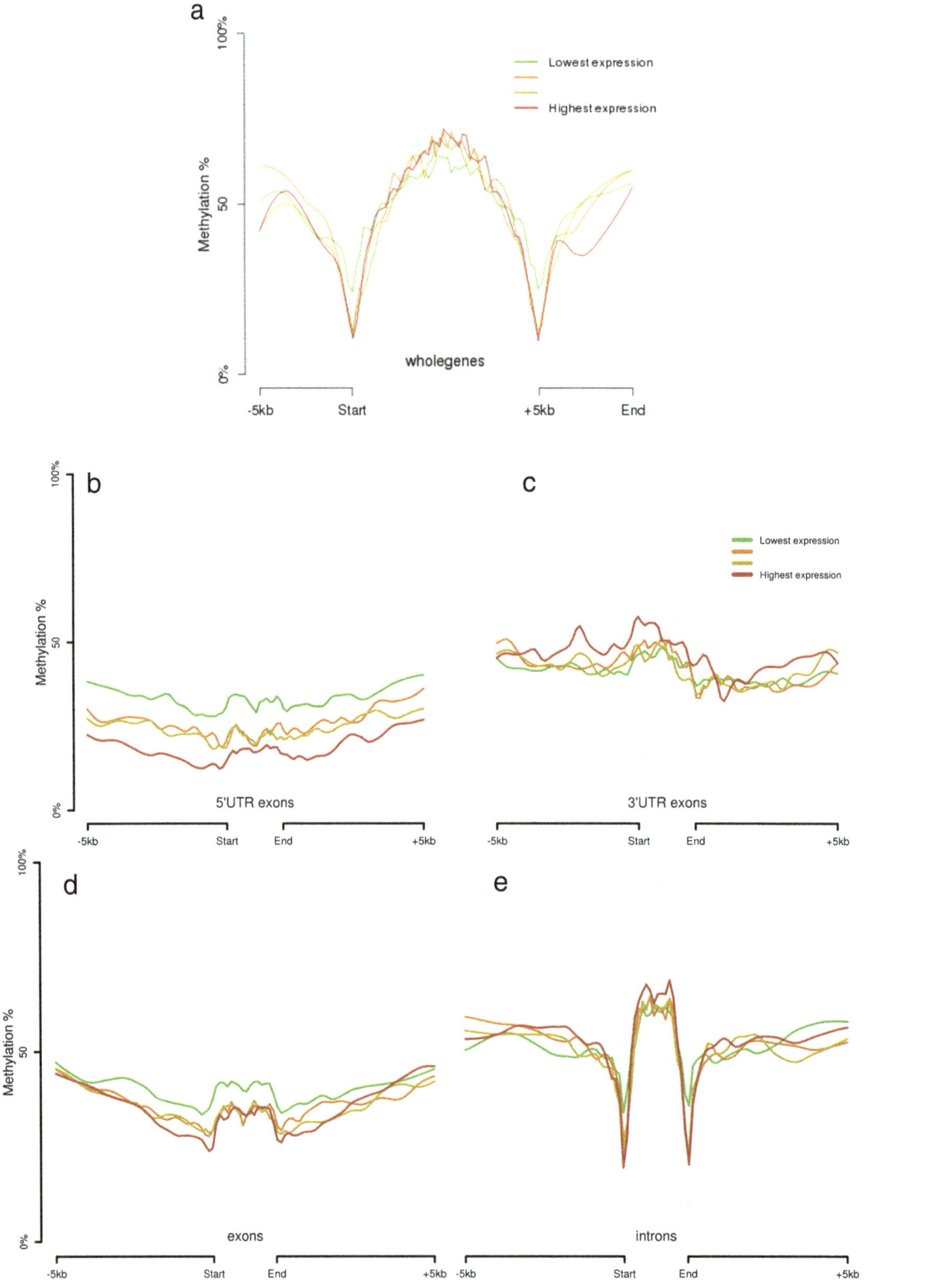

Fig. 5 Association between DNA methylation and expression in CLL samples. **a** Local regression showing methylation levels of whole genes stratified by expression quartiles in CLL samples. **b** Local regression showing methylation levels within 5′ and 3′UTRs for different transcripts stratified by expression quartiles. **c** Methylation levels within exons and introns for transcripts in different expression quartiles. **d** Methylation levels at exon boundary in different expression quartiles. **e** Methylation levels at intron boundary in different expression quartiles

(corr = −0.02; *p* value = 6.2E-2). Also, we identified a very clear distinction in methylation patterns from different expression quartiles in exons specifically from 5'UTRs (Fig. 5b). Overall, 5'UTRs had a negative correlation between methylation and expression (corr = −0.2; *p* value <2.2E-16). Conversely, exons from 3'UTRs had the opposite methylation pattern (Fig. 5c). 3'UTR exons from the highest expression quartile genes had the highest methylation (Fig. 5d, Figure S8 in Additional file 1) and overall, they had weak but positive correlation (corr = 0.1; *p* value = 2.4E-3). In summary, we observed different methylation effects on expression for different genic regions, particularly within exons from 5'UTR and 3'UTR that related to methylation changes at widespread genomic locations in CLL.

Correlation module analysis

In order to further investigate the role of 3'UTR methylation change on expression, we used both expression and methylation data to construct co-expression and co-differential methylation network modules, respectively. These modules were generated using the weighted gene correlation network analysis (WGCNA) framework [40]. For this, we selected 1780 transcripts from 19 matching CLL samples, from which both expression and average 3'UTR methylation data were available.

WGCNA identified 21 co-expression modules with sizes ranging from 41 to 181 transcripts from the expression data and 17 co-differential methylation modules with sizes ranging from 37 to 284 transcripts from the methylation data (average of all CpGs within 3'UTRs). Methylation values of transcripts in each CLL sample were compared against methylation of transcripts from one common control sample, individually. Differential methylation values for all transcripts in all CLL samples were thus obtained. Correlation network modules in each dataset were obtained using hierarchical clustering of pairwise gene correlation structures using WGCNA. WGCNA does not use gene ontology information but clusters the interconnected genes defined as branches of a hierarchical cluster tree. Hence, modules are initially labeled by arbitrary integers and then coded by colors for each dataset. Since clustering for module generation has no gene annotation or functional information, functional interpretation for each module in each dataset was further obtained by conducting a GO enrichment analysis. GO enrichment analyses revealed unique and significant enrichment of various GO terms, providing evidence of a functional role for each module as a whole (Additional file 7; Tables S2, S3, S8, and S9 in Additional file 1). Overall, different biological processes for different modules implied biological significance of clustering transcripts in separate modules in both expression and methylation data.

Next, to investigate the relationship between expression and methylation modules, these modules were matched by pairwise comparison of each methylation module to each expression module using two methods. First, they were compared to measure a statistically significant overlap of genes in each pair. Second, we used network-based statistics to assess whether the density and connectivity patterns of genes were also preserved in a two-paired set of modules with significant gene overlaps. The second method generated a composite statistic value, i.e., $Z_{summary}$, using a permutation test to measure the strength of methylation module and expression module preservation. Also, knowing the $Z_{summary}$ statistic bias towards a module with a large size, a rank-based statistic *medianRank* was used in the second method to measure their relative preservation irrespective of module size. The medianRank is the statistic calculated from observed preservation values and does not conduct any permutation test against background gene modules.

From network preservation tests, we found that expression and differential methylation modules in general exhibited relatively few overlapping genes (Additional file 7) although some of the overlaps were statistically significant. The most significant overlaps (p.adj < 0.05) were observed between large co-expression modules and co-differential methylation modules, enriched for same GO terms (Table 1 and Additional file 7; Table S4 in Additional file 1). Figure 6a reports the number of common genes resulting from pairwise module overlap analysis. The statistical significance of each pair as shown by a color scale was computed to see if the numbers of common genes were obtained according to an iterative pattern and not by chance. WGCNA arbitrarily color-code modules for visual identification, so all color-module associations described here do not have any additional meaning outside of this specific analysis. The most significant overlap as shown in Fig. 6a was for "turquoise" color-coded expression module with "magenta," "yellow", and "midnight blue" methylation module. The turquoise expression module also had the highest $Z_{summary}$ ($Z_{summary} = 28$) and median rank from network-based statistic method (Fig. 6b). GO enrichment analysis of the turquoise expression module showed enrichment of "*TNFR*," "cell adhesion," "leukocyte proliferation," and "apoptosis/cell death." All the overlapping methylation modules which were color-coded in magenta (enriched for "*EGF*" p.adj = 1.60E-02), yellow (enriched for "focal adhesion and kinases"), midnight blue (enriched for "cofactor and ion binding") were enriched for growth factor and regulation of "Ras protein signal transduction," "kinase activity," and "ion binding." Hence, we see that the most significantly overlapping and preserved modules in CLL samples were the ones involved in cancer development. This also indicates the regulatory role of 3′UTR methylation on expression change in cancer.

Also, "green," "pink," "blue," "black," and "grey60" color-coded expression modules were the other top

Table 1 Significant overlap and preserved modules in WGCNA of 3′UTR methylation and expression

Methylation module (size)	Expression module (size)	Overlap count (*p* value)	$Z_{summary}$	Median rank	Functional annotation	Gene symbols
Magenta (79)	Turquoise (181)	20 (6.17E-05)	28	6	Regulation of Ras protein signal transduction	*ABCC3,ALS2CL,ATG16L2,COG8,DNASE1, DOCK9,ESPL1,PDE4D,TMEM63C,TNFAIP2, TNFRSF4,TTLL1,UQCC1,ZNF385A*
Red (101)	Grey60 (52)	9 (2.04E-03)	13	19	Cell division and chromosome partitioning/cytoskeleton	*CHID1,FDXR,HERC2,HERC6,MYO9B, SEPT5,UBXN7*
Yellow (165)	Turquoise (181)	28 (3.18E-03)	28	6	Kinases	*ATG16L2,BMP1,C1orf159,CLUH,COL6A2, CRTC1,DAGLA,DNAH3,ENTHD2,EPHA10, FAM101B,FAM53A,GPR56,IGF1R,LAMC3, NLRP2,NR3C2,OPLAH,PITPNM2,PPP2R2B, PRKCA,PTPRK,RASGRF1,STK32C,THNSL2*
Turquoise (284)	Blue (176)	41 (4.83E-03)	13	18	Signaling and apoptosis, cell cycle checkpoint	*ACOXL,ANKH,ARHGEF18,B3GAT3,CCAR1, CCDC137,CKB,CREM,DDX39A,DFFB,DNAJB12, FAIM3,HUS1,ITPK1,KIAA0930,LRPAP1,MGRN1, MRPS24,NADK,NRARP,NUBPL,NUP155, OSBPL7,PHF14,PIP5K1A,PPFIA3,PSTPIP1, PTMA,RALBP1,RIN3,RPS6KB2,SH3BP2,SH3TC1, TP53I3,TRAF4,TRIB2,TSSC1,USP42*
Brown (197)	Light green (49)	12 (5.48E-03)	9.8	9	Apoptosis/cell death	*UEVLD,UNC13B,DTNB,BANP,IRF7,CCNL2, INTS9,FNTA,RBM19,DNASE1,GRB7*
Midnightblue (45)	Turquoise (181)	10 (1.24E-02)	28	6	Ion binding	*ABLIM2,ACE,COMMD1,ELFN2,GLT1D1, HAUS7,TOM1*
Turquoise (284)	Midnight blue (55)	15 (2.11E-02)	12	2	Nucleotide binding	*ADCY9,AGTRAP,BSDC1,INO80E,MCHR1, MTHFSD,NADK,P4HB,PDE8A,POR,RAB3A, RPS19BP1,SMUG1,SOX12,STX8*

modules showing a strong preservation ($Z_{summary}$ >10) and low median rank (Fig. 6b). All these four modules were again enriched for "zinc ion binding," "regulation of transcription," and "apoptosis". They overlapped with "light cyan," "midnight blue," "black," and "turquoise" methylation modules. Biological processes like "cell division," "chromosome partitioning/cytoskeleton," and "GTPase regulator activity" were enriched in both "grey60" (second least rank = 5, $Z_{summary}$ = 13) expression module along with its overlapping red methylation module (Additional file 7). An additional network analysis was carried out using expression and average methylation of whole genes (not just 3′UTRs) that are non-coding (i.e., transcripts that do not encode a protein product) along with 3′UTR methylation. Results from this analysis can be accessed in Additional file 7. This non-coding RNA analysis also gave results similar to the 3′UTRs, including overlap of modules enriched for similar cancer-related terms. Hence, we see that significantly preserved expression and methylation modules were enriched for similar cancer-related biological processes like leukocyte proliferation, apoptosis, signal transduction, and cell-cycle regulation. Our observation from network preservation of expression and 3′UTR methylation change provides clues for a better understanding of the contribution made by the regulatory role imposed by 3′UTR methylation overexpression.

Next, a correlation analysis between methylation and expression modules was conducted using module *eigengene* (aka *eigennode*) that is intuitively understood as a weighted average of the variable profiles in a module. Although the composition of co-expression and co-differential methylation modules can vary, we observed multiple strong Pearson correlations between many expression and methylation module eigengenes as shown in Fig. 7, and Tables S6 and S12 in Additional file 7. For example, in our non-coding gene analysis, eigengenes of "red" methylation module was highly negatively correlated (corr = −0.97, *p* value = 5.75E-12) to a "brown" expression module. The red methylation module was enriched for "regulation of cell cycle" and "intracellular signal cascade" and "brown" expression module for apoptosis and leukocyte proliferation as per GO analysis, showcasing complimentary functional annotations involved in cancer regulation (Tables S8 and S9 in Additional file 7). Similarly, eigengenes of the blue methylation module were significantly and positively correlated (corr = 0.95, *p* value = 1.22E-09) to the "dark red" expression module, both of which were enriched for "protein localization" or "intracellular transport" (Figure S6 in Additional file 7). Also, we saw both significantly positive and negative correlations in 3′ UTR methylation to expression modules and occasionally for the same module. For example, red expression module (enriched for "kinases and nucleotide binding") was negatively correlated with "green" (enriched for "nucleotide binding" and "positive regulation of apoptosis") and positively correlated with "midnight blue" and "tan" (both enriched for "nucleotide binding")

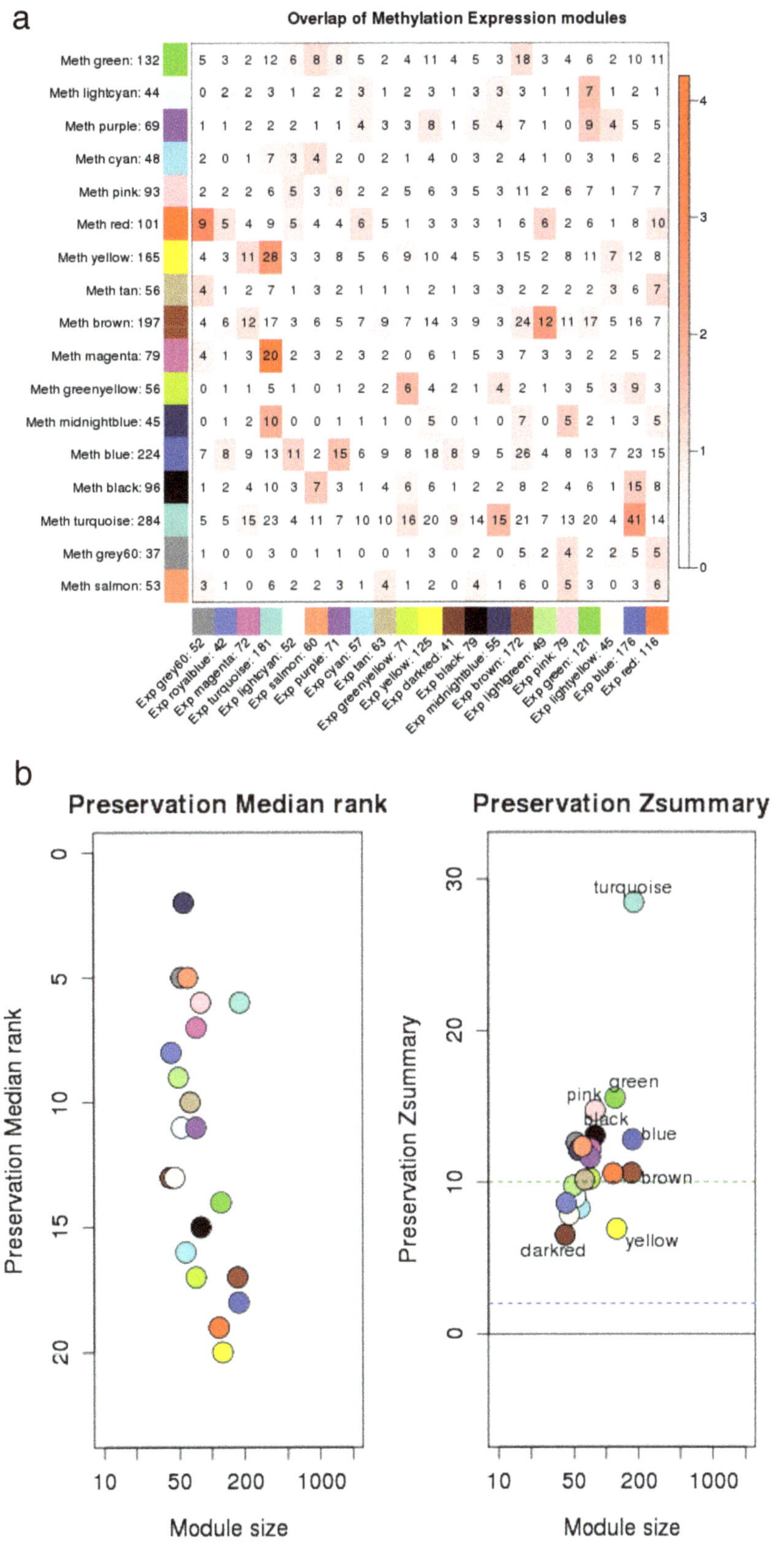

Fig. 6 (See legend on next page.)

(See figure on previous page.)

Fig. 6 Module preservation. **a** Table showing gene overlap between each pair of methylation and expression modules. Each *row* of the table corresponds to one methylation module (labeled by color as well as text), and each *column* corresponds to one expression module. *Numbers* in the table indicate gene counts in the intersection of the corresponding modules. *Coloring* of the table encodes – log(*p*), with *p* being the Fisher's exact test *p* value for the overlap of the two modules. The stronger the *red color*, the more significant the overlap is between a methylation module for 3′UTR and an expression module. **b** Plot showing statistical analysis results for module preservation test to check preservation of 3′ UTR methylation modules against expression modules based on the density and connectivity patterns of genes in each module. The *left panel* shows the medianRank of the observed preservation statics and the *right panel* shows the distribution of $Z_{summary}$ statistics obtained from a permutation analysis for each methylation module. A module with a lower median rank tends to exhibit stronger observed preservation statistics than a module with a higher median rank. The $Z_{summary}$ statistic of a given module summarizes the evidence that the network connections of the module are more significantly preserved than those of random set of genes of equal size. The significance thresholds for $Z_{summary}$ are $Z_{summary} < 2$ implies no evidence that the module is preserved, $2 < Z_{summary} < 10$ implies weak to moderate evidence, and $Z_{summary} > 10$ implies strong evidence for module preservation between co-expression module and 3′UTR methylation module

3′UTR methylation modules. All together within the 3′UTR methylation correlations, we observed a majority of positive correlated modules of lower significance compared to negative correlated modules of high significance. Correlation in different directions can be assumed to be due to location of methylation differences within exons or introns, as we saw in our previous analysis and the direction of methylation change. Overall, we observed significant correlations in modules enriched for cancer-related terms, giving evidence of the role of methylation change in 3′UTRs towards tumorigenesis.

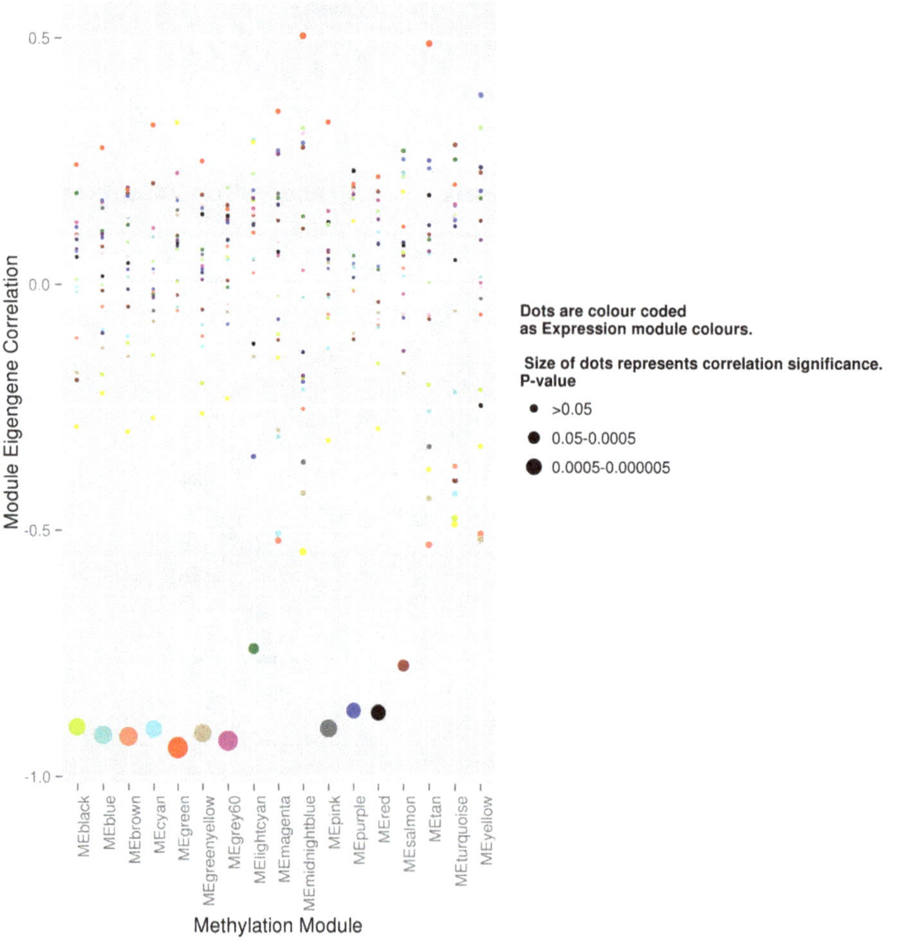

Fig. 7 Pairwise correlation between each methylation module to each expression module. Plot showing correlation between eigengenes of each 3′ UTR methylation and expression modules. X-axis shows all 17 differential methylation modules, and Y-axis shows the module eigengene correlation value for each of the 21 different color-coded dots representing 21 expression modules. Statistical significance of each correlation was calculated and represented by dot size for each corresponding methylation module

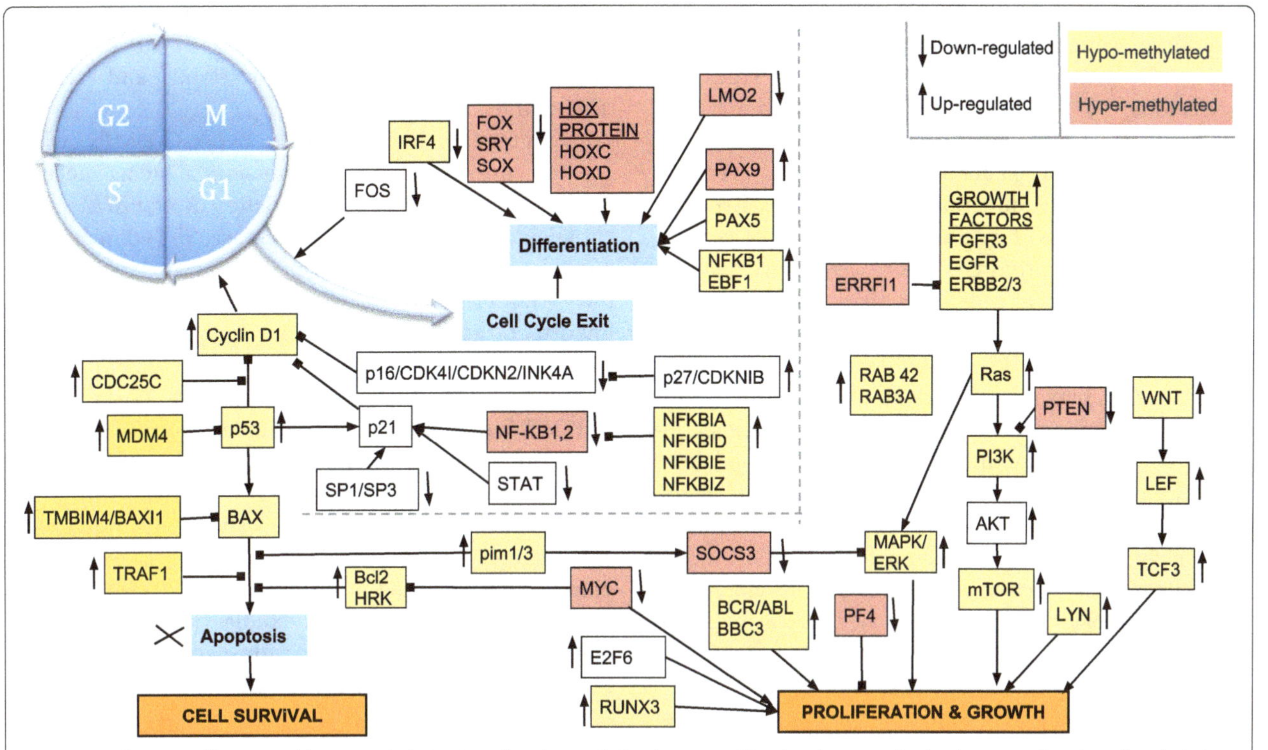

Fig. 8 Coordination of hypo- and hypermethylation in cell-cycle regulation in cancer. Plot showing coordination between direction of methylation and expression change in cancer regulation. Each gene is colored showing their methylation change along with *up or down arrow* showing how their expression changes. Genes that are not marked by color or arrow shows no corresponding data recorded

Interplay between hypo- and hypermethylation

Also, while describing the importance of hypomethylation in CLL, we described the overall interplay among hyper/hypomethylation and gene expression change. Figure 8 shows both methylation and expression change information together for key cancer and cell cycle-regulating genes. Genes are marked as hypo- or hypermethylated if any of the respective C-DMRs overlap on them. As observed from all our enrichment analyses, Fig. 8 shows that growth and proliferation is dominated by hypomethylation whereas hypermethylation blocks cell-cycle exiting and differentiation. We can see many instances where opposite methylation changes target genes in the same process but still coordinate with each other towards cancer development. Both hyper- and hypomethylation changes were found within the same network based on functional role or direction of target gene in the network. For instance, although, all genes involved in cell growth and proliferation are targeted by hypomethylation and have activated transcription, *PF4*—which is known to be involved in inhibition of hematopoiesis and *PTEN*, is hypermethylated. *PF4* negatively regulates the *PI3K-AKT/PKB* signaling pathway and acts as a tumor-suppressor and hence, hypermethylated and repressed. Similarly, in order to drive the cell cycle forward to progress through subsequent phases of cell cycle and escape cell-cycle exit, Fig. 8 shows much complementary coordination of opposite methylation changes. We can see how the *FOS* gene, which is involved in cell-cycle exit is repressed in CLL samples but *CyclinD1* and its other genes, which are required for G1-S phase transition in cell-cycle progression are hypomethylated. Hypomethylation of genes involved in G1-S transition, thereby enables uncontrolled cell division. Also, all genes involved in inhibiting apoptosis are hypomethylated leading to their transcription activation. These examples show how hypo- and hypermethylation coordinate with each other to impose a double negative effect towards the same goal of cancer development in CLL.

Discussion

Role of hypomethylation in cell-cycle regulation, histone modification, and transcription activation in CLL

Hypermethylation at the promoter region of tumor suppressors and their subsequent silencing is a well-studied mechanism of tumorigenesis. In contrast, hypomethylation, potentially leading to upregulation of oncogenes, is not fully understood. Also, genic hypomethylation is often considered as a random and non-consistent process due to a particularly predominant demethylation process in mature B cells in CLL samples. In this study, we showed that consistent hypomethylated regions (referred to here as hypo-C-DMRs) account for a significant pattern of methylation changes in CLL with a distinctive pattern of gene expression and regulatory associations.

In particular, we observed that both hypo- and hyper-C-DMRs were enriched for similar biological processes but in an opposite direction. For example, hyper-C-DMRs were enriched for "positive regulation of cell differentiation", but hypo-C-DMRs were enriched for "negative regulation of cell differentiation." We also observed a significant enrichment of *BCR* signaling associated with hypo-C-DMRs. This further strengthens the importance of hypomethylation in CLL since *BCR* is a central pathogenic mechanism in B cell malignancies, including CLL [41]. In addition, GO annotations relate to transcription regulation, chromatin modification, apoptosis, cell proliferation, leukocyte differentiation, and signal transduction were enriched for hypo-C-DMR, which also defines their functional role in cancer development.

Also, the most significantly enriched TFBS for hypo-C-DMRs was *EBF1*, which is a transcription factor that is critical for both B lymphopoiesis and B cell function [42]. *EBF1*, in collaboration with a hierarchy of partner proteins, including E2A, Runx1, and Pax5 (also enriched in motif analysis) activates the B cell transcriptome and represses programs of alternate hematopoietic lineages. DNA binding by *EBF1* has also been linked to changes in epigenetic marks on their target genes. Binding of *EBF1* and other factors including *E2A* have also been correlated with H3K4me1 at target genes, which is also the most enriched histone modification mark in our analysis. H3K4me1 is in fact known to facilitate additional epigenetic modifications necessary for transcription [43]. *RUNX3, TCF3, PU.1*, and *PAX5* are also key transcription factors in B lymphopoiesis and cell proliferation. Other TFBS enriched for hypo-C-DMRs were *POL2, CHD2, WHIP*, and *TBLR1*. *CHD2* is a DNA-binding helicase that specifically binds to the promoter of target genes, leading to chromatin remodeling and promoting their expression [44]. WHIP is a protein that binds to DNA polymerase delta and increases the initiation frequency of DNA polymerase delta-mediated DNA synthesis [45]. *TBLR1* is a key regulator of different properties of the BCL-3 [46] that acts as an oncogenic protein through multiple mechanisms that include the induction of cyclin D1 expression and also inhibits cell apoptosis through induction of the E3 ligase of *p53, MDM2* [47, 48]. Among other enriched histone modifications, H3K79 di-methylation is known for regulating the initiation of DNA replication [49], and H3K36me3 is found in actively transcribed gene bodies of genes involved in G1/S transition in a cell cycle [50]. Presence of hypo-C-DMR overlapping enhancers and weak promoters further emphasize their role in activation of transcription. Overall, both enriched TFBS and histone modifications are known to relate to B lymphopoiesis, transcription activation, and cancer development.

In contrast to hypo-C-DMRs, hyper-C-DMRs, which are known to regulate the expression silencing mechanism, were implicated by the enrichment of *EZH2*. *EZH2* contains a histone methyltransferase SET domain that methylates histone tails on gene promoters to repress their transcription initiation, and this domain is an important component of the polycomb repressive complex 2 (PRC2). The *PRC2* protein *EZH2* is also known to preferentially methylate Lysine 27 on histone 3 (H3K27) [51] and also H3K9 under certain conditions. H3K27me3 and H3K9me3 were both enriched for hyper-LSDMRs in our analysis as well. H3K4me3, H3K9me3, and H3K27me3 co-localizes with most polycomb target proteins like *SUZ12, CTBP2*, and *EZH2*-binding sites enriched in hyper-C-DMRs (Additional file 1; Figure S5). Several other studies [51, 52] have reported DNA methylation and tumor suppressors in cancers marked with polycomb proteins enriched with *EZH2* and H3K27me3. This study also elucidates the known mechanism of hyper-C-DMR in gene silencing and promoting cancer development. Further, enrichment of repressor chromatin region for hyper-C-DMRs confirms their role in silencing the expression of target genes.

Our motif enrichment analysis showed hypermethylation enriched for motifs like homeobox and TATAbox, which are usually present in promoter regions and thus silence many key genes. In contrast, hypomethylation was enriched in motifs of transcription activator binding genes, such as *ETS* [38], *ZFX* [37], *cMYC* [39] (Table 1), which are again involved in cell growth, apoptosis, and metabolism, processes necessary for tumor progression. Enriched transcription factor motifs like *Ikaros (IKZF)* and *PU.1* govern B cell lineage priming, which involves changes in histone modifications and chromatin structure of genes encoding molecules important for the establishment of a B cell program [53]. Other significant classes of motifs enriched in hypo-C-DMRs were motifs containing ETS domain in genes like *Elk1* and *Fli* and RHD domain in genes like *NFAT* and *NFkB-p65*. These genes are downstream nuclear targets of *Ras-MAP* kinase signaling and are also known as oncogenic transcription activators, specific to [54] cell survival and proliferation.

Methylation pattern in exons, introns, and 3′UTRs

In addition to evidence of transcription activation, we observed that hypomethylation in CLL mostly targets intronic, intergenic, and 3′UTR regions. Regarding the relationship between methylation and expression change with respect to genic locations, we found negative correlation for methylation in exons and whole transcript expression within 30 CLL samples. But, this correlation within exons was inconsistent in UTRs. Exons in 5′UTRs seem to act more like promoters, but exons in 3′UTRs had the opposite effect on expression. Hence, these findings suggest that in contrast to a gene expression-inhibiting role of increasing methylation associated with 5′UTR exons, methylation in 3′UTR exons is in fact required in the normal transcription process.

Regulation of expression by 3′UTR methylation pattern

Our co-expression and co-methylation network analysis revealed that both transcriptome and methylome can be organized into modules. Genes in co-methylation and co-expression modules were found highly enriched for specific gene ontology categories, underscoring their functional importance. Many 3′ UTR modules associated with methylation changes were found to have moderate to strong preservation with expression modules. Also, the most preserved module had functional annotations related to signaling and growth and proliferation. Hence, preserved 3′ UTR methylation and expression modules revealed the ability of 3′UTR methylation to dictate their expression. The regulatory behavior of methylation change could, therefore, be detected—not only in 5′ UTR, promoters, and gene bodies—but also in 3′ UTRs in CLL. Also, significantly correlated 3′UTR methylation and expression modules were enriched for biologically important pathways involved in signaling cascade, apoptosis, and cell proliferation. These results provide a fine-grained look at the interaction among 3′UTR co-methylation and co-expression modules altered in CLL.

In summary, we report that hypomethylation of DNA appears to facilitate the aberrant expression of proto-oncogenes/oncogenes, potentially stimulating cell proliferation in CLL. We observed that apart from global hypomethylation of repeat sequences, there also exists site-specific hypomethylation of certain genes and genic regions, especially in genes linked with signaling pathways (e.g., *BCR*, *LYN RAB8A*, *NFKBIB*), chromatin modifications (e.g., *CHD2*, *CHD3*, *SMARCB1*), cell growth and development (e.g., *EBF1*, *EGR1*, *EGFR*, *ERBB2*, *MYC*), apoptosis inhibition (e.g., *BCL2*, *TRAF1*), and promoting cell proliferation (e.g., *CCND1*, *LYN*, *BCL3*). We observed 3′UTRs to possess a high percentage of hypo-DMRs consistent in the majority of our test samples. We report genes with 3′UTR consistent hypomethylation in CLL like *LIF* and *PIM3*. Along with that, we also report genes with consistent hypermethylation in CLL in 3′UTRs like *HMX2* and other genic regions. We also observed that methylation changes at 3′UTR had significant correlation with expression along with overlapping network modules in both datasets. Our findings, thus, suggest that hypomethylation in different genic regions might exhibit a significant deleterious effect on gene expression that results in malignant transformation and/or tumor progression.

Conclusions

We observed that hypomethylated regions were less consistent over the genome among different samples, in contrast to hypermethylation loci. However, some hypomethylated regions were highly consistent in most of the samples, and their functional analysis revealed their potential biological significance in CLL.

We observed hypomethylation at many genes containing key TFBS involved in cell growth and development, histone remodeling, apoptosis, and cellular proliferation. We found hypomethylation in many key signaling regulators consistent in majority of samples, which do not appear to be random events or a non-specific part of global hypomethylation. In addition, this study contributes to our understanding about the relationship between methylation and expression levels in CLL samples. Results from positional analyses for genic location indicate that the conventional model of methylation regulating expression in an antagonistic manner is most common. However, we also uncovered an interesting and conflicting relationship between methylation and expression for methylation occurring in exons of 3′ UTRs. Specifically, we found evidence of a loss of DNA methylation that not only causes genomic instability but also potentially activates many genes mainly in signaling pathways like *BCR* in CLL. Finally, we showed that 3′UTR methylome and transcriptome are organized into biologically meaningful modules with significant correlations and strong-to-moderate preservation of their density and connections between two datasets. The preserved modules were also found as functionally related indicating the role of 3′UTR methylation in expression regulation.

Methods

Data sources

Publicly available reduced representation bisulfite sequencing (RRBS) methylation for 30 CLL and three control samples were obtained from the GEO website (http://www.ncbi.nlm.nih.gov/geo/query/acc.cgi?acc=GSE66121). Control samples were CD19+ B cells isolated from peripheral blood of normal controls. Human genome annotation data from the UCSC genome browser (hg19 genome assembly), such as Refseq and

UCSC genes, CpG islands, Vista Enhancers, ENCODE Transcription Factor ChIP-Seq, and RepeatMasker Tracks, were used to annotate differentially methylated regions of interest. For genes with multiple isoforms, the longest one was used as the reference. Promoter regions were selected from −2 kb upstream to the transcription start site of each gene.

Read mapping and % methylation

The bisulfite-treated sequencing reads in DNA methylation data for CD19+ B cells were mapped to bisulfite-converted human genome using Bismark [55] (using Bowtie). Bismark was used also to obtain the genome-wide cytosine methylation calls at a base resolution in the CpG context. Additional file 8 provides read mapping count tables for each sample.

Sequencing reads from RNA-seq experiments were mapped using Bowtie with known ENSEMBL transcripts as gene models. After mapping, FPKM values for each gene/transcript were calculated by Cufflinks [56] and differentially expressed (DE) genes were defined by abs(ln(fold-change)) > 1.5. FDR-corrected $p < 0.05$ for all DE genes were calculated by Cuffdiff [57]. Next, the over enriched GO categories were obtained based on a .05 FDR cutoff using the GO-seq R package.

DMR calculation

Considering the high correlation between methylation of adjacent CpGs, the methylation information obtained from RRBS data was summarized on 1000 bp tiling windows (step-size 1000 bp) with minimum 3 CpGs and minimum 10 reads mapped on each CpG using the R package, *methylKit* [58]. For DMR calculation, pairwise comparison of 1000 bp tiles in each of the 30 tumor samples against each control normal sample was performed using Fisher's exact test. From each such test, differential methylation values were obtained only for the regions that were common between CLL and control sample. Thirty such tests were conducted for each control sample. Next, in order to ensure comparable statistics, only those regions that had differential values from each of the 30 tests were used. This gave us 41,421 common regions obtained from the first control sample comparison tests. Similarly, 39,327 and 41,359 regions were obtained from each of the other two control samples.

Entropy calculation

Also, the methylation entropy across all CLL samples was calculated in order to see probability distribution of methylation changes for each 1000 bp region across all samples. Entropy for each sample was computed as follows:

The methylation vector m_r of region r across N samples was defined as,

$$m_r = m_{r,1}, m_{r,2}, \ldots, m_{r,5}, \ldots, m_{r,N}$$

where $m_{r,s}$ represents the methylation level in sample s. The sum of methylation levels of region r in samples $(\Sigma_{S=1}^{N} m_{r,s})$ was treated as a total methylation value. The ratio of methylation level of region in sample relative to the total value was defined as the relative methylation probability, $p_{s/r} = m_{r,s}/\Sigma_{S=1}^{N} m_{r,s}$. The original Shannon entropy of the region can be calculated as $H_o = -\sum_{S=1}^{N} p_{\frac{s}{r}} \log_2\left(p_{s/r}\right)$.

Enrichment analysis

Enrichment analysis of genes overlapped by C-DMRs for GO categories and KEGG pathways was performed using GOStats R package [59]. Gene set enrichment for gene symbols overlapping hypo-C-DMRs was also performed using GeneDecks [60] to highlight shared descriptors between pairs of genes based on annotations within the GeneCards compendium of human genes.

The epigenomic enrichment analysis of C-DMRs was performed using Genome Runner [61]. Briefly, genomic coordinates of hyper- and hypo-C-DMRs were collected and tested for co-localization with three groups of genome annotation datasets: (1) chromatin state segmentation by HMM from ENCODE/Broad, (2) histone modifications by ChIP-seq from ENCODE/Broad Institute and ENCODE/Stanford/Yale/USC/Harvard, and (3) experimentally validated transcription factor binding sites from ENCODE/Broad Institute and ENCODE/Stanford/Yale/USC/Harvard. Genomic regions annotated by the ENCODE with any functional/regulatory information (~80 % of the whole genome) were used as a "background" to estimate co-localizations that can occur by chance. p values were calculated using Chi-square test and corrected for multiple testing using FDR.

Motif analysis was also carried out using Homer [62] software after retrieving sequences around each DMR CpG along with those around non-DMR CpGs randomly chosen as a background.

Expression in relation to methylation analysis

To associate gene expression changes with methylation differences, all CpG average methylation values were paired with the average expression of transcripts they overlap in all CLL samples. Estimated expression profiles of all transcripts were divided into four expression quartiles and referred to as lowest to highest expression groups within all transcripts. The positional enrichment analysis for each gene region was performed using Homer, and R scripts were used to calculate and plot smoothened density estimates. Locfit library was used for fitting local regression, likelihood models, and related smoothing procedures.

Correlation of whole transcript expression to methylation of CpGs within each specific gene region was calculated by using the Pearson correlation coefficient. For correlation calculation average methylation of CpGs (across all CLL samples) in a specific gene region and average expression of the whole transcript corresponding to these CpGs were used.

Correlation module analysis

From 19 matching CLL samples from both methylation and expression data, we obtained differential methylation and differential expression (FPKM) for 3′UTRs of 1780 transcripts. For this, whole transcript expression and average methylation for all CpGs in each of its 3′ UTRs were used. Differential expression and 3′UTR methylation for each transcript was then computed by comparing each CLL sample individually against one common control sample.

We then used differential expression and methylation value matrices to identify co-expression and co-differential methylation network modules through the WGCNA R package (see Additional file 7 for more details), individually on each dataset. WGCNA computes networks by calculating each gene-to-gene pairwise correlation and interconnection strength by checking number of shared neighbors. It then finally generates modules using hierarchical clustering. Tables S1 and S2 in Additional file 7 provide a list of 10 top hub genes (genes with most significant module membership) in each module, and Additional file 9 consists of module membership values for all genes in each expression and methylation module.

After constructing modules in each dataset, we checked to see if any of the modules in one dataset were preserved in any of the modules from the other data set using two approaches: cross tabulation and network-based statistics. In cross tabulation, overlaps of the constituent genes in each pair of modules from the two data sets were calculated and Fisher's exact test was used to assign a p value to each overlap. In the second method, we used network module preservation statistics (NP) described in and implemented in [63] the WGCNA R package. The NP method not only assesses the significant overlap of genes, but also whether the density and connectivity patterns of modules defined in a reference data set are preserved in a test data set. We considered expression data as reference data and methylation data as test data. This NP statistic test calculates statistic values based on density and connectivity preservation within reference and test modules. From calculated statistic values, the NP test in the WGCNA package module was used to obtain two values, (1) the median rank, which is the rank for the average of the observed preservation static values and (2) a composite module preservation statistic referred to as $Z_{summary}$ using a permutation test. Thus, we reported a $Z_{summary}$ for each expression module in the methylation modules.

Also, since WGCNA groups together highly correlated variables to generate modules, we summarized the variable profiles in each module to a single representative, i.e., the module eigengene. The module eigengene, which is defined as the first principal component of the standardized matrix containing variables in the module was used to calculate the correlation between expression and methylation within non-coding genes and 3′UTRs.

Also, since non-coding genes do not translate and do not undergo post-transcription changes (i.e., stripping 3′ UTRs) with no defined UTR or a gene body region (or in other words—whole portion can be identified as UTR), we also conducted the same network analysis by including non-coding genes.

Additional files

Additional file 1: Additional Figures, Tables and Methods. This is a "docx" file, which includes various additional figures, tables and methods that are referred in the main text supporting this research.

Additional file 2: List of C-DMRs. This is an "xls" file providing coordinates for hyper- and hypo-C-DMRs common across all control tests in separate excel sheets, respectively.

Additional file 3: Gene lists for C-DMRs. This is an "xls" file providing a list of genes overlapped by common hyper and hypo-C-DMRs in separate excel sheets, respectively. It also consists of excel sheets for genes overlapping different gene regions for hypo- and hyper-C-DMRs, respectively.

Additional file 4: KEGG and GO enrichment analysis results. This is an "xls" format file that provides enrichment test results from GOStats package for KEGG pathways and GO biological processes for both hyper- and hypo-C-DMRs and DMRs from pooled sample analysis in separate excel sheets, respectively.

Additional file 5: Phenotype enrichment analysis results. This is an "xls" format file that provides enrichment results for phenotype with different phenotype descriptors, their enrichment p values along with their count and names of their corresponding genes sharing that descriptor for both hypo- and hyper-C-DMRs in separate excel sheet, respectively.

Additional file 6: ENCODE enrichment results. This is an "xls" file that provides the ENCODE epi-genomic mark enrichment analysis results from Gm12878 cell line with the name and the description of the datasets, enrichment p values that are adjusted for multiple testing using FDR, for hypo/hyper-C-DMRs in separate excel sheets, respectively, along with the name of the regulatory mark. It also consists of enrichment analysis results from all ENCODE cell lines for each regulatory mark in hypo- and hyper-C-DMRs.

Additional file 7: WGCNA. This is a "docx" file that describes correlation modules in details, together with the step-by-step description of WGCNA analysis. WGCNA description includes data cleaning and preprocessing, adjacency topological overlap matrix construction, module detection, calculation of various module measures, and description of preservation statistics methods used. It includes tables and figures for both 3′UTR methylation and non-coding gene data, and their relation with expression of genes analysis.

Additional file 8: Read mapping details. This file provides the mapping statistics for all the samples in both RRBS and RNA-seq datasets. Table S1 lists the number of RRBS reads obtained, their % that is uniquely mapped on human genome (hg19) along with total number of CpGs analyzed from each sample. Table S2 lists the number of RNA-seq reads obtained and their % that is uniquely mapped on human genome (hg19) for each sample.

Additional file 9: Gene module membership. This is an "xls" file that provides the matrix for transcript's module membership or eigengene-based connectivity measure of each transcript for each methylation and expression module for 3′UTRs in separate excel sheet, respectively.

Competing interests
The authors declare that they have no competing interests.

Authors' contributions
GK developed the hypothesis and performed all the analyses and drafted the manuscript. MD and JDW performed epigenomic enrichment analysis, and contributed to figure preparation and writing of the manuscript. JQ contributed and verified the statistical testing used in the project. HS contributed datasets and conceptualization of the project. DX and HS contributed to the development of the method, data analysis, and manuscript writing along with jointly directing the project. All authors read and approved the final manuscript.

Acknowledgements
We thank Drs. Andrew Smith, Kristen Taylor, Jeffrey Bryan, Michael Wang, and Joseph L. Wiemels for their helpful discussions.

Declarations
This article has been published as part of *Human Genomics* Volume 10 Supplement 2, 2016: From genes to systems genomics: human genomics. The full contents of the supplement are available online at http://humgenomics.biomedcentral.com/articles/supplements/volume-10-supplement-2.

Funding
This work was supported in part by the National Institute of Health (Grants CA134304 and DA025779).

Author details
[1]Christopher S. Bond Life Sciences Center, University of Missouri, Columbia, MO 65211, USA. [2]Informatics Institute, University of Missouri, Columbia, MO 65211, USA. [3]Department of Biostatistics, Virginia Commonwealth University, Richmond, VA 23225, USA. [4]Arthritis and Clinical Immunology Program, Oklahoma Medical Research Foundation, Oklahoma City, OK 73104, USA. [5]Department of Applied Economics & Statistics, University of Delaware, Newark, DE 19716, USA. [6]GRU Cancer Center, Georgia Regents University, Augusta, GA 30912, USA. [7]Department of Biochemistry and Molecular Biology, Georgia Regents University, Augusta, GA 30912, USA. [8]Department of Computer Science, University of Missouri, Columbia, MO 65211, USA.

References

1. Feinberg AP, Vogelstein B. Hypomethylation distinguishes genes of some human cancers from their normal counterparts. Nature. 1983;301(5895):89–92.
2. Cadieux B, Ching TT, VandenBerg SR, Costello JF. Genome-wide hypomethylation in human glioblastomas associated with specific copy number alteration, methylenetetrahydrofolate reductase allele status, and increased proliferation. Cancer Res. 2006;66(17):8469–76. doi:10.1158/0008-5472.CAN-06-1547.
3. Widschwendter M, Jiang G, Woods C, Muller HM, Fiegl H, Goebel G, et al. DNA hypomethylation and ovarian cancer biology. Cancer Res. 2004;64 (13):4472–80. doi:10.1158/0008-5472.CAN-04-0238.
4. Brothman AR, Swanson G, Maxwell TM, Cui J, Murphy KJ, Herrick J, et al. Global hypomethylation is common in prostate cancer cells: a quantitative predictor for clinical outcome? Cancer Genet Cytogenet. 2005;156(1):31–6. doi:10.1016/j.cancergencyto.2004.04.004.
5. Wahlfors J, Hiltunen H, Heinonen K, Hamalainen E, Alhonen L, Janne J. Genomic hypomethylation in human chronic lymphocytic leukemia. Blood. 1992;80(8):2074–80.
6. Kulis M, Heath S, Bibikova M, Queiros AC, Navarro A, Clot G, et al. Epigenomic analysis detects widespread gene-body DNA hypomethylation in chronic lymphocytic leukemia. Nat Genet. 2012;44(11):1236–42. doi:10.1038/ng.2443.
7. Lin CH, Hsieh SY, Sheen IS, Lee WC, Chen TC, Shyu WC, et al. Genome-wide hypomethylation in hepatocellular carcinogenesis. Cancer Res. 2001;61(10): 4238–43.
8. Kim YI, Giuliano A, Hatch KD, Schneider A, Nour MA, Dallal GE, et al. Global DNA hypomethylation increases progressively in cervical dysplasia and carcinoma. Cancer. 1994;74(3):893–9.
9. Feinberg AP, Gehrke CW, Kuo KC, Ehrlich M. Reduced genomic 5-methylcytosine content in human colonic neoplasia. Cancer Res. 1988;48 (5):1159–61.
10. Ehrlich M, Jiang G, Fiala E, Dome JS, Yu MC, Long TI, et al. Hypomethylation and hypermethylation of DNA in Wilms tumors. Oncogene. 2002;21(43): 6694–702. doi:10.1038/sj.onc.1205890.
11. De Smet C, Lurquin C, Lethe B, Martelange V, Boon T. DNA methylation is the primary silencing mechanism for a set of germ line- and tumor-specific genes with a CpG-rich promoter. Mol Cell Biol. 1999;19(11):7327–35.
12. Li M, Balch C, Montgomery JS, Jeong M, Chung JH, Yan P, et al. Integrated analysis of DNA methylation and gene expression reveals specific signaling pathways associated with platinum resistance in ovarian cancer. BMC Med Genet. 2009;2:34. doi:10.1186/1755-8794-2-34.
13. Pulukuri SM, Estes N, Patel J, Rao JS. Demethylation-linked activation of urokinase plasminogen activator is involved in progression of prostate cancer. Cancer Res. 2007;67(3):930–9. doi:10.1158/0008-5472.can-06-2892.
14. Jackson K, Yu MC, Arakawa K, Fiala E, Youn B, Fiegl H, et al. DNA hypomethylation is prevalent even in low-grade breast cancers. Cancer Biol Ther. 2004;3(12):1225–31.
15. Ateeq B, Unterberger A, Szyf M, Rabbani SA. Pharmacological inhibition of DNA methylation induces proinvasive and prometastatic genes in vitro and in vivo. Neoplasia (New York, NY). 2008;10(3):266–78.
16. Denda A, Rao PM, Rajalakshmi S, Sarma DS. 5-azacytidine potentiates initiation induced by carcinogens in rat liver. Carcinogenesis. 1985;6(1):145–6.
17. Qu G, Dubeau L, Narayan A, Yu MC, Ehrlich M. Satellite DNA hypomethylation vs. overall genomic hypomethylation in ovarian epithelial tumors of different malignant potential. Mutat Res. 1999;423(1-2):91–101.
18. Rodriguez J, Vives L, Jorda M, Morales C, Munoz M, Vendrell E, et al. Genome-wide tracking of unmethylated DNA Alu repeats in normal and cancer cells. Nucleic Acids Res. 2008;36(3):770–84. doi:10.1093/nar/gkm1105.
19. Su M, Han D, Boyd-Kirkup J, Yu X, Han JD. Evolution of Alu elements toward enhancers. Cell Rep. 2014;7(2):376–85. doi:10.1016/j.celrep.2014.03.011.
20. Gribben JG. How I treat CLL up front. Blood. 2010;115(2):187–97. doi:10.1182/blood-2009-08-207126.
21. Crespo M, Bosch F, Villamor N, Bellosillo B, Colomer D, Rozman M, et al. ZAP-70 expression as a surrogate for immunoglobulin-variable-region mutations in chronic lymphocytic leukemia. N Engl J Med. 2003;348(18): 1764–75. doi:10.1056/NEJMoa023143.
22. Damle RN, Wasil T, Fais F, Ghiotto F, Valetto A, Allen SL, et al. Ig V gene mutation status and CD38 expression as novel prognostic indicators in chronic lymphocytic leukemia. Blood. 1999;94(6):1840–7.
23. Hamblin TJ, Davis Z, Gardiner A, Oscier DG, Stevenson FK. Unmutated Ig V(H) genes are associated with a more aggressive form of chronic lymphocytic leukemia. Blood. 1999;94(6):1848–54.
24. Kanduri M, Cahill N, Goransson H, Enstrom C, Ryan F, Isaksson A, et al. Differential genome-wide array-based methylation profiles in prognostic subsets of chronic lymphocytic leukemia. Blood. 2010;115(2):296–305. doi:10.1182/blood-2009-07-232868.
25. Rush LJ, Raval A, Funchain P, Johnson AJ, Smith L, Lucas DM, et al. Epigenetic profiling in chronic lymphocytic leukemia reveals novel methylation targets. Cancer Res. 2004;64(7):2424–33.
26. Raval A, Tanner SM, Byrd JC, Angerman EB, Perko JD, Chen SS, et al. Downregulation of death-associated protein kinase 1 (DAPK1) in chronic lymphocytic leukemia. Cell. 2007;129(5):879–90. doi:10.1016/j.cell.2007.03.043.
27. Liu TH, Raval A, Chen SS, Matkovic JJ, Byrd JC, Plass C. CpG island methylation and expression of the secreted frizzled-related protein gene family in chronic lymphocytic leukemia. Cancer Res. 2006;66(2):653–8. doi:10.1158/0008-5472.can-05-3712.

28. Chen SS, Claus R, Lucas DM, Yu L, Qian J, Ruppert AS, et al. Silencing of the inhibitor of DNA binding protein 4 (ID4) contributes to the pathogenesis of mouse and human CLL. Blood. 2011;117(3):862–71. doi:10.1182/blood-2010-05-284638.
29. Seeliger B, Wilop S, Osieka R, Galm O, Jost E. CpG island methylation patterns in chronic lymphocytic leukemia. Leuk Lymphoma. 2009;50(3):419–26. doi:10.1080/10428190902756594.
30. Raval A, Lucas DM, Matkovic JJ, Bennett KL, Liyanarachchi S, Young DC, et al. TWIST2 demonstrates differential methylation in immunoglobulin variable heavy chain mutated and unmutated chronic lymphocytic leukemia. J Clin Oncol Off J Am Soc Clin Oncol. 2005;23(17):3877–85. doi:10.1200/jco.2005.02.196.
31. Lipsanen V, Leinonen P, Alhonen L, Janne J. Hypomethylation of ornithine decarboxylase gene and erb-A1 oncogene in human chronic lymphatic leukemia. Blood. 1988;72(6):2042–4.
32. Hanada M, Delia D, Aiello A, Stadtmauer E, Reed JC. bcl-2 gene hypomethylation and high-level expression in B-cell chronic lymphocytic leukemia. Blood. 1993;82(6):1820–8.
33. Ernst J, Kheradpour P, Mikkelsen TS, Shoresh N, Ward LD, Epstein CB, et al. Mapping and analysis of chromatin state dynamics in nine human cell types. Nature. 2011;473(7345):43–9. doi:10.1038/nature09906.
34. Ashburner M, Ball CA, Blake JA, Botstein D, Butler H, Cherry JM, et al. Gene ontology: tool for the unification of biology. The Gene Ontology Consortium. Nat Genet. 2000;25(1):25–9. doi:10.1038/75556.
35. Kanehisa M, Goto S, Furumichi M, Tanabe M, Hirakawa M. KEGG for representation and analysis of molecular networks involving diseases and drugs. Nucleic Acids Res. 2010;38(Database issue):D355–60. doi:10.1093/nar/gkp896.
36. Birney E, Stamatoyannopoulos JA, Dutta A, Guigo R, Gingeras TR, Margulies EH, et al. Identification and analysis of functional elements in 1 % of the human genome by the ENCODE pilot project. Nature. 2007;447(7146):799–816. doi:10.1038/nature05874.
37. Filion GJ, Zhenilo S, Salozhin S, Yamada D, Prokhortchouk E, Defossez PA. A family of human zinc finger proteins that bind methylated DNA and repress transcription. Mol Cell Biol. 2006;26(1):169–81. doi:10.1128/mcb.26.1.169-181.2006.
38. Hogart A, Lichtenberg J, Ajay SS, Anderson S, Margulies EH, Bodine DM. Genome-wide DNA methylation profiles in hematopoietic stem and progenitor cells reveal overrepresentation of ETS transcription factor binding sites. Genome Res. 2012;22(8):1407–18. doi:10.1101/gr.132878.111.
39. Miller DM, Thomas SD, Islam A, Muench D, Sedoris K. c-Myc and cancer metabolism. Clin Cancer Res. 2012;18(20):5546–53. doi:10.1158/1078-0432.ccr-12-0977.
40. Langfelder P, Horvath S. WGCNA: an R package for weighted correlation network analysis. BMC Bioinf. 2008;9:559. doi:10.1186/1471-2105-9-559.
41. Chiorazzi N, Ferrarini M. B cell chronic lymphocytic leukemia: lessons learned from studies of the B cell antigen receptor. Annu Rev Immunol. 2003;21:841–94. doi:10.1146/annurev.immunol.21.120601.141018.
42. Hagman J, Ramirez J, Lukin K. B lymphocyte lineage specification, commitment and epigenetic control of transcription by early B cell factor 1. Curr Top Microbiol Immunol. 2012;356:17–38. doi:10.1007/82_2011_139.
43. Robertson AG, Bilenky M, Tam A, Zhao Y, Zeng T, Thiessen N, et al. Genome-wide relationship between histone H3 lysine 4 mono- and tri-methylation and transcription factor binding. Genome Res. 2008;18(12):1906–17. doi:10.1101/gr.078519.108.
44. Hazan RB, Qiao R, Keren R, Badano I, Suyama K. Cadherin switch in tumor progression. Ann N Y Acad Sci. 2004;1014:155–63.
45. Tsurimoto T, Shinozaki A, Yano M, Seki M, Enomoto T. Human Werner helicase interacting protein 1 (WRNIP1) functions as a novel modulator for DNA polymerase delta. Genes to cells : devoted to molecular & cellular mechanisms. 2005;10(1):13–22. doi:10.1111/j.1365-2443.2004.00812.x.
46. Yoon HG, Chan DW, Huang ZQ, Li J, Fondell JD, Qin J, et al. Purification and functional characterization of the human N-CoR complex: the roles of HDAC3, TBL1 and TBLR1. The EMBO journal. 2003;22(6):1336–46. doi:10.1093/emboj/cdg120.
47. Kashatus D, Cogswell P, Baldwin AS. Expression of the Bcl-3 proto-oncogene suppresses p53 activation. Genes Dev. 2006;20(2):225–35. doi:10.1101/gad.1352206.
48. Massoumi R, Chmielarska K, Hennecke K, Pfeifer A, Fassler R. Cyld inhibits tumor cell proliferation by blocking Bcl-3-dependent NF-kappaB signaling. Cell. 2006;125(4):665–77. doi:10.1016/j.cell.2006.03.041.
49. Fu H, Maunakea AK, Martin MM, Huang L, Zhang Y, Ryan M, et al. Methylation of histone H3 on lysine 79 associates with a group of replication origins and helps limit DNA replication once per cell cycle. PLoS Genet. 2013;9(6), e1003542. doi:10.1371/journal.pgen.1003542.
50. Sims 3rd RJ, Reinberg D. Processing the H3K36me3 signature. Nat Genet. 2009;41(3):270–1. doi:10.1038/ng0309-270.
51. Cao R, Wang L, Wang H, Xia L, Erdjument-Bromage H, Tempst P, et al. Role of histone H3 lysine 27 methylation in Polycomb-group silencing. Science. 2002;298(5595):1039–43. doi:10.1126/science.1076997.
52. Reddington JP, Perricone SM, Nestor CE, Reichmann J, Youngson NA, Suzuki M, et al. Redistribution of H3K27me3 upon DNA hypomethylation results in de-repression of Polycomb target genes. Genome Biol. 2013;14(3):R25. doi:10.1186/gb-2013-14-3-r25.
53. Ng SY, Yoshida T, Zhang J, Georgopoulos K. Genome-wide lineage-specific transcriptional networks underscore Ikaros-dependent lymphoid priming in hematopoietic stem cells. Immunity. 2009;30(4):493–507. doi:10.1016/j.immuni.2009.01.014.
54. Fujita T, Nolan GP, Liou HC, Scott ML, Baltimore D. The candidate proto-oncogene bcl-3 encodes a transcriptional coactivator that activates through NF-kappa B p50 homodimers. Genes Dev. 1993;7(7B):1354–63.
55. Krueger F, Andrews SR. Bismark: a flexible aligner and methylation caller for Bisulfite-Seq applications. Bioinformatics (Oxford, England). 2011;27(11):1571–2. doi:10.1093/bioinformatics/btr167.
56. Trapnell C, Williams BA, Pertea G, Mortazavi A, Kwan G, van Baren MJ, et al. Transcript assembly and quantification by RNA-Seq reveals unannotated transcripts and isoform switching during cell differentiation. Nat Biotechnol. 2010;28(5):511–5. doi:10.1038/nbt.1621.
57. Trapnell C, Hendrickson DG, Sauvageau M, Goff L, Rinn JL, Pachter L. Differential analysis of gene regulation at transcript resolution with RNA-seq. Nat Biotechnol. 2013;31(1):46–53. doi:10.1038/nbt.2450.
58. Akalin A, Kormaksson M, Li S, Garrett-Bakelman FE, Figueroa ME, Melnick A, et al. methylKit: a comprehensive R package for the analysis of genome-wide DNA methylation profiles. Genome Biol. 2012;13(10):R87. doi:10.1186/gb-2012-13-10-r87.
59. Falcon S, Gentleman R. Using GOstats to test gene lists for GO term association. Bioinformatics (Oxford, England). 2007;23(2):257–8. doi:10.1093/bioinformatics/btl567.
60. Stelzer G, Inger A, Olender T, Iny-Stein T, Dalah I, Harel A, et al. GeneDecks: paralog hunting and gene-set distillation with GeneCards annotation. OMICS. 2009;13(6):477–87. doi:10.1089/omi.2009.0069.
61. Dozmorov MG, Cara LR, Giles CB, Wren JD. GenomeRunner: automating genome exploration. Bioinformatics (Oxford, England). 2012;28(3):419–20. doi:10.1093/bioinformatics/btr666.
62. Heinz S, Benner C, Spann N, Bertolino E, Lin YC, Laslo P, et al. Simple combinations of lineage-determining transcription factors prime cis-regulatory elements required for macrophage and B cell identities. Mol Cell. 2010;38(4):576–89. doi:10.1016/j.molcel.2010.05.004.
63. Langfelder P, Luo R, Oldham MC, Horvath S. Is my network module preserved and reproducible? PLoS Comput Biol. 2011;7(1), e1001057. doi:10.1371/journal.pcbi.1001057.

11

The up-regulation of Myb may help mediate EGCG inhibition effect on mouse lung adenocarcinoma

Hong Zhou[1*], Joseph Manthey[1], Ekaterina Lioutikova[1], William Yang[2], Kenji Yoshigoe[2], Mary Qu Yang[2*] and Hong Wang[3]

Abstract

Background: Green tea polyphenol epigallocatechin-3-gallate (EGCG) has been demonstrated to inhibit cancer in experimental studies through its antioxidant activity and modulations on cellular functions by binding specific proteins. By means of computational analysis and functional genomic approaches, we previously identified a set of protein coding genes and microRNAs whose expressions were significantly modulated in response to the EGCG treatment in tobacco carcinogen-induced lung adenocarcinoma in A/J mice. However, to what degree these genes are involved in the cancer inhibition of EGCG remains unclear.

Results: In this study, we further employed statistical methods and literature research to analyze these data in combination with The Cancer Genome Atlas (TCGA) lung adenocarcinoma datasets for additional data mining. Under the assumption that, if a gene mediates EGCG's cancer inhibition, its expression level change caused by EGCG should be opposite to what occurred in the carcinogenesis, we identified Myb and Peg3 as the primary putative genes involved in the cancer inhibitory activity. Further analysis suggested that the regulation of Myb could be mediated through an EGCG-upregulated microRNA, miR-449c-5p.

Conclusions: Although the actions of EGCG involve multiple targets/pathways, further analysis by mining the existing genomic datasets revealed that the upregulations of Myb and Peg3 are likely the key anti-cancer events of EGCG in vivo.

Background

Green tea polyphenol epigallocatechin-3-gallate (EGCG) has been shown to have preventive effect for several diseases including cancer [1–4]. A substantial number of studies have been conducted to uncover the cancer preventive mechanisms of EGCG at the cellular and molecular levels including experimental studies using animal models. The results from these studies support that the treatment with EGCG or EGCG-rich tea extract leads to a wide range of responses and that the cancer prevention activities are most likely to be mediated through multiple mechanisms resulted from direct scavenging of stress molecules such as reactive oxygen species (ROS) and/or the physical interactions of EGCG with specific proteins to modulate gene expression and cellular signaling. However, most experimental evidence supporting anti-cancer mechanisms of EGCG are obtained from in vitro studies. Whether or not these mechanisms play significant roles in the cancer prevention/inhibition in vivo remains to be determined.

The tobacco carcinogen-induced lung carcinogenesis in A/J mice is a well-characterized animal model. It has been shown using this animal model that tumor multiplicity and size are effectively inhibited when mice are fed an experimental diet containing EGCG [2, 5]. Using this animal model, our recent study has demonstrated that cellular changes in lung cancer cells treated with EGCG are associated with alterations in both messenger RNA (mRNA) and microRNA (miRNA) expressions [6]. Computational analysis on microarray data revealed that

* Correspondence: hzhou@usj.edu; mqyang@ualr.edu
[1]Department of Mathematical Science, School of Health and Natural Sciences, University of Saint Joseph, 1678 Asylum Avenue, West Hartford, CT 06117, USA
[2]Joint Bioinformatics Ph.D. Program, University of Arkansas at Little Rock and University of Arkansas for Medical Sciences, 2801 S. University Avenue, Little Rock, AR 72204, USA

the EGCG-induced expression changes of some genes also involved miRNA-mediated gene regulation [6].

It is well-recognized that EGCG treatment can cause a wide range of responses at both the cellular and molecular levels [2]. Using "EGCG" as the keyword to search through NIH's TOXNET databases, specifically the Comparative Toxicogenomics Database (CTD) which provides scientific data describing relationships between chemicals, genes, and human diseases, we found that EGCG treatment or co-treatment with other agents can impact the expression of about 2000 genes in both humans and mice. Our recent study also showed that, in the carcinogen-induced lung tumor in A/J mice, EGCG treatment induces the expression level change of 367 genes (at least onefold change) [6]. Since the large group of genes up- or down-regulated by EGCG includes genes which are not related to lung carcinogenesis [7, 8], identifying the relevant genes would advance our understanding of the cancer inhibition mechanism of EGCG.

In this study, we employed statistical approaches and literature research and combined the data from The Cancer Genome Atlas (TCGA) [9] to further determine the candidate genes, including miRNA, which participate in the EGCG inhibition mechanism. We focused on exploring the lung cancer-related genes and identifying the ones that could potentially play predominant roles in mediating the cancer inhibition by EGCG in the carcinogen-induced A/J mouse lung cancer model.

Methods

Microarray data of mRNA expression and miRNA expression were obtained from two sources. The first was from our previous study that compared the mRNA and miRNA expression profiles in A/J mice bearing 4-(methylnitrosamino)-1-(3-pyridyl)-1-butanone (NNK)-induced lung tumor fed on the diet containing 0.4 % EGCG or the control AIN93M diet [6]. In this dataset, mRNA expression profiles include 3 microarray results of lung tumors collected from 3 control mice and 3 EGCG-treated mice, and the miRNA expression profiles include microarray results of lung tumors collected from 8 control mice and 8 EGCG-treated mice. The second source was the gene expression profile batch 37 of lung adenocarcinoma obtained from TCGA data matrix [9]. The filter settings used to obtain this dataset include Data Level = 3, Availability = Available, Center/Platform = All, Access Tier = Public, and Tumor/Normal = Tumor-matched.

When performing statistical analysis on the microarray datasets, we made the following assumptions.

(1) There are random variations in gene expression among samples which are independent of the treatments. These random variations in gene expression represent the normal variations of individuals in a group of experimental animals.
(2) When treated with EGCG, the expression changes of responsive genes are expected to be statistically significant and consistent among all treated samples compared to the control.

To analyze the mRNA expression profiles, within the 3 controls and the 3 EGCG-treated samples, we first removed those genes whose expression in the 3 EGCG treatments were not consistently up or down compared to the average of the 3 controls. This means that we only selected those genes whose expressions were consistently up-regulated or down-regulated in all the 3 EGCG-treated samples compared to the average of the 3 controls. Then, we computed the difference between the averaged expression levels of the 3 controls and the 3 treatments for each gene. The standard deviation was calculated for the difference distribution, and z-scores were obtained for each gene. Only those genes whose z-scores were ≥3.00 or ≤−3.00 were considered genes that were impacted significantly by EGCG treatment.

To analyze the miRNA profiles, with the 8 controls and 8 EGCG treatments, the difference between averaged control and treatment was obtained for each miRNA. The standard deviation was calculated for the differences, and z-scores were obtained for each miRNA. We first selected those miRNAs whose z-scores were ≥2.00 or ≤−2.00. Then, among those selected miRNAs, we conducted an independent sample *t* test between the 8 controls and the 8 EGCG samples. Only those miRNAs with *p* values of the *t* test less than 0.05 were considered as miRNAs that were responsive to EGCG treatment.

From TCGA database, we obtained microarray gene expression data for 21 human lung adenocarcinoma samples (batch 37) publically released by Michael Topal and Katherine Hoadley from the University of North Carolina at Chapel Hill on February 10, 2009 [9]. These 21 datasets represent the normalized gene expression differences between lung adenocarcinoma and a normal cell line. Although there are another 11 sets of such data in batch 52, some gene expressions are null in batch 52, and batch 52 was not used in this study. After the standard deviation was calculated based on the average of the 21 datasets, z-scores were computed for each gene. Only those genes whose expression levels are all up or all down in the 21 sets and whose z-scores were ≥3.00 or ≤−3.00 were selected.

Gene pathway analyses were conducted using iPathwayGuide (https://apps.advaitabio.com/ipg/home). The only adjustable setting of iPathwayGuide is its DE threshold. The settings used were as follows: Fold Change (log) = 1.0 and Adjusted *p* value = 0.01. Gene interaction analysis was conducted using the PCViz web tool http://www.pathwaycommons.org.

Results

In the comparison of the microarray results of mRNA expression profiles of the 3 controls and 3 EGCG samples, mRNAs whose expression levels are not consistently up or down between the controls and EGCG-treated samples were removed. We selected only these consistent data records because they tend to be more reliable. Fourteen thousand seven hundred sixty-five records were selected. Z-scores were computed for every mRNA (gene). Only those genes whose z-scores were ≥3.00 or ≤3.00 were considered genes that are impacted significantly by EGCG treatment, i.e., the expression changes of these genes between the control and the sample are likely a result of the EGCG treatment. There were 225 unique genes selected (see Additional file 1). The large number of genes impacted by EGCG treatment is expected as EGCG treatment induces a wide range of biological responses [1–3].

In the A/J mouse lung carcinogenesis model, the tumor multiplicity and size are effectively inhibited when mice are fed a diet containing EGCG [2, 5]. Apoptosis was induced and pro-proliferation signalings were reduced in tumors after a long-term treatment with EGCG [10, 11]. The gene expression profiles showed that cell cycle regulation and inflammation were the most impacted pathways by a long-term EGCG treatment (~20 weeks) [12]. Since a long-term EGCG treatment may cause multiple waves of responses which can disguise the targeted genes or pathways of EGCG, we preferred a short-term treatment experiment for elucidating the earlier responses, as described in our recent study in which EGCG was applied for only 1 week [6]. Although it is somewhat surprising that none of the 17 signature genes identified by Lu et al. [12] were found among the 225 genes, such a discrepancy indicates that the short-term treatment causes a wider range of early responses while the result induced by the long-term treatment represents the overall consequence post the early response. Thus, the result of short treatment offers better chance to identify the mechanism.

By analyzing the 225 genes using iPathwayGuide, the only pathway approaching statistical significance (p = 0.08) is the Kyoto Encyclopedia of Genes and Genomes (KEGG) chemokine pathway [13]. This pathway is associated with multiple cellular functions such as cellular growth and differentiation, cell survival, migration, apoptosis, chemotaxis, and ROS production [14–26]. Indeed, this is consistent with what was reported previously, either with a long-term or short-term EGCG treatment [6, 10–12]. This result supports that the anti-cancer mechanism of EGCG is mediated through the regulation of cellular growth, apoptosis, differentiation, and migration.

By applying the same statistical selection process on the 21 lung adenocarcinoma datasets collected from the TCGA database, 478 genes were selected from the TCGA LUAD datasets since they displayed significantly up-regulated or down-regulated expression levels in the lung adenocarcinoma tissues. Comparing with the 225 genes selected from EGCG treatment, 16 genes were found to be in both groups. We postulated that if EGCG is truly inhibiting the lung carcinogenesis, then it should reverse the expression levels of some genes that were over-expressed or under-expressed in lung cancer tissues. Thus, we were searching for those genes whose expression levels were reversed in the EGCG-treated samples when compared with the TCGA LUAD datasets. In the overlapped genes between the 478 genes selected from the TCGA LUAD datasets and the 225 genes selected from EGCG-treated group, only Myb, Peg3, and Myl4 display a reverse expression pattern (Table 1). While Myl4 was not found to be related to carcinogenesis based on the existing literature, both Myb and Peg3 were reported to be involved in carcinogenesis [27–30]. Although Myb has been considered as an oncogene [31, 32], its down-regulation in human lung cancer suggests that it may have dual functions. Nevertheless, this comparison suggested that EGCG's inhibition on mouse lung carcinogenesis reversed the carcinogenesis-associated changes, and Myb and Peg3 are the putative genes that mediate such inhibition effect.

Using the functional annotation tool of David Bioinformatics Resources 6.7 (http://david.abcc.ncifcrf.gov/) to

Table 1 Genes whose expression levels were significantly altered and were found in both the EGCG experiment and the TCGA dataset

Genes	From normal to LUAD	From control to EGCG treatment
Cox7a1	Up	Up
Myh11	Up	Up
Fmo3	Up	Up
Myb	Down	Up
Cxcl13	Up	Up
Scgb3a1	Up	Up
F13a1	Up	Up
Peg3	Down	Up
Acta2	Up	Up
Fabp4	Up	Up
Clic6	Up	Up
Myl4	Down	Up
S100a9	Up	Up
Col8a2	Up	Up
Bank1	Up	Up
Mmp9	Up	Up

analyze these overlapped genes also identified F13a1, Fmo3, Mmp9, and Myh11 as related to cancer. Among these genes, Mmp9 is specifically related to lung cancer [33–36]. However, these genes including Mmp9 are less likely to be related to the inhibition function of EGCG since they do not exhibit a reversed expression pattern.

In order to assess the possible roles of Myb, Peg3, and Myl4, we employed the PCViz network visualization tool (www.pathwaycommons.org), a web tool to construct gene interaction network based on information mined from published literature and to analyze the possible gene interactions for Myb, Peg3, and Myl4. We found that there are no identified gene interactions for both Peg3 and Myl4, while Myb has the potential to control the expression of a large number of genes including Myc, Nras, and Bcl2 that are well-characterized for their role in tumorigenesis (Fig. 1). This suggests that Myb might play a much more critical role than Peg3 in mediating the anti-cancer activity of EGCG.

A further analysis on those genes that were identified by the PCViz network to be affected by Myb shows that there are 29 mRNA genes whose expressions were affected by EGCG treatment. However, there are only 3 genes, Col1a2, Ccnb1, and Copa, whose expression levels could be considered to be significantly impacted by EGCG treatment. Col1a2 was up-regulated by 1.8-fold, while Ccnb1 and Copa were down-regulated by 2.4- and 3.4-fold, respectively. Clearly, much more studies are required before any conclusion can be drawn on how Myb mediates EGCG's anti-cancer activities.

In our previous study, we demonstrated that miRNAs can mediate the gene regulation by EGCG [6]. Here, we used statistical methods to further investigate the possible roles of miRNA in EGCG treatments, especially if miRNA can possibly mediate the regulation of Myb and/or Peg3 by EGCG. We first used statistical methods to identify those miRNAs whose expression levels were significantly modified by EGCG treatment. The selection of such miRNAs is a two-step process. In step 1, the averaged miRNA expression levels were computed for both the 8 controls and 8 samples. The averaged difference was then calculated for each miRNA. By treating the pool of the averaged differences as normally distributed, z-scores were computed for each miRNA. Only those

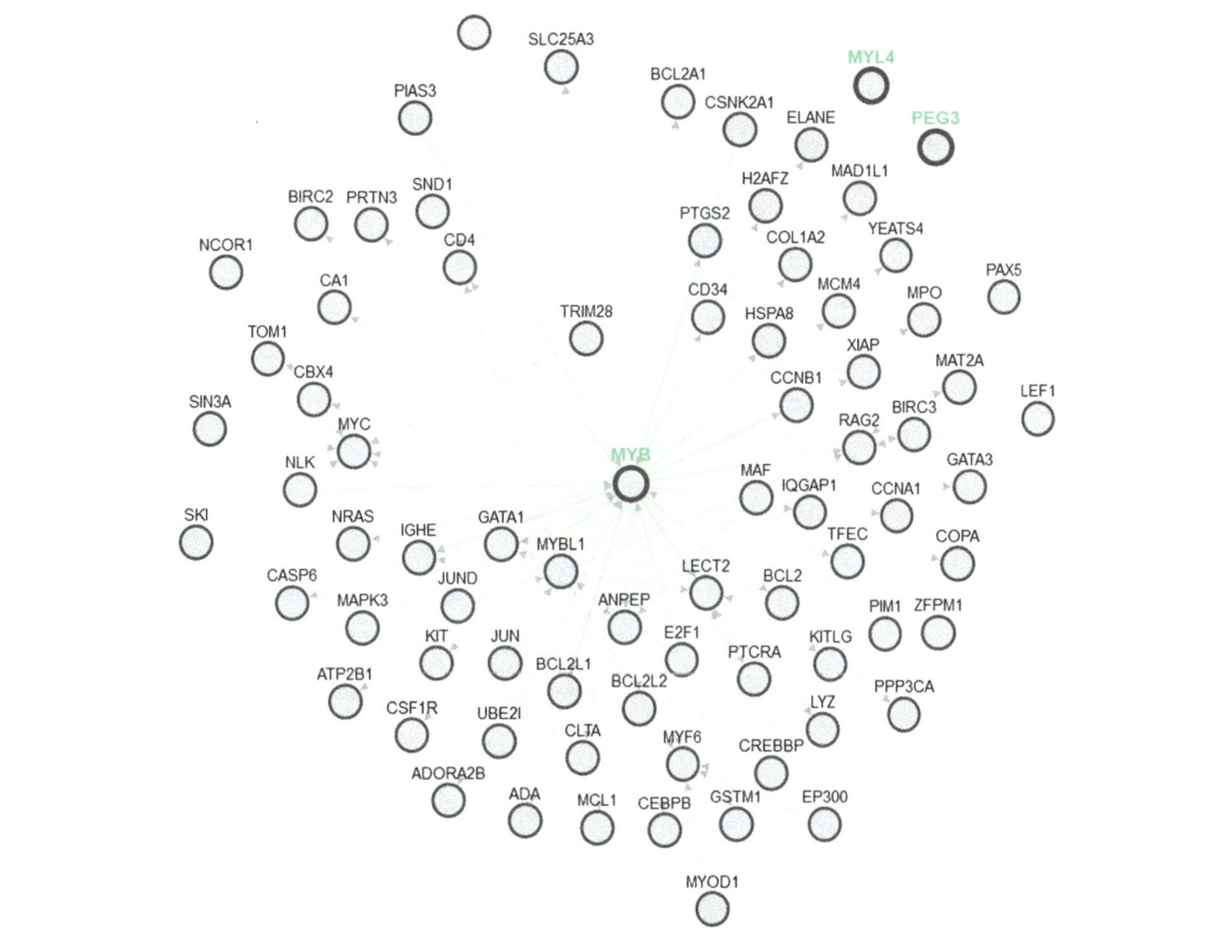

Fig. 1 The gene interaction network of Myb, Peg3, and Myl4. There are 76 genes and 88 interactions for Myb, while none for Peg3 or Myl4

miRNAs for which $|z| \geq 2.00$ were selected. In step 2, an independent sample t test (two tails) was conducted between the 8 controls and 8 EGCG-treated samples for each selected miRNA. Those miRNAs that did not show a statistically significant difference ($p \leq 0.05$) between the controls and samples were removed. Using this selection process, 27 miRNAs were selected as shown in Table 2.

Among the 27 miRNAs, 20 were up-regulated. Since the function of miRNA is to suppress the maturation of its targeting mRNAs, up-regulated expression of miRNA usually result in down-regulated mRNA expression and vice versa. Using both Diana microT-CDS v3.0 and miRDB microRNA target prediction tools, we collected a number of potential microRNA target genes for the 27 miRNAs in Table 2. Based on the up/down-regulated expression levels of these 27 miRNAs, we only selected a protein coding gene as a target of a microRNA if (1) its expression change is opposite to the change of the miRNA expression and (2) it exists in the 225 gene groups. The results are summarized in Table 3.

Thirty genes were found to be candidates targeted by the 27 miRNAs. It is interesting to notice that of the 30 genes, only Fbp1 has its expression level up-regulated; and of the 27 miRNAs, only 6 were found to regulate gene expressions significantly. In this candidate gene list,

Table 2 miRNAs that display a statistically significant difference between the controls and EGCG treatments

Up-regulated miRNAs	Down-regulated miRNAs
mmu-miR-2137	mmu-miR-1199-3p
mmu-miR-5131	mmu-miR-218-5p
mmu-miR-680	mmu-miR-7a-5p
mmu-miR-5130	mmu-miR-374c-5p
mmu-miR-144	mmu-miR-449c-5p
mmu-miR-486	mmu-miR-450a-2-3p
mmu-miR-711	mmu-miR-696
mmu-miR-449a	
mmu-miR-193	
mmu-miR-34c-5p	
mmu-miR-2861	
mmu-miR-211-3p	
mmu-miR-763	
mmu-miR-128-2-5p	
mmu-miR-542-5p	
mmu-miR-3473	
mmu-miR-511-3p	
mmu-miR-34c-5p	
mmu-miR-143-5p	
mmu-miR-5115	

Table 3 Genes regulated by EGCG potentially mediated through miRNA

Targeted gene	Gene expression change	miRNA(s)	miRNA expression change
Rsph4a	Up	mmu-miR-374c-5p	Down
Rbm24	Up	mmu-miR-374c-5p	Down
DCN	Up	mmu-miR-374c-5p	Down
Acta2	Up	mmu-miR-374c-5p	Down
Zfp182	Up	mmu-miR-374c-5p	Down
KLHL4	Up	mmu-miR-374c-5p	Down
ART3	Up	mmu-miR-374c-5p	Down
GAS1	Up	mmu-miR-374c-5p, mmu-miR-449c-5p	Down
Myb	Up	mmu-miR-449c-5p	Down
Elmod1	Up	mmu-miR-449c-5p	Down
Ldb3	Up	mmu-miR-449c-5p	Down
Calcb	Up	mmu-miR-449c-5p	Down
ZFHX4	Up	mmu-miR-449c-5p, mmu-miR-450a-2-3p	Down
IGFBP5	Up	mmu-miR-450a-2-3p	Down
Bnc1	Up	mmu-miR-450a-2-3p	Down
GABRP	Up	mmu-miR-450a-2-3p	Down
Cd19	Up	mmu-miR-450a-2-3p	Down
AQP4	Up	mmu-miR-450a-2-3p	Down
VCAN	Up	mmu-miR-450a-2-3p	Down
Cnr1	Up	mmu-miR-218-5p, mmu-miR-374c-5p	Down
EBF1	Up	mmu-miR-218-5p, mmu-miR-374c-5p	Down
LASP1	Up	mmu-miR-218-5p	Down
Gm3008	Up	mmu-miR-218-5p	Down
Gstm6	Up	mmu-miR-218-5p	Down
BICD1	Up	mmu-miR-218-5p, mmu-miR-374c-5p	Down
ACSL1	Up	mmu-miR-218-5p, mmu-miR-449c-5p	Down
Six4	Up	mmu-miR-218-5p, mmu-miR-7a-5p	Down
AACS	Up	mmu-miR-218-5p, mmu-miR-7a-5p	Down
Pfn2	Up	mmu-miR-7a-5p	Down
Fbp1	Down	mmu-miR-34c-5p	Up

Myb gene is shown as a target of mmu-miR-449c-5p, indicating that the miRNA such as miR-449c-5p may play an important role in the inhibitory activity of EGCG.

Discussion

Since EGCG treatment causes a wide range of responses at both cellular and molecular levels, it is difficult to elucidate how EGCG unleashes its anti-cancer effects, especially in an in vivo model like the carcinogen-induced lung adenocarcinoma in A/J mice. One possible approach is to apply the genomic studies with bioinformatics analysis integrated with literature research. We demonstrated that this is a feasible approach in this study.

A critical assumption in this study is that most genes have small variations on their expressions as a random phenomenon, while genes impacted by EGCG treatment would exhibit larger variations, i.e., statistically significant variations. Though the distribution of the mRNA expression differences between the averaged control and EGCG treatment is not a normal distribution, the large size of the sample (14,765 gene records) allows us to make this assumption. We made a similar assumption on the miRNA expression alterations caused by EGCG treatment. However, the sample size of miRNAs is only 656, much smaller than that of mRNAs. To ensure the significance of the miRNAs selected from our statistical approach, we used a two-step process. In the first step, z-score of 2.0 was used as the cutoff. A z-score of 2.0 was used instead of a z-score of 3.0 due to the relatively small sample size of miRNA genes. In addition, the independent sample *t* test used in the second step further ensures the significance of the selected miRNAs. After identifying 225 mRNAs and 27 miRNAs whose altered expression levels are statistically significant, we assumed that some of these selected genes, either mRNA or miRNA, may be related to EGCG's anti-cancer mechanism.

While the pathway analysis showed that this group of 225 genes is likely to be involved in the chemokine pathway which plays an important role in migration, cell growth and differentiation, apoptosis, and chemotaxis [13], it did not reveal the genes related to anti-cancer activity of EGCG. The TCGA lung adenocarcinoma (LUAD) datasets contain the normalized gene expression microarray data which records the fold changes between lung adenocarcinoma tissues and a normal cell line. These datasets serve as a good supplemental control to our experiment. We expect that if a gene mediates the anti-cancer activity of EGCG, then its expression level change in our EGCG treatment experiment should be opposite to its expression level change in the TCGA LUAD datasets. Three genes, Myb, Peg3, and Myl4, were found to match this criterion, and their expression level changes are statistically significant. While our literature research has not found any role of Myl4 in carcinogenesis, Peg3 has been reported to act like a tumor suppressor gene [29, 30].

As a transcription factor, Myb gene has been reported to be involved in the progression of different types of cancer including lung cancer and has recently been considered as an oncogene because of its critical role in cell proliferation and differentiation [27, 28, 31, 32]. However, its expression which is reduced in TCGA LUAD datasets suggests that Myb expression decrement is necessary for human lung carcinogenesis. Although we do not understand the reason, one possibility is that Myb may have dual functions or tissue specific function. If so, our result here supports that Myb is necessary for EGCG to exert its anti-cancer effect. Interestingly, our result further showed that Myb could be regulated by EGCG down-regulated miRNA, miR-449c-5p. Again, if Myb does not act as oncogene but mediates the cancer inhibitory activity of EGCG, this result suggests that miRNA-mediated gene regulation is an important action of EGCG although these miRNAs may not be directly regulated by EGCG as we discussed previously [6].

Conclusions

EGCG treatment leads to the expression level changes of a large number of genes, causing a wide range of biological responses. However, it is unlikely that majority of these regulated genes mediate the anti-cancer activity of EGCG. Our analysis on the whole transcriptome integrated with TCGA datasets on human lung cancer revealed that EGCG reverses the lung carcinogenesis-associated changes of Myb and Peg3, suggesting that Myb and Peg3 play key roles in the anti-cancer activity of EGCG. In addition, our analysis of the miRNA profiles suggests that the up-regulation of Myb by EGCG could be achieved by EGCG-induced down-regulation of miRNA mmu-miR-449c-5p, supporting a role of miRNA in the anti-cancer activity of EGCG.

Competing interests

The authors declare that they have no competing interests.

Authors' contributions

HZ and MQY conceived the project and all authors participated in the analysis of the data, interpretation of the results, and review of the paper. HZ, HW, JM, EL, WY, KY and MQY performed the data analysis, HW helped conduct the experiments. HZ, HW and JM drafted the paper. All authors read and approved the final version of the manuscript.

Acknowledgements

HZ received TLC faculty research fund and publication fund from the University of Saint Joseph. MQY and KY were supported by NIH 1R15GM114739. Funding for open-access publication of this article came from NIH 1R15GM114739.

Declarations

This article has been published as part of *Human Genomics* Volume 10 Supplement 2, 2016: From genes to systems genomics: human genomics. The full contents of the supplement are available online at http://humgenomics.biomedcentral.com/articles/supplements/volume-10-supplement-2.

Author details

[1]Department of Mathematical Science, School of Health and Natural Sciences, University of Saint Joseph, 1678 Asylum Avenue, West Hartford, CT 06117, USA. [2]Joint Bioinformatics Ph.D. Program, University of Arkansas at Little Rock and University of Arkansas for Medical Sciences, 2801 S. University Avenue, Little Rock, AR 72204, USA. [3]Susan L. Cullman Laboratory for Cancer Research, Department of Chemical Biology and Centre for Cancer Prevention Research, Ernest Mario School of Pharmacy, Rutgers, The State University of New Jersey, 164 Frelinghuysen Road, Piscataway, NJ 08854, USA.

References

1. Khan N, Afaq F, Saleem M, Ahmad N, Mukhtar H. Targeting multiple signaling pathways by green tea polyphenol (-)-epigallocatechin-3-gallate. Cancer Res. 2006;66:2500–5.
2. Yang CS, Wang X, Lu G, Picinich SC. Cancer prevention by tea: animal studies, molecular mechanisms and human relevance. Nat Rev Cancer. 2009; 9:429–39.
3. Yang CS, Wang H, Li GX, Yang Z, Guan F, Jin H. Cancer prevention by tea: evidence from laboratory studies. Pharmacol Res. 2011;64:113–22.
4. Kitamura M, Nishino T, Obata Y, Furusu A, Hishikawa Y, Koji T, Kohno S. Epigallocatechin gallate suppresses peritoneal fibrosis in mice. Chem Biol Interact. 2012;195:95–104.
5. Ju J, Lu G, Lambert JD, Yang CS. Inhibition of carcinogenesis by tea constituents. Semin Cancer Biol. 2007;17:395–402.
6. Zhou H, Chen J, Yang CS, Yang M, Deng Y, Wang H. Gene regulation mediated by microRNAs in response to green tea polyphenol EGCG in mouse lung cancer. BMC Genomics. 2014;15 suppl 11:S3.
7. Kim HS, Quon MJ, Kim J. New insights into the mechanisms of polyphenols beyond antioxidant properties; lessons from the green tea polyphenol, epigallocatechin-3-gallate. Redox Biol. 2014;2:187–95.
8. El-Telbany A, Ma PC. Cancer genes in lung cancer: racial disparities: are there any? Genes Cancer. 2012;3:467–80.
9. https://tcga-data.nci.nih.gov/tcga/dataAccessMatrix.htm?mode=ApplyFilter, accessed on 13 Nov 2014.
10. Lu G, Liao J, Yang G, Reuhl KR, Hao X, Yang CS. Inhibition of adenoma progression to adenocarcinoma in a 4-(methylnitrosamino)-1-(3-pyridyl)-1-butanone-induced lung tumorigenesis model in A/J mice by tea polyphenols and caffeine. Cancer Res. 2006;66:11494–501.
11. Li GX, Chen YK, Hou Z, Xiao H, Jin H, Lu G, Lee MJ, Liu B, Guan F, Yang Z, et al. Pro-oxidative activities and dose-response relationship of (-)-epigallocatechin-3-gallate in the inhibition of lung cancer cell growth: a comparative study in vivo and in vitro. Carcinogenesis. 2010;31:902–10.
12. Lu Y, Yao R, Yan Y, Wang Y, Hara Y, Lubet RA, You M. A gene expression signature that can predict green tea exposure and chemopreventive efficacy of lung cancer in mice. Cancer Res. 2006;66:1956–63.
13. http://www.genome.jp/kegg/pathway.html. Accessed on 24 Nov 2014.
14. Mellado M, Rodriguez-Frade JM, Mañes S, Martinez-A C. Chemokine signaling and functional responses: the role of receptor dimerization and TK papthway activation. Annu Rev Immunol. 2001;19:397–421.
15. Wong MM, Fish EN. Chemokines: attractive mediators of the immune response. Semin Immunol. 2003;15:5–14.
16. Curnock AP, Logan MK, Ward SG. Chemokine signaling: pivoting around multiple phosphoinostitide 3-kinases. Immunology. 2002;105:125–36.
17. Busillo JM, Benovic JL. Regulation of CXCR4 signaling. Biochim Biophys Acta. 1768;2007:952–63.
18. Olson TS, Ley K. Chemokines and chemokine receptors in leukocyte trafficking. Am J Physiol Regul Integr Comp Physiol. 2002;283:R7–28.
19. Knall C, Young S, Nick JA, Buhl AM, Worthen GS, Johnson GL. Interleukin-8 regulation of the Ras/Raf/mitogen-activated protein kinase pathway in human neutrophils. J Biol Chem. 1996;271:2832–8.
20. Hauck CR, Klingbeil CK, Schlaepfer DD. Focal adhesion kinase functions as a receptor-proximal signaling component required for directed cell migration. Immunol Res. 2000;21:293–303.
21. Chandrasekar B, Bysani S, Mummidi S. CXCL16 signals via Gi, phosphatidylinositol 3-kinase, Akt, I kappa B kinase, and nuclear factor-kappa B and induces cell-cell adhesion and aortic smooth muscle cell proliferation. J Biol Chem. 2004;279:3188–96.
22. Schwartzberg PL, Finkelstein LD, Readinger JA. TEC-family kinases: regulators of T-helper-cell differentiation. Nat Rev Immunol. 2005;5:284–95.
23. Ticcioni M, Essafi M, Jeandel PY, Davi F, Cassuto JP, Deckert M, Bernard A. Hemeostatic chemokines increase survival of B-chronic lymphocytic leukemia cells through inactivation of transcription factor FOXO3a. Oncegene. 2007;26:7081–91.
24. Johnson Z, Power CA, Weiss C, Rintelen F, Ji H, Ruckle T, Camps M, Wells TN, Schwarz MK, Proudfoot AE, Rommel C. Chemokine inhibition—why, when, where, which and how? Biochem Soc Trans. 2004;32:366–77.
25. Bach TL, Chen QM, Kerr WT, Wang Y, Lian L, Choi JK, Wu D, Kazanietz MG, Koretzky GA, Zigmond S, Abrams CS. Phospholipase cbeta is critical for T cell chemotaxis. J Immunol. 2007;179:2223–7.
26. Hornstein I, Alcover A, Katzav S. Vav proteins, masters of the world of cytoskeleton organization. Cell Signal. 2004;16:1–11.
27. George OL, Ness SA. Situational awareness: regulation of the Myb transcription factor in differentiation, the cell cycle and oncogenesis. Cancers. 2014;6:2049–71.
28. Stenman G, Andersson MK, Andrén Y. New tricks from an old oncogene gene fusion and copy number alterations of MYB in human cancer. Cell Cycle. 2010;9:2986–95.
29. Kohda T, Asai A, Kuroiwa Y, Kobayashi S, Aisaka K, Nagashima G, Yoshida MC, Kondo Y, Kagiyama N, Kirino T, Kaneko-Ishino T, Ishino F. Tumor suppressor activity of human imprinted gene PEG3 in a glioma cell line. Genes Cells. 2001;6(3):237–47.
30. Feng W, Marquez RT, Lu Z, Liu J, Lu KH, Issa JP, Fishman DM, Yu Y, Bast RC. Jr. Imprinted tumor suppressor genes ARHI and PEG3 are the most frequently down-regulated in human ovarian cancers by loss of heterozygosity and promoter methylation. Cancer. 2008;112(7):1489–502.
31. Ramsay RG, Gonda TJ. MYB function in normal and cancer cells. Nat Rev Cancer. 2008;8(7):523–34.
32. Introna M, Golay J. How can oncogenic transcription factors cause cancer: a critical review of the myb story. Leukemia. 1999;13(9):1301–6.
33. Li L, Tan J, Zhang Y, Han N, Di X, Xiao T, Cheng S, Gao Y, Liu Y. DLK1 promotes lung cancer cell invasion through upregulation of MMP9 expression depending on notch signaling. PLoS ONE. 2014;9(3):e91509.
34. Bayramoglu A, Gunes HV, Metintas M, Değirmenci I, Mutlu F, Alatas F. The association of MMP-9 enzyme activity, MMP-9 C1562T polymorphism, and MMP-2 and -9 and TIMP-1,-2,-3, and -4 gene expression in lung cancer. Genet Test Mol Biomarkers. 2009;13(5):671–8.
35. Wang RJ, Wu P, Cai GX, Wang ZM, Xu Y, Peng JJ, Sheng WQ, Lu HF, Cai SJ. Down-regulated MYH11 expression correlates with poor prognosis in stage II and III colorectal cancer. Asian Pac J Cancer Prev. 2014;15(17):7223–8.
36. Morrissey C, True LD, Roudier MP, Coleman IM, Hawley S, Nelson PS, Coleman R, Wang YC, Corey E, Langge PH, Higano CS, Vessella RL. Differential expression of angiogenesis associated genes in prostate cancer bone, liver and lymph node metastases. Clin Exp Metastasis. 2008;25(4):377–88.

12

A genomic case study of desmoplastic small round cell tumor: comprehensive analysis reveals insights into potential therapeutic targets and development of a monitoring tool for a rare and aggressive disease

Elisa Napolitano Ferreira[1], Bruna Durães Figueiredo Barros[1], Jorge Estefano de Souza[2], Renan Valieris Almeida[1], Giovana Tardin Torrezan[1], Sheila Garcia[1], Ana Cristina Victorino Krepischi[3], Celso Abdon Lopes de Mello[4], Isabela Werneck da Cunha[5], Clóvis Antonio Lopes Pinto[5], Fernando Augusto Soares[5], Emmanuel Dias-Neto[1], Ademar Lopes[4], Sandro José de Souza[6] and Dirce Maria Carraro[1*]

Abstract

Background: Genome-wide profiling of rare tumors is crucial for improvement of diagnosis, treatment, and, consequently, achieving better outcomes. Desmoplastic small round cell tumor (DSRCT) is a rare type of sarcoma arising from mesenchymal cells of abdominal peritoneum that usually develops in male adolescents and young adults. A specific translocation, t(11;22)(p13;q12), resulting in *EWS* and *WT1* gene fusion is the only recurrent molecular hallmark and no other genetic factor has been associated to this aggressive tumor. Here, we present a comprehensive genomic profiling of one DSRCT affecting a 26-year-old male, who achieved an excellent outcome.

Methods: We investigated somatic and germline variants through whole-exome sequencing using a family based approach and, by array CGH, we explored the occurrence of genomic imbalances. Additionally, we performed mate-paired whole-genome sequencing for defining the specific breakpoint of the EWS-WT1 translocation, allowing us to develop a personalized tumor marker for monitoring the patient by liquid biopsy.

Results: We identified genetic variants leading to protein alterations including 12 somatic and 14 germline events (11 germline compound heterozygous mutations and 3 rare homozygous polymorphisms) affecting genes predominantly involved in mesenchymal cell differentiation pathways. Regarding copy number alterations (CNA) few events were detected, mainly restricted to gains in chromosomes 5 and 18 and losses at 11p, 13q, and 22q. The deletions at 11p and 22q indicated the presence of the classic translocation, t(11;22)(p13;q12). In addition, the mapping of the specific genomic breakpoint of the EWS-WT1 gene fusion allowed the design of a personalized biomarker for assessing circulating tumor DNA (ctDNA) in plasma during patient follow-up. This biomarker has been used in four post-treatment blood samples, 3 years after surgery, and no trace of EWS-WT1 gene fusion was detected, in accordance with imaging tests showing no evidence of disease and with the good general health status of the patient.
(Continued on next page)

* Correspondence: dirce.carraro@cipe.accamargo.org.br
[1]International Research Center/CIPE, A.C. Camargo Cancer Center, São Paulo, SP, Brazil
Full list of author information is available at the end of the article

(Continued from previous page)

Conclusions: Overall, our findings revealed genes with potential to be associated with risk assessment and tumorigenesis of this rare type of sarcoma. Additionally, we established a liquid biopsy approach for monitoring patient follow-up based on genomic information that can be similarly adopted for patients diagnosed with a rare tumor.

Keywords: Desmoplastic small round cell tumor, Genomic profiling, Whole-exome sequencing, EWS-WT1 gene fusion, Personalized biomarker, Liquid biopsy

Background

Comprehensive molecular profiling is an especially important tool to gain insights on the biological pathways involved in tumor onset and to improve the management and treatment of rare tumors. Desmoplastic small round cell tumor (DSRCT) is a very rare type of sarcoma, with an age-adjusted incidence rate of 0.3 cases/million [1], which typically arises from the abdominal or pelvic peritoneum and occurs mainly in male adolescents and young adults (peak incidence at 20–24 years of age) [1]. Current therapeutic approaches involve the use of multimodal therapeutic regimen, including aggressive polychemotherapy, debulking surgery, and whole abdominal radiation [2].

A specific translocation, t(11;22)(p13;q12), is detected in DSRCT cases, juxtaposing the Ewing's sarcoma gene (*EWSR1*) to the Wilm's tumor gene (*WT1*). The chimeric transcript containing the 5′ region of the *EWSR1*, which includes the N-terminal transactivation domain of EWS, and the 3′ sequence of *WT1* containing 2–4 zinc finger domains have been shown to upregulate EGR-1 [3] and induce the expression of PDGFA [4] and IGF1R [5].

Apart from this translocation, no other recurrent genomic alteration has been reported in DSRCT cases. Silva et al. [6] detected a somatic amplification involving *AURKB* and *MCL1* genes in one patient, and La Starza et al. [7] found specific genomic imbalances, including gain at chromosome 3 reported in two cases and chromosome 5 polysomy in one case. In terms of point mutations, the data is even scarcer. Variants of unknown clinical significance were reported in *ARID1A* and *RUNX1* genes in one patient [6], whereas in another study, no mutations were detected in a panel of 29 genes evaluated in a cohort of 24 DSRCT cases [8]. This limited genomic information about DSRCT impairs new and more efficient therapeutic opportunities for the young patients affected with this rare tumor.

Here, aiming to contribute with the knowledge of the genomic abnormalities that underlies DSRCT, we performed a comprehensive genomic profiling using a family based approach in one case of DSRCT diagnosed in a young male patient with pelvic tumor, who presented excellent outcome sustained for above 3 years. We identified somatic mutations in a genomic background of rare germline variants either homozygous or as compound heterozygous inheritance, which can improve the understanding of the genetic basis of this rare tumor. We have also generated the profile of genomic imbalances, which was confirmed by whole-exome sequencing. In addition, as we were able to define the precise genomic breakpoints of the EWS-WT1 translocation by whole-genome and Sanger sequencing, we managed to establish a personalized strategy for tracking DNA tumor traces in plasma, allowing an accurate monitoring of tumor recurrence.

Overall, our analysis revealed potential genes and pathways associated with this rare sarcoma and demonstrated the feasibility of using genomic profiling for the benefit of patients affected by rare tumors by developing a personalized monitoring strategy.

Methods

DNA extraction

Tumor tissues and blood samples were collected following the technical and ethical procedures of A.C. Camargo Tumor Bank, registered at National Council for Ethics in Research by the number B001 [9]. Genomic DNA and plasma DNA were extracted in DNA and RNA Bank [10] using QIASymphony DNA Mini kit (QIAGEN, Hilden, Germany) for tumor and leukocyte DNA and QIAamp DNA blood Midi kit (QIAGEN, Hilden, Germany) for plasma DNA, following standard procedures.

Target sequencing

Target sequencing was performed using the Ion AmpliSeq™ Comprehensive Cancer Panel, which comprises all exons from 409 genes associated with different types of tumors (AmpliSeq, Ion Torrent™). This panel, based on multiplex PCR, was performed with as little as 40 ng of DNA from the tumor sample. Library was prepared based on Ion AmpliSeq™ Library Preparation protocol and sequenced at Ion Proton™ platform (Ion Torrent™), according to the manufacturer's instructions.

Whole-exome sequencing

Whole-exome sequencing of the tumor and leukocyte DNA samples from the patient and his mother were performed using the TargetSeq™ Exome Enrichment Kit (Life Technologies), followed by paired-end sequencing (75 × 50) in SOLiD 5500xl System (Life Technologies). Leukocyte

DNA sample from his father was submitted for whole-exome sequencing using Ion Xpress™ Plus Fragment Library kit and Ion TargetSeq™ Exome Enrichment Kit (Life Technologies), followed by sequencing at Ion Proton™ platform (Ion Torrent™), according to the manufacturer's instructions. Single-end sequencing was performed on an Ion PI™ Chip v2 with 200 pb sequencing kit (Ion Torrent™).

Whole-genome sequencing

Whole-genome sequencing was performed by mate-paired DNA libraries prepared using the 5500 SOLiD™ Mate-Paired Library Construction Kit (Life Technologies), following the manufacturer's instructions. Briefly, genomic DNA from tumor and leukocyte of the patient was sheared with a Covaris sonicator into approximately 2 Kb fragments, circularized with mate-paired adaptors, nick-translated and digested, incorporated with sequencing adaptors and individual barcodes (distinct barcodes were used for the tumor and leukocyte DNA), and submitted to emulsion PCR. Mate-paired sequencing (60 × 60) was performed in a SOLiD 5500xl System (Life Technologies).

Sanger sequencing

For validation, primers were designed flanking the variants, in order to generate fragments of nearly 400 bp. PCR reactions were performed using GoTaq® Green Master Mix (Promega, Madison, WI, USA), using 15 ng of DNA, with 300 nM of each primer, for a final reaction volume of 20 μL. Approximately 200 ng of PCR-amplified fragments were purified with ExoSAP-IT (USB Corporation, Cleveland, OH, USA) and sequenced in both directions. All alterations were evaluated in all four samples (mother, father, and patient's leukocyte and tumor). Products were analyzed using an ABI 3130xl DNA sequencer (Applied Biosystems, Foster City, CA, USA), and sequences were aligned with the respective gene reference sequence using CLC Genomics Workbench Software (QIAGEN, Hilden, Germany).

Comparative genome hybridization based on microarrays (array CGH)

Comparative genomic hybridization based on microarrays was performed in a commercial whole-genome 180 K platform containing 180,000 oligonucleotide probes (Agilent Technologies; design 22060), using DNA from the tumor sample. Reference DNA was a commercially available human pool of samples from multiple anonymous healthy donors (Promega Corporation). Technical procedures are described in Torrezan et al. [11]. Hybridization and washing were performed as recommended by the manufacturer. Scanned images were processed using Feature Extraction 10.7.3.1 software (Agilent Technologies), and array CGH analysis was conducted with Nexus Copy Number software 7.0 (Biodiscovery). We used the FASST2 segmentation algorithm, according to the following settings: minimum of five consecutive probes (effective resolution of ~70 Kb for CNA calling), significance threshold set at 10^{-8}, and threshold $\log_2$ Cy3/Cy5 of 0.33 and −0.3 for gains for loss, respectively, and 1.2 and −1.1 for high copy number gains and homozygous losses, respectively. All copy number alterations are reported in the Database of Genomic Variants [12].

Bioinformatics analysis

Comprehensive cancer panel

Sequencing reads from Ion Proton™ were mapped to the reference genome (GRCh37/hg19) with TMAP (torrent mapper 4.2.18). Sequence variants (SNVs and indels) were identified with Torrent Variant Caller 4.0-5, followed by confirmation by GATK protocol vs3.2-2-gec30cee [13]. Variants were annotated using SnpEff version 3.5d (build 2014-03-05) [14].

Whole-exome sequencing

Sequencing reads from SOLiD 5500xl System were mapped to the reference genome (GRCh37/hg19) with Lifescope (LifeScope™ Genomic Analysis Software v2.5.1). Sequencing reads from Ion Proton™ were mapped to the reference genome (GRCh37/hg19) with TMAP (torrent mapper 4.2.18). Sequence variants (SNVs and indels) were identified following the GATK protocol vs3.2-2-gec30cee [13] for SOLiD 5500XL System and with Torrent Variant Caller 4.0-5, followed by GATK protocol vs3.2-2-gec30cee for Ion Proton reads. Variants were annotated using SnpEff version 3.5d (build 2014-03-05) [14] and an in-house developed script. Identified variants were compared to dbNSFP version 2.4 [15, 16]; COSMIC v69 [17]; 1000 Genomes [18]; NHLBI GO Exome Sequencing Project version ESP6500SI-V2 [19]; HapMap [20]; and dbSNP version 138 [21, 22] for further annotation. Somatic variants were defined for regions with a minimum coverage of 10× for both tumor and leukocyte sample from the patient and minimum variant frequency of 20% in the tumor only. De novo variants were defined with a minimum coverage of 10× for leukocyte samples of the patient and his parents and with a minimum variant frequency of 30%. To identify rare polymorphisms inherited in homozygosity, we selected variants with a minimum coverage of 10× for leukocyte samples of the patient and his parents, detected in heterozygosis in both parents and homozygosis in the patient presenting a minor allele frequency ≤10% in the public databases (1000 Genome [18], NHLBI GO Exome Sequencing Project [19], and HapMap [20]). To identify germline compound heterozygosis cases, we identified genes with two distinct heterozygous mutations in the patient, where each variant was exclusively present in one of his parents in heterozygosity and detected in regions with a minimum coverage of 10× for all leukocyte samples. We discarded variants that are detected with a minor allele frequency above 10% in the 1000 Genome Project [18]. Copy number alterations were detected using the bioinformatics packages Excavator (version 2.2) [23] and cn.mops (version 1.8.9) [24] by comparing exome data from the tumor to leukocyte from the patient. For visualization, we used circos 0.67-7 package [25].

Whole-genome sequencing

For detecting structural variations, mate-pair reads obtained by SOLiD 5500xl System were analyzed by svdetect (version r0.8b) [26].

Ingenuity Pathway Analysis

We applied the core analysis of Ingenuity Pathway Analysis (IPA) system (QIAGEN, Germantown, MD, USA) to identify gene interaction networks.

Digital droplet PCR

Digital droplet PCR assays were carried out using the QX200™ Droplet Digital™ (ddPCR™) System (Bio-Rad). A primer-probe assay labeled with FAM was designed for the amplification of wild-type *WT1* gene and a primer-probe assay labeled with HEX was designed for the amplification of the gene fusion event (EWS-WT1). For the amplification reaction, we used 1× ddPCR Supermix, 1× primer-probe assay (FAM), 1× primer-probe assay (HEX), and 4 µl of DNA. Droplet generation, PCR amplification, and droplet counting were performed following the manufacturer's recommendations.

DNA samples from tumor tissue (60 ng–6 pg) and from leukocytes (6 ng) were used as positive and negative controls, respectively. We loaded 4 µl of 30 µl (1/8) of cfDNA samples from the patient. We also used DNA and cell-free DNA extracted from leukocytes and plasma, respectively, from healthy donors as negative controls and performed non-template control. All reactions were performed with at least two replicates.

Results

In this study, we performed a comprehensive genomic profiling of one case of desmoplastic small round cell tumor (DSRCT) by a combination of targeted sequencing, array CGH, whole genome, and whole exome applied in a family based format. The patient studied here is a 26-year-old male, who presented at A.C. Camargo Cancer Center in November, 2011, with a large abdominal mass and a small nodule on the pelvic region. Staging images showed that the disease was limited to the abdominal cavity. He underwent a CT-guided biopsy that revealed a desmoplastic small round cell tumor (DSRCT), showing positivity for EMA, desmin, and nuclear staining for WT1 (carboxy-terminus antibody). FISH analysis was positive for EWS translocation.

The patient started systemic treatment with 4 cycles of vincristine, cyclophosphamide, and doxorubicin (VAC) and alternated with ifosfamide, carboplatin, and etoposide (ICE). After 4 cycles, the best response was stable disease, with minor reduction in the tumor dimensions. He underwent complete surgical cytoreduction, with resection of the large mass and resection of peritoneal implant on the pelvic region, and hyperthermic intraperitoneal chemotherapy (HIPEC), with cisplatin and doxorubicin. The patient presented a complete recovery from these procedures. After that, the patient received four more cycles of chemotherapy and total abdominal irradiation (total of 30 Gy). After a follow-up of 48 months since surgery, the patient is asymptomatic, with no signs of disease (Additional file 1: Figure S1).

The comprehensive genomic profiling was carried out in multiple fronts. To identify actionable mutations, we carried out targeted sequencing of the most important actionable genes in the tumor sample. Further, to identify genes and mutations possibly involved with tumor onset and predisposition, we performed whole exome sequencing, using the DSRCT tumor sample and blood samples from the patient and his both parents (Additional file 2: Table S1). Array CGH was performed in tumor sample to identify structural rearrangements and copy number imbalances. Whole-genome sequencing defined one tumor marker used to precisely monitor patient after treatment.

Producing a portrait of somatically acquired variants

To identify actionable mutations or pathways related to DSRCT in this patient, we initially performed targeted sequencing using a cancer-oriented gene panel composed of 409 genes in the tumor sample (Comprehensive Cancer Panel – Thermo Scientific). Since no actionable mutation for targeted therapy was detected in the tumor, we investigated the complete landscape of somatic mutations by whole-exome sequencing (WES) the tumor and the patient's leukocyte. The analysis of the tumor revealed 15 somatic acquired mutations, 12 of which were protein-affecting variants (validated by capillary sequencing) including one non-sense mutation in the *ZNF808* gene, one nucleotide change at the 3' splice site of *RIMS4*, and 10 missense mutations considered disease associated by at least one pathogenicity prediction program (Table 1).

Gene ontology enrichment analysis of the 12 genes harboring protein-affecting somatic mutations revealed several biological processes such as muscle tissue/organ development (*ZFPM2* and *MEGF10*), which is related to the mesothelium origin of this tumor, cell adhesion (*DPP4, CDH9, CNTNAP4, MEGF10*), response to mechanic stimulus (*MEIS2, TRPA4*), and response to abiotic

Table 1 Description of somatically acquired point mutations detected in the DSRCT by whole-exome sequencing

Chromosome position	Gene symbol	Variant description	Variant type	Frequency (tumor coverage)	Coverage of leukocyte DNA	dbSNP	PolyPhen	Sift	Mutation taster
chr3:436494	*CHL1*	c.3033A>G, p.A111A	Synonymous	35% (55×)	53×	–	–	–	–
chr6:134305546	*TBPL1*	c.315T>G, p.V105V	Synonymous	23% (31×)	28×	–	–	–	–
chr12:34179763	*ALG10*	c.1335A>T, p.A445A	Synonymous	43% (82×)	66×	–	–	–	–
chr1:45808899	*TOE1*	c.1058C>T, p.P353L	Missense	20% (15×)	18×	rs145913038	Benign	Damaging	Polymorphism
chr2:162875307	*DPP4*	c.1352C>T, p.P451L	Missense	37% (41×)	46×	–	Deleterious	Tolerated	Disease causing
chr5:126753368	*MEGF10*	c.1169G>C, p.G390C	Missense	22% (82×)	39×	–	Deleterious	Damaging	Disease causing
chr5:26915867	*CDH9*	c.394G>C, p.D132Y	Missense	25% (71×)	75×	–	Deleterious	–	Disease causing
chr6:123319098	*CLVS2*	c.176G>A, p.R59Q	Missense	40% (25×)	20×	–	Deleterious	Damaging	Disease causing
chr8:106813312	*ZFPM2*	c.1002T>A, p.S334R	Missense	28% (36×)	44×	–	Deleterious	Tolerated	Disease causing
chr8:72983969	*TRPA1*	c.245T>C, p.I82T	Missense	36% (45×)	35×	–	Deleterious	Damaging	Disease causing
chr15:37385900	*MEIS2*	c.521G>A, p.R86Q	Missense	26% (31×)	23×	–	Possible damaging	Damaging	Disease causing
chr16:76495948	*CNTNAP4*	c.1210G>T, p.A404S	Missense	33% (42×)	43×	–	Benign	Tolerated	Disease causing
chr17:10300120	*MYH8*	c.4362G>T, p.K1454N	Missense	26% (38×)	33×	–	Deleterious	–	Disease causing
chr19:53057457	*ZNF808*	c.1288G>T, p.E430Ter	Nonsense	43% (30×)	27×	–	–	Tolerated	Polymorphism
chr20:43385680	*RIMS4*	c.455-2T>A	3′ splice site	28% (29×)	37×	–	–	–	–

stimulus (*DPP4, MEIS2, TRPA1*) (Additional file 3: Table S2). Intriguingly, biological network analysis obtained using Ingenuity Pathway Analysis (IPA) interconnected the 15 genes harboring somatic mutations in a single network associated with cell death and survival, cell damage or degeneration, and nervous system development and function (Fig. 1a).

Searching for germline variants associated with DSRCT

In an attempt to identify de novo germline mutations and inherited variants potentially associated with DSRCT, we performed whole-exome sequencing of the leukocyte DNA from the patient's parents (Additional file 2: Table S1). For selecting genetic variants, a minimum coverage of 10× in all samples with at least 30% frequency of the variant allele was considered. Based on these criteria, no de novo variants were found.

Next, we explored the possibility of finding genetic variants associated with DSRCT in an autosomal recessive model of inheritance. First, we searched for polymorphisms (MAF ≤10%) occurring in homozygosity in the patient that were inherited from both heterozygous parents. Four polymorphisms inherited in homozygosis were found in *ADAMTS12, RASSF1, VEZT,* and *ISX* genes (population frequency ranging from 2.0 to 7.8%). All polymorphisms lead to missense alterations, two of them reported as possibly disease associated by at least one pathogenicity prediction program (Table 2). Interestingly, biological network analysis showed an interconnection between the four genes in a single network from IPA, showing association with cell cycle and digestive system development and function (Fig. 1b).

Next, to identify candidate genes affected by compound heterozygosity, we looked for genes containing two distinct variants inherited independently from each parent. We could confirm 11 genes affected by germline compound heterozygous mutations, in which one variant allele was inherited from the mother and the other variant allele was inherited from the father (MAF ≤10%) (Table 3). We speculate that these genes could be associated with risk to DSRCT development in an autosomal recessive model of inheritance.

Gene ontology analysis of these 11 genes showed enrichment of biological processes related to muscle tissue development (*LAMB2, SYNE1,* and *TTN*), morphogenesis (*C2CD3* and *TTN*), and cell cycle (*RSPH1, TTN,* and *SPICE1*) (Additional file 4: Table S4). Functional analysis of IPA revealed that 9 of the 11 genes are interconnected in a single network related to cancer, organismal injury and abnormalities, and gastrointestinal disease.

Copy number alterations

Genomic copy number alterations (CNA) were investigated in the DSRCT tumor sample using array CGH in a 180-K platform. Few copy number alterations were detected (Fig. 2a), including aneuploidies such as gain of chromosomes 5 and 18, and 11p, 13q, and 22q deletions. Only one small focal homozygous deletion was identified in a segment of ~1.3 Mb at 9p22.2 (chr9:17,106,384-18,449,088; hg19), encompassing the *CNTLN* and *SH3GL2* genes.

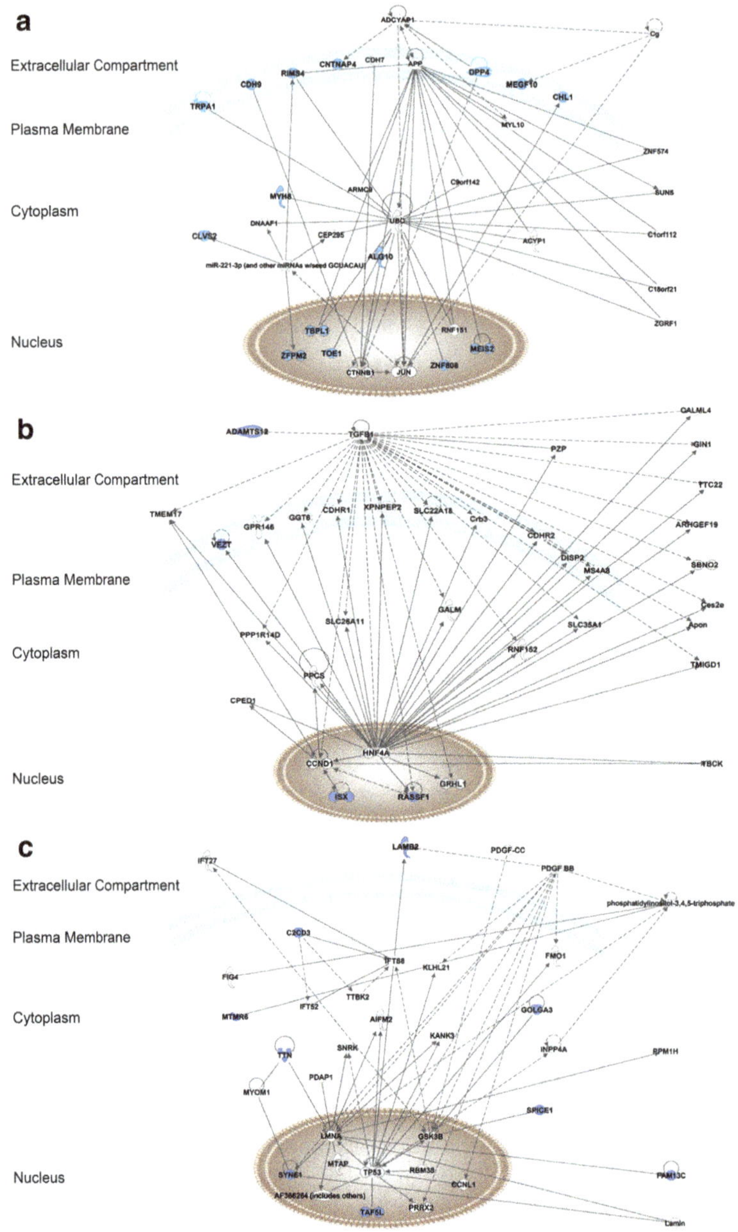

Fig. 1 Network analysis by IPA. **a** Interaction network of genes harboring protein-affecting somatic mutations (network score = 45) is associated with the top disease and functions: cell death and survival, nervous system development and function, cellular compromise. **b** Interaction network of genes harboring rare polymorphisms detected in homozygosis in the patient (network score = 12) is associated with the top disease and functions: cell cycle, digestive system development and function, hair and skin development and function. **c** Interaction network of genes affected by compound heterozygous variants (network score = 25) is associated with the top disease and functions: cancer, organismal injury, abnormalities, and gastrointestinal disease. Continuous and dashed lines indicate direct and indirect interactions between molecules, respectively. Blue molecules represent the genes encountered in our analysis and blank molecules represent other genes automatically included by IPA. Molecules are displayed by various shapes depending on the functional class of the gene product, according to IPA Path designer shapes (Additional file 7)

The detection of copy number losses affecting terminal segments of 11p and 22q suggested the presence of the chromosomal translocation t(11;22)(p13;q12) involving *EWSR1* and *WT1* genes.

Additionally, we used NGS data from the WES of the tumor and patient's leukocyte to search for CNAs, and 98.4% of the events detected by array CGH were validated, demonstrating the efficacy of WES for identification of a

Table 2 Description of rare polymorphisms detected in homozygosity in the DSRCT patient. All variants were validated by sanger sequencing

Gene symbol	cDNA change	Protein change	Type	dbSNP (MAF)	Patient (Frequency/ Coverage)	Mother (Frequency/ Coverage)	Father (Frequency/ Coverage)	Polyphen	Sift	Mutation Taster
VEZT	c.1486G > A	p.V496I	Missense	rs10507051 (0.0302)	100% / 17	17.9% / 28	35.0% / 80	PD	T	DC
ISX	c.248G > A	p.R83Q	Missense	rs8140287 (0.0308)	100% / 13	37.5% / 24	50.0% / 70	PrD	T	DC
RASSF1	c.409G > T	p.A137S	Missense	rs2073498 (0.0711)	83.3% / 12	27.5% / 40	53.1% / 32	B	T	P
ADAMTS12	c.3529 T > C	p.W1177R	Missense	rs3813474 (0.0513)	100% / 51	42.0% / 88	45.0% / 40	B	T	P

MAF Minor allele frequency, *PrD* Probably damaging, *B* Benign, *PD* Possibly damaging, *D* Damaging, *T* Tolerated, *DC* Disease causing, *P* Polymorphism. (*) low confidence prediction

wide range of somatic events, besides point mutations and indels (Fig. 2b; Additional file 5: Table S3).

Establishment of a personalized monitoring strategy based on detection of circulating tumor DNA (ctDNA)

The genomic translocation t(11;22)(p13;q12), which is considered the molecular hallmark of this tumor type, was initially detected by FISH analysis for diagnostic purposes. Furthermore, the same translocation was also detected in the array CGH and confirmed by whole-genome sequencing. The mate-pair approach used for whole-genome sequencing followed by validation by PCR and Sanger sequencing allowed the precise delimitation of the chromosomal breakpoints (Fig. 3). This somatic fusion event was then used as a tumor biomarker for monitoring the patient along the follow-up period using a liquid biopsy-based approach. We searched for traces of circulating tumor DNA in plasma samples collected 17, 36, 42, and 47 months after surgery. No signs of the translocation in any of the post-treatment plasma samples were detected (Fig. 3) using digital droplet PCR (ddPCR). The absence of the biomarker in any of the post-treatment plasma samples is in agreement with favorable clinical response of the patient, showing long-term disease-free survival and no sign of disease recurrence. As a positive control, we confirmed the presence of cell-free circulating DNA by detecting non-rearranged *WT1* gene in all plasma samples.

Despite the unavailability of plasma samples at the moment of diagnosis and before treatment (neoadjuvant/adjuvant chemotherapy and surgery) to be used as a baseline positive control, we carried out stringent control assays. We tested the robustness of the approach by evaluating six different amounts of tumor DNA, ranging from 60 ng to 6 pg, and searched for both the tumor-specific fusion event and for the non-rearranged *WT1* gene. We achieved a linear quantification of tumor marker and wild-type DNA, and we were able to discriminate the presence of the fusion event even in extremely low quantity of DNA (6 pg) (Fig. 3d). To test the specificity of the ddPCR assay, we used leukocyte sample of the patient and also DNA from plasma and leukocyte samples of healthy donors, and the absence of detection of tumor-specific fusion confirmed the assay specificity for tumor DNA, without false positive signals (Additional file 6: Figure S2). Further, we mimicked a situation of circulating tumor DNA in body fluid by mixing 1 part of tumor DNA to 100 and 1000 parts of leukocyte DNA, then screened for the fusion event using 1 ng of this DNA mix. Typically, the detection of circulating tumor DNA has been reported as a fraction between 0.1 and 90% of plasma DNA for cancer patients, depending on tumor type and patient characteristics [27]. Here, we were able to detect the fusion event in the 1.0 and 0.1% fractions, supporting the reliability of our established approach for patient surveillance based on liquid-biopsy screening.

Discussion

DSRCT is an aggressive tumor not yet broadly investigated with the powerful genomic tools available. Mainly due to the rarity of this disease, only a few studies investigated molecular alterations in this tumor type. Shukla et al. [8] screened the occurrence of 275 COSMIC mutations in 29 oncogenes and found no alterations in any of the 24 DSRCT samples investigated. More recently, a study based on targeted exome sequencing of six adult patients with pediatric-type malignancies found *AURKB* and *MCL1* amplifications and variants of unknown clinical significance in *ARID1A* and *RUNX1* genes in one DSRCT [6].

Here, by performing a comprehensive screening of the genomic alterations in a family based approach, we identified somatic and germline variants possibly associated with DSRCT. In our study, the use of a commercially available gene panel did not show to be an adequate strategy. Based on this finding, one can argue that screening by commercially available gene panels is not an effective approach for most cases of rare tumors, since the targeted genes represented in these panels are usually those well characterized in common solid tumors. On the other hand, the use of WES not only revealed mutated genes but also showed robustness for detecting DNA copy number alterations. Concordance rates between WES and

Table 3 Description of compound heterozygous variants detected in the DSRCT patient. Each one of the variants was exclusively inherited by one of the parents. The genotype and variant frequency were obtained by leukocyte DNA sequencing. All variants were validated by Sanger sequencing

Gene	cDNA change	Protein change	dbSNP (MAF)	Mother		Father		Patient		Polyphen	Sift	Mutation Taster
				Genotype	Variant Frequency	Genotype	Variant Frequency	Genotype	Variant Frequency			
C2CD3	c.5653 T > C	p.S1885P	rs142277857 (0.001)	T/C	43.1	T/T	-	T/C	53.57	PrD	D	P
	c.3223A > C	p.S1075R	-	A/A	-	A/C	50.91	A/C	41.67	PrD	D	DC
FAM13C	c.1361G > A	p.R454H	rs369226393	G/A	56.4	G/G	-	G/A	50	B	T	P
	c.439C > T	p.P147S	rs73299227 (0.0092)	C/C	-	C/T	51,43	C/T	36.36	PD	D*	DC
GOLGA3	c.209G > A	p.G70E	rs2291256 (0.0581)	G/A	52.3	G/G	-	G/A	47.06	B	D*	P
	c.3728G > A	p.R1243Q	rs140646528 (0.0134)	G/G	-	G/A	60	G/A	25	B	T	P
LAMB2	c.1424G > A	p.R475Q	rs370565848	G/A	36.4	G/G	-	G/A	60	PrD	T	P
	c.5293G > A	p.A1765T	rs74951356 (0.0130)	G/G	-	G/A	55.81	G/A	41.18	B	T	DC
MTMR6	c.685C > G	p.P229A	rs149526134 (0.0002)	C/G	60.9	C/C	-	C/G	26.32	B	T	P
	c.1795G > A	p.A599T	rs62619824 (0.0571	G/G	-	G/A	35.09	G/A	51.85	B	T	DC
RSPH1	c.742G > A	p.G248R	rs117385282 (0.0839)	G/A	50	G/G	-	G/A	31.25	B	T	P
	c.733G > A	p.G245R	rs151158140 (0.0026)	G/G	-	G/A	50.77	G/A	58.33	PD	T	P
SLC9A9	c.1765A > G	p.I589V	rs2289491 (0.0290)	A/G	31.1	A/A	-	A/G	28	B	T	P
	c.1618A > G	p.I540V	rs16853300 (0.0066)	A/A	-	A/G	48.62	A/G	36.36	B	T	P
SPICE1	c.2470A > C	p.T824P	rs57006145 (0.0313)	A/C	40.4	A/A	-	A/C	62.16	PrD	T	DC
	c.850G > A	p.V284M	rs73239152 (0.0078)	G/G	-	G/A	47.54	G/A	29.27	B	D	DC
SYNE1	c.16277C > T	p.T5426M	rs2306914 (0.0463)	C/T	39.1	C/C	-	C/T	41.07	B	T	P
	c. 12442G > C	p.D4148H	rs117501809 (0.0124)	G/G	-	G/C	49.15	G/C	28.57	PrD	D	P
TAF5L	c.721G > A	p.V241I	rs55655740 (0.0042)	G/A	36.0	G/G	-	G/A	48	B	-	DC
	c.1123A > G	p.T375A	rs41304137 (0.0008)	A/A	-	A/G	20	A/G	40	PrD	T	P
TTN	c.106619 T > C	p.I35540T	rs55880440 (0.0046)	T/C	40.0	T/T	-	T/C	57.69	-	-	P
	c.65147C > T	p.S21716L	rs13021201 (0.0108)	C/C	-	C/T	42.86	C/T	58.14	-	-	P

MAF Minor allele frequency, *PrD* Probably damaging, *B* Benign, *PD* Possibly damaging, *D* Damaging, *T* Tolerated, *DC* Disease causing, *P* Polymorphism. (*) low confidence prediction

array CGH (the gold standard for CNA screening) were above 98% (Fig. 2). Among the CNAs not detected in the WES analysis, two of them were mapped to regions not covered by the library probes and five were low-level mosaic alterations (Additional file 3: Table S2). Thus, if we consider CNAs mapping to WES target regions and non-mosaic CNAs, concordance rates were above 99.8%.

In total, 38 somatically acquired alterations, including point mutations (15) and CNAs (23), were detected. The small number of somatic alterations identified here is in agreement with what is expected for pediatric tumors [28]. Moreover, given the occurrence of the driver EWS-WT1 fusion protein, additional oncogenic mutations for tumor onset is probably less necessary.

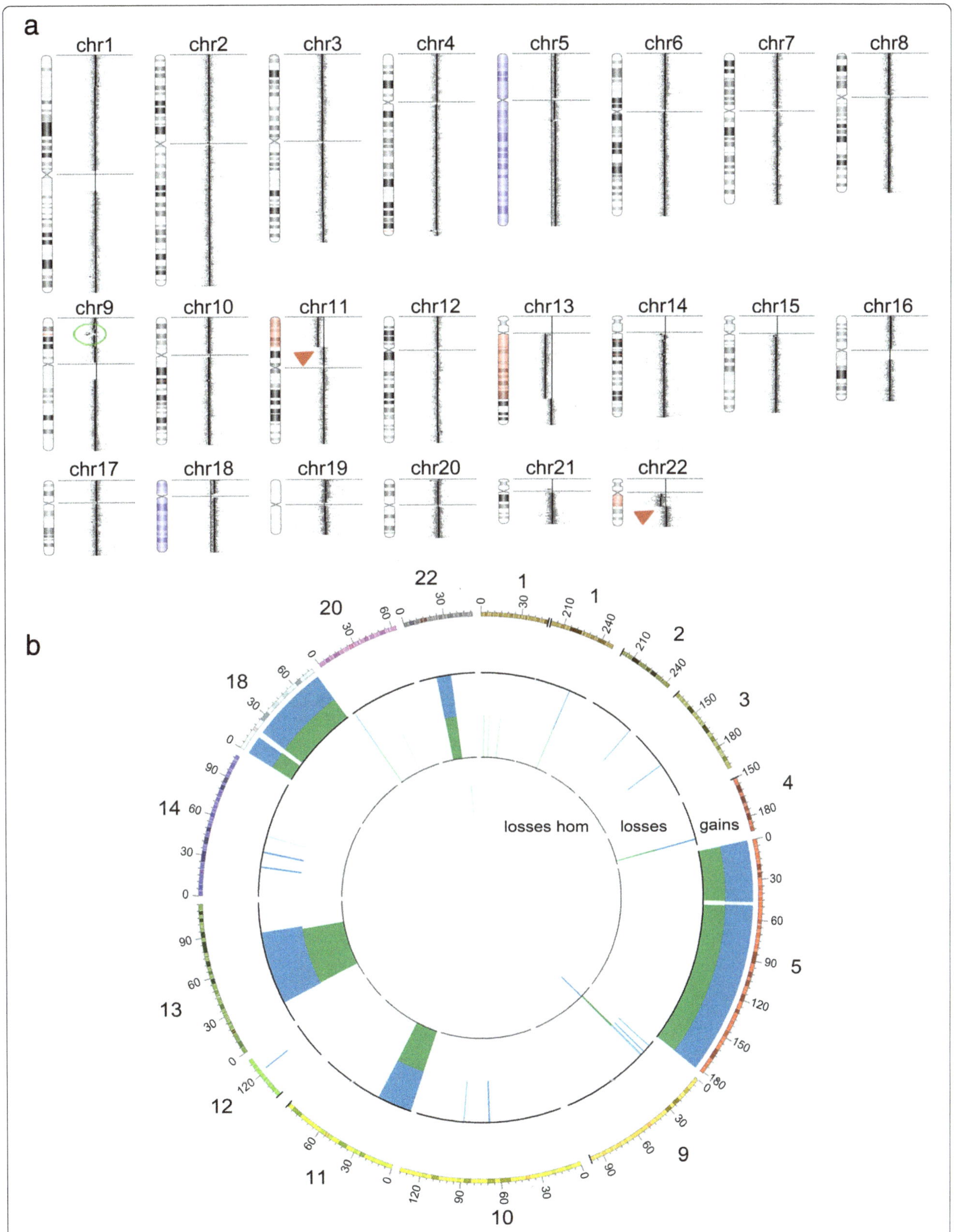

Fig. 2 (See legend on next page.)

(See figure on previous page.)

Fig. 2 Array CGH profile showing the pattern of somatic copy number alterations detected in the DSRCT genome. **a** Copy number alterations detected by array CGH analysis using a 180-K platform with an effective resolution of ~70 Kb: aneuploidy of chromosomes 5 and 18 (gains, *in blue*), and partial losses of chromosome 13q, 11p, and 22q (*in red*). The *green circle* indicates the focal deletion of a segment of 1.3 Mb at 9p24.1. *Arrows* indicate chromosome 11 and chromosome 22 breakpoints, 11p13 and 22q12.2, respectively. **b** *Circus* plot shows the copy number alterations detected by array CGH and WES. Only the genomic regions affected by CNA events are represented. The numbers on each chromosome region are described in megabases. In *blue*, data from array CGH and in *green* data from WES. A great overlap of CNA detection can be observed using both approaches

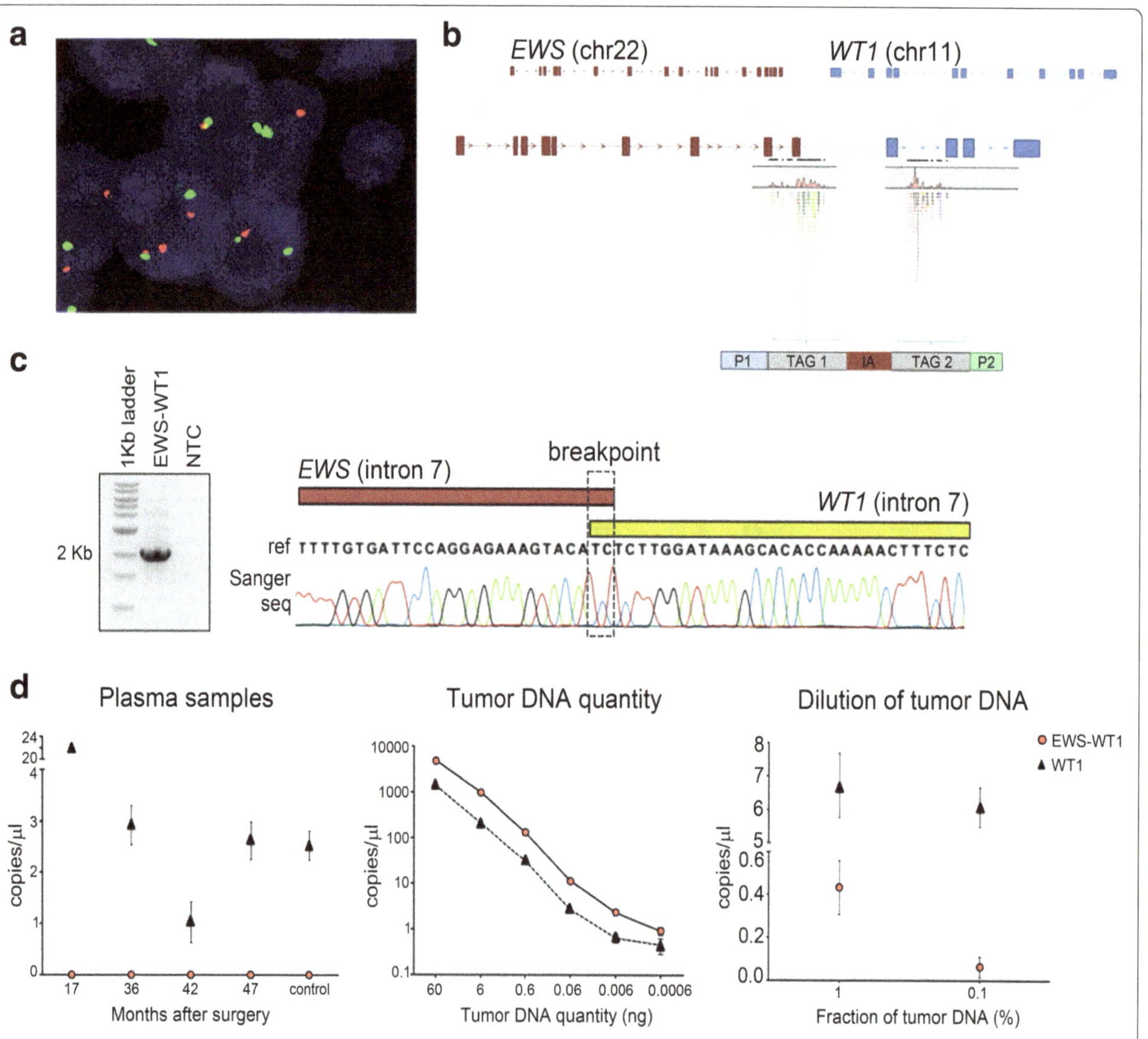

Fig. 3 Use of the chromosomal translocation t(11;22)(p13;q12) as a personalized tool for patient monitoring along follow-up. **a** FISH analysis shows break apart probes for *WT1* gene, indicating the occurrence of the fusion. **b** Mate-pair whole-genome sequencing detected paired reads mapping to *EWS* and *WT1* genes. **c** PCR amplification followed by Sanger sequencing confirmed the breakpoint region involving intronic regions of *EWS* and *WT1* genes. **d** Digital droplet PCR assays for detection of the somatic rearrangement EWS-WT1. *Left panel*—Screening of ctDNA from plasma samples collected serially along patient follow-up by ddPCR. No gene fusion was detected in ctDNA from the patient collected in four different time points after surgery, suggesting no relapse, recurrence, or progression of the disease. Presence of cell-free DNA is shown by detection of non-rearranged WT1 probes in the plasma samples from the patient and from control plasma sample. *Middle panel*—Serial dilutions of tumor DNA to check the sensibility of the approach in detecting the fusion event, starting from 60 ng of input following five dilution series of tenfold as indicated. *Right panel*—Detection of somatic rearrangement in different tumor DNA fractions, 1.0 and 0.1%

We identified 12 genes affected by somatic mutations possibly involved with the disease. These genes are involved with cellular development and morphology that are pathways in which *WT1* gene plays an important role. Similarly, the genes affected by compound heterozygous mutations showed enrichment in biological processes of muscle tissue development and morphogenesis. Altogether, these data suggests that disruption of the embryonic cellular development process is involved with DSRCT onset, which is commonly seen in pediatric tumors.

Another interesting finding is that among the set of somatically mutated genes, 8 showed to be mutated in desmoplastic melanoma samples from TCGA project [29, 30], in frequencies ranging from 5 to 25% of the 20 samples interrogated. This data suggests that mutation in these genes might be involved with the desmoplastic phenotype, seen in both tumor types.

Additionally, 7 out of 15 genes harboring somatic mutations (*CHL1, MEGF10, MEIS2, MYH8, RIMS4, TBPL1,* and *ZFPM2*) are regulated by the same transcription factor, LEF1 ($p < 0.001$ by enrichment analysis), which, in turn, is regulated by WT1 [31]. We therefore postulate that DSRCT tumors presenting increased activity of WT1 due to EWS-WT1 fusion might upregulate the expression of several genes mediated by LEF1 transcription factor. However, the accumulation of mutations in this set of genes regulated by LEF1 activation and its interrelation with the EWS-WT1 fusion protein remains to be addressed.

Finally, the definition of the precise genomic breakpoint of the t(11;22)(p13;q12) translocation by whole-genome and Sanger sequencing enabled the development of a personalized tool to precisely monitor the presence of ctDNA in plasma samples during the patient's follow-up. Detection of tumor-specific genomic rearrangements has been shown as a sensitive and specific method for monitoring of disease status of cancer patients [32–35] and has clear advantages over point mutations concerning the specificity of detection [33]. Here, we applied ctDNA screening in plasma samples collected in three clinical appointments during 3 years after surgery and, up to now, we did not detect the presence of this tumor marker. These results are in agreement with imaging exams (CT scan and PET scan) showing no signs of disease and also with good overall clinical condition of the patient and highlight the applicability of using genomic rearrangement for building personalized tool for patient surveillance. After defining the genomic breakpoint of EWS-WT1 fusion, DSRCT patients can benefit from a highly specific test that has the advantage of a rapid turnaround time and potentially higher sensitivity in detecting disease progression earlier than imaging exams or other cancer antigens measurements, as reported for other tumor types [36, 37]. Monitoring through liquid biopsy is particularly attractive for solid tumors, which cannot be repeatedly sampled without more invasive procedures. Considering the rarity of this subtype of sarcoma and the lack of effective treatment, the detection of specific tumor marker and the monitoring of its persistence can improve the identification of patients with worse prognosis to tailor the treatment more properly. Thus, the perspective is to employ the approach used here for new patients and improve the outcome for those with worse prognosis.

Conclusion

To our knowledge, this is the first comprehensive genomic characterization of one DSRCT case. Continuous efforts to establish the genomic landscape of rare diseases, frequently neglected in large sequencing consortiums, are highly significant to improve the knowledge of defective pathways involved with tumor onset in general, in addition to the strong potential of revealing druggable targets for clinical use.

Additional files

Additional file 1: Figure S1. Patient medical history and sample collection time points. Chemotherapy treatment marked in green consisted of 4 cycles of vincristine, cyclophosphamide, and doxorubicin (VAC) alternated with ifosfamide, carboplatin, and etoposide (ICE). Chemotherapy treatment marked in red consisted of hyperthermic intraperitoneal chemotherapy (HIPEC) with cisplatin and doxorubicin. Abdominal irradiation total of 30 Gy.

Additional file 2: Table S1. Statistics of sequencing results. Sequence coverage by Comprehensive Cancer Panel (Thermo Scientific), Whole Exome Sequencing (Thermo Scientific) and Whole Genome Sequencing (Mate-Paired approach) (Thermo Scientific).

Additional file 3: Table S2. Gene Ontology enriched categories of genes affected by somatic mutations. Biological processes with a p-value <0,001 was considered based on Webgestalt annotation tool [38, 39].

Additional file 4: Table S4. Gene Ontology-enriched categories of genes affected by compound heterozygous mutations. Biological processes with a *p* value <0.001 was considered based on WebGestalt annotation tool [38, 39].

Additional file 5: Figure S3. Copy Number Alterations detected by array CGH and confirmed by WES.

Additional file 6: Figure S2. Screening of ctDNA in leukocyte samples. Pre-surgery sample collected at day of surgery. Post-surgery sample collected at 22 months after diagnosis (17 months after surgery).

Additional file 7: Description of the functional class of each molecule shape used by IPA.

Abbreviations

CGH: Comparative genomic hybridization; CNA: Copy number alterations; COSMIC: Catalogue of Somatic Mutations in Cancer; CT: Computed tomography; ctDNA: Circulating tumor DNA; ddPCR: Digital droplet PCR; DSRCT: Desmoplastic small round cell tumor; GATK: Genome Analysis Toolkit; HIPEC: Hyperthermic intraperitoneal chemotherapy; ICE: Ifosfamide, carboplatin, and etoposide; Indel: Small insertions and deletions; IPA: Ingenuity pathway analysis; MAF: Minor allele frequency; PET: Positron emission tomography; SNP: Simple nucleotide polymorphism; TCGA: The cancer genome atlas; VAC: Vincristine, cyclophosphamide, and doxorubicin; WES: Whole-exome sequencing

Acknowledgements
The authors thank the patient and his parents for their collaboration, the A.C. Camargo Cancer Center Biobank for providing the tumor sample, and Louise D. C. Mota for the technical support for plasma DNA collection and extraction.

Funding
This work was supported by São Paulo Research Foundation—FAPESP (2013/23277-8)—and by the National Council of Technological and Scientific Development—CNPq (483775/2012-6).

Authors' contributions
ENF, BDFB, and GTT carried out the sequencing experiments, and BDFB and SG performed the validation experiments. ENF performed and analyzed the ddPCR assays. ACVK performed and analyzed the CGH array experiments and revised the manuscript. JES and RVA conducted the bioinformatics analyses, and SJS supervised the bioinformatics analysis. CCF and AL were responsible for patient treatment and care. IWC, CP, and FAS supervised immunohistochemical reactions and performed the histopathological analyses. SJS and EDN contributed to the analysis of the results and revised the manuscript. DMC and ENF designed the study, analyzed the results, and wrote the initial manuscript. DMC conceived and supervised the study. All authors read and approved the final manuscript.

Competing interests
The authors declare that they have no competing interests.

Consent for publication
Written informed consent for publication of their clinical details was obtained from the patient.

Author details
[1]International Research Center/CIPE, A.C. Camargo Cancer Center, São Paulo, SP, Brazil. [2]Instituto Metrópole Digital, Federal University of Rio Grande do Norte, Natal, RN, Brazil. [3]Institute of Biosciences, University of São Paulo, São Paulo, SP, Brazil. [4]Departament of Abdominal Surgery, A.C. Camargo Cancer Center, São Paulo, SP, Brazil. [5]Department of Anatomic Pathology, A.C. Camargo Cancer Center, São Paulo, SP, Brazil. [6]Federal University of Rio Grande do Norte, Natal, RN, Brazil.

References
1. Lettieri CK, Garcia-Filion P, Hingorani P. Incidence and outcomes of desmoplastic small round cell tumor: results from the surveillance, epidemiology, and end results database. J Cancer Epidemiol. 2014;2014:680126.
2. Zhang S, Zhang Y, Yu YH, Li J. Results of multimodal treatment for desmoplastic small round cell tumor of the abdomen and pelvis. Int J Clin Exp Med. 2015;8:9658–66.
3. Liu J, Nau MM, Yeh JC, Allegra CJ, Chu E, Wright JJ. Molecular heterogeneity and function of EWS-WT1 fusion transcripts in desmoplastic small round cell tumors. Clin Cancer Res. 2000;6:3522–9.
4. Lee SB, Kolquist KA, Nichols K, Englert C, Maheswaran S, Ladanyi M, Gerald WL, Haber DA. The EWS-WT1 translocation product induces PDGFA in desmoplastic small round-cell tumour. Nat Genet. 1997;17:309–13.
5. Karnieli E, Werner H, Rauscher 3rd FJ, et al. The IGF-I receptor gene promoter is a molecular target for the Ewing's sarcoma-Wilms' tumor 1 fusion protein. J Biol Chem. 1996;271:19304–9.
6. Silva JG, Corrales-Medina FF, Maher OM, Tannir N, Huh WW, Rytting ME, Subbiah V. Clinical next generation sequencing of pediatric-type malignancies in adult patients identifies novel somatic aberrations. Oncoscience. 2015;2:187–92.
7. La Starza R, Barba G, Nofrini V, Pierini T, Pierini V, Marcomigni L, Perruccio K, Matteucci C, Storlazzi CT, Daniele G, Crescenzi B, Giansanti M, Giovenali P, Dal Cin P, Mecucci C. Multiple EWSR1-WT1 and WT1-EWSR1 copies in two cases of desmoplastic round cell tumor. Cancer Genet. 2013;206:387–92.
8. Shukla N, Ameur N, Yilmaz I, Nafa K, Lau CY, Marchetti A, Borsu L, Barr FG, Ladanyi M. Oncogene mutation profiling of pediatric solid tumors reveals significant subsets of embryonal rhabdomyosarcoma and neuroblastoma with mutated genes in growth signaling pathways. Clin Cancer Res. 2012;18:748–57.
9. Campos AH, Silva AA, Mota LD, Olivieri ER, Prescinoti VC, Patrão D, Camargo LP, Brentani H, Carraro DM, Brentani RR, Soares FA. The value of a tumor bank in the development of cancer research in Brazil: 13 years of experience at the A C Camargo hospital. Biopreserv Biobank. 2012;10:168–73.
10. Olivieri EH, Franco Lde A, Pereira RG, Mota LD, Campos AH, Carraro DM. Biobanking practice: RNA storage at low concentration affects integrity. Biopreserv Biobank. 2014;12:46–52.
11. Torrezan GT, da Silva FC, Santos EM, Krepischi AC, Achatz MI, Aguiar Jr S, Rossi BM, Carraro DM. Mutational spectrum of the APC and MUTYH genes and genotype-phenotype correlations in Brazilian FAP, AFAP, and MAP patients. Orphanet J Rare Dis. 2013;8:54.
12. Database of genomic variants. http://projects.tcag.ca/variation/.
13. McKenna A, et al. The genome analysis toolkit: a MapReduce framework for analyzing next-generation DNA sequencing data. Genome Res. 2012;20:1297–303.
14. Cingolani P, Platts A, le Wang L, Coon M, Nguyen T, Wang L, Land SJ, Lu X, Ruden DM. A program for annotating and predicting the effects of single nucleotide polymorphisms, SnpEff: SNPs in the genome of Drosophila melanogaster strain w1118; iso-2; iso-3. Fly (Austin). 2012;6:80–92.
15. Liu X, Jian X, Boerwinkle E. dbNSFP: a lightweight database of human non-synonymous SNPs and their functional predictions. Hum Mutat. 2011;32:894–9.
16. Liu X, Jian X, Boerwinkle E. dbNSFP v2.0: a database of human non-synonymous SNVs and their functional predictions and annotations. Hum Mutat. 2013;34:E2393–402.
17. Forbes SA, Bindal N, Bamford S, Cole C, Kok CY, Beare D, Jia M, Shepherd R, Leung K, Menzies A, Teague JW, Campbell PJ, Stratton MR, Futreal PA. COSMIC: mining complete cancer genomes in the catalogue of somatic mutations in cancer. Nucleic Acids Res. 2011;39:D945–50.
18. 1000 Genomes Project Consortium, Auton A, Brooks LD, Durbin RM, Garrison EP, Kang HM, Korbel JO, Marchini JL, McCarthy S, McVean GA, Abecasis GR. A global reference for human genetic variation. Nature. 2015;526:68–74.
19. Exome Variant Server, NHLBI GO Exome Sequencing Project (ESP), Seattle. http://evs.gs.washington.edu/EVS/. Version: ESP6500SI-V2.
20. International HapMap Consortium. The International HapMap Project. Nature. 2003;426:789–96.
21. Sherry ST, Ward MH, Kholodov M, Baker J, Phan L, Smigielski EM, Sirotkin K. dbSNP: the NCBI database of genetic variation. Nucleic Acids Res. 2001;29:308–11.
22. Database of Single Nucleotide Polymorphisms (dbSNP). Bethesda: National Center for Biotechnology Information, National Library of Medicine. (dbSNP Build ID: 138). Available from: http://www.ncbi.nlm.nih.gov/SNP/.
23. Magi A, Tattini L, Cifola I, et al. EXCAVATOR: detecting copy number variants from whole-exome sequencing data. Genome Biol. 2013;14:R120.
24. Klambauer G, Schwarzbauer K, Mayr A, Clevert DA, Mitterecker A, Bodenhofer U, Hochreiter S. cn.MOPS: mixture of Poissons for discovering copy number variations in next-generation sequencing data with a low false discovery rate. Nucleic Acids Res. 2012;40:e69.
25. Krzywinski M, Schein J, Birol I, Connors J, Gascoyne R, Horsman D, Jones SJ, Marra MA. Circos: an information aesthetic for comparative genomics. Genome Res. 2009;19:1639–45.
26. Zeitouni B, Boeva V, Janoueix-Lerosey I, Loeillet S, Legoix-ne P, Nicolas A, Delattre O, Barillot E. SVDetect: a tool to identify genomic structural variations from paired-end and mate-pair sequencing data. Bioinformatics. 2010;26:1895–6.
27. Taniguchi K, Uchida J, Nishino K, Kumagai T, Okuyama T, Okami J, Higashiyama M, Kodama K, Imamura F, Kato K. Quantitative detection of EGFR mutations in circulating tumor DNA derived from lung adenocarcinomas. Clin Cancer Res. 2011;17:7808–15.
28. Vogelstein B, Papadopoulos N, Velculescu VE, Zhou S, Diaz Jr LA, Kinzler KW. Cancer genome landscapes. Science. 2013;339:1546–58.

29. Gao J, Aksoy BA, Dogrusoz U, Dresdner G, Gross B, Sumer SO, Sun Y, Jacobsen A, Sinha R, Larsson E, Cerami E, Sander C, Schultz N. Integrative analysis of complex cancer genomics and clinical profiles using the cBioPortal. Sci Signal. 2013;6:l1.
30. Cerami E, Gao J, Dogrusoz U, Gross BE, Sumer SO, Aksoy BA, Jacobsen A, Byrne CJ, Heuer ML, Larsson E, Antipin Y, Reva B, Goldberg AP, Sander C, Schultz N. The cBio cancer genomics portal: an open platform for exploring multidimensional cancer genomics data. Cancer Discov. 2012;2:401–4.
31. Gao Y, Toska E, Denmon D, Roberts SG, Medler KF. WT1 regulates the development of the posterior taste field. Development. 2014;141:2271–8.
32. McBride DJ, Orpana AK, Sotiriou C, Joensuu H, Stephens PJ, Mudie LJ, Hämäläinen E, Stebbings LA, Andersson LC, Flanagan AM, Durbecq V, Ignatiadis M, Kallioniemi O, Heckman CA, Alitalo K, Edgren H, Futreal PA, Stratton MR, Campbell PJ. Use of cancer-specific genomic rearrangements to quantify disease burden in plasma from patients with solid tumors. Genes Chromosomes Cancer. 2010;49:1062–9.
33. Leary RJ, Sausen M, Kinde I, Papadopoulos N, Carpten JD, Craig D, O'Shaughnessy J, Kinzler KW, Parmigiani G, Vogelstein B, Diaz Jr LA, Velculescu VE. Detection of chromosomal alterations in the circulation of cancer patients with whole-genome sequencing. Sci Transl Med. 2012;4:162ra154.
34. Donnard ER, Carpinetti PA, Navarro FC, Perez RO, Habr-Gama A, Parmigiani RB, Camargo AA, Galante PA. ICRmax: an optimized approach to detect tumor-specific interchromosomal rearrangements for clinical application. Genomics. 2015;105:265–72.
35. Olsson E, Winter C, George A, Chen Y, Howlin J, Tang MH, Dahlgren M, Schulz R, Grabau D, van Westen D, Fernö M, Ingvar C, Rose C, Bendahl PO, Rydén L, Borg Å, Gruvberger-Saal SK, Jernström H, Saal LH. Serial monitoring of circulating tumor DNA in patients with primary breast cancer for detection of occult metastatic disease. EMBO Mol Med. 2015;7:1034–47.
36. Dawson SJ, Tsui DW, Murtaza M, Biggs H, Rueda OM, Chin SF, Dunning MJ, Gale D, Forshew T, Mahler-Araujo B, Rajan S, Humphray S, Becq J, Halsall D, Wallis M, Bentley D, Caldas C, Rosenfeld N. Analysis of circulating tumor DNA to monitor metastatic breast cancer. N Engl J Med. 2013;368:1199–209.
37. Pereira E, Camacho-Vanegas O, Anand S, Sebra R, Catalina Camacho S, Garnar-Wortzel L, Nair N, Moshier E, Wooten M, Uzilov A, Chen R, Prasad-Hayes M, Zakashansky K, Beddoe AM, Schadt E, Dottino P, Martignetti JA. Personalized circulating tumor DNA biomarkers dynamically predict treatment response and survival in gynecologic cancers. PLoS One. 2015;10:e0145754.
38. Zhang B, Kirov SA, Snoddy JR. WebGestalt: an integrated system for exploring gene sets in various biological contexts. Nucleic Acids Res. 2005;33:W741–8.
39. Wang J, Duncan D, Shi Z, Zhang B. WEB-based GEne SeT AnaLysis Toolkit (WebGestalt): update 2013. Nucleic Acids Res. 2013;41:W77–83.

13

The *NF1* somatic mutational landscape in sporadic human cancers

Charlotte Philpott, Hannah Tovell, Ian M. Frayling, David N. Cooper and Meena Upadhyaya*

Abstract

Background: Neurofibromatosis type 1 (NF1: Online Mendelian Inheritance in Man (OMIM) #162200) is an autosomal dominantly inherited tumour predisposition syndrome. Heritable constitutional mutations in the *NF1* gene result in dysregulation of the RAS/MAPK pathway and are causative of NF1. The major known function of the *NF1* gene product neurofibromin is to downregulate RAS. NF1 exhibits variable clinical expression and is characterized by benign cutaneous lesions including neurofibromas and café-au-lait macules, as well as a predisposition to various types of malignancy, such as breast cancer and leukaemia. However, acquired somatic mutations in *NF1* are also found in a wide variety of malignant neoplasms that are not associated with NF1.

Main body: Capitalizing upon the availability of next-generation sequencing data from cancer genomes and exomes, we review current knowledge of somatic *NF1* mutations in a wide variety of tumours occurring at a number of different sites: breast, colorectum, urothelium, lung, ovary, skin, brain and neuroendocrine tissues, as well as leukaemias, in an attempt to understand their broader role and significance, and with a view ultimately to exploiting this in a diagnostic and therapeutic context.

Conclusion: As neurofibromin activity is a key to regulating the RAS/MAPK pathway, *NF1* mutations are important in the acquisition of drug resistance, to BRAF, EGFR inhibitors, tamoxifen and retinoic acid in melanoma, lung and breast cancers and neuroblastoma. Other curiosities are observed, such as a high rate of somatic *NF1* mutation in cutaneous melanoma, lung cancer, ovarian carcinoma and glioblastoma which are not usually associated with neurofibromatosis type 1. Somatic *NF1* mutations may be critical drivers in multiple cancers. The mutational landscape of somatic *NF1* mutations should provide novel insights into our understanding of the pathophysiology of cancer. The identification of high frequency of somatic *NF1* mutations in sporadic tumours indicates that neurofibromin is likely to play a critical role in development, far beyond that evident in the tumour predisposition syndrome NF1.

Keywords: NF1, Sporadic tumours, Somatic mutations, Cancer, Melanoma, Lung cancers, Glioblastoma, Leukaemia, Breast cancer, Phaeochromocytoma

Background

Neurofibromatosis type 1 (NF1: Online Mendelian Inheritance in Man (OMIM) #162200) is an autosomal dominantly inherited tumour predisposition syndrome. Affecting 1/3000–4000 individuals worldwide, it results from constitutional mutations of the *NF1* gene, lo\cated on the long arm of human chromosome 17 [1–4]. A variety of characteristic clinical features are associated with NF1, including hyperpigmentary abnormalities of the skin (café-au-lait macules (CALMs) and inguinal/axillary freckling, iris hamartomas (Lisch nodules) and the growth of benign peripheral nerve sheath tumours (neurofibromas) in the skin. Neurofibromas can be divided into several different subtypes and are associated with a variety of clinical complications. Cutaneous neurofibromas are small, discrete dermal tumours observed in most, but not all, adult NF1 patients [5]. The generally much larger plexiform neurofibromas (PNFs), a more diffuse tumour type, are present in 30–50% of NF1 patients. Importantly, some 10–15% of these benign PNFs subsequently develop into aggressive malignant peripheral nerve sheath tumours (MPNSTs) which are the main cause of morbidity in NF1 [6–8]. A number of other tumours are also associated with NF1, including optic gliomas, juvenile myelomonocytic leukaemia (JMML), benign

* Correspondence: Upadhyaya@cardiff.ac.uk
Division of Cancer and Genetics, Institute of Medical Genetics, Cardiff University, Heath Park, Cardiff CF14 4XN, UK

or malignant phaeochromocytomas, gastrointestinal stromal tumours, glomus tumours, juvenile xanthogranulomas, rhabdomyosarcomas and lipomas.

NF1 is a tumour suppressor gene; in order for a particular cell to become cancerous, both alleles of a tumour suppressor gene must be mutated. This concept, known as the 'two-hit' hypothesis, was first proposed by Knudson, and the majority of NF1-associated tumours exhibit biallelic inactivation of *NF1* [9, 10].

The *NF1* gene is spread over a large locus (350 kbp) at 17q11.2. It contains 61 exons, including four alternatively spliced exons, and is transcribed into a 12 kbp messenger RNA (mRNA) containing an open reading frame of 8454 nucleotides [11]. Curiously, intron 27b, the largest intron of *NF1* at 61 kbp, contains three embedded genes, *OMGP*, *EVI2B* and *EVI2A*, that are all transcribed in the opposite orientation to *NF1* but whose protein products appear to have little or no interaction with neurofibromin [11].

Neurofibromin: the *NF1* gene product

Neurofibromin is a 2818 amino acid, multidomain protein. Although ubiquitously expressed, its highest levels are to be found in cells of the central nervous system (CNS), where it is often found in association with tubulin. Neurofibromin is a member of a large family of evolutionarily conserved proteins: the mammalian Ras-GTPase-activating protein (GAP)-related proteins, and its most highly conserved region is the centrally located GAP-related domain (GRD), which is encoded by exons 20–27a. The best understood function of neurofibromin is its role in tightly regulating cellular levels of activated RAS proteins. All RAS proteins exist in two cellular states, the majority being found in their inactive GDP-bound form, with only a very small fraction present in their metabolically active GTP-bound form. Only in their GTP-bound form are RAS proteins able to upregulate the many downstream effector proteins that form part of the RAS/RAF/MAPK signalling pathway [12–16]. The key role of neurofibromin is to downregulate the activated GTP-bound RAS by stimulating the low intrinsic GTPase activity of the RAS proteins themselves, thereby promoting the conversion of active RAS-GTP into its inactive RAS-GDP state. Hence, any loss of neurofibromin functionality, due to inactivating mutations in *NF1*, will result in sustained intracellular levels of active RAS-GTP, resulting in prolonged activation of the RAS/RAF/MAPK signalling pathway and ultimately a loss of growth control and increased cellular proliferation.

Increased active RAS-GTP levels also stimulate the PI3K/AKT/mTOR signalling pathway which protects cells from apoptosis. In the absence of functional neurofibromin, the pathway can become constitutively activated resulting in an increase in cell proliferation and survival. The RAF/MAPK and PI3K/AKT pathways both activate mTOR signalling, a process found to be highly regulated in neurofibromas whereby mTOR pathway activation occurs in the absence of growth factors, in both NF1 tumours and neurofibromin-deficient cultured cells. Indeed, the mTOR pathway is constitutively activated in neurofibromin-deficient primary cells and tumours, and is regulated by phosphorylation and inactivation of the *TSC2*-encoded protein tuberin by AKT, ERK and RSK [13, 17]. It has also been suggested that increased RAS activity in brain cells may be associated with NF1-related learning deficiencies; it may result in long-term impairment as a result of increased GABA-mediated inhibition [18]. Neurofibromin levels and therefore Ras signalling can also be affected by mechanisms other than *NF1* mutation including ubiquitination [19].

Neurofibromin is known to associate with a large number of proteins, including tubulin, kinesin, protein kinases A and C, syndecan, caveolin, cytokeratin intermediate filaments and the amyloid precursor protein, although the biological significance of these protein-protein interactions is largely unknown. The diversity of protein associations does however emphasize the point that neurofibromin is likely to have many functions other than merely functioning as a GAP protein [14, 20]. Nonetheless, to date, only the function of the GAP-related domain of neurofibromin is fully understood, so it is to be hoped that new molecular studies will reveal additional functional properties of neurofibromin [21].

Mutation analysis of the *NF1* gene

The germline mutation rate of *NF1* is some 10-fold higher than that observed for most other inherited disease genes, with more than half of NF1 cases attributed to de novo mutations [7]. Currently, over 2600 different inherited mutations in *NF1* have been reported in the Human Gene Mutation Database (HGMD®) as a cause of NF1, varying in size from large genomic deletions spanning several megabases to single base-pair substitutions that alter an encoded amino acid or the function of a splice site [22–26]. There is, however, no evidence of any localized mutation clustering within *NF1*. Whilst the constitutional *NF1* mutational spectrum is well defined with missense/nonsense (27.7%), splicing (16.3%), microdeletions (26.9%), microinsertions (11.1%), indels (2.0%), gross deletions (>20 bp; 13.3%), gross insertions (>20 bp; 2.0%), complex rearrangements (0.6%) and a couple of putative regulatory mutations, there is no evidence of any localized mutation clustering within *NF1* [27, 28]. The majority (>80%) of constitutional *NF1* mutations are inactivating, predicted to result in almost complete absence of the transcript or protein [25]. Approximately 5–10% of all heritable *NF1* mutations involve gross DNA alterations, mainly genomic deletions spanning the whole gene and flanking region, as well as intragenic multi-exon rearrangements [29]. Constitutional mutations have not been identified in any of the four alternatively spliced exons in research studies, but this may be due to ascertainment bias, as the majority of clinical laboratories that analyse *NF1* do not screen these alternative exons for mutations.

A subset of the many *NF1* splicing mutations, i.e. deep intronic mutations, result in the creation of novel acceptor/donor splice sites. These may give rise to the inclusion of a novel cryptic exon into the transcribed mRNA, leading to the production of an aberrant neurofibromin protein. Such mutations account for ~2% of all reported constitutional *NF1* mutations [30].

To date, only three NF1 families with gonadal or germline mosaicism have been reported [31–33]. In such families, only a small proportion of the germ cells, whether sperm or ova, will carry the new *NF1* mutation, but this can nevertheless result in more than one affected child being produced by clinically normal parents [34].

A major challenge for clinicians and geneticists dealing with NF1 is the successful identification and characterization of causative *NF1* mutations in their patients. This problem relates to a number of features of the *NF1*, including its large genomic size (~350 kbp) and complexity (61 exons), the absence of any obvious mutational hotspots or recurrent mutations, and the wide spectrum of mutation types observed. Indeed, the lack of mutational clustering and the paucity of recurrent mutations necessitates analysis of the entire *NF1* gene in the search for potential pathogenic mutations. Furthermore, given the broad spectrum of known *NF1* mutations, no single mutation detection test can, as yet, successfully identify all such mutation types [35]. Furthermore, some 30% of all *NF1* mutations are predicted to cause aberrant splicing, and for this reason, the analysis of both RNA and DNA from patients in mutation screening protocols is clearly required [25]. Whilst the majority of *NF1* splicing mutations occur within consensus acceptor and donor splice site sequences, a number of missense, nonsense, and even 'silent' mutations may also result in aberrant splicing, which are often only identifiable by screening a patient's RNA [25]. As well as the challenges in collection and analysis of patient mRNA, a frequent issue is the difficulty in interpreting the clinical diagnostic significance of putative *NF1* missense mutations, as this may require a family segregation study and/or in vitro functional analysis to determine the pathogenicity (or otherwise) of the variant in question [25, 36].

Furthermore, many highly homologous *NF1* pseudogene sequences are scattered throughout the human genome and can often interfere with PCR-based diagnostic tests. This emphasizes the need for the careful selection of PCR primers to avoid non-specific amplification of these pseudogene sequences.

The spatial distribution of *NF1* microdeletions is strongly influenced by the presence of a number of low-copy repeats (LCRs) spanning the 17q11.2 region that encompasses the *NF1* gene. Indeed, studies into *NF1* microdeletions have provided a general model to understand the different mutational mechanisms underlying large genomic rearrangements associated with inherited diseases [37].

The *NF1* mutation detection rate in classical NF1 patients can be up to 95%. However, somatic mutation detection is more challenging, largely because of the cellular heterogeneity which is characteristic of tumour tissue [38]. Mutations in multiple genes encoding the components of the RAS/MAPK pathway predispose patients to develop clinical features that overlap with those of NF1, e.g. Legius syndrome, Noonan syndrome inter alia, and the majority of these conditions are associated with tumours [39].

Tumour biology

All cancers originate from a single cell that starts to behave abnormally due to acquired somatic mutations in its genome. These somatic mutations may be the consequence of impaired DNA replication machinery, exogenous or endogenous mutagen exposures, enzymatic modification of DNA or defective DNA repair.

A subset of these somatic changes, termed 'driver mutations', confer a selective growth advantage and are implicated in cancer development, whereas the remainder are considered to be 'passengers' [40]. The Cancer Genome Atlas (TCGA), International Cancer Genome Consortium (ICGC), Catalogue of Somatic Mutations in Cancer (COSMIC) and cBioPortal for Cancer Genomics collectively represent the results of large-scale sequencing of cancers, thereby capturing many of the genomic alterations driving malignancy [41–44]. The cBio Cancer Genomics Portal is an open-access resource for the interactive exploration of multidimensional cancer genomics data sets, currently providing access to data from more than 5000 tumour samples from 147 cancer studies [44–46]. It contains data on somatic *NF1* mutations in different types of tumour including melanoma (desmoplastic, skin cutaneous and uveal), breast carcinoma, neuroendocrine prostate cancer, glioblastoma, lung adenocarcinoma and squamous cell carcinoma, urothelial carcinoma, uterine carcinoma, adenoid and ovarian serous cystadenocarcinoma, paraganglioma, phaeochromocytoma, pancreatic cancer, adrenocortical carcinoma, stomach adenocarcinoma, sarcoma, oesophageal cancer, rhabdomyosarcoma and many more. In this review, we detail the frequency of somatic *NF1* mutations in many non-NF1-associated sporadic cancers including melanoma, glioblastoma, neuroblastoma, breast cancer, ovarian serous carcinoma, paraganglioma and phaeochromocytoma, lung adenocarcinoma, lung squamous cell carcinoma, bladder, colorectal and leukaemia. Further, it is anticipated that with the advent of powerful sequencing technologies, combined with precise microdissection of tissue, somatic *NF1* mutations will be identified in additional tumour types. Somatic *NF1* mutations are important not only because they may be drivers but also because they may contribute to resistance to therapy [47]. Elucidation of the mutational landscape of somatic *NF1* mutations in a large number of sporadic tumours, their role in the initiation and progression of tumours and how they can confer resistance or sensitivity to a therapeutic intervention may provide further insight into the mechanisms underlying tumour development and ultimately aid the development and targeting of therapies.

The frequency of somatic *NF1* mutations in different sporadic tumour types derived from the literature is given in Table 1. The cBioPortal for Cancer Genomics provides a web resource for exploring, visualizing and analysing multidimensional cancer genomics data and provides graphical summaries of gene-level data from multiple platforms, shown in Fig. 1 [45].

Main body

Melanoma

Melanoma is a skin cancer that arises from melanocytes. Although the precise causes of melanomas are still not fully understood, environmental exposure to ultraviolet (UV) radiation from sunlight or tanning lamps certainly increases the risk of developing melanoma. Although NF1 is associated with pigmentary abnormalities such as CALMs, malignant melanoma is not a tumour type associated with NF1.

Table 1 Frequency of somatic *NF1* mutations in different human neoplasms

Neoplasm	Frequency of somatic *NF1* mutations	References
Cutaneous melanoma	12–30%	[49–51, 58]
Desmoplastic melanoma	45–90%	[60, 61]
Lung adenocarcinoma	7–11.8%	[65–67, 166, 176, 177]
Lung squamous cell carcinoma	10.3–11%	[72, 177]
Acute myeloid leukaemia	3.5–23.6%	[82–85]
T cell acute lymphoblastic leukaemia	3%	[88]
Breast cancer	2.5–27.7%	[106, 177]
Ovarian carcinoma	12–34.4%	[113, 115, 170, 177–180]
Paraganglioma/ phaeochromocytoma	21–26%	[121, 124, 177]
Neuroblastoma	2.2–6%	[130]
Glioblastoma	14–23%	[132, 134, 177]
Colon adenocarcinoma	3.8–6.25%	[143, 177]
Bladder transitional cell carcinoma	6–14%	[149, 167, 177]

Somatic mutation analysis of melanoma by next-generation sequencing has been performed at multiple centres leading to the identification of several different pathways thought to be involved in the initiation and progression of melanoma.

The direct involvement of *NF1* in melanoma was first reported by Andersen and colleagues in 1993 who identified a homozygous *NF1* deletion in one of eight malignant melanoma cell lines which resulted in the loss of detectable *NF1* mRNA and neurofibromin protein [48]. Furthermore, the apparent absence of neurofibromin and *NF1* mRNA was recorded in a primary melanoma. This led to their proposal that *NF1* may function as a tumour suppressor gene in the development or progression of malignant melanoma. Many subsequent studies have identified additional somatic *NF1* mutations in melanoma in 12–30% of cases [45, 49–55].

RAS/MAPK pathway dysregulation has been identified as a key culprit in non-familial melanoma, leading to the discovery of *BRAF* and *NRAS* as the most commonly mutated genes [56]. Indeed, *BRAF* mutations occur in 50–70% of all cutaneous malignant melanomas, whilst *NRAS* alterations only occur in 19–28% of tumours. In both cases, these gene lesions result in constitutive activation of the MAPK pathway and are believed to be early somatic events associated with melanoma initiation [56, 57]. The high frequency of *BRAF* and *NRAS* mutations in melanomas has recently been confirmed by high-throughput next-generation sequencing (NGS) analysis which also identified additional driver mutations, including a recurrent *RAC* mutation, which is the third most frequent activating mutation in sun-exposed melanomas after *BRAF* and *NRAS* mutations [50, 51].

Inactivating *NF1* mutations have been detected in approximately 13% of melanomas, alongside mutations in other tumour suppressor genes, including *TP53*, *ARID2*, *PTEN*, *CDKN2A*, *MAP2K1* and *RB1* [51]. The impact on *NRAS* is however non-uniform, with some *NF1* mutant melanomas exhibiting full *NRAS* activation (i.e. the same activation level as oncogenic *NRAS* mutations), whereas others exhibit only partial activation [51]. In a mouse melanoma model, *NF1* mutations cooperate with *BRAF* mutations in the pathogenesis of melanoma by preventing oncogene-induced senescence, an indication that NF1 plays a key role in early melanoma development [58]. In both mouse tumour models and A375 human melanoma cell lines, Maertens and colleagues have shown that resistance to treatment was enhanced by further suppression of *NF1* by small hairpin RNA (shRNA). Furthermore, they observed that resistance to the BRAF inhibitor PLX4720 was attenuated by reconstitution of

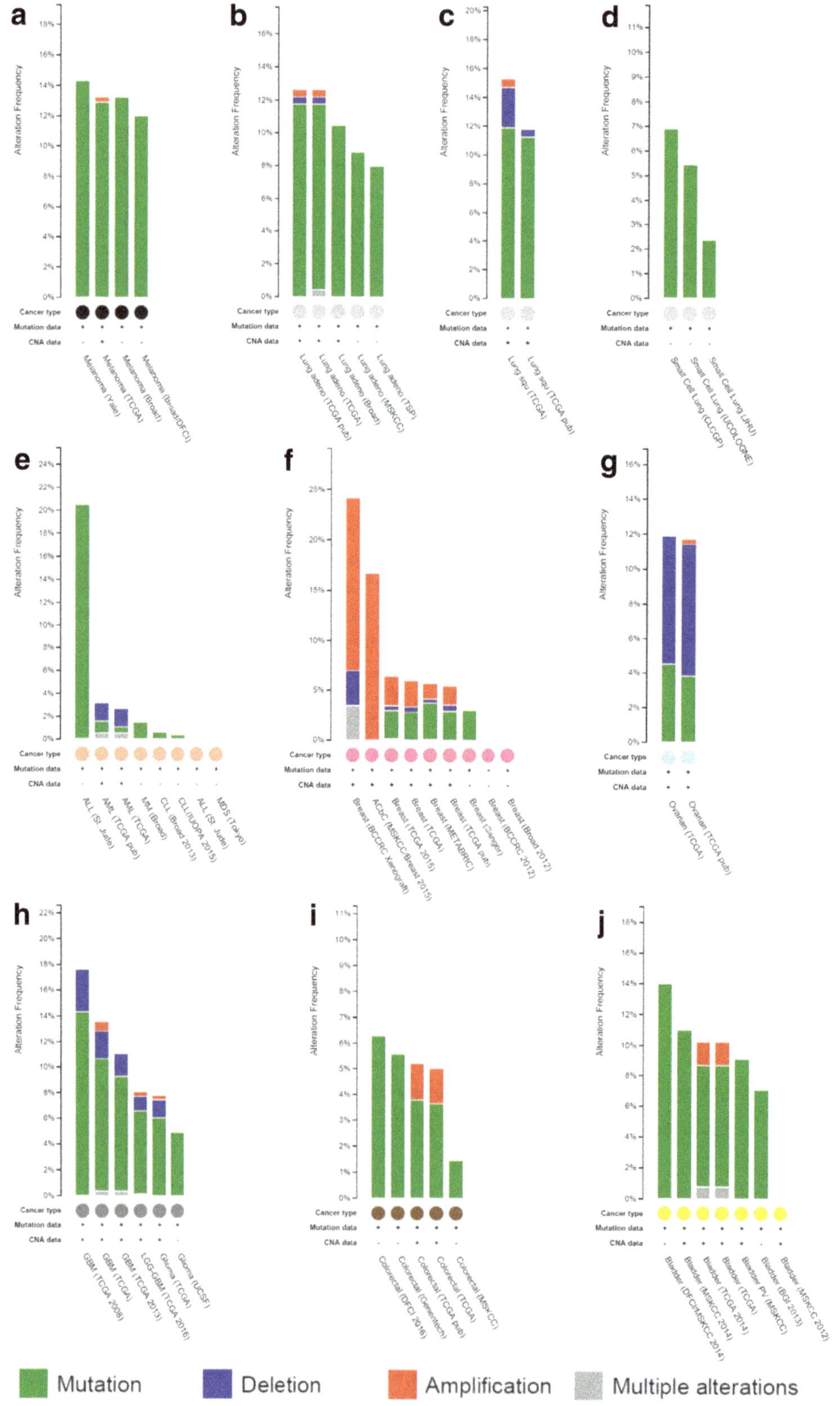

Fig. 1 (See legend on next page.)

(See figure on previous page.)
Fig. 1 The frequency and nature of somatic *NF1* mutations in different cancer types derived from the cBio dataset. **a** Malignant melanoma. **b** Lung adenocarcinoma. **c** Lung squamous cell carcinoma. **d** Small cell lung carcinoma. **e** Acute lymphocytic leukaemia (*ALL*). Acute myeloid leukaemia (*AML*), chronic lymphocytic leukaemia (*CLL*), malignant myeloma (*MM*) and myelodysplastic syndrome (*MDS*). **f** Breast carcinoma. **g** Serous ovarian carcinoma. **h** Brain glioma, including glioblastoma multiforme (*GBM*). **i** Colorectal carcinoma. **j** Bladder transitional cell carcinoma. Mutations = single base-pair substitutions, in-frame microdeletions/insertions, frameshift microdeletions/insertions, splice site mutations (including those that can create in-frame deletions via exon skipping), nonsense mutations and frameshift insertions/deletions (shown in *green*); deletions = gross, multi-exonic and whole gene deletion identified as copy number changes (shown in *blue*); amplification = multi-exonic, whole gene duplications identified as copy number changes (shown in *red*); multiple alterations = some combination of mutations, deletions and/or amplification (shown in *grey*) [44–46]

NF1 in these cells [58]. Using RNA interference (RNAi) screening techniques, Whittaker and colleagues confirmed that *NF1* mutation is a key mechanism in BRAF inhibitor resistance. An RNAi screen, targeting more than 16,500 genes in a BRAF inhibitor-sensitive melanoma cell line, identified NF1 as the highest ranking protein affected by BRAF inhibition, and that, *NF1* knockdown abrogated the growth inhibitory effects of BRAF inhibition [53]. Indeed, it was found that *NF1* suppression led to a 31-fold increase in resistance to PLX4720, as well as a partial (7-fold) resistance to MEK inhibition, demonstrating that human melanoma samples with innate resistance to BRAF inhibition and sensitivity to a MEK inhibitor harboured *NF1* mutations [53].

Importantly, *NF1* mutations have been found in melanomas that lack both *BRAF* and *NRAS* mutations, with 25–30% of such melanomas found to harbour deleterious *NF1* mutations, thus implying that *NF1* inactivation has conferred aberrant MAPK pathway activation in these tumours [50, 51]. *BRAF/NRAS* wild-type and *NF1* mutant melanomas are strongly associated with UV damage, as evidenced clinically by the higher degree of solar elastosis and, at a molecular level, by a high proportion of C > T transitions at pyrimidine dimers and more frequent tandem CC>TT transitions [59].

A recent study based on 213 human melanoma samples identified three frequently mutated genes: *BRAF*, *NRAS* and *NF1*, with frequencies of 38.5, 28.6 and 12.2%, respectively [49]. Whilst known recurrent activating mutations were identified in *BRAF* and *NRAS*, a high number of inactivating mutations were identified in *NF1*. Notably, almost half (26/56) of *BRAF* and *NRAS* wild-type melanomas had an *NF1* mutation, most identified by loss of heterozygosity (LOH). Furthermore, *NF1* mutation-containing melanomas also harboured significantly more somatic mutations across all loci and occurred in significantly older patients, although they were associated with similar overall patient survival rates as compared to *BRAF* or *RAS* mutant or *BRAF-RAS-NF1* wild-type melanoma. In addition, all 26 *NF1* mutant *BRAF-RAS* wild-type melanomas carried mutations in other known RASopathy genes, including *RASA2*, *PTPN11*, *SOS1*, *RAF1* and *SPRED1* [49]. In contrast to Whittaker and colleagues, Krauthammer et al. also found that 6/10 *NF1* mutant cell lines were highly sensitive to a MEK inhibitor, whereas the other four were highly resistant, clearly indicating that *NF1* suppression is not always associated with either sensitivity or resistance to MEK inhibitor [49, 53].

Desmoplastic melanoma

The highest frequency of somatic *NF1* mutations were found in desmoplastic melanomas (14/15) [60]. These melanomas are characterized by their higher propensity for local recurrence and less frequent metastatic spread to regional lymph nodes. The high frequency of *NF1* mutations in desmoplastic melanomas appears to indicate an important role for neurofibromin in the specific biology of this type of melanoma. Another recent study screened 20 desmoplastic melanomas by exome sequencing for alterations in the MAPK and PI3K signalling pathways, i.e. mutations in *CBL*, *ERBB2*, *MAP2K1*, *MAP3K1*, *BRAF*, *EGFR*, *PTPN11*, *MET*, *RAC1*, *SOS2*, *NRAS* and *PIK3C*, which were found in 15/20 (75%), with *NF1* mutations being found in 9/20 (45%) [61].

Uveal melanoma

Melanoma of the uveal tract (i.e. iris, ciliary body and choroid) is rarer than cutaneous melanoma but is nevertheless the most common primary intraocular malignancy in adults, with inactivating mutations found in approximately 60% (23/38) of uveal melanomas [62]. Intriguingly, whilst not malignant, the Lisch nodules characteristic of NF1 is hamartomatous uveal melanocytic proliferations of the iris.

Mucosal melanoma

Mucosal melanoma differs from cutaneous melanoma in terms of its molecular profile, with less frequent *BRAF* and more frequent *KIT* mutations but also has a poor prognosis. In a recent study [63] of a cohort of 75 tumours from patients with a mucosal melanoma, *NF1* and *RAS* mutations were identified in 18.3 and 16.9% samples, respectively, whereas 8.4 and 7% of tumour samples harboured *BRAF* and *KIT* mutations [63]. This study demonstrates that *NF1* is the most frequently occurring driver mutation in mucosal melanoma.

Lung cancer

Lung cancer is responsible for about 10% of all cancer cases worldwide; the vast majority of which has been attributed to tobacco smoking [64]. The two main types are non-small cell lung cancer (NSCLC) in 80–90% cases and small cell lung cancer (SCLC) found in 10–15% of patients. NSCLC has multiple subtypes, including adenocarcinoma (ADC), squamous cell carcinoma (SqCC) and undifferentiated (large cell) lung carcinoma.

Adenocarcinoma

Approximately 40% of NSCLC are ADC, and several studies have reported somatic *NF1* mutations in some 7–11% of ADC [65–68]. The high mortality rate characteristic of this tumour type is due in part to the frequent presentation of such tumours at a locally advanced or metastatic stage and the lack of an effective advanced stage treatment [65, 69]. A number of potential novel therapeutic targets have been identified, including the activating mutations in *KRAS, BRAF, ERBB2* and *PIK3CA*; the translocations in *RET* and *ROS1*; and the loss of function or deletions of *TP53, NF1, CDKN2A* and *KEAP1* [65, 70]. Whilst *NF1* mutations were only found in 7% (13/188) of sporadic lung ADC [65], further analysis found that biallelic inactivation at the *NF1* locus may be present in as many as 23% (3/13), although it is not known whether these lesions occurred in *cis* or in *trans* [65]. Similarly, Imielinski et al. identified somatic *NF1* mutations in 10.9% (20/183) of lung ADC, of which half were found to be truncating mutations, resulting in a complete loss of function [66].

In addition to *NF1* being recurrently mutated in a subset of sporadic lung ADC patients, the MAPK pathway also appears to be an important regulatory pathway involved in tumorigenesis [65]. The TCGA research network examined the genomes, RNA and some protein from 230 previously untreated lung ADC and matched normal samples [41, 67]. In three quarters of the samples, the group identified mutations in *NF1* and other genes that activate the RTK/RAS/RAF cell signalling pathway. This study not only identified loss-of-function *NF1* defects but also demonstrated that *NF1* mutations (as well as *KEAP1* and *TP53* mutations) are far more frequent in the *BRAF-RAS* oncogene-negative subset of lung ADC. Additionally, TCGA and other groups have identified genes such as *TP53, KRAS, STK11* (*LKB1*), *EGFR* and *NF1* to be significantly mutated in ADC [67].

Markedly reduced *NF1* mRNA expression in ADC has been found to confer both an intrinsic and an acquired resistance to EGFR inhibitors [71]. By performing a genome-wide siRNA screen of both a human lung cancer cell line and a murine mutant EGFR-driven lung ADC, this revealed reduced *NF1* mRNA expression in both, and furthermore, whilst the EGFR inhibitor erlotinib failed to fully inhibit RAS-ERK signalling when neurofibromin levels were reduced, treatment of neurofibromin-deficient lung cancers with MEK inhibitor restored sensitivity to erlotinib [71].

In a recent study of 591 NSCLC, 60 had *NF1* mutations (10%) whilst 141 (24%) harboured *KRAS* mutations [68]. Approximately 25% of the *NF1* mutations co-occurred with mutations in known oncogenes: *BRAF, ERBB2, KRAS, HRAS* and *NRAS*. Therapeutic strategies targeting *KRAS* activation, including the use of inhibitors of MAP kinase signalling, may warrant investigation in *NF1* mutant tumours. Additional tumour suppressor inactivation pattern studies may help to inform novel treatment strategies.

Squamous cell carcinoma

According to the TCGA, somatic *NF1* changes are present in approximately 12% of squamous cell lung cancers (SqCC), of which four distinct subtypes have been identified: classical, primitive, basal and secretory expression [72]. The basal expression subtype was found to harbour *NF1* alterations, suggesting a potential direction for the treatment of such tumours. The information from the TCGA studies has highlighted the involvement of *NF1* in both lung ADC and SqCC and served to improve our understanding of the genetic pathways that lead to lung cancer [72].

Transcriptome analysis of 153 tumour samples, including ADC, SqCC, large cell lung cancer, adenoid cystic carcinomas and derived cell lines, has been integrated with the data from The Cancer Genome Atlas and other published sources [73]. This confirms the previously reported *CD74-NRG1* fusion and also suggests that the *NRG1, NF1* and Hippo pathway fusions may play important roles in tumours without known driver mutations and that this prognostic factor may be associated with poor survival [73]. Several different gene fusions, viz. *NF1-GOSR1, NF1-PSMD11, NF1-NLK, NF1-DRG2* and *NF1-MYO15A*, were also detected by transcriptome sequencing of lung cancers [73]. Interestingly, both lung ADC and SqCC DNA displayed a significantly increased frequency of guanine (cytosine) to thymine (adenine) mutations, a type of mutation associated with exposure to tobacco smoke [68]. Lung ADC genomes also manifest regional heterogeneity in terms of the distribution of mutations with sequencing data from lung cancer studies clearly indicating that lung cancer, at the molecular level, is a highly heterogeneous disease. Indeed, the mutational landscape of lung ADC is substantially different from that of SqCC of the lung or SCLC [74], with frequent receptor tyrosine kinase mutations found in lung ADC, that are rarely encountered in either SqCC or SCLC [75].

Mutations in *TP53, KRAS, LKB1, NF1* and *RBM10* are enriched in transversion-high tumours, whilst mutations in *EGFR, RB1* and *PIK3CA* and in-frame insertions in the receptor tyrosine kinases *EGFR* and *ERBB2* are enriched in transversion-low tumours [75]. The transversion-high group was found to be strongly associated with past or present smoking ($P < 2.2 \times 10^{-16}$) [72, 74, 75].

To compare lung ADC and SqCC and to identify new drivers of lung carcinogenesis, Campbell and colleagues examined the exome sequences and copy number profiles of 660 lung ADC and 484 lung SqCC tumour normal pairs [74]. They observed median somatic mutation rates of 8.7 mutations/Mbp and 9.7 mutations/Mbp for lung ADC and SqCC, respectively. At least 38 genes were significantly mutated in lung ADC and 20 genes in SqCC; however, only six genes, *TP53, RB1, ARIDIA, CDKN2A, PIK3CA* and *NF1*, were significantly mutated in both tumour types, and of these, *TP53, CDKN2A* and *PIK3CA* mutations had a significantly higher frequency in lung SqCC. Recurrent alterations in lung SqCC were more similar to those of other squamous carcinomas than to alterations in lung ADCs, whilst the significantly mutated genes in lung ADC were most similar to those associated with glioblastoma and colorectal cancer.

Small cell lung cancer

Although there is a paucity of data for small cell lung cancer (SCLC), the frequency of *NF1* mutations in SCLC was found to be 2.4 and 6.9% in two independent studies [76, 77]. In a subsequent study of 98 SCLC, DNA was sequenced to a high, uniform coverage and analysed for all classes of genomic alterations [78]. Of the seven most commonly altered genes identified, only one (*RICTOR*) was considered to be actionable in terms of treatment. The most common non-actionable genomic alterations were found in *TP53* (86% of SCLC cases), *RB1* (54%) and *MLL2* (17%), with *NF1* mutations identified in only 3% of SCLC, consistent with the earlier studies.

Myeloid malignancies

Myeloid malignancies are clonal disorders characterized by acquired somatic mutations in various haematopoietic progenitors. Constitutional *NF1* mutations are known to predispose individuals to myeloid malignancies such as chronic myelomonocytic leukaemia (CMML), JMML and acute myeloid leukaemia (AML) [79]. Somatic 17q11 deletions encompassing *NF1* have been described in many adult myeloid malignancies [80]. More generally, the RAS signalling pathway has been found to be fundamental in the development of myeloid malignancies, with somatic activating mutations in *NRAS* and *KRAS* genes estimated to be present in 20 to 40% of diagnosed cases of AML, CMML and JMML [81]. Recent advances in understanding the genetic basis of myeloid malignancies have provided important insights into the pathogenesis of AML. Whilst somatic *KRAS* and *NRAS* mutations are frequently found in AML, mutations in other RAS signalling pathway genes, including *NF1*, occur at lower frequencies, although the reported frequency for *NF1* somatic mutations ranges quite widely from 3.5 to 23.6% [79, 82–85].

Parkin and colleagues identified *NF1* mutations in 7% of cases with AML, with a further 12% displaying copy number alterations (CNAs) involving *NF1*, mainly heterozygous deletions [85]. The absence of *NF1* expression was observed in 7% of adult AML associated with an increased RAS-GTP level. In another study of AML with CBHB-MYHII rearrangements, 16% of the samples harboured *NF1* deletions [84]. However, high-resolution studies have failed to provide any evidence for frequent *NF1* alterations in de novo AML, although they suggested that *NF1* mutations may contribute to tumour progression [82]. In this study, the authors screened a total of 488 previously untreated de novo AML patients for the *NF1* deletion using either array comparative genomic hybridization (aCGH) or real-time quantitative PCR/fluorescence in situ hybridization approaches. Using aCGH, a small ~0.3 Mbp minimally deleted region involving *NF1* was defined; the overall frequency of *NF1* deletion was 3.5% (17/485). Furthermore, *NF1* deletion was significantly associated with abnormal cytogenetics and a monosomal karyotype, whilst only one of five *NF1*-deleted patients acquired a coding mutation in the remaining allele. This study indicates that *NF1* microlesions are infrequent in de novo AML and may be secondary events in leukemic progression.

Myelodysplastic syndrome

The frequency of *NF1* changes in myelodysplastic syndrome has been found to vary between 0 and 9% [86, 87].

T cell acute lymphoblastic leukaemia

T cell acute lymphoblastic leukaemia (T-ALL) is a variant of acute lymphoblastic leukaemia (ALL), with features similar to some types of lymphoma. It accounts for about 15 and 25% of ALL in paediatric and adult cohorts, respectively.

T-ALL is a highly aggressive malignancy, characterized by rapid progression and high relapse rates [79]. Somatic mutations in a number of established T-ALL drivers such as *KRAS, NRAS, PIK3CA, PTEN, NOTCH1, PHF6* and *NF1* have been identified in T-ALL cell lines and patient samples [88]. Somatic *NF1* mutations have been found in 27.3% (9/33) of the T-ALL cohort; however, only 12.1% (4/33) were non-synonymous mutations [88]. The type 1 *NF1* microdeletion (1.4 Mb) was reported in 2.9% (3/103) of T-ALL patients [79]. None of these three individuals with the microdeletion exhibited any clinical characteristics of NF1.

Juvenile myelomonocytic leukaemia

JMML is a myeloproliferative neoplasm (MPN) of childhood, occurring when too many immature white blood cells (myelocytes and monocytes) are made in the bone marrow. In 1997, Side and colleagues reported constitutional *NF1* mutations in 15% of JMML patients [89]. JMML generally carries a very poor prognosis, with the only curative treatment being haematopoietic stem cell transplantation.

JMML was once considered a unique example of RAS-driven oncogenesis because it was thought to be initiated by mutually exclusive mutations in the RAS genes (*NRAS* or *KRAS*) or in several RAS pathway regulators (*PTPN11*, *NF1* or *CBL*) [90].

In an exploration of the somatic mutation landscape of 30 patients with syndromic ($n = 8$) or sporadic ($n = 22$) JMML, a combination of genome-wide DNA array analysis, whole-exome sequencing and targeted sequencing was used in paired germline and tumour samples [90]. In total, 85 somatically acquired genetic alterations were found in 83% (25/30) of patients in this sub-cohort. Genes containing somatic variants detected by whole-exome sequencing, or previously reported to be mutated in JMML, were then sequenced in the full cohort of 118 JMML cases. A total of 122 secondary clonal abnormalities, in addition to initiating RAS pathway mutations, were identified in 49% (58/118) of patients [90]. In addition, sequencing of isolated myeloid colonies demonstrated the coexistence of multiple RAS hits in the same myeloid progenitors in three of the JMML cases tested, challenging the concept of mutually exclusive RAS pathway mutations.

The polycomb recessive complex 2 (PRC2) is involved in cellular differentiation, maintenance of cell identity and proliferation as well as stem cell plasticity [91] and also drives myeloid malignancies. *Nf1/Kras* double-mutant mice have been shown to develop myeloid malignancies with reduced latency and increased severity in comparison to mice with only one of the two defects because copy number variations (CNVs) in *Nf1/Kras* mutant mice frequently resulted in haploinsufficiency for PRC2 core subunits (*SUZ12* or *EZH2*) or PRC2-associated factors necessary for optimal PRC2 activity (*AEBP2*, *CDYL* or *JARID2*) [92]. In addition, haploinsufficiency for multiple genes that regulate PRC2 function can cooperate in myeloid transformation, and other mutations in JMML target a small number of pathways specifically, including components of the RAS and PRC2 networks [93, 94]. Thus, RAS activation is a major player, and other pathways such as PRC2 are also important. Notably, PRC2 also plays a role in the development of MPNSTs. Loss of function of PRC2 (due to mutations in *EED* or *SUZ12*) is also found in the vast majority of sporadic, NF1-associated, and radiotherapy-associated MPNSTs (where PRC2 loss amplifies Ras-driven transcription) [95, 96].

In a recent study focussing on characterization of serial samples from JMML patients at diagnosis and then beyond through relapse and transformation to AML, mutations were found in *NF1*, *NRAS*, *KRAS*, *PTPN11* or *CBL* in 85% of patients, as well as recurrent mutations in other genes involved in signal transduction, splicing, PRC2 and transcription. The number of somatic alterations present at diagnosis appeared to be important for the outcome of JMML [97].

Breast cancer

The *NF1* gene is reported to be frequently mutated in sporadic breast cancers, although in only a few studies has mutation frequency been published. NF1 patients have an increased risk of developing breast cancer as compared to the general population [8, 98]. In particular, women under the age of 50 with NF1 have an increased (4–5-fold) risk of developing breast cancer (standardized incidence ratio for women under 50) and also a 3.5-fold increased fatality risk (proportionate mortality ratio) [98–100]. A predisposition to breast cancer in NF1 patients has led researchers to postulate the potential involvement of somatic *NF1* mutations in initiating and driving the malignant transformation and progression of sporadic breast cancer. A number of breast cancer genome sequencing studies have identified *NF1* as one of a number of novel, recurrently mutated genes in sporadic tumours which could potentially be targeted in a therapeutic context [101, 102].

It was Ogata and colleagues, working with established breast cancer cell lines in 2001, who first identified a role for *NF1* in the malignant transformation of mammary cells [103]. Further analysis of the *NF1* deletion-bearing tumours revealed significantly higher levels of active RAS, indicating that RAS signal transduction pathway dysregulation, through *NF1* loss, may be responsible for driving malignancy in these cells. Neurofibromin was found to be below detectable levels in the highly malignant and treatment-resistant MB-231 breast cancer cell line as compared with four other less aggressive cell lines. Additionally, the MB-231 cells exhibited a 10-fold increase in pMAPK levels as a result of activated Ras, despite there being no changes in p120^{GAP}. Hence, this study suggested that under-expression of *NF1* and reduced neurofibromin activity may have a direct influence on malignant transformation and resistance to anti-cancer agents [103]. This is consistent with other studies and goes some way towards accounting for the presence of the somatic *NF1* mutations found in sporadic breast tumours.

The mouse model *Chaos3* is characterized by the spontaneous development of mammary tumours, due to a mutation in *Mcm4* leading to chromosomal instability through disruption of the MCM2-7 complex [104, 105]. Somatic *NF1* deletions were found in almost all (59/60) of the mammary tumours studied in this mouse model, and upon subsequent examination of TCGA data, it was noted that *NF1* is somatically mutated or deleted in 27.7% of human breast cancers [105, 106].

Large-scale NGS to compare primary and recurrent breast cancer has found mutations in recurrent tumours which were not present in matched primary tissue [107]. However, the difficulties inherent in studying recurrent tumours mean that the sample size was necessarily small in this study, with only 74 matched tumours from 43 patients across the various breast cancer subtypes. So, the precise role for *NF1* in breast cancer is still unclear and further studies are required.

CNAs dominate the breast cancer genome, with *NF1* gene amplification being a particular feature not seen in the other tumour types in which *NF1* mutations are observed (Fig. 1), suggesting that gain of neurofibromin function is especially important in breast cancer biology. In contrast, genes generally mutated in breast cancers are subject to a low frequency of somatic mutations, including single nucleotide mutations and indels in driver genes [105, 106].

Large-scale efforts by the TCGA and ICGC have contributed greatly towards determining the identity of genes mutated in breast cancer, but analysis of clinical associations in these data sets is limited by the scarcity of long-term patient follow-up data and the stringent criteria used for sample selection (e.g. tumour size, malignant cellularity) [41, 42].

In a recent study based on 2433 molecular profiles of breast cancer, it was noted that high levels of intra-tumour heterogeneity was generally associated with a worse clinical outcome, with one exception: highly aggressive breast tumours with 11q13–14 amplification had low levels of intra-tumour heterogeneity [108, 109]. Inactivating *NF1* mutations were also found to be associated with breast cancer severity score in oestrogen receptor-negative tumours.

As with melanoma and neuroblastoma, inactivation of *NF1* in breast cancer is associated with resistance to drug therapy. A potential mechanism for *NF1* and drug resistance in breast adenocarcinoma has been suggested following analysis of the MCF-7 breast cancer cell line [110]. Silencing of *NF1*, amongst several other genes, has been shown to confer a tamoxifen-resistant phenotype, although it was noted that resistance- or sensitivity-specific gene expression patterns may give a better prediction of treatment outcome as compared to single genes [111]. This is potentially of great clinical importance, of course, as, although tamoxifen is one of the most widely used anti-breast cancer agents, it is now apparent that up to ~40% of early-stage breast cancer patients who receive tamoxifen as an adjuvant therapy will ultimately develop tamoxifen resistance and relapse [111, 112].

Ovarian cancer

High-grade serous ovarian carcinoma (HGOSC) is the most common and malignant form of ovarian tumours accounting for up to 70% of all ovarian cancer cases. Some serous cancers may initiate in cells at the distal end of the fallopian tube, then spread to the ovary. There are different subtypes of epithelial ovarian cancer including mucinous, endometrioid, clear cell, undifferentiated or unclassifiable; therefore, HGOSC is a molecularly and clinically heterogeneous disease which accounts for the majority of ovarian cancer deaths.

More than a third of all ovarian serous carcinomas (OSCs) harbour somatic *NF1* mutations, identifying an alternative target for treatment and an additional prognostic marker. This is of particular importance when considering the disease heterogeneity, high relapse and fatality rates [113, 114].

A role for *NF1* in ovarian serous carcinoma (OSC) was first proposed by Sangha et al. in 2008 [113]. Genome-wide microarray analysis of 36 primary OSC identified homozygous *NF1* deletions in two tumours. This group subsequently screened 18 ovarian carcinoma-derived cell lines and 41 primary OSC for additional *NF1* alterations, with 8/18 cell lines exhibiting marked reduction or no expression of *NF1*. Homozygous *NF1* gene deletions and *NF1* splicing mutations were identified in 9/41 primary OSC. Additionally, tumours and cell lines with *NF1* lesions were found to lack *KRAS* and *BRAF* mutations, whilst exhibiting Ras pathway activation [113].

The Cancer Genome Atlas project analysed the expression of mRNA and microRNA, promoter methylation and DNA copy number in 489 HGOSC and performed genomic DNA analysis in 316 tumours. Loss of *NF1* function was identified in 12% (37/316) of samples, and of these, 24 had deletions, one had a duplication and the remaining (12) samples harboured other somatic mutations. The Australian Ovarian Cancer Study (AOCS) specifically examined CNAs and reported regions of copy number loss at the *NF1* locus in 34% (137/398) of ovarian cancer samples, comprising 157 serous adenocarcinomas from the TCGA cohort and a further 241 samples, of both endometrioid and serous subtypes [115].

HGOSC shows a simple mutational profile, with *TP53* nearly always mutated, but with other genes, including *NF1*, mutated at a low frequency [116]. Approximately 50% of all HGSOCs exhibit homologous recombination

(HR) deficiency, with such tumours being highly sensitive to PARP inhibitors [117]. However, *NF1* mutations identified in advanced HGOSC are associated with resistance to treatment because of the acquisition of different new mutations within the gene [116–118].

Paragangliomas and phaeochromocytomas

Phaeochromocytomas are rare tumours (annual incidence of 1–6 million per year) that develop from neural crest-derived chromaffin cells and produce excess catecholamine, resulting in hypertension and flushing. Despite being rare in the general population, the frequency of occurrence amongst NF1 patients is much higher, with 0.1–6% developing a phaeochromocytoma [119, 120].

NF1 is one of a number of known paraganglioma and phaeochromocytoma susceptibility genes, constitutional mutations in which are responsible for inherited tumour syndromes. Somatic *NF1* mutations occurred in 35/161 (21.7%) of sporadic phaeochromocytomas, with the majority exhibiting LOH and low *NF1* mRNA expression [121–123], whilst somatic mutations in the susceptibility genes *NF1, MAX, RET, VHL, SDHA, SDHB, SDHC, SDHD, SDHAF2, KIF1Bβ* and *TMEM127* are present in 11–19% of sporadic cases [124–126]. It has also been demonstrated that the majority (83%, 35/42) of sporadic phaeochromocytomas harbour a CNA in at least one of these susceptibility genes, thereby altering respective protein expression levels [123]. This is in addition to the 26% (11/42) of sporadic paragangliomas and phaeochromocytomas that have lost one *NF1* allele, associated with a reduction in *NF1* mRNA level. Furthermore, 10 of 11 tumours were also observed to harbour a somatic protein-truncating *NF1* mutation in the second allele [121]. This study also identified a correlation between *NF1* mutations and a biochemical phenotype: paragangliomas and phaeochromocytomas harbouring a somatic *NF1* mutation were found to display higher plasma levels of normetanephrine ($P = 0.005$) and metanephrine ($P = 0.0025$), markers for catecholamine-secreting tumours [121]. This could be of significance as plasma catecholamine levels are used in the diagnosis of phaeochromocytoma and paraganglioma; however, these findings were reported in only a small sample group and the biochemical data was non-centralized and incomplete, limiting their overall significance [123].

A large-scale analysis of a cohort of 202 paragangliomas and phaeochromocytomas, collected by the *Cortico et Médullosurrénale: les Tumeurs Endocrines* (COMETE) network, examined CNAs, somatic and constitutional mutations in known susceptibility genes [124]. Almost a quarter (25/119) of the sporadic phaeochromocytomas/paragangliomas carried an inactivating *NF1* mutation, of which 21/25 were associated with the loss of the wild-type allele. Of all the somatic mutations identified in the study, 56% were located in *NF1*, showing that *NF1* is frequently mutated in phaeochromocytomas/paragangliomas [124].

Neuroblastoma

Neuroblastoma is a neuroendocrine tumour that originates from neural crest cells of the sympathetic nervous system, with most tumours developing in the abdomen. Neuroblastoma is the second most common solid tumour in childhood and accounts for 8% of all childhood cancers. The treatment for neuroblastoma includes surgery, chemotherapy, radiation and bone marrow transplantation. Familial neuroblastoma cases comprise only a small fraction (~1–2%) of all neuroblastoma cases, and their genetic aetiology is relatively well understood [127, 128]. In contrast, far less is known of the genetic aetiology of sporadic neuroblastomas, despite their accounting for the majority of cases.

It was a quarter of a century ago when *NF1* was first reported to play a role in the development of neuroblastoma. In this study, 4/10 neuroblastoma cell lines were observed to express either a reduced level or a complete absence of neurofibromin, with *NF1* mutations being identified in two of these cell lines [129]. Furthermore, it was demonstrated that the introduction of a normal human chromosome 17 into a neuroblastoma cell line suppressed its tumorigenicity. Several *NF1*-deficient neuroblastoma cell lines exhibited only moderately elevated *Ras*–GTP levels, in contrast to *NF1* tumour cells, indicating that neurofibromin can contribute differently to the negative regulation of RAS in different cell types [130, 131].

Somatic *NF1* mutations in neuroblastomas have been correlated with reduced expression of neurofibromin and poor patient prognosis, whilst higher levels of expression are associated with longer progression-free survival [130, 131]. Hölzel and colleagues also reported a loss of neurofibromin expression in 8/25 neuroblastoma cell lines and that a further SNP analysis of 20 neuroblastoma cell lines detected 50% (10/20) with abnormal *NF1* alleles [130]. Genomic aberrations in *NF1* were also found in primary neuroblastomas but at a lower frequency of 6% (5/83).

A large-scale RNAi screen revealed an association of *NF1* loss in neuroblastoma cell lines with resistance to retinoic acid (RA) treatment which is used as targeted therapy in the treatment of neuroblastomas. Loss of *NF1* activates RAS-MEK signalling, which in turn represses *ZNF423*, a critical transcriptional coactivator of the retinoic acid receptors; neuroblastomas with low levels of both *NF1* and *ZNF423* have an extremely poor outcome. However, inhibition of MEK signalling downstream of *NF1* restores responsiveness to RA, suggesting a potential therapeutic strategy to overcome RA resistance in *NF1*-deficient neuroblastomas [130].

Glioblastoma

Glioblastomas are tumours that arise from astrocytes that comprise the supportive tissue of the brain. These tumours are usually aggressive as the cells divide rapidly and are also supported by a large network of blood vessels. The most aggressive subtype is glioblastoma multiforme (GBM) which is the most frequent form of brain cancer in adults, renowned for its lethality and poor prognosis and is thus an important target of study [132, 133].

Glioblastoma-associated *NF1* somatic mutations are well described [132, 134, 135], with recurrent driver mutations being identified in *NF1* and a number of other candidate genes (*IDH1, TP53, CDK4, EGFR, PI3KR1, PIK3CA, PTEN, RB1* and *CDNK2A*) in GBM [132]. *NF1* mutations were identified in at least 15% (16/105) of all GBM by Parsons and colleagues, although chromosomal translocations or epigenetic changes were not tested in this cohort [132].

A TCGA analysis assessed levels of gene expression, CNAs and DNA methylation in a cohort of 206 glioblastoma tumour samples, with recurrent mutations in *NF1, AKT3, PRK3R1* and *PARK2* being identified, and with 14% (13/91) of samples found to contain at least one somatic *NF1* mutation. Verhaak and colleagues subsequently performed large-scale genomic analysis of these TCGA data, dividing glioblastoma cases into four subtypes: proneural, neural, classical and mesenchymal [136]. They found that GBM with *NF1* and *PTEN* alterations had a distinct mesenchymal-like expression profile, with 53% of mesenchymal cases having an *NF1* mutation. The mutual exclusivity of *NF1* and *BRAF* mutations in GBM has also been reported [134].

In animal models, inactivation of *TP53* and *PTEN* may cooperate with *NF1* loss in the development of glioblastoma [137]. Haploinsufficiency of *NF1* is also reported to increase astrocyte proliferation and enhancement of angiogenesis in $Nf1^{+/-}$ heterozygous mouse models [138, 139].

Colorectal cancer

Colorectal cancer (CRC) is one of the leading causes of cancer-related deaths in the western world, with at least 50% of CRCs exhibiting dysregulation of the RAS/MAPK pathway. Reports of the type of *NF1* mutations in CRC vary widely, with *NF1* LOH first reported in 14–57%, and reported gains in part of, or even a complete duplication of, the *NF1* gene in 17% of CRC [140–142]. The 2012 TCGA genome-scale analysis of 212 CRC found that 24 genes were predominantly mutated, including *NF1* in approximately 5.6% (11/212) of cases [143]. Subsequent studies have confirmed this, with *NF1* mutations being identified in 5.6% (4/72) and 5.8% of cases (39/619), respectively [144, 145].

Several critical genes and pathways, such as WNT, RAS/MAPK, PI3K, TGF-β, P53 and DNA mismatch repair, are recognized in the initiation and progression of CRC [146, 147]. Although genetic alterations in the PI3K and RAS/MAPK pathways are common in CRC and *NF1* alterations have been detected in 5–6% of cases, it remains unclear as to whether *NF1* mutations in CRC are related to chemotherapeutic effect.

Urinary tract transitional cell carcinoma

The best documented molecular factors involved in urothelial transitional cell carcinoma (TCC) are the *RAS* proto-oncogene activation and *TP53* mutations. Alterations in *NF1* gene expression in TCC were first reported in 1999 [148], where decreased *NF1* gene expression was observed in 83% (23/29) of TCC specimens (as estimated by immunohistochemistry), whilst *NF1* mRNA levels were markedly lower in TCC tissue as compared with those in adjacent non-neoplastic urothelium. Neurofibromin levels were also decreased in high-grade TCC, suggesting that alterations of *NF1* gene expression might be involved in urinary TCC carcinogenesis. Whole genomic analysis performed on 35 stage IV urothelial cancers that had relapsed and progressed after primary surgery and conventional chemotherapy revealed *NF1* mutations in two cases (6%) [149]. Integrated analysis of 131 urothelial carcinomas showed recurrent mutations in 32 genes, with 14% of tumours having *NF1* mutations.

Other malignant tumours

There are a number of other malignant tumour types that have been found to harbour *NF1* alterations including neuroendocrine prostate cancer (24%), myxofibrosarcomas (10.5%) and pleomorphic liposarcomas (8%), pancreatic cancer (11%), gastric adenocarcinoma (10%) and rhabdomyosarcoma (7%) [44, 45]. Somatic *NF1* mutations have also been detected in 41–72% of sporadic MPNSTs, showing that *NF1* inactivation plays a major role in the development of this tumour type [96].

General discussion

Neurofibromatosis type 1, caused by constitutional inactivating mutations in the tumour suppressor gene *NF1*, is a neurodegenerative disorder predisposing individuals to both benign and malignant tumours [150–152]. Additionally, somatic mutations of *NF1* are also frequent in desmoplastic, cutaneous and mucosal melanoma, high-grade serous ovarian cancer, breast cancer, phaeochromocytomas and paragangliomas, glioblastoma multiforme, myeloid malignancies, neuroblastoma, and colorectal and urinary bladder transitional cell carcinoma (Table 1). Aberrations in neurofibromin result in the dysregulation of the RAS/MAPK pathway leading to unregulated cell growth and proliferation. The related mTOR pathway and other downstream activators and effectors of RAS including PI3K are also involved in cancer [17, 153].

Mutations (chromosomal aberrations, nucleotide substitutions and epigenetic aberrations) in a subset of candidate genes are likely to confer a growth advantage resulting in the development of cancer. Cancer encompasses more than 100 different diseases, the study of which provides insight into both the commonalities and differences between and amongst various types and subtypes of cancer [147]. In order to understand this complex disease and to develop novel targeted therapeutics, it is essential to characterize the somatic mutational spectra in each cancer genome in order to facilitate our understanding of the biological processes underlying the cancer as well as the pathways of evolutionary progression. The availability of the human genome reference sequence enabled the rapid resequencing of cancer genomes, leading to the discovery of many additional cancer genes, revealing for the first time the molecular heterogeneity of cancer genomes and identifying therapeutic targets. To improve the diagnosis and treatment of cancer patients, several large-scale cancer genomics projects, e.g. the TCGA, ICGC, cBioPortal and COSMIC, have been undertaken in recent years [41–44]. These pan-cancer projects have generated high-throughput data which provide valuable opportunities to understand the biology, initiation and progression of human cancers. One caveat, however, is distinguishing artefactual DNA damage from the bona fide mutations that actually occurred in the tumour, given that it has been reported that mutagenic damage accounts for the majority of the erroneous identification of variants with low to moderate (1 to 5%) frequency in whole (cancer) genome sequencing studies [154].

Generally, a large number of mutations occur in cancer genomes, such as somatic mutations, CNAs, methylation aberrations and histone modifications. It is critical to distinguish driver mutations and driver genes (which contribute to the progression of cancer from normal to malignant states) from passenger mutations and passenger genes (which accumulate in cells but do not contribute to cancer development). There is a subtle difference between a driver gene and a driver gene mutation. A driver gene harbours driver gene mutations but may also harbour passenger gene mutations. A driver mutation typically confers upon a tumour only a very small growth advantage, which may be as low as a 0.4% increase in the difference between cell birth and death rates [155]. More recently, Bozic and colleagues have shown that the first, and hence most abundant, passenger mutations are influenced both by the mutation rate and by the death-birth ratio of the cancer cells [156]. It should be appreciated that whilst passenger mutations do not, by definition, exert a strong selective growth advantage, they are not entirely neutral. Indeed, many are deleterious in terms of their effect on cellular proliferation and cancer progression [157, 158]. It should also be appreciated that whilst the damaging effect of a non-synonymous passenger mutation is on average 100 times smaller than the effect of a driver mutation, passengers are 100 times more numerous than drivers [158]. The paucity of drivers in a sea of passenger mutations represents a challenge to identifying the former. This task is made all the more daunting by the possibility that drivers and passengers are not discrete entities but rather lie along a continuum which includes latent driver mutations which 'behave as passengers but coupled with other emerging mutations, drive cancer development and drug resistance' [159].

In 2004, Futreal and colleagues published a 'Census of human cancer genes' which aimed to list all genes that are causally implicated in tumorigenesis. This census has been kept up to date and currently includes 602 entries [43, 160]. This implies that more than 2% of all human genes are implicated in cancer. Of these, approximately 90% have somatic mutations in cancer; 20% have germline mutations that predispose to cancer; and 10% harbour both somatic and germline mutations. A second resource, the Network of Cancer Genes (NCG) contains a total of 1053 'cancer genes' whose possible involvement in cancer has been inferred by statistical means [161]. The number of genes recognized as being cancer-associated is likely to increase as new techniques are devised to identify the function of the associated proteins [162, 163].

Cooperativity and exclusivity of *NF1* somatic mutations

Mitogen-activated protein kinases (MAPK) and phosphoinositide-3 kinase (PI3K) pathways are key cellular growth regulators. In a normal cell, these control cell growth and survival but are often disrupted in a malignant cell with a deregulated MAPK or PI3K pathway. It is now well recognized that the focus should be upon cellular pathways rather than on individual genes to achieve a full understanding of cancer biology. Therefore, defining driver pathways is an important step to understanding the molecular mechanisms underlying cancer. Previous studies have focussed mainly on identifying the alterations in cancer genomes at the individual gene or single pathway level. However, a great deal of evidence indicates that multiple pathways often function cooperatively in carcinogenesis and other key biological processes. A common and restricted number of driver genes and pathways are probably responsible for most common forms of cancer [40, 147].

In general, mutations of the genes in one pathway usually exhibit mutual exclusivity, because a single mutation is usually enough to disturb one pathway and any further hits in other components of that pathway confer no added selectable advantage. Thus, sporadic tumours with *NF1* mutations are mutually exclusive for mutations in

MAPK kinase 1 (*MAP2K1*) or *NRAS*. Strongly activating 'canonical' mutations in oncogenes (for example G12D or G12V mutations in KRAS) can drive cancer formation on their own and are known to be epistatic in relation to other canonical mutations within the same pathway [164]. However, whether there are, for example, 'non-canonical' mutations that weakly activate oncogenes or only partially inactivate tumour suppressor activity and yet can drive cancer formation is less clear. Examination of genomic data from the Cancer Cell Line Encyclopedia (CCLE) and TCGA has indicated that whilst canonical *KRAS* mutations do not occur with increased frequency in the context of *NF1* mutations, non-canonical *KRAS* mutations certainly do, suggesting that such pairs of mutations might act together to confer a selective advantage in human tumours [164]. Activation of RAS guanine nucleotide exchange factors (RAS-GEFs) was predicted to have similar effects to neurofibromin loss and that non-canonical *KRAS* mutations co-occur with RAS-GEF mutations in TCGA and CCLE data [164]. Furthermore, increased frequencies of mutations in both *NF1* and other RAS pathway activators or effectors have been found which suggests that this principle could apply more broadly to other genes in the RAS network and possibly to other oncogenic signalling pathways [58]. Subsequently, *NF1* loss has been described as a key mediator of acquired and intrinsic *BRAF* inhibitor resistance following a high-throughput short hairpin RNA screening approach [53]. Furthermore, on the basis of analyses of somatic co-mutation patterns in the TCGA data sets (cBio Portal for Cancer Genomics), 9.6% of melanomas with *NF1* mutations also have mutations in *BRAF*, *NRAS* or *RAF1* [47]. But, whilst mutant *NF1* is known to cooperate with RASopathy genes (*RASA2*, *PTPN11*, *SOS1*, *RAF1* and *SPRED1*) in melanoma and although *NF1* is found to be frequently mutated (25–30%) in melanomas harbouring wild-type *BRAF* and *NRAS*, it is curious that melanoma is not a tumour type associated with NF1 [8, 49–51].

The capacity of *NF1* mutations to act both cooperatively and exclusively without *BRAF* and *NRAS* mutations in melanoma may be mediated through pathways other than the MAPK pathway. Maertens and colleagues have identified increased activation of the PI3K/AKT/mTOR pathway in *BRAF*/*NF1* double mutants, and a combinatorial MEK marker and mTOR inhibitor treatment has proven effective in many MEK inhibitor-resistant neoplasms [58]. In a glioblastoma animal model, *NF1* cooperates with both *TP53* and *PTEN*, but no co-occurrence of *NF1* and *BRAF* mutations is seen [137]. Moreover, whilst simultaneous inactivation of *Nf1* and expression of K-Ras^{G12D} in mouse haematopoietic cells results in AML that was fatal in primary mice within 4 weeks, in ovarian serous carcinomas, cooperation between mutant *TP53* and *NF1* results in a poor prognosis [92, 117]. In addition, an association between inactivated *NF1* and *ZNF423* levels in neuroblastomas has been identified as a putative prognostic marker [130].

It should be appreciated that the same gene can function in completely opposite ways in different cell types. In melanomas harbouring *BRAF* V600E mutations, a BRAF inhibitor induces remission of the tumour; however, the same drug is ineffective in colorectal cancer cells harbouring identical mutations. This has been attributed to the expression of EGFR which occurs in some colorectal cancers, but not in melanomas [165].

Despite all the cancer genome information available regarding *NF1*, it remains unclear why NF1 patients are predisposed only to certain types of tumours. Why, for example, are NF1 patients not predisposed to lung tumours given that at least 10% of all sporadic lung cancers have *NF1* mutations [8, 65, 72, 166]?

NF1 and drug resistance

The RAS/MAPK pathway, with an important role in cancer biology, is a prime target for anti-cancer agents; however, the presence of an *NF1* mutation, resulting in reduced expression of neurofibromin, confers resistance to several therapeutic drugs. Furthermore, *NF1*-associated drug resistance to RAF and EGFR inhibitors, tamoxifen and retinoic acid, has been observed in melanoma, lung cancers, breast cancers and neuroblastoma, respectively, and melanoma cells with *BRAF*/*NF1* mutations develop resistance to BRAF inhibitors [58, 111, 130, 167]. It is not clear whether the specific nature of the mutations could have exerted an influence on the sensitivity of the drug, as complete inactivation of *NF1* has been noted to confer sensitivity to rapamycin in AML [85].

Mutational spectrum

Large constitutional *NF1* deletions, encompassing the *NF1* gene and many adjacent genes, occur in 5–10% of NF1 cases and are often associated with a more severe phenotype including learning disabilities and increased susceptibility to MPNSTs [168, 169]. Intriguingly, such mutations resulting in heterozygous or homozygous loss of *NF1* expression are found to occur more often as sporadic events in AML and ovarian carcinoma, based on cBioPortal data [45]. An *NF1* microdeletion in combination with an abnormal karyotype is an indicator of poor prognosis in AML; 7.6% of ovarian serous cystadenocarcinomas, 2.8% of lung squamous cell carcinomas, 3.3% of glioblastomas and 1.9% of phaeochromocytomas/paragangliomas harboured deletions [45, 82, 84].

NF1 amplification, and presumably increased neurofibromin expression and hence activity, has been identified in many cancers, including breast (17%), pancreatic (21.5%), uterine endometrial (1.8%) and neuroendocrine prostate cancer (21.5%) [45].

The pathological significance of sporadic *NF1* point mutations, especially putative missense mutations that have been identified in many sporadic tumours, is often unclear. Constitutional *NF1* missense mutations represent about 15% of all *NF1* mutations, but their frequency in sporadic tumours ranges widely from 15 to 71% [24, 25, 45, 72, 106, 143, 167, 170–172]. The characterization of such missense mutations has yielded new insights into the structure and function of neurofibromin. For example, through analysis of missense mutations, the arginine finger loop of the neurofibromin GRD has been found to be crucial for stabilizing the transition state of the GTPase reaction, and many missense mutations in the GRD have been found to exert a significant, pathological effect on Ras activity levels [36, 173, 174].

Conclusion

Somatic *NF1* mutations are present in tumours associated with NF1 and in a range of sporadic tumours, in different cell types and at various frequencies (Table 1). The frequency and temporal occurrence of somatic mutations and the range of histological types in which they occur therefore imply an important role for neurofibromin function in cancer development and progression. Whilst it is unclear whether the biallelic loss of *NF1* is common or if only heterozygous mutations of *NF1* contribute to tumour progression in sporadic tumours, mouse cells heterozygous for *Nf1* mutations show abnormal growth and invasion [138, 175].

Somatic *NF1* mutations may be critical drivers in multiple cancers as well as contributing to resistance to therapy. The mutational landscape of somatic *NF1* mutation should provide new insights into our understanding of the pathophysiology of cancer.

The introduction of a molecular genomics approach to cancer biology represents a major shift in our approach to the diagnosis and treatment of malignancy. The vast amount of genomic data generated over the last 10 years, which continues to be generated, is providing invaluable insights into the complexities of cancer genome structure, function and evolution. With recent advances in sequencing technology and high-throughput drug discovery, the increasing availability of more sophisticated animal models and the application of the state-of-the-art tumour imaging techniques and the diagnosis and treatment of cancer can only improve. The identification of somatic *NF1* mutations in such a wide spectrum of tumours, including types not associated with NF1, indicates that neurofibromin is likely to play a key role in cancer, far beyond that evident in the tumour predisposition syndrome NF1.

Abbreviations

ADC: Adenocarcinoma; AML: Acute myeloid leukaemia; AOCS: The Australian Ovarian Cancer Study; CCLE: Cancer Cell Line Encyclopedia; CMML: Chronic myelomonocytic leukaemia; CNS: Central nervous system; COSMIC: Catalogue of Somatic Mutations in Cancer; HGOSC: High-grade serous ovarian carcinoma; HR: Homologous recombination; ICGC: International Cancer Genome Consortium; JMML: Juvenile myelomonocytic leukaemia; MAPK: Mitogen-activated protein kinases; MPNST: Malignant peripheral nerve sheath tumour; NF1: Neurofibromatosis type 1; NSCLC: Non-small cell lung cancer; OSC: Ovarian serous carcinoma; PI3K: Phosphoinositide-3 kinase; RAS-GEFs: RAS guanine nucleotide exchange factors; SCLC: Small cell lung cancer; SqCC: Squamous cell lung cancer; T-ALL: T cell acute lymphoblastic Leukaemia; TCC: Urothelial transitional cell carcinoma; TCGA: The Cancer Genome Atlas

Acknowledgements
Not applicable.

Funding
We thank Sheila and Clive Owen for the financial support.

Authors' contributions
MU initiated the study, supported by CP, HT, IMF and DNC. All authors contributed to the writing and review of the manuscript. All authors read and approved the final manuscript.

Competing interests
The authors declare that they have no competing interests.

Consent for publication
Not applicable.

References

1. Bennett E, Thomas N, Upadhyaya M. Neurofibromatosis type 1: its association with the Ras/MAPK pathway syndromes. J Pediatr Neurol. 2009; 7(2):105–15.
2. Cooper DN, Upadhyaya M. The germline mutational spectrum in neurofibromatosis type 1 and genotype-phenotype correlations, Chapter 10. In: Upadhyaya M, Cooper DN, editors. Neurofibromatosis Type 1, vol. Chapter 10. Berlin: Springer Verlag; 2012. p. 115–34.
3. Huson SM, Compston DA, Clark P, Harper PS. A genetic study of von Recklinghausen neurofibromatosis in south east Wales. I. Prevalence, fitness, mutation rate, and effect of parental transmission on severity. J Med Genet. 1989;26(11):704–11.
4. Lammert M, Friedman JM, Kluwe L, Mautner VF. Prevalence of neurofibromatosis 1 in German children at elementary school enrollment. Arch Dermatol. 2005;141(1):71–4.
5. Upadhyaya M, Huson SM, Davies M, Thomas N, Chuzhanova N, Giovannini S, Evans DG, Howard E, Kerr B, Griffiths S, et al. An absence of cutaneous neurofibromas associated with a 3-bp inframe deletion in exon 17 of the NF1 gene (c.2970-2972 delAAT): evidence of a clinically significant NF1 genotype-phenotype correlation. Am J Hum Genet. 2007;80(1):140–51.
6. Upadhyaya M. Genetic basis of tumorigenesis in NF1 malignant peripheral nerve sheath tumors. Front Biosci (Landmark Ed). 2011;16:937–51.
7. Upadhyaya M, Kluwe L, Spurlock G, Monem B, Majounie E, Mantripragada K, Ruggieri M, Chuzhanova N, Evans DG, Ferner R, Thomas N, Guha A, Mautner V. Germline and somatic NF1 gene mutation spectrum in NF1-associated malignant peripheral nerve sheath tumors (MPNSTs). Hum Mutat. 2008;29(1):74–82.

8. Walker L, Thompson D, Easton D, Ponder B, Ponder M, Frayling I, Baralle D. A prospective study of neurofibromatosis type 1 cancer incidence in the UK. Br J Cancer. 2006;95(2):233–8.
9. Brems H, Beert E, de Ravel T, Legius E. Mechanisms in the pathogenesis of malignant tumours in neurofibromatosis type 1. Lancet Oncol. 2009;10(5):508–15.
10. Knudson Jr AG. Mutation and cancer: statistical study of retinoblastoma. Proc Natl Acad Sci U S A. 1971;68(4):820–3.
11. Viskochil D, Buchberg AM, Xu G, Cawthon RM, Stevens J, Wolff RK, Culver M, Carey JC, Copeland NG, Jenkins NA, et al. Deletions and a translocation interrupt a cloned gene at the neurofibromatosis type 1 locus. Cell. 1990;62(1):187–92.
12. Cichowski K, Jacks T. NF1 tumor suppressor gene function: narrowing the GAP. Cell. 2001;104(4):593–604.
13. McClatchey AI. Neurofibromatosis. Annu Rev Pathol. 2007;2:191–216.
14. Welti S, D'Angelo I, Scheffzek K. Structure and function of neurofibromin. In: Neurofibromatoses. Basel: Karger; 2008:113–28.
15. Scheffzek K, Welti S. Pleckstrin homology (PH) like domains—versatile modules in protein-protein interaction platforms. FEBS Lett. 2012;586(17):2662–73.
16. Scheffzek K, Welti S. Neurofibromin: protein domains and functional characteristics. In: Upadhyaya M, Cooper DN, editors. Neurofibromatosis Type 1. Berlin Heidelberg: Springer; 2012. p. 305–26.
17. Johannessen CM, Reczek EE, James MF, Brems H, Legius E, Cichowski K. The NF1 tumor suppressor critically regulates TSC2 and mTOR. Proc Natl Acad Sci U S A. 2005;102(24):8573–8.
18. Shilyansky C, Lee YS, Silva AJ. Molecular and cellular mechanisms of learning disabilities: a focus on NF1. Annu Rev Neurosci. 2010;33:221–43.
19. Hollstein PE, Cichowski K. Identifying the ubiquitin ligase complex that regulates the NF1 tumor suppressor and Ras. Cancer Discov. 2013;3(8):880–93.
20. Peltonen S, Kallionpaa RA, Peltonen J. Neurofibromatosis type 1 (NF1) gene: beyond cafe au lait spots and dermal neurofibromas. Exp Dermatol. 2016. doi:10.1111/exd.13212.
21. Gutmann DH, Parada LF, Silva AJ, Ratner N. Neurofibromatosis type 1: modeling CNS dysfunction. J Neurosci. 2012;32(41):14087–93.
22. Neurofibromin (NF1). https://grenada.lumc.nl/LOVD2/mendelian_genes/home.php?select_db=NF1. Accessed Mar 2017.
23. Griffiths S, Thompson P, Frayling I, Upadhyaya M. Molecular diagnosis of neurofibromatosis type 1: 2 years experience. Fam Cancer. 2007;6(1):21–34.
24. Messiaen LM, Callens T, Mortier G, Beysen D, Vandenbroucke I, Van Roy N, Speleman F, Paepe AD. Exhaustive mutation analysis of the NF1 gene allows identification of 95% of mutations and reveals a high frequency of unusual splicing defects. Hum Mutat. 2000;15(6):541–55.
25. Messiaen LM, Wimmer K. NF1 Mutational spectrum. In: neurofibromatoses. Kaufmann D, editor. Basel: Karger; 2008:63–77.
26. van Minkelen R, van Bever Y, Kromosoeto JN, Withagen-Hermans CJ, Nieuwlaat A, Halley DJ, van den Ouweland AM. A clinical and genetic overview of 18 years neurofibromatosis type 1 molecular diagnostics in the Netherlands. Clin Genet. 2014;85(4):318–27.
27. Stenson PD, Mort M, Ball EV, Evans K, Hayden M, Heywood S, Hussain M, Phillips AD, Cooper DN. The Human Gene Mutation Database: towards a comprehensive repository of inherited mutation data for medical research, genetic diagnosis and next-generation sequencing studies. Hum Genet. 2017. doi:10.1007/s00439-017-1779-6 [Epub ahead of print].
28. Evans DG, Bowers N, Burkitt-Wright E, Miles E, Garg S, Scott-Kitching V, Penman-Splitt M, Dobbie A, Howard E, Ealing J, et al. Comprehensive RNA analysis of the NF1 gene in classically affected NF1 affected individuals meeting NIH criteria has high sensitivity and mutation negative testing is reassuring in isolated cases with pigmentary features only. EBioMedicine. 2016;7:212–20.
29. Mautner VF, Kluwe L, Friedrich RE, Roehl AC, Bammert S, Hogel J, Spori H, Cooper DN, Kehrer-Sawatzki H. Clinical characterisation of 29 neurofibromatosis type-1 patients with molecularly ascertained 1.4 Mb type-1 NF1 deletions. J Med Genet. 2010;47(9):623–30.
30. Pros E, Gomez C, Martin T, Fabregas P, Serra E, Lazaro C. Nature and mRNA effect of 282 different NF1 point mutations: focus on splicing alterations. Hum Mutat. 2008;29(9):E173–193.
31. Bottillo I, Torrente I, Lanari V, Pinna V, Giustini S, Divona L, De Luca A, Dallapiccola B. Germline mosaicism in neurofibromatosis type 1 due to a paternally derived multi-exon deletion. Am J Med Genet A. 2010;152A(6):1467–73.
32. Colman SD, Rasmussen SA, Ho VT, Abernathy CR, Wallace MR. Somatic mosaicism in a patient with neurofibromatosis type 1. Am J Hum Genet. 1996;58(3):484–90.
33. Lazaro C, Ravella A, Gaona A, Volpini V, Estivill X. Neurofibromatosis type 1 due to germ-line mosaicism in a clinically normal father. N Engl J Med. 1994;331(21):1403–7.
34. Messiaen L, Vogt J, Bengesser K, Fu C, Mikhail F, Serra E, Garcia-Linares C, Cooper DN, Lazaro C, Kehrer-Sawatzki H. Mosaic type-1 NF1 microdeletions as a cause of both generalized and segmental neurofibromatosis type-1 (NF1). Hum Mutat. 2011;32(2):213–9.
35. Wimmer K, Yao S, Claes K, Kehrer-Sawatzki H, Tinschert S, De Raedt T, Legius E, Callens T, Beiglbock H, Maertens O, et al. Spectrum of single- and multiexon NF1 copy number changes in a cohort of 1,100 unselected NF1 patients. Genes Chromosomes Cancer. 2006;45(3):265–76.
36. Thomas L, Richards M, Mort M, Dunlop E, Cooper DN, Upadhyaya M. Assessment of the potential pathogenicity of missense mutations identified in the GTPase-activating protein (GAP)-related domain of the neurofibromatosis type-1 (NF1) gene. Hum Mutat. 2012;33(12):1687–96.
37. Kehrer-Sawatzki H, Vogt J, Mussotter T, Kluwe L, Cooper DN, Mautner VF. Dissecting the clinical phenotype associated with mosaic type-2 NF1 microdeletions. Neurogenetics. 2012;13(3):229–36.
38. Upadhyaya M. Neurofibromatosis type 1: diagnosis and recent advances. Expert Opin Med Diagn. 2010;4(4):307–22.
39. Tidyman WE, Rauen KA. Pathogenetics of the RASopathies. Hum Mol Genet. 2016;25(R2):R123–32.
40. Stratton MR, Campbell PJ, Futreal PA. The cancer genome. Nature. 2009; 458(7239):719–24.
41. The Cancer Genome Atlas (TCGA). http://cancergenome.nih.gov/. Accessed Sept 2016.
42. International Cancer Genome Consortium (ICGC). http://icgc.org/. Accessed Sept 2016.
43. Catalogue of Somatic Mutations in Cancer (COSMIC). http://cancer.sanger.ac.uk/cosmic. Accessed Sept 2016.
44. cBioPortal for Cancer Genomics. http://www.cbioportal.org/. Accessed Sept 2016.
45. Cerami E, Gao J, Dogrusoz U, Gross BE, Sumer SO, Aksoy BA, Jacobsen A, Byrne CJ, Heuer ML, Larsson E, et al. The cBio cancer genomics portal: an open platform for exploring multidimensional cancer genomics data. Cancer Discov. 2012;2(5):401–4.
46. Gao J, Aksoy BA, Dogrusoz U, Dresdner G, Gross B, Sumer SO, Sun Y, Jacobsen A, Sinha R, Larsson E, et al. Integrative analysis of complex cancer genomics and clinical profiles using the cBioPortal. Sci Signal. 2013;6(269):l1.
47. Ratner N, Miller SJ. A RASopathy gene commonly mutated in cancer: the neurofibromatosis type 1 tumour suppressor. Nat Rev Cancer. 2015;15(5): 290–301.
48. Andersen LB, Fountain JW, Gutmann DH, Tarle SA, Glover TW, Dracopoli NC, Housman DE, Collins FS. Mutations in the neurofibromatosis 1 gene in sporadic malignant melanoma cell lines. Nat Genet. 1993;3(2):118–21.
49. Krauthammer M, Kong Y, Bacchiocchi A, Evans P, Pornputtapong N, Wu C, McCusker JP, Ma S, Cheng E, Straub R, et al. Exome sequencing identifies recurrent mutations in NF1 and RASopathy genes in sun-exposed melanomas. Nat Genet. 2015;47(9):996–1002.
50. Krauthammer M, Kong Y, Ha BH, Evans P, Bacchiocchi A, McCusker JP, Cheng E, Davis MJ, Goh G, Choi M, et al. Exome sequencing identifies recurrent somatic RAC1 mutations in melanoma. Nat Genet. 2012;44(9):1006–14.
51. Hodis E, Watson IR, Kryukov GV, Arold ST, Imielinski M, Theurillat JP, Nickerson E, Auclair D, Li L, Place C, et al. A landscape of driver mutations in melanoma. Cell. 2012;150(2):251–63.
52. Nissan MH, Pratilas CA, Jones AM, Ramirez R, Won H, Liu C, Tiwari S, Kong L, Hanrahan AJ, Yao Z, et al. Loss of NF1 in cutaneous melanoma is associated with RAS activation and MEK dependence. Cancer Res. 2014;74(8):2340–50.
53. Whittaker SR, Theurillat JP, Van Allen E, Wagle N, Hsiao J, Cowley GS, Schadendorf D, Root DE, Garraway LA. A genome-scale RNA interference screen implicates NF1 loss in resistance to RAF inhibition. Cancer Discov. 2013;3(3):350–62.
54. Akbani R, Ng PK, Werner HM, Shahmoradgoli M, Zhang F, Ju Z, Liu W, Yang JY, Yoshihara K, Li J, et al. Corrigendum: a pan-cancer proteomic perspective on The Cancer Genome Atlas. Nat Commun. 2015;6:4852.
55. Akbani R, Ng PK, Werner HM, Shahmoradgoli M, Zhang F, Ju Z, Liu W, Yang JY, Yoshihara K, Li J, et al. A pan-cancer proteomic perspective on The Cancer Genome Atlas. Nat Commun. 2014;5:3887.
56. Hill VK, Gartner JJ, Samuels Y, Goldstein AM. The genetics of melanoma: recent advances. Annu Rev Genomics Hum Genet. 2013;14:257–79.
57. Garnett MJ, Marais R. Guilty as charged: B-RAF is a human oncogene. Cancer Cell. 2004;6(4):313–9.
58. Maertens O, Johnson B, Hollstein P, Frederick DT, Cooper ZA, Messiaen L, Bronson RT, McMahon M, Granter S, Flaherty K, et al. Elucidating distinct roles for NF1 in melanomagenesis. Cancer Discov. 2013;3(3):338–49.

59. Mar VJ, Wong SQ, Li J, Scolyer RA, McLean C, Papenfuss AT, Tothill RW, Kakavand H, Mann GJ, Thompson JF, et al. BRAF/NRAS wild-type melanomas have a high mutation load correlating with histologic and molecular signatures of UV damage. Clin Cancer Res. 2013;19(17):4589–98.
60. Wiesner T, Kiuru M, Scott SN, Arcila M, Halpern AC, Hollmann T, Berger MF, Busam KJ. NF1 mutations are common in desmoplastic melanoma. Am J Surg Pathol. 2015;39(10):1357–62.
61. Shain AH, Yeh I, Kovalyshyn I, Sriharan A, Talevich E, Gagnon A, Dummer R, North J, Pincus L, Ruben B, et al. The genetic evolution of melanoma from precursor lesions. N Engl J Med. 2015;373(20):1926–36.
62. Foster WJ, Fuller CE, Perry A, Harbour JW. Status of the NF1 tumor suppressor locus in uveal melanoma. Arch Ophthalmol. 2003;121(9):1311–5.
63. Cosgarea I, Ugurel S, Sucker A, Livingstone E, Zimmer L, Ziemer M, Utikal J, Mohr P, Pfeiffer C, Pfohler C, et al. Targeted next generation sequencing of mucosal melanomas identifies frequent NF1 and RAS mutations. Oncotarget. 2017.
64. Stewart B, Wild CP. World Cancer Report 2014. International Agency for Research on Cancer. Lyons: WHO Press; 2014.
65. Ding L, Getz G, Wheeler DA, Mardis ER, McLellan MD, Cibulskis K, Sougnez C, Greulich H, Muzny DM, Morgan MB, et al. Somatic mutations affect key pathways in lung adenocarcinoma. Nature. 2008;455(7216):1069–75.
66. Imielinski M, Berger AH, Hammerman PS, Hernandez B, Pugh TJ, Hodis E, Cho J, Suh J, Capelletti M, Sivachenko A, et al. Mapping the hallmarks of lung adenocarcinoma with massively parallel sequencing. Cell. 2012;150(6):1107–20.
67. Cancer Genome Atlas Research N. Comprehensive molecular profiling of lung adenocarcinoma. Nature. 2014;511(7511):543–50.
68. Redig AJ, Capelletti M, Dahlberg SE, Sholl LM, Mach S, Fontes C, Shi Y, Chalasani P, Janne PA. Clinical and molecular characteristics of NF1-mutant lung cancer. Clin Cancer Res. 2016;22(13):3148–56.
69. Jemal A, Bray F, Center MM, Ferlay J, Ward E, Forman D. Global cancer statistics. CA Cancer J Clin. 2011;61(2):69–90.
70. Lipson D, Capelletti M, Yelensky R, Otto G, Parker A, Jarosz M, Curran JA, Balasubramanian S, Bloom T, Brennan KW, et al. Identification of new ALK and RET gene fusions from colorectal and lung cancer biopsies. Nat Med. 2012;18(3):382–4.
71. de Bruin EC, Cowell C, Warne PH, Jiang M, Saunders RE, Melnick MA, Gettinger S, Walther Z, Wurtz A, Heynen GJ, et al. Reduced NF1 expression confers resistance to EGFR inhibition in lung cancer. Cancer Discov. 2014;4(5):606–19.
72. Cancer Genome Atlas Research N. Comprehensive genomic characterization of squamous cell lung cancers. Nature. 2012;489(7417):519–25.
73. Dhanasekaran SM, Balbin OA, Chen G, Nadal E, Kalyana-Sundaram S, Pan J, Veeneman B, Cao X, Malik R, Vats P, et al. Transcriptome meta-analysis of lung cancer reveals recurrent aberrations in NRG1 and Hippo pathway genes. Nat Commun. 2014;5:5893.
74. Campbell JD, Alexandrov A, Kim J, Wala J, Berger AH, Pedamallu CS, Shukla SA, Guo G, Brooks AN, Murray BA, et al. Distinct patterns of somatic genome alterations in lung adenocarcinomas and squamous cell carcinomas. Nat Genet. 2016;48(6):607–16.
75. Devarakonda S, Morgensztern D, Govindan R. Genomic alterations in lung adenocarcinoma. Lancet Oncol. 2015;16(7):e342–351.
76. Rudin CM, Durinck S, Stawiski EW, Poirier JT, Modrusan Z, Shames DS, Bergbower EA, Guan Y, Shin J, Guillory J, et al. Comprehensive genomic analysis identifies SOX2 as a frequently amplified gene in small-cell lung cancer. Nat Genet. 2012;44(10):1111–6.
77. Peifer M, Fernandez-Cuesta L, Sos ML, George J, Seidel D, Kasper LH, Plenker D, Leenders F, Sun R, Zander T, et al. Integrative genome analyses identify key somatic driver mutations of small-cell lung cancer. Nat Genet. 2012; 44(10):1104–10.
78. Ross JS, Wang K, Elkadi OR, Tarasen A, Foulke L, Sheehan CE, Otto GA, Palmer G, Yelensky R, Lipson D, et al. Next-generation sequencing reveals frequent consistent genomic alterations in small cell undifferentiated lung cancer. J Clin Pathol. 2014;67(9):772–6.
79. Balgobind BV, Van Vlierberghe P, van den Ouweland AM, Beverloo HB, Terlouw-Kromosoeto JN, van Wering ER, Reinhardt D, Horstmann M, Kaspers GJ, Pieters R, et al. Leukemia-associated NF1 inactivation in patients with pediatric T-ALL and AML lacking evidence for neurofibromatosis. Blood. 2008;111(8):4322–8.
80. Fioretos T, Strombeck B, Sandberg T, Johansson B, Billstrom R, Borg A, Nilsson PG, Van Den Berghe H, Hagemeijer A, Mitelman F, et al. Isochromosome 17q in blast crisis of chronic myeloid leukemia and in other hematologic malignancies is the result of clustered breakpoints in 17p11 and is not associated with coding TP53 mutations. Blood. 1999;94(1):225–32.
81. Braun BS, Shannon K. Targeting Ras in myeloid leukemias. Clin Cancer Res. 2008;14(8):2249–52.
82. Boudry-Labis E, Roche-Lestienne C, Nibourel O, Boissel N, Terre C, Perot C, Eclache V, Gachard N, Tigaud I, Plessis G, et al. Neurofibromatosis-1 gene deletions and mutations in de novo adult acute myeloid leukemia. Am J Hematol. 2013;88(4):306–11.
83. Garcia-Orti L, Cristobal I, Cirauqui C, Guruceaga E, Marcotegui N, Calasanz MJ, Castello-Cros R, Odero MD. Integration of SNP and mRNA arrays with microRNA profiling reveals that MiR-370 is upregulated and targets NF1 in acute myeloid leukemia. PLoS One. 2012;7(10):e47717.
84. Haferlach C, Grossmann V, Kohlmann A, Schindela S, Kern W, Schnittger S, Haferlach T. Deletion of the tumor-suppressor gene NF1 occurs in 5% of myeloid malignancies and is accompanied by a mutation in the remaining allele in half of the cases. Leukemia. 2012;26(4):834–9.
85. Parkin B, Ouillette P, Wang Y, Liu Y, Wright W, Roulston D, Purkayastha A, Dressel A, Karp J, Bockenstedt P, et al. NF1 inactivation in adult acute myelogenous leukemia. Clin Cancer Res. 2010;16(16):4135–47.
86. Misawa S, Horiike S, Kaneko H, Kashima K. Genetic aberrations in the development and subsequent progression of myelodysplastic syndrome. Leukemia. 1997;11 Suppl 3:533–5.
87. Kolquist KA, Schultz RA, Furrow A, Brown TC, Han JY, Campbell LJ, Wall M, Slovak ML, Shaffer LG, Ballif BC. Microarray-based comparative genomic hybridization of cancer targets reveals novel, recurrent genetic aberrations in the myelodysplastic syndromes. Cancer Genet. 2011;204(11):603–28.
88. Kalender Atak Z, De Keersmaecker K, Gianfelici V, Geerdens E, Vandepoel R, Pauwels D, Porcu M, Lahortiga I, Brys V, Dirks WG, et al. High accuracy mutation detection in leukemia on a selected panel of cancer genes. PLoS One. 2012;7(6):e38463.
89. Side L, Taylor B, Cayouette M, Conner E, Thompson P, Luce M, Shannon K. Homozygous inactivation of the NF1 gene in bone marrow cells from children with neurofibromatosis type 1 and malignant myeloid disorders. N Engl J Med. 1997;336(24):1713–20.
90. Caye A, Strullu M, Guidez F, Cassinat B, Gazal S, Fenneteau O, Lainey E, Nouri K, Nakhaei-Rad S, Dvorsky R, et al. Juvenile myelomonocytic leukemia displays mutations in components of the RAS pathway and the PRC2 network. Nat Genet. 2015;47(11):1334–40.
91. Margueron R, Reinberg D. The Polycomb complex PRC2 and its mark in life. Nature. 2011;469(7330):343–9.
92. Cutts BA, Sjogren AK, Andersson KM, Wahlstrom AM, Karlsson C, Swolin B, Bergo MO. Nf1 deficiency cooperates with oncogenic K-RAS to induce acute myeloid leukemia in mice. Blood. 2009;114(17):3629–32.
93. Abdel-Wahab O, Tefferi A, Levine RL. Role of TET2 and ASXL1 mutations in the pathogenesis of myeloproliferative neoplasms. Hematol Oncol Clin North Am. 2012;26(5):1053–64.
94. Abdel-Wahab O, Dey A. The ASXL-BAP1 axis: new factors in myelopoiesis, cancer and epigenetics. Leukemia. 2013;27(1):10–5.
95. De Raedt T, Beert E, Pasmant E, Luscan A, Brems H, Ortonne N, Helin K, Hornick JL, Mautner V, Kehrer-Sawatzki H, et al. PRC2 loss amplifies Ras-driven transcription and confers sensitivity to BRD4-based therapies. Nature. 2014;514(7521):247–51.
96. Lee W, Teckie S, Wiesner T, Ran L, Prieto Granada CN, Lin M, Zhu S, Cao Z, Liang Y, Sboner A, et al. PRC2 is recurrently inactivated through EED or SUZ12 loss in malignant peripheral nerve sheath tumors. Nat Genet. 2014; 46(11):1227–32.
97. Stieglitz E, Taylor-Weiner AN, Chang TY, Gelston LC, Wang YD, Mazor T, Esquivel E, Yu A, Seepo S, Olsen SR, et al. The genomic landscape of juvenile myelomonocytic leukemia. Nat Genet. 2015;47(11):1326–33.
98. Sharif S, Moran A, Huson SM, Iddenden R, Shenton A, Howard E, Evans DG. Women with neurofibromatosis 1 are at a moderately increased risk of developing breast cancer and should be considered for early screening. J Med Genet. 2007;44(8):481–4.
99. Evans DG, O'Hara C, Wilding A, Ingham SL, Howard E, Dawson J, Moran A, Scott-Kitching V, Holt F, Huson SM. Mortality in neurofibromatosis 1: in North West England: an assessment of actuarial survival in a region of the UK since 1989. Eur J Hum Genet. 2011;19(11):1187–91.
100. Madanikia SA, Bergner A, Ye X, Blakeley JO. Increased risk of breast cancer in women with NF1. Am J Med Genet A. 2012;158A(12):3056–60.
101. Sjoblom T, Jones S, Wood LD, Parsons DW, Lin J, Barber TD, Mandelker D, Leary RJ, Ptak J, Silliman N, et al. The consensus coding sequences of human breast and colorectal cancers. Science. 2006;314(5797):268–74.

102. Stephens PJ, Tarpey PS, Davies H, Van Loo P, Greenman C, Wedge DC, Nik-Zainal S, Martin S, Varela I, Bignell GR, et al. The landscape of cancer genes and mutational processes in breast cancer. Nature. 2012;486(7403):400–4.
103. Ogata H, Sato H, Takatsuka J, De Luca LM. Human breast cancer MDA-MB-231 cells fail to express the neurofibromin protein, lack its type I mRNA isoform and show accumulation of P-MAPK and activated Ras. Cancer Lett. 2001;172(2):159–64.
104. Shima N, Alcaraz A, Liachko I, Buske TR, Andrews CA, Munroe RJ, Hartford SA, Tye BK, Schimenti JC. A viable allele of Mcm4 causes chromosome instability and mammary adenocarcinomas in mice. Nat Genet. 2007;39(1):93–8.
105. Wallace MD, Pfefferle AD, Shen L, McNairn AJ, Cerami EG, Fallon BL, Rinaldi VD, Southard TL, Perou CM, Schimenti JC. Comparative oncogenomics implicates the neurofibromin 1 gene (NF1) as a breast cancer driver. Genetics. 2012;192(2):385–96.
106. Cancer Genome Atlas N. Comprehensive molecular portraits of human breast tumours. Nature. 2012;490(7418):61–70.
107. Meric-Bernstam F, Frampton GM, Ferrer-Lozano J, Yelensky R, Perez-Fidalgo JA, Wang Y, Palmer GA, Ross JS, Miller VA, Su X, et al. Concordance of genomic alterations between primary and recurrent breast cancer. Mol Cancer Ther. 2014;13(5):1382–9.
108. Pereira B, Chin SF, Rueda OM, Vollan HK, Provenzano E, Bardwell HA, Pugh M, Jones L, Russell R, Sammut SJ, et al. Erratum: the somatic mutation profiles of 2,433 breast cancers refine their genomic and transcriptomic landscapes. Nat Commun. 2016;7:11908.
109. Pereira B, Chin SF, Rueda OM, Vollan HK, Provenzano E, Bardwell HA, Pugh M, Jones L, Russell R, Sammut SJ, et al. The somatic mutation profiles of 2,433 breast cancers refines their genomic and transcriptomic landscapes. Nat Commun. 2016;7:11479.
110. Cui XY, Guo YJ, Yao HR. Analysis of microRNA in drug-resistant breast cancer cell line MCF-7/ADR. Nan Fang Yi Ke Da Xue Xue Bao. 2008;28(10):1813–5.
111. Mendes-Pereira AM, Sims D, Dexter T, Fenwick K, Assiotis I, Kozarewa I, Mitsopoulos C, Hakas J, Zvelebil M, Lord CJ, et al. Genome-wide functional screen identifies a compendium of genes affecting sensitivity to tamoxifen. Proc Natl Acad Sci U S A. 2012;109(8):2730–5.
112. Ring A, Dowsett M. Mechanisms of tamoxifen resistance. Endocr Relat Cancer. 2004;11(4):643–58.
113. Sangha N, Wu R, Kuick R, Powers S, Mu D, Fiander D, Yuen K, Katabuchi H, Tashiro H, Fearon ER, et al. Neurofibromin 1 (NF1) defects are common in human ovarian serous carcinomas and co-occur with TP53 mutations. Neoplasia. 2008;10(12):1362–72. following 1372.
114. Heintz AP, Odicino F, Maisonneuve P, Quinn MA, Benedet JL, Creasman WT, Ngan HY, Pecorelli S, Beller U. Carcinoma of the ovary. FIGO 26th Annual Report on the Results of Treatment in Gynecological Cancer. Int J Gynaecol Obstet. 2006;95 Suppl 1:S161–192.
115. Gorringe KL, George J, Anglesio MS, Ramakrishna M, Etemadmoghadam D, Cowin P, Sridhar A, Williams LH, Boyle SE, Yanaihara N, et al. Copy number analysis identifies novel interactions between genomic loci in ovarian cancer. PLoS One. 2010;5(9):e11408.
116. Cooke SL, Ng CK, Melnyk N, Garcia MJ, Hardcastle T, Temple J, Langdon S, Huntsman D, Brenton JD. Genomic analysis of genetic heterogeneity and evolution in high-grade serous ovarian carcinoma. Oncogene. 2010;29(35):4905–13.
117. Mittempergher L. Genomic characterization of high-grade serous ovarian cancer: dissecting its molecular heterogeneity as a road towards effective therapeutic strategies. Curr Oncol Rep. 2016;18(7):44.
118. Kulkarni-Datar K, Orsulic S, Foster R, Rueda BR. Ovarian tumor initiating cell populations persist following paclitaxel and carboplatin chemotherapy treatment in vivo. Cancer Lett. 2013;339(2):237–46.
119. Koch CA, Vortmeyer AO, Huang SC, Alesci S, Zhuang Z, Pacak K. Genetic aspects of pheochromocytoma. Endocr Regul. 2001;35(1):43–52.
120. Walther MM, Herring J, Enquist E, Keiser HR, Linehan WM. von Recklinghausen's disease and pheochromocytomas. J Urol. 1999;162(5):1582–6.
121. Welander J, Larsson C, Backdahl M, Hareni N, Sivler T, Brauckhoff M, Soderkvist P, Gimm O. Integrative genomics reveals frequent somatic NF1 mutations in sporadic pheochromocytomas. Hum Mol Genet. 2012;21(26):5406–16.
122. Opocher G, Schiavi F. Genetics of pheochromocytomas and paragangliomas. Best Pract Res Clin Endocrinol Metab. 2010;24(6):943–56.
123. Welander J, Soderkvist P, Gimm O. The NF1 gene: a frequent mutational target in sporadic pheochromocytomas and beyond. Endocr Relat Cancer. 2013;20(4):C13–17.
124. Burnichon N, Buffet A, Parfait B, Letouze E, Laurendeau I, Loriot C, Pasmant E, Abermil N, Valeyrie-Allanore L, Bertherat J, et al. Somatic NF1 inactivation is a frequent event in sporadic pheochromocytoma. Hum Mol Genet. 2012;21(26):5397–405.
125. Fishbein L, Nathanson KL. Pheochromocytoma and paraganglioma: understanding the complexities of the genetic background. Cancer Genet. 2012;205(1-2):1–11.
126. Galan SR, Kann PH. Genetics and molecular pathogenesis of pheochromocytoma and paraganglioma. Clin Endocrinol (Oxf). 2013;78(2):165–75.
127. Deyell RJ, Attiyeh EF. Advances in the understanding of constitutional and somatic genomic alterations in neuroblastoma. Cancer Genet. 2011;204(3):113–21.
128. Shojaei-Brosseau T, Chompret A, Abel A, de Vathaire F, Raquin MA, Brugieres L, Feunteun J, Hartmann O, Bonaiti-Pellie C. Genetic epidemiology of neuroblastoma: a study of 426 cases at the Institut Gustave-Roussy in France. Pediatr Blood Cancer. 2004;42(1):99–105.
129. The I, Murthy AE, Hannigan GE, Jacoby LB, Menon AG, Gusella JF, Bernards A. Neurofibromatosis type 1 gene mutations in neuroblastoma. Nat Genet. 1993;3(1):62–6.
130. Holzel M, Huang S, Koster J, Ora I, Lakeman A, Caron H, Nijkamp W, Xie J, Callens T, Asgharzadeh S, et al. NF1 is a tumor suppressor in neuroblastoma that determines retinoic acid response and disease outcome. Cell. 2010;142(2):218–29.
131. Han D, Spengler BA, Ross RA. Increased wild-type N-ras activation by neurofibromin down-regulation increases human neuroblastoma stem cell malignancy. Genes Cancer. 2011;2(11):1034–43.
132. Parsons DW, Jones S, Zhang X, Lin JC, Leary RJ, Angenendt P, Mankoo P, Carter H, Siu IM, Gallia GL, et al. An integrated genomic analysis of human glioblastoma multiforme. Science. 2008;321(5897):1807–12.
133. Louis DN. Molecular pathology of malignant gliomas. Annu Rev Pathol. 2006;1:97–117.
134. Brennan CW, Verhaak RG, McKenna A, Campos B, Noushmehr H, Salama SR, Zheng S, Chakravarty D, Sanborn JZ, Berman SH, et al. The somatic genomic landscape of glioblastoma. Cell. 2013;155(2):462–77.
135. Jones DT, Hutter B, Jager N, Korshunov A, Kool M, Warnatz HJ, Zichner T, Lambert SR, Ryzhova M, Quang DA, et al. Recurrent somatic alterations of FGFR1 and NTRK2 in pilocytic astrocytoma. Nat Genet. 2013;45(8):927–32.
136. Verhaak RG, Hoadley KA, Purdom E, Wang V, Qi Y, Wilkerson MD, Miller CR, Ding L, Golub T, Mesirov JP, et al. Integrated genomic analysis identifies clinically relevant subtypes of glioblastoma characterized by abnormalities in PDGFRA, IDH1, EGFR, and NF1. Cancer Cell. 2010;17(1):98–110.
137. Zhu Y, Guignard F, Zhao D, Liu L, Burns DK, Mason RP, Messing A, Parada LF. Early inactivation of p53 tumor suppressor gene cooperating with NF1 loss induces malignant astrocytoma. Cancer Cell. 2005;8(2):119–30.
138. Gutmann DH, Loehr A, Zhang Y, Kim J, Henkemeyer M, Cashen A. Haploinsufficiency for the neurofibromatosis 1 (NF1) tumor suppressor results in increased astrocyte proliferation. Oncogene. 1999;18(31):4450–9.
139. Wu M, Wallace MR, Muir D. Nf1 haploinsufficiency augments angiogenesis. Oncogene. 2006;25(16):2297–303.
140. Ahlquist T, Bottillo I, Danielsen SA, Meling GI, Rognum TO, Lind GE, Dallapiccola B, Lothe RA. RAS signaling in colorectal carcinomas through alteration of RAS, RAF, NF1, and/or RASSF1A. Neoplasia. 2008;10(7):680–6. 682 p following 686.
141. Cawkwell L, Lewis FA, Quirke P. Frequency of allele loss of DCC, p53, RBI, WT1, NF1, NM23 and APC/MCC in colorectal cancer assayed by fluorescent multiplex polymerase chain reaction. Br J Cancer. 1994;70(5):813–8.
142. Leggett B, Young J, Buttenshaw R, Thomas L, Young B, Chenevix-Trench G, Searle J, Ward M. Colorectal carcinomas show frequent allelic loss on the long arm of chromosome 17 with evidence for a specific target region. Br J Cancer. 1995;71(5):1070–3.
143. Cancer Genome Atlas N. Comprehensive molecular characterization of human colon and rectal cancer. Nature. 2012;487(7407):330–7.
144. Giannakis M, Mu XJ, Shukla SA, Qian ZR, Cohen O, Nishihara R, Bahl S, Cao Y, Amin-Mansour A, Yamauchi M, et al. Genomic correlates of immune-cell infiltrates in colorectal carcinoma. Cell Rep. 2016;17(4):1206.
145. Seshagiri S, Stawiski EW, Durinck S, Modrusan Z, Storm EE, Conboy CB, Chaudhuri S, Guan Y, Janakiraman V, Jaiswal BS, et al. Recurrent R-spondin fusions in colon cancer. Nature. 2012;488(7413):660–4.
146. Fearon ER. Molecular genetics of colorectal cancer. Annu Rev Pathol. 2011;6:479–507.
147. Vogelstein B, Papadopoulos N, Velculescu VE, Zhou S, Diaz Jr LA, Kinzler KW. Cancer genome landscapes. Science. 2013;339(6127):1546–58.
148. Aaltonen V, Bostrom PJ, Soderstrom KO, Hirvonen O, Tuukkanen J, Nurmi M, Laato M, Peltonen J. Urinary bladder transitional cell carcinogenesis is associated with down-regulation of NF1 tumor suppressor gene in vivo and in vitro. Am J Pathol. 1999;154(3):755–65.

149. Ross JS, Wang K, Al-Rohil RN, Nazeer T, Sheehan CE, Otto GA, He J, Palmer G, Yelensky R, Lipson D, et al. Advanced urothelial carcinoma: next-generation sequencing reveals diverse genomic alterations and targets of therapy. Mod Pathol. 2014;27(2):271–80.
150. Bader JL. Neurofibromatosis and cancer. Ann N Y Acad Sci. 1986;486:57–65.
151. Knudson AG. Antioncogenes and human cancer. Proc Natl Acad Sci U S A. 1993;90(23):10914–21.
152. Matsui I, Tanimura M, Kobayashi N, Sawada T, Nagahara N, Akatsuka J. Neurofibromatosis type 1 and childhood cancer. Cancer. 1993;72(9):2746–54.
153. Wullschleger S, Loewith R, Hall MN. TOR signaling in growth and metabolism. Cell. 2006;124(3):471–84.
154. Chen L, Liu P, Evans Jr TC, Ettwiller LM. DNA damage is a pervasive cause of sequencing errors, directly confounding variant identification. Science. 2017; 355(6326):752–6.
155. Bozic I, Antal T, Ohtsuki H, Carter H, Kim D, Chen S, Karchin R, Kinzler KW, Vogelstein B, Nowak MA. Accumulation of driver and passenger mutations during tumor progression. Proc Natl Acad Sci U S A. 2010;107(43):18545–50.
156. Bozic I, Gerold JM, Nowak MA. Quantifying clonal and subclonal passenger mutations in cancer evolution. PLoS Comput Biol. 2016;12(2):e1004731.
157. McFarland CD, Korolev KS, Kryukov GV, Sunyaev SR, Mirny LA. Impact of deleterious passenger mutations on cancer progression. Proc Natl Acad Sci U S A. 2013;110(8):2910–5.
158. McFarland CD, Mirny LA, Korolev KS. Tug-of-war between driver and passenger mutations in cancer and other adaptive processes. Proc Natl Acad Sci U S A. 2014;111(42):15138–43.
159. Nussinov R, Tsai CJ. 'Latent drivers' expand the cancer mutational landscape. Curr Opin Struct Biol. 2015;32:25–32.
160. Futreal PA, Coin L, Marshall M, Down T, Hubbard T, Wooster R, Rahman N, Stratton MR. A census of human cancer genes. Nat Rev Cancer. 2004;4(3): 177–83.
161. Network of Cancer Genes (NCG). http://ncg.kcl.ac.uk/. Accessed Sept 2016.
162. Lawrence MS, Stojanov P, Mermel CH, Robinson JT, Garraway LA, Golub TR, Meyerson M, Gabriel SB, Lander ES, Getz G. Discovery and saturation analysis of cancer genes across 21 tumour types. Nature. 2014;505(7484):495–501.
163. Lawrence MS, Stojanov P, Polak P, Kryukov GV, Cibulskis K, Sivachenko A, Carter SL, Stewart C, Mermel CH, Roberts SA, et al. Mutational heterogeneity in cancer and the search for new cancer-associated genes. Nature. 2013; 499(7457):214–8. doi:10.1038/nature12213.
164. Seton-Rogers S. Oncogenes: one of these things is not like the others. Nat Rev Cancer. 2016;16(1):5.
165. Prahallad A, Sun C, Huang S, Di Nicolantonio F, Salazar R, Zecchin D, Beijersbergen RL, Bardelli A, Bernards R. Unresponsiveness of colon cancer to BRAF(V600E) inhibition through feedback activation of EGFR. Nature. 2012;483(7387):100–3.
166. Furukawa K, Yanai N, Fujita M, Harada Y. Novel mutations of neurofibromatosis type 1 gene in small cell lung cancers. Surg Today. 2003;33(5):323–7.
167. Cancer Genome Atlas Research N. Comprehensive molecular characterization of urothelial bladder carcinoma. Nature. 2014;507(7492):315–22.
168. De Raedt T, Brems H, Wolkenstein P, Vidaud D, Pilotti S, Perrone F, Mautner V, Frahm S, Sciot R, Legius E. Elevated risk for MPNST in NF1 microdeletion patients. Am J Hum Genet. 2003;72(5):1288–92.
169. Pasmant E, Sabbagh A, Spurlock G, Laurendeau I, Grillo E, Hamel MJ, Martin L, Barbarot S, Leheup B, Rodriguez D, et al. NF1 microdeletions in neurofibromatosis type 1: from genotype to phenotype. Hum Mutat. 2010; 31(6):E1506–1518.
170. Cancer Genome Atlas Research N. Integrated genomic analyses of ovarian carcinoma. Nature. 2011;474(7353):609–15.
171. Cancer Genome Atlas Research N. Comprehensive genomic characterization defines human glioblastoma genes and core pathways. Nature. 2008; 455(7216):1061–8.
172. Messiaen L, Yao S, Brems H, Callens T, Sathienkijkanchai A, Denayer E, Spencer E, Arn P, Babovic-Vuksanovic D, Bay C, et al. Clinical and mutational spectrum of neurofibromatosis type 1-like syndrome. JAMA. 2009;302(19):2111–8.
173. Ahmadian MR, Kiel C, Stege P, Scheffzek K. Structural fingerprints of the Ras-GTPase activating proteins neurofibromin and p120GAP. J Mol Biol. 2003; 329(4):699–710.
174. Ahmadian MR, Wiesmuller L, Lautwein A, Bischoff FR, Wittinghofer A. Structural differences in the minimal catalytic domains of the GTPase-activating proteins p120GAP and neurofibromin. J Biol Chem. 1996;271(27):16409–15.
175. Ding H, Shannon P, Lau N, Wu X, Roncari L, Baldwin RL, Takebayashi H, Nagy A, Gutmann DH, Guha A. Oligodendrogliomas result from the expression of an activated mutant epidermal growth factor receptor in a RAS transgenic mouse astrocytoma model. Cancer Res. 2003;63(5):1106–13.
176. Kan Z, Jaiswal BS, Stinson J, Janakiraman V, Bhatt D, Stern HM, Yue P, Haverty PM, Bourgon R, Zheng J, et al. Diverse somatic mutation patterns and pathway alterations in human cancers. Nature. 2010;466(7308):869–73.
177. Kandoth C, McLellan MD, Vandin F, Ye K, Niu B, Lu C, Xie M, Zhang Q, McMichael JF, Wyczalkowski MA, et al. Mutational landscape and significance across 12 major cancer types. Nature. 2013;502(7471):333–9.
178. Bashashati A, Ha G, Tone A, Ding J, Prentice LM, Roth A, Rosner J, Shumansky K, Kalloger S, Senz J, et al. Distinct evolutionary trajectories of primary high-grade serous ovarian cancers revealed through spatial mutational profiling. J Pathol. 2013;231(1):21–34.
179. Kanchi KL, Johnson KJ, Lu C, McLellan MD, Leiserson MD, Wendl MC, Zhang Q, Koboldt DC, Xie M, Kandoth C, et al. Integrated analysis of germline and somatic variants in ovarian cancer. Nat Commun. 2014;5:3156.
180. Ross JS, Ali SM, Wang K, Palmer G, Yelensky R, Lipson D, Miller VA, Zajchowski D, Shawver LK, Stephens PJ. Comprehensive genomic profiling of epithelial ovarian cancer by next generation sequencing-based diagnostic assay reveals new routes to targeted therapies. Gynecol Oncol. 2013;130(3):554–9.

14

Evaluating somatic tumor mutation detection without matched normal samples

Jamie K. Teer[1*], Yonghong Zhang[1], Lu Chen[2], Eric A. Welsh[1], W. Douglas Cress[2], Steven A. Eschrich[1] and Anders E. Berglund[1]

Abstract

Background: Observations of recurrent somatic mutations in tumors have led to identification and definition of signaling and other pathways that are important for cancer progression and therapeutic targeting. As tumor cells contain both an individual's inherited genetic variants and somatic mutations, challenges arise in distinguishing these events in massively parallel sequencing datasets. Typically, both a tumor sample and a "normal" sample from the same individual are sequenced and compared; variants observed only in the tumor are considered to be somatic mutations. However, this approach requires two samples for each individual.

Results: We evaluate a method of detecting somatic mutations in tumor samples for which only a subset of normal samples are available. We describe tuning of the method for detection of mutations in tumors, filtering to remove inherited variants, and comparison of detected mutations to several matched tumor/normal analysis methods. Filtering steps include the use of population variation datasets to remove inherited variants as well a subset of normal samples to remove technical artifacts. We then directly compare mutation detection with tumor-only and tumor-normal approaches using the same sets of samples. Comparisons are performed using an internal targeted gene sequencing dataset (n = 3380) as well as whole exome sequencing data from The Cancer Genome Atlas project (n = 250). Tumor-only mutation detection shows similar recall (43–60%) but lesser precision (20–21%) to current matched tumor/normal approaches (recall 43–73%, precision 30–82%) when compared to a "gold-standard" tumor/normal approach. The inclusion of a small pool of normal samples improves precision, although many variants are still uniquely detected in the tumor-only analysis.

Conclusions: A detailed method for somatic mutation detection without matched normal samples enables study of larger numbers of tumor samples, as well as tumor samples for which a matched normal is not available. As sensitivity/recall is similar to tumor/normal mutation detection but precision is lower, tumor-only detection is more appropriate for classification of samples based on known mutations. Although matched tumor-normal analysis is preferred due to higher precision, we demonstrate that mutation detection without matched normal samples is possible for certain applications.

Keywords: Somatic mutation, Cancer genomics, Next-generation sequencing, Precision medicine

Background

Methods for massively parallel sequencing analysis have matured, even as sequencing technologies have undergone continued, rapid improvement. Detection of somatic mutations in cancer samples has proven to be challenging due to the presence of inherited germline variants, sample heterogeneity, and genomic instability. Somatic mutations can be identified from massively parallel sequencing data by directly comparing the DNA sequence from tumor samples with their matched normal samples. This allows subtraction of the germline variants shared by all cells in an individual, leaving only acquired somatic mutations. Somatic mutations include the important driver mutations that give a cell the growth advantage leading to tumorigenesis [1]. The paired tumor/normal approach to precisely identify somatic mutations has been used in landscape studies that have identified commonly mutated positions and genes in a wide variety of cancers, including recent publications by The Cancer Genome Atlas consortium (for review, see Watson et al. [2]). There are several

* Correspondence: Jamie.Teer@moffitt.org
[1]Department of Biostatistics and Bioinformatics, H. Lee Moffitt Cancer Center and Research Institute, Tampa, FL 33612, USA
Full list of author information is available at the end of the article

implementations, including VarScan [3, 4], Shimmer [5], SomaticSniper [6], Strelka [7], and MuTect [8]. However, this approach effectively doubles the number of samples that must be sequenced and analyzed and limits investigation to those tumor samples for which a matched normal tissue sample is available. This approach is theoretically sound and widely used, and many methods have been compared and evaluated, including in the crowdsourced DREAM challenge [9] and others [10]. However, the efficacy of somatic mutation detection without matched normal samples has not been widely studied. Recently, Jones et al. reported that tumor-only mutation detection resulted in large numbers of false positive detections and concluded that tumor-only detection should be used with caution, even though the approach is common in clinical testing [11].

As part of the Total Cancer Care® (TCC) project [12], we have developed a large tumor bank consisting of 26,473 frozen tumor samples. Through collaboration with a pharmaceutical partner, Merck & Co., 3917 samples from 3380 unique individuals were subjected to targeted gene sequencing (TGS) covering 1321 genes of interest. Here, we describe and evaluate a detailed approach for somatic mutation detection without matched normal samples based on a Genome Analysis ToolKit (GATK) [13, 14] pipeline. Although GATK is built on a model assuming a diploid genome that is often not applicable in tumor samples, the tool is widely used for somatic mutation detection. We therefore deliberately choose to evaluate this approach because of the disconnect between theoretical concerns and widespread use. We describe the effect of various filters on mutation detection rates and compare tumor-only mutation detection to paired tumor-normal comparison approaches using TGS data and whole exome sequencing (WES) data from the TCGA project (250 samples from 5 diseases). This study expands on the findings of Jones et al. to allow for a better understanding of the limitations and potential utility of tumor-only mutation detection. We finally describe the detailed pipeline built for this evaluation from publically available analysis tools, allowing researchers to evaluate and utilize tumor-only mutation detection themselves.

Methods

Experimental design

The objectives of this study were to define a specific methodology to detect somatic mutations without matched normal samples and to evaluate its performance. As a subset of tumor samples did have a matched normal sample, mutations were also directly compared between tumor-only and tumor-normal mutation detection strategies to calculate precision and recall.

Study cohorts

A cohort of samples from 3380 unique individuals (2575 primary solid tumors, 675 metastatic solid tumor, and 130 hematologic malignancies) from the TCC project was utilized in this study (Fig. 1a). Samples were classified according to site of tumor origin (Additional file 1: Table S1). The sites with the highest number of samples include the lung, large bowel, breast, kidney, ovary, and skin. These samples were subjected to TGS across the protein coding exons of 1321 genes covering 3.8 megabases (Additional file 2: Table S2). The median number of reads aligning per sample was 15,283,830. The read depth was consistent across tissue sites of origin with a median depth coverage of 141× (Additional file 3: Figure S1d). The median percentage of targeted bases which covered ≥ 10× across samples was 93.7%. Altogether, 53.4 million reads were generated, for a total of 4.8 trillion bases.

To identify potential batch effects or other confounding factors, a principal component analysis (PCA) was performed on various sequence metrics, including missing values, mutation counts, read counts, and transition/

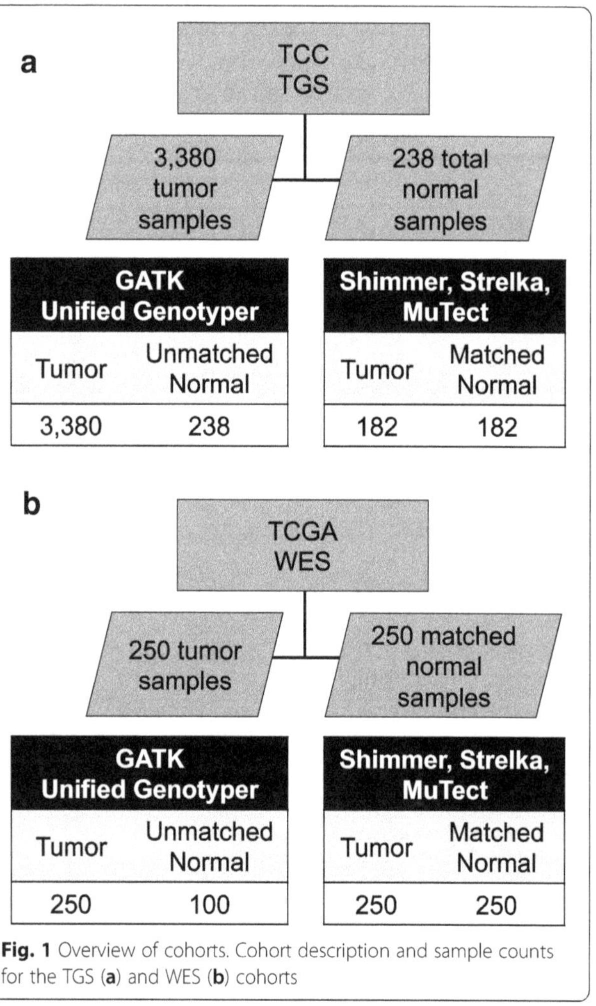

Fig. 1 Overview of cohorts. Cohort description and sample counts for the TGS (**a**) and WES (**b**) cohorts

transversion ratios. The majority of samples were grouped together, with two smaller subgroups showing some deviation (Additional file 3: Figure S1a). PCA loadings showed that the 1st component subgroup (tailing out to the right) was affected by missing values and the 2nd component subgroup (tailing to the bottom left) was affected by mutation counts (presumed to be samples with a hyper-mutator phenotype) (Additional file 3: Figure S1b) It was noted that the sites of origin did not cluster together, suggesting that the batch effects were not responsible for similarities between samples within a site of origin.

To assess the extent of potential sample issues using sequencing data and clinical metadata alone, the balance of sequence reads aligning to the X and Y chromosomes was examined to infer gender, which was then matched to clinical data for each patient. The ratio of sequence reads on chromosome X compared to chromosome Y varied over 7 logs, but formed a very distinct bi-modal pattern (Additional file 3: Figure S1c). The high ratio peak was inferred to be female, and empirical cutoffs were set to determine gender across the cohort (male ≤ 4, female ≥ 5.75). Of all samples with determined gender, 0.7% showed a discrepant gender call and were excluded from further analysis.

As a part of the TCC cohort, 238 adjacent normal tissue samples were available from individuals with cancer, which were used to create a normal pool for filtering purposes. Of these, 182 normal samples were paired with a primary tumor sample: matched tumor/normal mutation detection software was applied to these pairs for comparison to tumor-only mutation detection.

WES was also included from a cohort of 250 samples assembled from five different cancers characterized as part of The Cancer Genome Atlas (TCGA) project (Fig. 1b). Fifty tumors each were selected from acute myeloid leukemia (LAML), glioblastoma multiforme (GBM), lung adenocarcinoma (LUAD), ovarian serous cystadenocarcinoma (OV), and skin cutaneous melanoma (SKCM) (Additional file 4: Table S3). These samples each had a matched normal sample, which was used for the matched tumor/normal mutation identification methods. One hundred of these normal samples were selected for a normal pool, which was used for tumor-only mutation detection.

Tissue samples and consent

Tissue samples were collected according to the TCC methods and consent protocols detailed by Fenstermacher et al. [12].

TGS sequencing

DNA was subjected to solution-hybridization-selection using SureSelect technology (Agilent Technologies, Santa Clara, CA) targeting 1321 genes. Samples were then sequenced on GAIIx sequencers using a 90 bp, paired-end configuration (Illumina, Inc., San Diego, CA).

Analysis—alignment

Sequence reads were aligned to the human reference genome (hs37d5) using the Burrows-Wheeler Aligner (BWA) version 0.5.9-r16 [15]. Duplicate reads were marked with Picard-Tools 1.56 (http://broadinstitute.github.io/picard/). Indel realignment and base quality score recalibration were performed with GATK [13, 14]. GenomeAnalysisTKLite-2.2 was used as it was one of the last freely available versions and therefore usable by a wider audience. Samtools v0.1.16 was used for BAM file handling.

Analysis—tumor-only genotype determination

Multi-sample genotype determination was performed with GATK UnifiedGenotyper. Variant confidence/quality by depth (QD) metric was excluded from Variant Quality Score Recalibration (VQSR), as we have previously found this to penalize variants deviating from the expected 50% alternate allele frequencies. Further modifications to the pipeline are described in Additional file 5. Sequence variants were annotated with ANNOVAR [16], and additional information was included from 1000 Genomes [17] (20110521 release), ESP (http://evs.gs.washington.edu/EVS/ , version ESP6500SI-V2), and COSMIC [18] version 61.

Analysis—matched tumor/normal mutation detection

Tumor-normal mutation detection of SNVs and indels was performed with Shimmer [5] (–minqual 20 –mapqual 16), Strelka [7] (v1.0.13, default settings), and MuTect [8] (v1.1.4, –max_alt_alleles_in_normal_count 3 –max_alt_allele_in_normal_fraction 0.05). In the MuTect analysis, indels were called using GATK SomaticIndelDetector.

Analysis—secondary

BEDTools [19] was used for overlap calculations. The analysis pipeline, VCF filtering scripts, and other analysis scripts were written in Perl, bash, and R. Principal component analysis was performed using Evince (v2.5.5 (Prediktera AB, Umeå, Sweden)) (http://www.prediktera.se/).

Precision (positive predictive value) was calculated as follows: mutations observed in both test method (GATK tumor-only) and standard method (MuTect) (true positives) divided by total mutations called in test method.

$$\text{Precision} = \frac{tp}{tp + fp} = \frac{\text{mutations observed in test AND standard methods}}{\text{total mutations observed in test method}}$$

Recall (sensitivity) was calculated as follows: mutations observed in both test method and standard method (true positives) divided by total mutations called in standard method.

$$\text{Recall} = \frac{tp}{tp + fn}$$

$$= \frac{\text{mutations observed in test AND standard methods}}{\text{total mutations observed in standard method}}$$

Results

Genotype calling and VQSR tuning

Somatic mutations were identified from tumor samples using BWA [15] alignments and GATK [14] quality improvement and genotype determination. GATK's UnifiedGenotyper module has the ability to determine the exact genotype of each sample at every variant position when using the multi-sample detection mode. This returns not only a list of variants seen in each sample but also whether non-variant samples have the reference genotype or are "missing" at a position due to insufficient data. This approach is critical to ensure precise classification of samples as mutated or reference for downstream phenotype association analyses. We initially followed the best practices guidelines with several adjustments (see Additional file 5).

BWA-GATK mutation detection was applied to the TGS dataset, and VQSR FILTER status was examined. A high rate of PASS putative mutations was observed, with about 5% of variants being assigned the least specific "SNPto100" tranche. However, with near-default discovery and VQSR settings, only 3.8% of the COSMIC v61 [18] mutations seen more than five times had a value of PASS (Additional file 3: Figure S2b), while 60% were in the least specific tranche (SNPto100). Neither VQSR tuning (removing HaplotypeScore and percentBadVariants) nor adding a cancer mutation training set (COSMIC v61 mutations seen more than once) greatly increased PASS count. The variant list was then filtered on the target regions plus 25 flanking base pairs (total size = 4.9 megabases) before VQSR, resulting in a large increase in the number of final passing COSMIC variants, 86.4%. This also resulted in a greater proportion of all variants passing filter (Additional file 3: Figure S2a). Finally, the target-region pre-filtering was combined with cancer-specific VQSR settings and training, and a COSMIC pass rate of 98.0% was observed. The overall pass rate also increased to 95.5%, suggesting these settings may have reduced specificity (as fewer positions are filtered) but have allowed very high sensitivity for known cancer mutations.

WES samples were less impacted by GATK settings (Additional file 3: Figure S2c, d). The overall PASS rates were slightly higher than in the TGS data, and COSMIC mutations had a much higher PASS rate with default settings (66.3% in WES vs. 3.8% in TGS). No COSMIC mutations were observed in the SNPto100 tranche with any applied settings. Tuned settings applied to the TGS cohort above were also applied to the WES dataset and also increased the proportion of both COSMIC and all PASS mutations. As was observed in the TGS cohort, the highest PASS rate in the WES cohort occurred when the mutations were first target-filtered, and then, VQSR was run using COSMIC training. While less critical, tumor-specific settings benefit whole exome sequencing as well by ensuring known somatic mutations are not falsely removed.

Efficacy of various filtering strategies

Several strategies were applied to enrich for somatic mutations. A median of 3328 potential mutations per sample was detected with the tuned BWA-GATK pipeline (Fig. 2a, "All"). The 1000 Genomes project [17, 20] has cataloged common inherited genetic variation across many different populations around the globe. Variants seen in this dataset were excluded as a first-pass filter for inherited variation, which decreased the putative mutation rate to a median of 608 per sample (Fig. 2a, "minus 1000 Genomes"). The NHLBI Exome Sequencing Project (ESP) dataset, which includes 6503 individuals, was used for further filtering. Although we expected that the large increase in "control" sample numbers would result in the exclusion of many more rare inherited variants, the median mutation count dropped only to 526 (Fig. 2a, "minus ESP"). Several larger population databases have recently become available. We examined the efficacy of filtering with ExAC [21] and KAVIAR [22]. ExAC includes data from > 60,000 whole exomes, although we used the non-TCGA download to avoid filtering known somatic mutations. KAVIAR includes > 13,000 whole genomes and > 64,000 whole exomes (including the ExAC database) and excludes cancer genomes. Although cancer samples should be absent from these databases, we observed common somatic mutations in both, necessitating the use of an allele frequency cutoff. We found that removing variants present in these databases at ≥ 1% allele frequency further decreases the number of detected mutations (Additional file 3: Figure S3a).

Many putative variants are likely artifacts arising from improper sequence alignment [23, 24], and these artifacts tend to be common across samples. We reasoned that variants observed commonly in tumor samples and also in a pool of normal samples are not likely to be cancer driver mutations and are more likely artifacts, especially when common population variants have already been removed. Potential artifacts were identified in a pool of 238 normal samples using the tuned BWA-GATK pipeline. Although these were matched samples, they were treated as unmatched: any mutation observed in this normal pool dataset at greater than or equal to 5% population allele frequency was removed. This dramatically reduced the number of putative tumor mutations to a median of 109 per sample (Fig. 2a, "minus Normal ≥ 5%"). A stricter filter

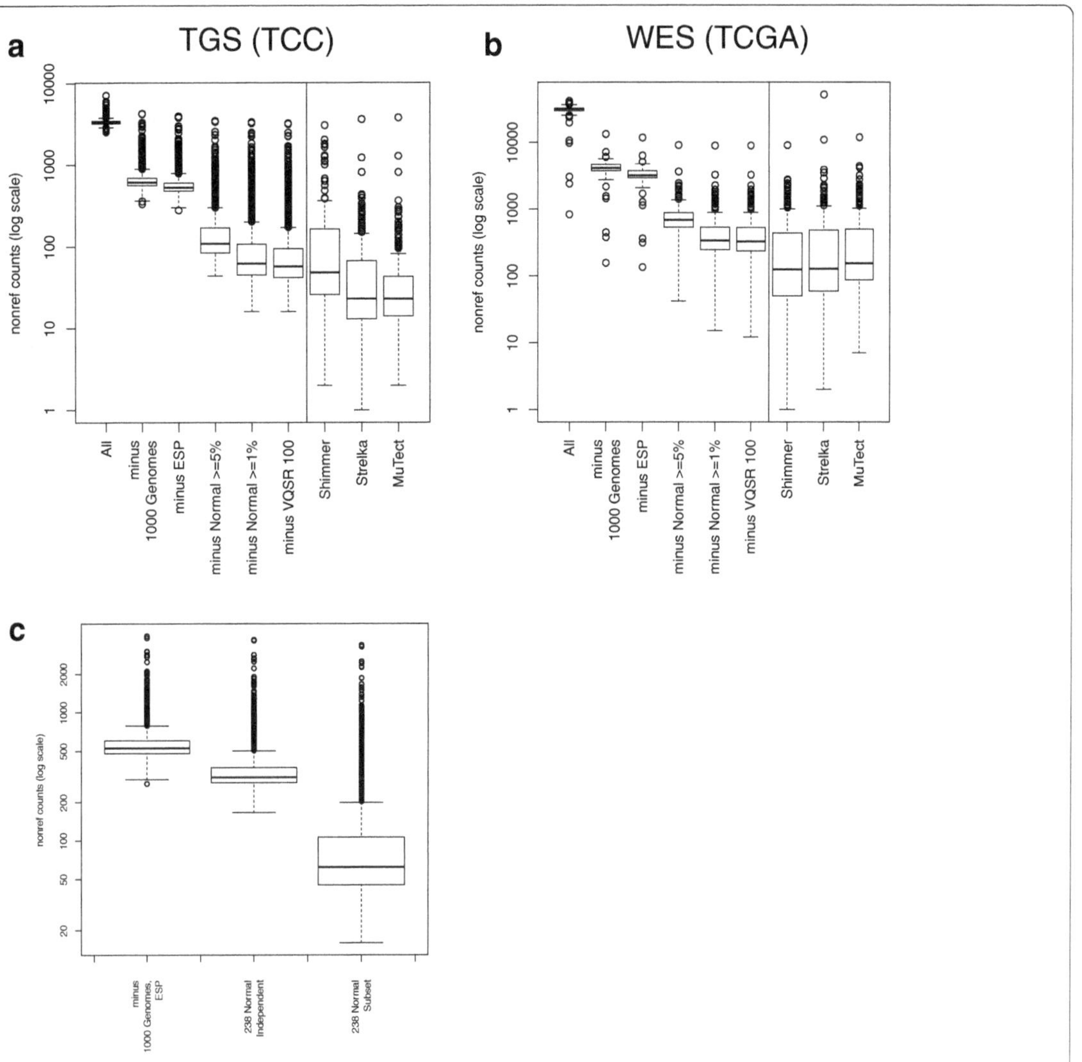

Fig. 2 Tumor-only mutation counts with filtering. **a** Boxplot showing numbers of mutations detected in the TGS cohort using tumor-only methods after each filtering step (left) and using matched tumor-normal methods on 182 sample pairs (right). **b** Boxplot showing numbers of mutations detected in the WES cohort using tumor-only methods after each filtering step (left) and using matched tumor-normal methods (right). **c** Boxplot demonstrating that in the TGS cohort, analyzing the normal samples independent of the tumor samples results in reduced ability to remove potential artifacts. GATK variant detection on all tumor and normal samples together, followed by isolation of the normal subset to annotate the tumor samples, results in the removal of more potential artifacts. Median counts are indicated by the dark line in the middle of the box. The bottom and top of the box are the first and third quartiles, respectively. The whiskers represent the most extreme points within 1.5 times the interquartile range. The *y*-axes are in a log scale

of no more than 1% normal allele frequency further reduced the median putative mutation count to 62 (Fig. 2a, Additional file 3: Figure S3a, "minusNormal ≥ 1%"). Finally, excluding the VQSR Tranche100 variants resulted in a final median mutation count of 57 ("minus VQSR 100"). This resulted in a final median mutation rate of 11.6/megabase investigated.

A subset of the TGS cohort also had matched adjacent normal samples, allowing for a direct comparison of matched tumor/normal mutation methods to our tumor-only pipeline. We applied three different commonly used algorithms for detection of mutations using matched tumor/normal pairs: Shimmer, Strelka, and MuTect. These methods have performed reasonably well in comparisons [9, 10] and are all capable of detecting single nucleotide and deletion/insertion mutations. Somatic mutations were identified in 182 matched primary tumor/normal pairs using Shimmer, Strelka, and MuTect, resulting in a median mutation count of 48.0 per sample (9.83/megabase), 23.0 per sample (4.71/megabase), and 23.0 per sample (4.71/megabase), respectively (Fig. 2a, right-hand side).

The same filtering strategy was applied to the WES cohort tumor-only analysis. As different TCGA Genome Sequencing Centers used different targeted capture designs, the refSeq coding exons (plus 25 flanking base pairs) were used as target regions. Although all 250 tumors had a matched normal sample in the TCGA dataset, a subset of 100 was selected for the normal pool and analyzed together with the tumor samples using the GATK tumor-only mutation detection strategy. Putative mutation counts were determined after each sequentially applied filter. Mutation counts were higher than the TGS cohort due to the larger target size (whole exome vs. 1321 genes). As observed for the TGS cohort, the median putative mutation count decreased with each additional filter (Fig. 2b, Additional file 3: Figure S3b): all detected (31,335), minus 1000 genomes (4099.5), minus ESP (3180.5), minus normal ≥ 5% (680), minus normal ≥ 1% (335), minus Tranche100 (327). A final mutation rate of 7.6/megabase was observed within the refSeq coding target (43.0 megabases, including 25 bp flanking regions). The difference between mutation rates of TGS and WES is most likely due to the differences in cohort makeup (the TGS cohort has more samples from the more highly mutated tumor types). Importantly, the pattern of putative mutation count decrease was similar in the TGS and WES cohorts: large initial decreases when removing 1000 genome variants; modest decreases after further excluding ESP, KAVIAR, and ExAC; and then large decreases after further filtering with a normal pool.

As the WES cohort used TCGA data, matched normal samples were available for all tumors, enabling a direct comparison of tumor-only and matched tumor/normal mutation detection. Similar to the results observed in the TGS cohort, mutation counts were lower with the matched tumor/normal methods (Fig. 2b, right-hand side): Shimmer 125 (2.9/megabase), Strelka 128 (3.0/megabase), and MuTect 154.5 (3.6/megabase).

Normal pools proved to be very effective in removing putative variants in both TGS and WES cohorts. Titration experiments were performed to determine filtering effectiveness using fewer normal samples. The resulting mutation counts were compared after filtering with decreasing numbers of normal samples: from 238 down to 12 (TGS cohort) and from 100 down to 20 (WES cohort). Surprisingly, the amount of putative mutations remaining after removing variants with normal sample allele frequency ≥ 1% was stable down to 25 samples (TGS) and 20 samples (WES) (Additional file 3: Figure S4a, b). Furthermore, the exact method of mutation detection in the normal pool affected the results. When the TGS normal samples were analyzed in a separate, independent GATK run, the number of putative artifacts removed was less then when the normal samples were analyzed together with the tumor samples (Fig. 3c). This is likely due to increased prior probability of detection when variants are observed in other samples using GATK multi-sample genotype detection. This suggests it is beneficial to analyze all samples together and then extract the normal samples for frequency calculations.

Precision, recall, and sensitivity for known tumor mutations

Mutation detection performance was examined by comparing results of each method at each mutated position. MuTect tumor/normal was used as a truth set due to its common usage in TCGA analyses, as well as its reasonable performance in evaluations of tumor/normal methods. Precision and recall were calculated for each sample against MuTect tumor/normal using GATK tumor-only, Strelka tumor/normal, and Shimmer tumor/normal (Fig. 3a, b). GATK tumor-only recall at all positions was similar to Shimmer and slightly decreased compared to Strelka in both TGS and WES datasets. However, the GATK tumor-only precision was much lower than the Strelka in TGS, and much lower than both Strelka and Shimmer in WES data. We also noted precision and recall heterogeneity across samples for each method. Precision and recall were calculated at subsequent filter levels, which demonstrated increasing precision and slightly decreasing recall with each additional filter (Additional file 3: Figures S5 and S6). Although many inherited variants are removed by population filters, precision only moderately increases due to the large number of remaining variants. This suggests it is not possible to precisely identify somatic mutations with current tumor-only methods and that both population filters and a normal pool are important to increase precision.

To further understand the differences between tumor-only and matched tumor-normal mutation detection methods, genotype calls were directly compared at each position. The agreement of calls was counted within each sample, and median values are displayed in Additional file 3: Figure S7. In both TGS and WES cohorts, the tumor-only method shows the most unique mutations. This was more pronounced in the WES dataset, which agrees with the earlier observation of a larger difference in mutation counts between tumor-only and tumor-normal methods (Fig. 2). Interestingly, Shimmer called many more unique mutations than other tumor-normal methods in the TGS dataset, but MuTect called many more unique mutations in the WES cohort. Positions at which all methods made the same mutation call were the more common (~ 5-fold) than any other combination of two or more methods. Despite this agreement, we noticed that many positions were called by some tumor/normal methods and not others (Additional file 3: Figure S8). Strelka had the highest degree of overlap with the other two methods in both cohorts.

Sensitivity for known cancer mutations was assessed by determining the fraction of COSMIC mutations observed in each dataset. 43.5% of those positions observed commonly in COSMIC (more than 20 times) were also observed in the tumor-only TGS analysis (Fig. 3c, right). This fraction decreased as the less common mutations were considered, likely due to the increased numbers of

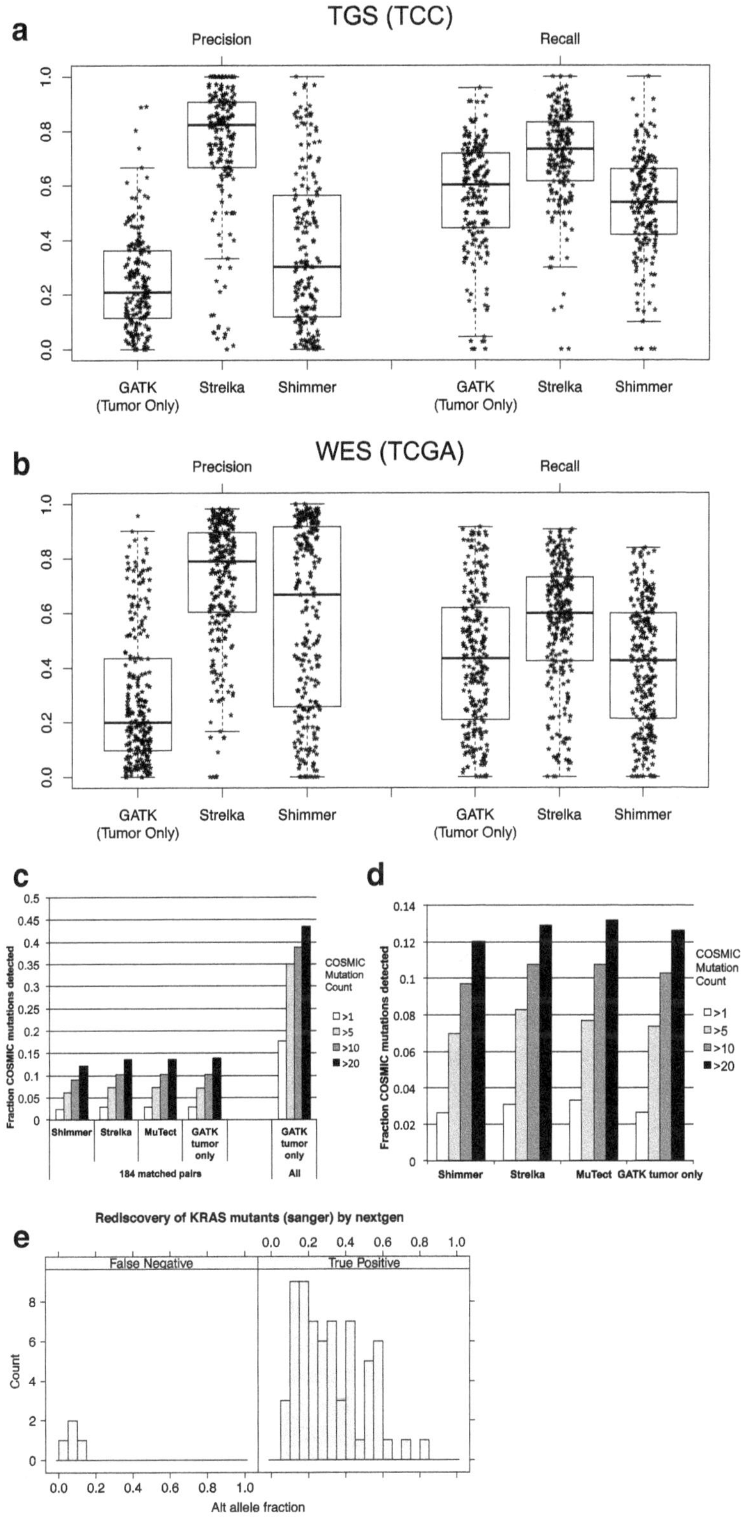

Fig. 3 Recall and precision of tumor-only and matched tumor-normal mutation detection. Recall and precision of methods compared to MuTect in TGS (**a**) and WES (**b**). Distributions are represented with box plots, and individual data points are plotted as asterisks. Fraction of COSMIC mutations detected by **c** matched tumor-normal and tumor-only methods within 182 TGS samples (left) and all TGS samples using tumor-only methods (right). **d** 250 WES samples. Shading indicates the number of times the mutation was observed in the COSMIC v61 database. **e** TGS alternate allele fraction and accuracy of *KRAS* G12/G13/Q61 mutations initially discovered by capillary sequencing. Not shown are the seven mutations detected in the TGS but not capillary sequencing

the more rare mutations as well as false positives (artifacts and common variants) in COSMIC. The fraction of COSMIC mutations detected in 182 TGS tumor/normal pairs was calculated from three different tumor-normal pair mutation detection methods (Shimmer, Strelka, MuTect) as well as from the GATK tumor-only method. The fraction of COSMIC bases observed was highly similar in all methods (Fig. 3c, left). Similar results were observed in the WES cohort: the tumor-only mutation detection method had similar sensitivity as the three different tumor-normal methods (Fig. 3d). This suggests the tumor-only approach has equivalent sensitivity to detect known cancer mutations.

Sample heterogeneity presents a specific challenge for sensitive detection of somatic mutations. The fraction of reads with a mutated base can be lower than expected due to normal sample contamination, mutational heterogeneity within the tumor, or chromosomal amplification. We therefore examined the sensitivity of our final tuned pipeline to detect low-frequency mutations. One hundred ninety of the lung samples that underwent TGS were also subjected to capillary sequencing at the G12/G13/Q61 *KRAS* loci. The capillary sequence data were analyzed with both automated genotype calling pipelines and extensive manual review of chromatograms in order to detect low-frequency mutations. Of the 70 mutations detected by capillary sequencing, 66 were also detected using the tumor-only method. Of the four mutations not detected, three had evidence of the variant, with allele frequencies less than 10% (Fig. 3e). Therefore, given the median overall target coverage of 141×, we observed a mutation allele frequency sensitivity limit of ~10%. In addition, seven mutations were detected only in TGS data (not in capillary), with allele frequencies ranging from 8 to 29% (mean = 18.0%, median = 15.6%).

Pan-cancer somatic mutation rates

Mutation rates detected by our tumor-only pipeline were calculated across different tumor sites of origin in TGS (sites with ≥50 samples) and WES cohorts. The frequencies observed using tumor-only mutation detection were higher than those from a matched tumor/normal large consortium sequencing project [25] (Fig. 4a, b). We observed a high variability in mutation rates in skin, uterus/endometrium, lung, and large bowel in agreement with the previous large consortium studies. Skin, uterus, and lung have the highest mutation rates in the "tumor-only" analyses; LAML and CLL have the lowest, mirroring other studies. This suggests that somatic mutations can be greatly enriched using tumor-only methods, but not as precisely identified as matched tumor/normal methods. Our observations have reproduced the overall mutation frequency patterns of large global consortium studies in a completely independent cohort.

Molecular associations with high mutation burden

Although the median mutation rate varies across tumor sites, every site has outlier tumors with very high mutation rates. To identify the potential molecular causes of high mutation rates, we examined DNA polymerase epsilon (*POLE*) exonuclease domain mutations (amino acids 268-471 and R494 in NP_006222). The recurrent *POLE* mutations almost always occur in the highly mutated outlier samples (Fig. 4c). Singleton *POLE* mutations fell into two groups: highly and moderately mutated tumors. Highly mutated samples with *POLE* mutations were primarily observed in tumors originating from the endometrium/uterus, large bowel, and ovary. One highly mutated sample with a *POLE* mutation was observed in breast and pancreatic cancers; the *POLE*-mutated sample was the most highly mutated in each site.

We have recently observed that the presence of homopolymer indels in both *TGFBR2* and *ACVR2A* is highly correlated with microsatellite instability (MSI) in TGS colorectal samples [26]. Here, we demonstrate that these samples have high mutation rates in the large bowel (Fig. 4d), strengthening the link between *ACVR2A+TGFBR2* mutation and MSI status. Additionally, several putative MSI samples in stomach (2), endometrium (3), and breast (1) tumors were observed. Notably, *ACVR2A+TGFBR2* mutations and *POLE* mutations only co-occurred once (singleton *POLE* mutation). These observations confirm and extend previously observed correlations of specific mutations and elevated mutation rates. Many highly mutated samples remained unexplained and require further analysis to identify mutational mechanisms.

Discussion

We have presented an analysis strategy for the detection of somatic mutations from tumor samples without matched normal samples (Fig. 5, Additional file 5). GATK modifications for detecting somatic mutations included (1) limiting putative mutations to targeted regions, (2) using a VQSR training set of known cancer mutations, and (3) tuning of settings (see Additional file 5) These modifications had a greater impact on reducing false negatives in smaller target sets. Tuning GATK also improved the filter quality of known mutations in whole exome data, although fewer false negatives were initially observed. The use of population genomic datasets (1000 Genomes) was effective at removing the vast majority of likely inherited variants, although the large number of remaining false positive mutations resulted in a small increase in precision. Interestingly, the addition of larger population-specific germline datasets (via the Exome Sequencing Project, ExAC, and KAVIAR) each only removed a modest fraction of additional common variants compared to decreases observed after filtering with a normal pool. Indeed, filtering with ExAC and KAVIAR after the normal pool resulted in removal of only

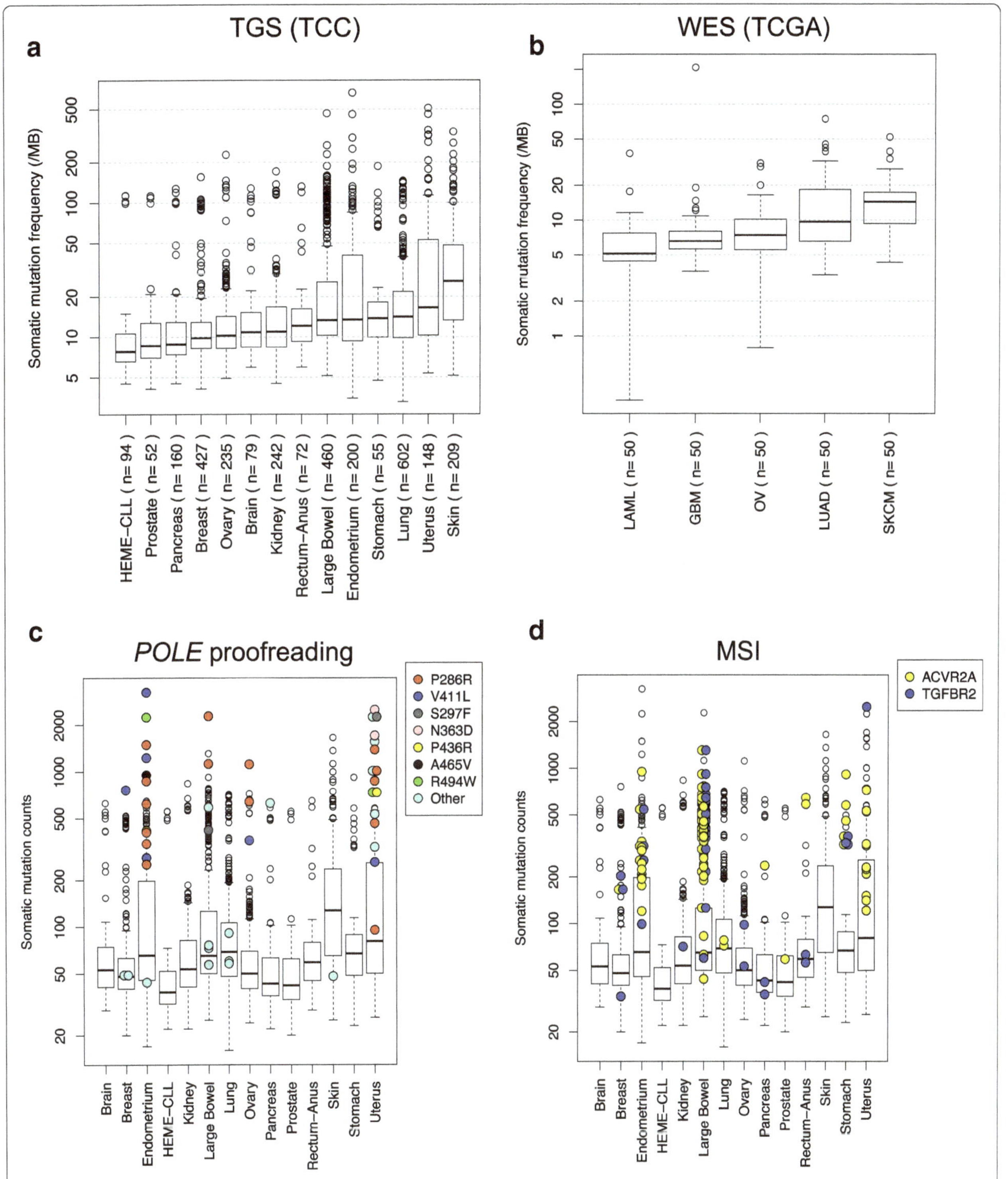

Fig. 4 Somatic mutation rates across different tissue types using the tumor-only method. Boxplot of mutation rates for tissue sites of origin in **a** TGS (sites with more than 50 samples, a total of 3035 samples) and **b** WES. **c** The colored dots identify the samples with the indicated *POLE* exonuclease domain mutation. **d** Homopolymer run mutations (the presence of *ACVR2A* and *TGFBR2* mutations side by side infers MSI status). The *y*-axes are in a log scale

a few variants (Additional file 3: Figure S3). While population databases are helpful in removing inherited variants, they often include overlapping samples and can contain known somatic mutations even when cancer samples have been removed. Therefore, investigators should review population datasets carefully before using them as a filter.

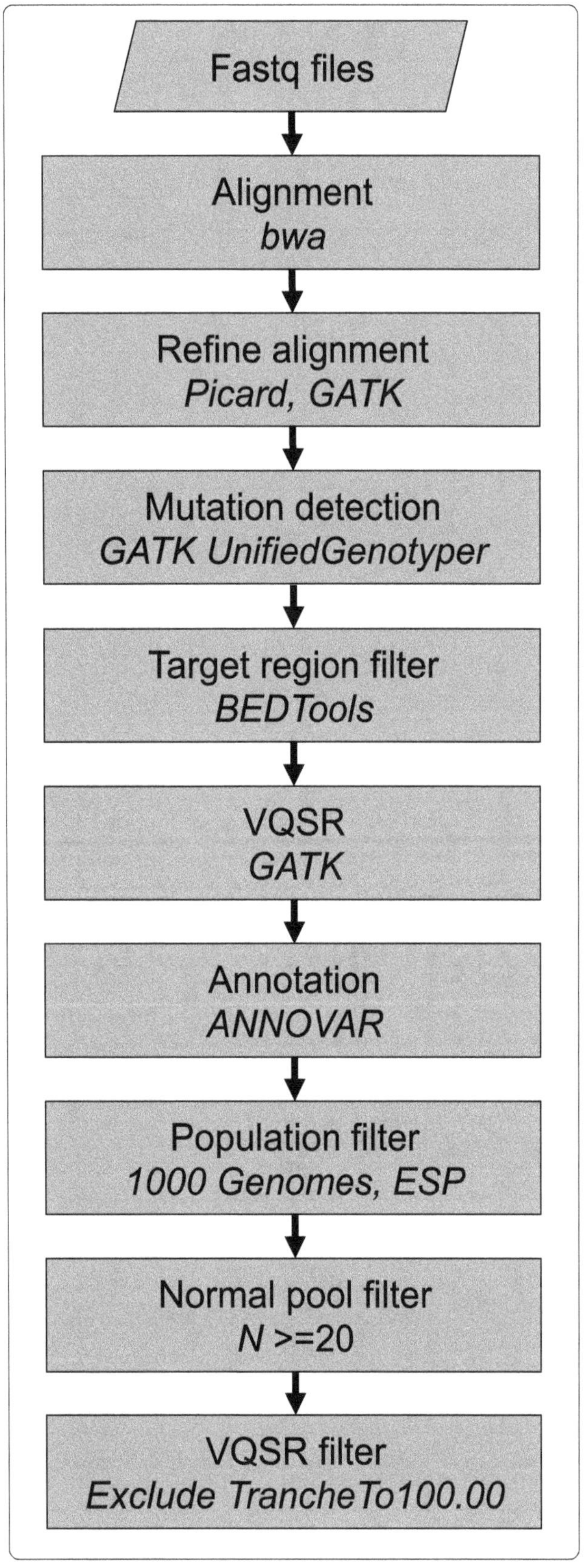

Fig. 5 Schematic of tumor-only mutation calling pipeline. Analytical pipeline overview for tumor mutation calling with a subset of matched normal samples. See Additional file 5 for details of commands, options, and settings

We demonstrated and quantitated the utility of excluding variants observed in a subset pool of normal samples to enrich for somatic mutations. Arbitrary normal pool variant frequency cutoffs of ≥ 5 and ≥ 1% were selected to ensure that known cancer mutations were not erroneously removed. Setting a normal pool allele frequency threshold is important: we observed common cancer mutations (*BRAF* V600E, *PTEN* truncation, *TP53* G245C) in a single normal sample each (TGS cohort). The TGS normal samples were the adjacent normal tissue from surgical resections, which may have contained infiltrating tumor cells. This risk is lessened with peripheral blood normal samples, but observations of circulating tumor cells or cell-free tumor DNA (reviewed in [27]) suggest that a normal pool allele frequency cutoff should be used to avoid false negatives. We also recommend examining the normal sample variants for any well-known cancer mutations to avoid erroneous exclusion. Although we describe mutation detection in tumors without matched normal samples as "tumor-only," the pool of normal samples is very important for reducing false positive variants and should be included in experimental design.

We observed a relatively small difference in the number of putative mutations removed using differently sized normal sample pools. Indeed, as few as 20 to 25 normal samples may be used to effectively remove many potential artifacts from a large tumor sequencing dataset. We also found that it was important to identify variants using GATK multi-sample genotype detection on the combined set of tumor and normal samples. Our final results show that more putative mutations were detected compared to that in three tumor/normal comparison methods. When compared to MuTect, a commonly used tumor/normal method, GATK tumor-only mutation detection, showed similar sensitivity/recall to tumor/normal methods. However, precision was much lower. Many of these "mutations" are likely to be very rare inherited variants that could only be removed by direct tumor/normal comparison, although future method improvements and larger population variant databases may improve precision. Interestingly, the overlap of calls among precise tumor/normal mutation detection was also imperfect, highlighting the challenge of somatic mutation detection in heterogeneous tumor samples. Although numerous filters were applied to increase mutation specificity, tumor-only sensitivity to detect known mutations was equivalent to tumor/normal pair mutation detection. Comparison with manually reviewed capillary sequencing data demonstrated high tumor-only sensitivity (down to 10% mutant allele frequency) in heterogeneous tumor samples. Therefore, tumor-only sequencing supplemented with a normal pool is an effective alternative to paired tumor/normal sequencing, with similar recall but reduced precision.

Recently, Jones et al. [11] described tumor-only sequencing in 58 targeted samples (111 genes) and 100 whole exomes. We have extended their observations by examining 3380 TGS samples (1321 genes) and 250 WES samples (drawn from 5 diseases included in TCGA). Our observations of high sensitivity for known mutations, but lower precision (especially in WES), agree with those of Jones et al.. We have additionally demonstrated significant non-overlap between three different matched tumor/normal methods. This suggests differences between tumor-only and tumor/normal methods may be due to inaccuracies in both analysis strategies. While Jones et al. conclude tumor-only methods may not be sufficient for high accuracy in the clinical setting, we find the high degree of sensitivity may be useful for tumor classification. Finally, we offer detailed methods to enable others to utilize tumor-only mutation detection.

The observed recall and precision of the tumor-only approach with a limited normal pool suggests that this method lends itself to specific use cases. It has been suggested [25] that there are still many cancer genes and mutations to be discovered, requiring sequencing of many more samples. Although the tumor-only approach results in almost half the cost to reach a target sample size (as each tumor no longer needs a matched normal sample), our analysis demonstrated much lower precision that would result in many more false positive mutations. We conclude that tumor-only approaches are not appropriate for novel mutation detection. However, given similar sensitivity to detect known cancer mutations in heterogeneous tumor samples with greatly reduced cost, the tumor-only detection method can be useful for characterization of known mutations. Indeed, we reproduced earlier observations of mutation rate patterns across diseases. We also identified mutations in the exonuclease domain of *POLE* and mutations associated with MSI as two mechanisms explaining highly mutated samples. MSI mutations were observed in large bowel but also occasionally in endometrium and stomach tumors. *POLE* mutations were observed in many tumor types: endometrium/uterus, large bowel, ovary, pancreas, and breast. Sample classification by known recurrent mutations enables the critical next step in cancer genomics: association of genomic alterations with clinical phenotype. The almost doubling of sample size at a given cost gained from omitting matched normal samples can dramatically improve power to associate mutations with phenotype, but researchers must consider the loss of precision that results when matched normal samples are not used.

Conclusions

Detection of somatic mutations using tumor samples and a smaller subset of normal samples is a valid strategy for cancer genomics studies. The use of population datasets (1000 Genomes) reduces the number of inherited variants and artifacts. However, filtering against a pool of normal samples captured and sequenced with the same technology increases precision noticeably and should be considered a required part of a "tumor-only" sequencing experiment. We find that recall across all observed mutations is similar to matched tumor/normal methods, and sensitivity for known cancer mutations is equivalent. However, the precision is lower: many putative mutations detected by the tumor-only method are not observed in matched tumor/normal methods. Therefore, tumor-only detection methods as described here are appropriate for characterization of known mutations in samples. Matched tumor/normal mutation detection is more appropriate for applications requiring high precision such as novel mutation detection and mutation signature analysis and remains the optimal approach, especially as sequencing costs continue to decrease.

Additional files

Additional file 1: Table S1. Sample counts by the site of tumor origin.

Additional file 2: Table S2. List of 1321 targeted genes.

Additional file 3: Figure S1. Large tumor dataset quality control metrics. A. Principal component analysis and B. loadings using sequencing metrics. Colors in A. represent the different tissue sites of origin. C. Ratio of sequence reads aligning to the X and Y chromosome and cutoffs used to infer gender. D. Histogram of average coverage over targeted bases (filtered, aligned reads). **Figure S2:** VQSR filtering effects on tumor-only mutation detection. A. Fraction of total putative TGS mutations falling in each GATK VQSR tranche (PASS being the most specific, SNPto100 being the least specific). B. Fraction of TGS mutations seen in COSMIC more than five times falling into each VQSR tranche. C. Fraction of total putative WES mutations falling in each GATK VQSR tranche (PASS being most specific, SNPto100 being least specific). D. Fraction of WES mutations seen in COSMIC more than five times falling into each VQSR tranche. **Figure S3:** Mutation counts after filtering with additional population databases. Boxplots showing numbers of mutations detected after filtering with KAVIAR, ExAC, or both (excluding AF $\geq$ 1%) in addition to 1000 Genomes and ESP. The rightmost columns show the minimal effect of filtering with KAVIAR and ExAC after the normal filter has been applied. A. TGS cohort, B. WES cohort. Median counts are indicated by the dark line in the middle of the box. The bottom and top of the box are the first and third quartiles, respectively. The whiskers represent the most extreme points within 1.5 times the interquartile range. The *y*-axes are in the log scale. **Figure S4:** Normal pool features affect the ability to remove variants. Boxplots showing the putative mutation counts after filtering with titrated sample counts in the normal pool for A. TGS cohort, B. WES cohort. **Figure S5:** Total nonref counts, precision, and recall with subsequent filters. Total nonref counts (left), precision compare to MuTect (middle), and recall compared to MuTect (right) for A. TGS and B. WES. All plots are in a linear scale. **Figure S6:** Precision-recall curve. Plot showing approximate precision vs recall for A. TGS and B. WES. Data point circles are area-proportional to the number of putative mutations at each filter level. Note the largest circle across the middle of the plots corresponds to precision = 0, recall = 1. Also note that data point circle sizes are scaled to fit, and the scaling factors are different for TGS and WES. The red line indicates performance of the random classifier based on positives (median number of MuTect call)/total positions (targeted bases). **Figure S7:** Overlap between mutation calls across four methods. Non-area-proportional Venn diagram showing median mutation counts across samples called by each combination of methods. The bold underlined values are the intersection of all the four methods. The underlined values are the counts unique to each method. A. TGS (TCC) cohort and B. WES (TCGA) cohort. **Figure S8:** Overlap between mutation calls across three matched tumor/normal methods. Non-area-proportional Venn diagram showing median mutation counts across samples called by each combination of methods. The bold underlined values are the intersection of all the three methods. The underlined values are the counts unique to each method. A. TGS (TCC) cohort and B. WES (TCGA) cohort.

Additional file 4: Table S3. List of TCGA samples used.

Additional file 5: Methods: A detailed description of the analysis methods used for the detection of somatic mutations with an unmatched pool of normal samples.

Acknowledgements
We thank the many patients who provided the data and tissue to the Total Cancer Care Consortium. Our study received valuable assistance from the Cancer Informatics Core and Collaborative Data Services Core at the H. Lee Moffitt Cancer Center & Research Institute, an NCI-designated Comprehensive Cancer Center, supported under the NIH grant P30-CA76292.

Funding
Total Cancer Care® is enabled, in part, by the generous support of the DeBartolo Family. This study was supported, in part, by the NIH grant P30-CA76292. The sequence data was generated in partnership with Merck & Co.

Authors' contributions
JKT, YZ, SAE, and AEB designed the experiments; JKT, YZ, LC, EAW, and WDC analyzed the data; and JKT, SAE, and AEB wrote and edited the manuscript. All authors read and approved the final manuscript.

Consent for publication
Not applicable

Competing interests
The authors declare that they have no competing interests.

Author details
[1]Department of Biostatistics and Bioinformatics, H. Lee Moffitt Cancer Center and Research Institute, Tampa, FL 33612, USA. [2]Department of Molecular Oncology, H. Lee Moffitt Cancer Center and Research Institute, Tampa, FL 33612, USA.

References
1. Stratton MR, Campbell PJ, Futreal PA. The cancer genome. Nature. 2009;458:719–24.
2. Watson IR, Takahashi K, Futreal PA, Chin L. Emerging patterns of somatic mutations in cancer. Nat Rev Genet. 2013;14:703–18.
3. Koboldt DC, Chen K, Wylie T, Larson DE, McLellan MD, Mardis ER, Weinstock GM, Wilson RK, Ding L. VarScan: variant detection in massively parallel sequencing of individual and pooled samples. Bioinformatics. 2009;25:2283–5.
4. Koboldt DC, Zhang Q, Larson DE, Shen D, McLellan MD, Lin L, Miller CA, Mardis ER, Ding L, Wilson RK. VarScan 2: somatic mutation and copy number alteration discovery in cancer by exome sequencing. Genome Res. 2012;22:568–76.
5. Hansen NF, Gartner JJ, Mei L, Samuels Y, Mullikin JC. Shimmer: detection of genetic alterations in tumors using next-generation sequence data. Bioinformatics. 2013;29:1498–503.
6. Larson DE, Harris CC, Chen K, Koboldt DC, Abbott TE, Dooling DJ, Ley TJ, Mardis ER, Wilson RK, Ding L. SomaticSniper: identification of somatic point mutations in whole genome sequencing data. Bioinformatics. 2012;28:311–7.
7. Saunders CT, Wong WS, Swamy S, Becq J, Murray LJ, Cheetham RK. Strelka: accurate somatic small-variant calling from sequenced tumor-normal sample pairs. Bioinformatics. 2012;28:1811–7.
8. Cibulskis K, Lawrence MS, Carter SL, Sivachenko A, Jaffe D, Sougnez C, Gabriel S, Meyerson M, Lander ES, Getz G. Sensitive detection of somatic point mutations in impure and heterogeneous cancer samples. Nat Biotechnol. 2013;31:213–9.
9. Ewing AD, Houlahan KE, Hu Y, Ellrott K, Caloian C, Yamaguchi TN, Bare JC, P'ng C, Waggott D, Sabelnykova VY, et al. Combining tumor genome simulation with crowdsourcing to benchmark somatic single-nucleotide-variant detection. Nat Methods. 2015;12:623–30.
10. Kroigard AB, Thomassen M, Laenkholm AV, Kruse TA, Larsen MJ. Evaluation of nine somatic variant callers for detection of somatic mutations in exome and targeted deep sequencing data. PLoS One. 2016;11:e0151664.
11. Jones S, Anagnostou V, Lytle K, Parpart-Li S, Nesselbush M, Riley DR, Shukla M, Chesnick B, Kadan M, Papp E, et al. Personalized genomic analyses for cancer mutation discovery and interpretation. Sci Transl Med. 2015;7:283ra253.
12. Fenstermacher DA, Wenham RM, Rollison DE, Dalton WS. Implementing personalized medicine in a cancer center. Cancer J. 2011;17:528–36.
13. McKenna A, Hanna M, Banks E, Sivachenko A, Cibulskis K, Kernytsky A, Garimella K, Altshuler D, Gabriel S, Daly M, et al. The Genome Analysis Toolkit: a MapReduce framework for analyzing next-generation DNA sequencing data. Genome Res. 2010;20:1297–303.
14. DePristo MA, Banks E, Poplin R, Garimella KV, Maguire JR, Hartl C, Philippakis AA, del Angel G, Rivas MA, Hanna M, et al. A framework for variation discovery and genotyping using next-generation DNA sequencing data. Nat Genet. 2011;43:491–8.
15. Li H, Durbin R. Fast and accurate short read alignment with Burrows-Wheeler transform. Bioinformatics. 2009;25:1754–60.
16. Wang K, Li M, Hakonarson H. ANNOVAR: functional annotation of genetic variants from high-throughput sequencing data. Nucleic Acids Res. 2010;38:e164.
17. Abecasis GR, Auton A, Brooks LD, DePristo MA, Durbin RM, Handsaker RE, Kang HM, Marth GT, McVean GA. An integrated map of genetic variation from 1,092 human genomes. Nature. 2012;491:56–65.
18. Forbes SA, Bhamra G, Bamford S, Dawson E, Kok C, Clements J, Menzies A, Teague JW, Futreal PA, Stratton MR. The Catalogue of Somatic Mutations in Cancer (COSMIC). Curr Protoc Hum Genet. 2008; Chapter 10:Unit 10 11.
19. Quinlan AR, Hall IM. BEDTools: a flexible suite of utilities for comparing genomic features. Bioinformatics. 2010;26:841–2.
20. Durbin RM, Abecasis GR, Altshuler DL, Auton A, Brooks LD, Gibbs RA, Hurles ME, McVean GA. A map of human genome variation from population-scale sequencing. Nature. 2010;467:1061–73.
21. Lek M, Karczewski KJ, Minikel EV, Samocha KE, Banks E, Fennell T, O'Donnell-Luria AH, Ware JS, Hill AJ, Cummings BB, et al. Analysis of protein-coding genetic variation in 60,706 humans. Nature. 2016;536:285–91.
22. Glusman G, Caballero J, Mauldin DE, Hood L, Roach JC. Kaviar: an accessible system for testing SNV novelty. Bioinformatics. 2011;27:3216–7.
23. Ng SB, Buckingham KJ, Lee C, Bigham AW, Tabor HK, Dent KM, Huff CD, Shannon PT, Jabs EW, Nickerson DA, et al. Exome sequencing identifies the cause of a mendelian disorder. Nat Genet. 2010;42:30–5.
24. Church DM, Schneider VA, Graves T, Auger K, Cunningham F, Bouk N, Chen HC, Agarwala R, McLaren WM, Ritchie GR, et al. Modernizing reference genome assemblies. PLoS Biol. 2011;9:e1001091.
25. Lawrence MS, Stojanov P, Mermel CH, Robinson JT, Garraway LA, Golub TR, Meyerson M, Gabriel SB, Lander ES, Getz G. Discovery and saturation analysis of cancer genes across 21 tumour types. Nature. 2014;505:495–501.

15

Update on the Kelch-like (KLHL) gene family

Bajinder S Dhanoa[1], Tiziana Cogliati[2], Akhila G Satish[2], Elspeth A Bruford[3] and James S Friedman[1*]

Abstract

The Kelch-like (KLHL) gene family encodes a group of proteins that generally possess a BTB/POZ domain, a BACK domain, and five to six Kelch motifs. BTB domains facilitate protein binding and dimerization. The BACK domain has no known function yet is of functional importance since mutations in this domain are associated with disease. Kelch domains form a tertiary structure of β-propellers that have a role in extracellular functions, morphology, and binding to other proteins. Presently, 42 KLHL genes have been classified by the HUGO Gene Nomenclature Committee (HGNC), and they are found across multiple human chromosomes. The KLHL family is conserved throughout evolution. Phylogenetic analysis of KLHL family members suggests that it can be subdivided into three subgroups with KLHL11 as the oldest member and KLHL9 as the youngest. Several KLHL proteins bind to the E3 ligase cullin 3 and are known to be involved in ubiquitination. KLHL genes are responsible for several Mendelian diseases and have been associated with cancer. Further investigation of this family of proteins will likely provide valuable insights into basic biology and human disease.

Keywords: KLHL, Kelch domain, BTB domain, Ubiquitination, Gene family, Evolution, Mendelian disease, Gene nomenclature, Cancer

Introduction

The KLHL (Kelch-like) gene family encodes proteins that constitute a subgroup at the intersection between the BTB/POZ domain and Kelch domain superfamilies. First identified in the vaccinia virus [1], the BTB motif was named based on a homologous domain of 115 amino acids in *Drosophila melanogaster* bric à brac 1, tramtrack, and broad-complex proteins (BTB) [2]. BTB domain-containing zinc finger proteins are conserved evolutionarily from *Drosophila* to humans and mice with more than 49 family members in the latter two [3]. The POZ domain was initially named after the 120 amino acid motifs present at the amino terminus in poxvirus proteins and zinc finger proteins [4]. The BTB/POZ domain facilitates protein binding [5] as reviewed in Perez-Torrado et al. [6]. Functions observed to be associated with other BTB-containing proteins involve a variety of cellular mechanisms such as control of cytoskeletal organization [7], ion channel gating [8], transcription suppression [9], and protein targeting for ubiquitination through cullin E3 ligases [10,11].

* Correspondence: james.friedman@ucdenver.edu
[1]Department of Ophthalmology, University of Colorado School of Medicine, Aurora, CO 80045, USA

The Kelch repeat or domain is also an evolutionarily conserved structure that can be found from *Drosophila melanogaster* to *Homo sapiens* [12]. Based on sequence identity, it has been suggested that each four-stranded β-sheet of the Kelch motif forms one blade of a β-propeller structure [12]. The Kelch superfamily of proteins can be subdivided into five groups. These subgroups include (1) N-propeller, C-dimer proteins, (2) N-propeller proteins, (3) propeller proteins, (4) N-dimer, C-propeller proteins, and (5) C-propeller proteins [12]. Kelch-containing proteins have roles in extracellular communication/interaction, cell morphology, gene expression, actin binding, and can be co-opted by virus post-infection [12]. KLHL family members belong to the N-dimer, C-propeller subclass of Kelch repeat proteins.

In addition to BTB/POZ and Kelch domains, the KLHL family members contain a BACK domain, first described as a 130-residue region of conservation observed amongst BTB-Kelch proteins [13]. Although no function has been assigned to the BACK domain, it is likely to be of functional significance because mutations in this region have been shown to cause human disease [14-19].

The BTB superfamily includes KLHL, KBTBD, and KLHDC subfamilies, which encompass structurally related molecules that differ in the types and numbers of their protein domains. In general, KLHL proteins contain one BTB/POZ domain, one BACK domain, and five to six Kelch motifs (BTB, BACK, 5/6 Kelch). KBTBD proteins have one BTB/POZ domain, occasionally a BACK domain, and two to four Kelch motifs (BTB/POZ, (BACK), 2/4 Kelch). Most KLHDC family members contain only three to seven Kelch motifs and usually do not have BTB or BACK domains (3/7 Kelch). Herein, we describe the evolutionary structure of the human KLHL family, discuss examples of KLHL family member biology, and present an overview of KLHL protein relationship to human disease.

Evolutionary structure of the human KLHL family

There are nine KBTBD genes in the human genome, and their encoded proteins typically possess a BTB and BACK domain and two to four Kelch motifs. Ten KLHDC genes have been defined by the HUGO Gene Nomenclature Committee (HGNC) in the human genome. KLHDC proteins generally do not have BTB or BACK domains and have three to seven Kelch motifs. These subfamilies will not be discussed further in this review.

KLHL proteins generally have a BTB/POZ domain, a BACK domain, and five to six Kelch domains. However, the domain composition for this family can appear to vary depending on the protein domain prediction program used to examine their protein sequences. The KLHL family protein structure is shown in Figure 1. It should be noted that KLHL29, KLHL31, KLHL40, and KLHL41 were previously assigned within the KBTBD family and were listed as KBTBD1 (KLHL31), KBTBD5 (KLHL40), KBTBD9 (KLHL29), and KBTBD10 (KLHL41). When these genes were originally named, they appeared to encode less than the five to six Kelch domains in the standard KLHL (BTB, BACK, 5/6 Kelch) structure. Therefore, they were classified as part of the KBTBD family; however, reannotation has shown that these genes do encode 5/6 Kelch domains. Likewise, the reannotation of KLHDC5 (KLHL42) has shown that it encodes the standard KLHL (BTB, BACK, 5/6 Kelch) structure. Consequently, they have since been placed within the KLHL family.

The HGNC presently defines 42 KLHL genes. They are spread over different chromosomes, though several are located on chromosomes 1, 4, and X (Additional file 1). The number of exons is not conserved and ranges from a single coding exon to 15 coding exons. However the number of KLHL genes is conserved between mammalian species (e.g., *Homo sapiens* and *Mus musculus*). ClustalO and phylogenetic analyses of KLHL family members suggest that they can be subdivided into multiple subgroups (Figure 2). KLHL11 appears the oldest to diverge, followed by KLHL42 and KLHL16. The most recent divergences appear to have happened for KLHL9 and KLHL13, followed by KLHL25 and KLHL37 (Figure 2).

Examples of KLHL family members

KEAP1 (KLHL19)

The *KEAP1* gene is clearly a member of the KLHL family. While the well-used KEAP1 symbol has been retained as the official gene nomenclature; it has also been assigned the KLHL19 synonym to clearly group it within the KLHL family. The human *KEAP1* (Kelch-like ECH-associated protein 1 gene is located on chromosome 19p13, and the mouse ortholog is located on chromosome 9. KEAP1 was originally identified as a nuclear factor erythroid 2-related factor 2 (NRF2) interacting protein. NRF2 is a transcription factor that is essential for the cellular reaction to electrophiles and binds to the antioxidant response element (ARE) present in promoters of genes involved in phase II detoxifying and oxidative stress enzyme response [24]. KEAP1 was shown to negatively control NRF2 transactivation potential [25]. Some of the genes controlled by NRF2 are important for cellular defense against harmful oxidative stresses that could result in carcinogenesis (as reviewed in Motohashi and Yamamoto [26]). NRF2 interacts as a heterodimer with Maf transcription factor protein that binds to the ARE and activates transcription through the Maf recognition element (MARE) (reviewed in Motohashi and Yamamoto [26]).

KEAP1's ability to repress NRF2's downstream target activation was demonstrated in zebrafish by gain-of-function and loss-of-function experiments in which transcriptional control by NRF2 of glutathione S-transferase gene (*gstp*) induction was tested in the absence and presence of KEAP1. NRF2-induced *gstp* expression was repressed when KEAP1 was also overexpressed [27]. KEAP1 was found to promote NRF2 degradation by targeting it for ubiquitination through the cullin 3 ligase complex [28,29], thus preventing NRF2 activity under normal cellular conditions [30]. Domain function analysis of KEAP1 revealed that NRF2 degradation requires both BTB and intervening domains [28].

KEAP1 is localized primarily in the cytoplasm of cells, with a minimal amount in the nucleus and endoplasmic reticulum [31]. KEAP1 scaffolding to the actin skeleton is crucial for effective sequestering of NRF2 into the cytoplasm [7]. Electrophiles promote the nuclear accumulation of NRF2 without altering the subcellular localization of KEAP1 [31]. Furthermore, KEAP1 appears to regulate both translational and post-translational responses to oxidative stress [32,33].

The crystal structure of mouse KEAP1 was resolved to reveal a six-bladed propeller tertiary structure encompassing the Kelch domain [34]. The analysis showed which bonds are needed for structural integrity and proper association between KEAP1 and NRF2 [34]. NRF2 has been suggested to be involved in susceptibility of lungs to cigarette smoke through the induction of antioxidant genes [35]. KEAP1's relationship with cancer is described below.

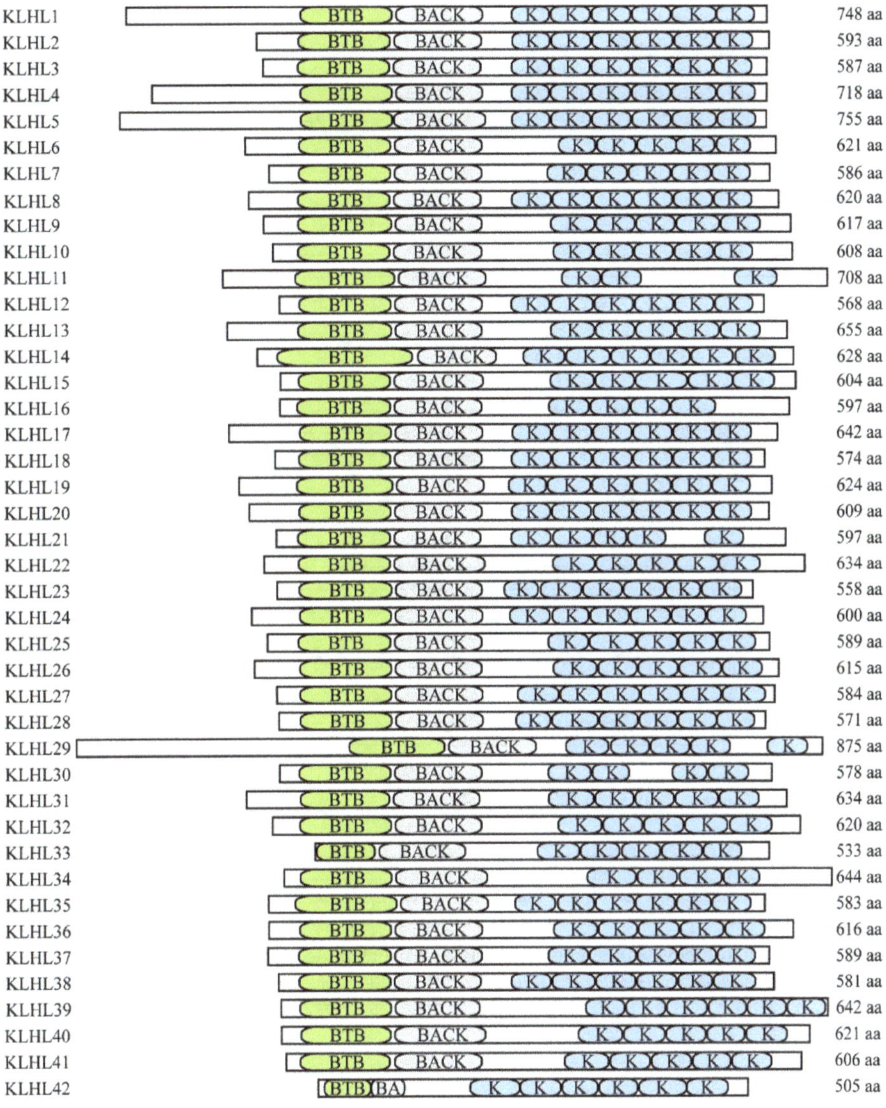

Figure 1 Schematic diagram of KLHL family members drawn to scale with amino acid numbers listed on the right. 'BTB,' 'BACK,' and 'K' indicate the BTB domain, BACK domain, and Kelch domains, respectively. In case of multiple isoforms, only the first one is depicted. Data was collected from [20] using a motif scan with Pfam HMMs (global or local models).

KLHL2 (Mayven)

KLHL2/Mayven is an actin-binding protein that shares 63% identity (77% similarity) with the *Drosophila* ring canal (Kelch) protein [36]. The human gene is localized on chromosome 4q21.1, and its murine ortholog is on chromosome 8 [36]. *KLHL2* RNA can be detected in developing and adult brain, heart, spleen, lung and liver, and adult kidney but most predominantly throughout the brain including the hippocampus, caudate nucleus, corpus callosum, and amygdala [36]. The KLHL2 protein has been shown to be constitutively expressed in developing and mature oligodendrocytes and neurons where it binds directly to F-actin through its Kelch repeats and plays an important role in the organization of the actin cytoskeleton [36,37]. In developing oligodendrocytes, KLHL2 is upregulated during differentiation [38], and it localizes to lamellipodia (but not filipodia) [39]. KLHL2 overexpression in oligodendrocyte progenitors accelerates neurite outgrowth and leads to longer processes. Conversely, downregulation inhibits process extension [37,38]. KLHL2 co-localizes and associates with FYN oncogene related to SRC, FGR, and YES (FYN) tyrosine kinase through its SH3-binding domain at the N-terminus. This interaction increases upon differentiation, suggesting a role in promoting oligodendrocyte process outgrowth and strengthening of the initial axonal-glial contact mediated by FYN signaling. Based on the type of interaction, it has been suggested that KLHL2 acts as a linker between FYN and actin [38]. Upon depolarization of primary hippocampal neurons with KCl, association of KLHL with actin is enhanced, resulting

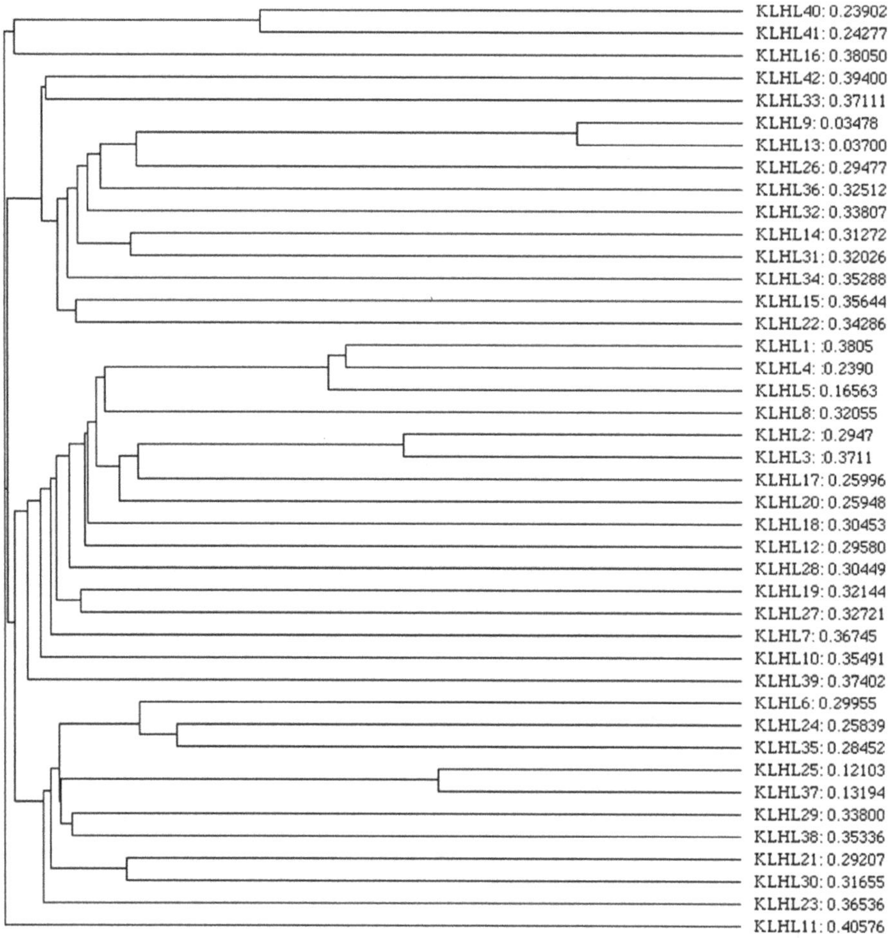

Figure 2 Phylogenetic tree of KLHL proteins with evolutionary distances shown next to each protein. Amino acid sequences were obtained from [21], and the alignment was created with ClustalO from [22]. The Cladogram was created using ClustalW2-Phylogeny from [23].

in re-distribution and translocation along the axonal processes [36]. The functional significance of these findings needs further investigation.

Recently, independent interactions with two different proteins have underscored KLHL2 involvement in ubiquitination. KLHL2 binds to nucleus accumbens-associated 1 (NACC1), a transcriptional repressor protein that interacts also with another KLHL family member, ectodermal-neural cortex 1 (ENC1/KLHL37). KLHL2 may form part of the ubiquitin complex through which NACC1 affects degradation of specific gene products and promotes proteasome activity and trafficking [40]. Finally, interactions of KLHL2 have been shown with neuronal pentraxin with chromo domain (NPCD, encoded by the *Npcd* gene in mouse which is a read-through between *Cbx6* and *Nptxr*) and with cullin 3. In this case, KLHL2 appears to function as a specific adapter for NPCD ubiquitination via cullin 3. Notably, overexpression of NPCD in hippocampal neurons leads to apoptosis [41].

KLHL family members and inherited disease

KLHL members associated with inherited forms of human disease include KLHL3, KLHL7, KLHL9, KLHL12, and GAN (KLHL16). Mutations in *KLHL3* have been identified in patients with familial hyperkalemic hypertension. Molecular analyses have shown that most mutations increase the activity of the Na^+Cl^- symporter in the distal convoluted tubule portion of the nephron. The increased activity causes more Na^+ and Cl^- reabsorption, increasing blood pressure and culminating in hypertension. Although mutations were identified in this familial disease, screening for single nucleotide polymorphisms (SNPs) in *KLHL3* did not reveal any significant association with blood pressure measurements in human subjects, indicating that common variants are not responsible for variations in blood pressure [19].

Patients with autosomal dominant retinitis pigmentosa (adRP), a neurodegenerative disease that leads to loss of rod and cone photoreceptors, carry mutations in *KLHL7*

[18]. Early and often rapid alteration of rod function is a characteristic of the classic form of adRP, but the phenotype observed in the *KLHL7* patients differs because of its late onset and preserved rod function in older family members [42,43]. Recent work suggests that KLHL7 protein binds to cullin 3 and that a single mutation in the BACK domain leads to reduced efficiency of cullin 3's ubiquitin ligase activity [44]. KLHL7 and KLHL12 have also been identified as autoantigens in Sjögren's syndrome, an autoimmune disease that causes damage to the salivary and lachrymal glands [45]. No significant immunological response to either KLHL7 or KLHL12 was observed in the sera of healthy individuals [45].

A missense mutation in *KLHL9* leads to the development of distal myopathy in human patients. Distal myopathy is a degenerative disease that initially causes atrophy of distal limb muscles and subsequently extends to proximal limbs [46]. Mutations in GAN (KLHL16), or gigaxonin, are linked to human giant axonal neuropathy, an autosomal recessive disorder [14]. Giant axonal neuropathy affects the central and peripheral nervous system that becomes populated with large, dysfunctional axons [16]. Compound heterozygous missense mutations in the Kelch-coding region of gigaxonin have recently been reported in Chinese cases [47].

KLHL family members and cancer

Four KLHL family members are associated with cancer: KLHL6, KEAP1 (KLHL19), KLHL20, and ENC1 (KLHL37). Mutations in *KLHL6* are recurrent in cases of chronic lymphocytic leukemia (CLL), a type of leukemia that is predominant in adults. Six mutations were identified within *KLHL6* in CLL patients, and all disrupt KLHL6 function in germinal center B cell formation [48,49]. Insertion, missense, frameshift, and missense mutations in *KEAP1* [17,35] have been identified in cancerous cells of the liver, gallbladder, and lung. Mutations that result in KEAP1 loss of function are thought to facilitate cancer cell expansion. Decreased KEAP1 expression releases the block on the transcriptional activity of NRF2, resulting in increased expression of oxidative stress enzymes and proteins that favor cancer cells survival and proliferation [33,50]. KLHL20 is an important KLHL family member related to cancer progression. KLHL20 is induced by HIF-1α protein and forms a KLHL20-cullin 3 complex that degrades the promyelocytic leukemia protein (PML) leading to prostate cancer progression [51]. Mutations in ENC1 (KLHL37), also called NRP/B, are associated with brain tumors. Mutations reported in KLHL37 are primarily located in the Kelch domain but also exist in the BTB and BACK domains [15]. KLHL37 protein is normally expressed in neurons but not in astrocytes; however, brain tumor cells that arise from astrocytes express KLHL37. It is hypothesized that mutated KLHL37 promotes cell growth, prevents apoptosis, and alters the cytoskeleton [15].

Conclusions

There are 42 KLHL family members encoded in the human genome, containing conserved BTB, BACK, and Kelch domains. KLHL proteins are known to be involved in the ubiquitination process, but the specific roles for each family member have not yet been elucidated. KLHL proteins will likely have multiple substrates. KEAP1 (KLHL19), for example, has at least three (NRF2, IKKβ and BCL-2) as reviewed in Tian et al. [52]. Similar protein motifs amongst substrates such as the ETGE region in NRF2 and IKKβ could be one way to explain how a KLHL protein can bind to more than one protein [52]. Another potential source of substrate diversity is possible through the BTB domain. BTB cross-dimerization between different KLHL proteins could theoretically allow for differential substrate binding depending on the spatial and temporal expression of KLHL proteins. Mutations in certain KLHL genes are detrimental and result in either Mendelian disease or human cancers. We anticipate that further studies will reveal that most, if not all, KLHL proteins have fundamental impacts on human biological processes and disease.

Competing interests
The authors declare that they have no competing interests.

Authors' contributions
BSD, TC, AGS, EAB, and JSF. drafted the manuscript. BSD, EAB, and JSF carried out sequence alignments and/or domain structure analyses. All authors read and approved the final manuscript.

Author details
[1]Department of Ophthalmology, University of Colorado School of Medicine, Aurora, CO 80045, USA. [2]Neurobiology-Neurodegeneration and Repair Laboratory (N-NRL), National Eye Institute, National Institutes of Health, Building 6/302, MSC 0610, 6 Center Drive, Bethesda, MD 20892, USA. [3]HUGO Gene Nomenclature Committee (HGNC), EMBL-EBI, Wellcome Trust Genome Campus, Hinxton, Cambridgeshire CB10 1SD, UK.

References

1. Koonin EV, Senkevich TG, Chernos VI: **A family of DNA virus genes that consists of fused portions of unrelated cellular genes.** *Trends Biochem Sci* 1992, **17**:213–214.
2. Zollman S, Godt D, Prive GG, Couderc JL, Laski FA: **The BTB domain, found primarily in zinc finger proteins, defines an evolutionarily conserved family that includes several developmentally regulated genes in Drosophila.** *Proc Natl Acad Sci USA* 1994, **91**:10717–10721.
3. Siggs OM, Beutler B: **The BTB-ZF transcription factors.** *Cell Cycle* 2012, **11**:3358–3369.

4. Bardwell VJ, Treisman R: **The POZ domain: a conserved protein-protein interaction motif.** *Genes Dev* 1994, **8:**1664–1677.
5. Albagli O, Dhordain P, Deweindt C, Lecocq G, Leprince D: **The BTB/POZ domain: a new protein-protein interaction motif common to DNA- and actin-binding proteins.** *Cell Growth Differ* 1995, **6:**1193–1198.
6. Perez-Torrado R, Yamada D, Defossez PA: **Born to bind: the BTB protein-protein interaction domain.** *Bioessays* 2006, **28:**1194–1202.
7. Kang MI, Kobayashi A, Wakabayashi N, Kim SG, Yamamoto M: **Scaffolding of Keap1 to the actin cytoskeleton controls the function of Nrf2 as key regulator of cytoprotective phase 2 genes.** *Proc Natl Acad Sci USA* 2004, **101:**2046–2051.
8. Minor DL, Lin YF, Mobley BC, Avelar A, Jan YN, Berger JM: **The polar T1 interface is linked to conformational changes that open the voltage-gated potassium channel.** *Cell* 2000, **102:**657–670.
9. Melnick A, Ahmad KF, Arai S, Polinger A, Ball H, Borden KL, Carlile GW, Prive GG, Licht JD: **In-depth mutational analysis of the promyelocytic leukemia zinc finger BTB/POZ domain reveals motifs and residues required for biological and transcriptional functions.** *Mol Cell Biol* 2000, **20:**6550–6567.
10. Furukawa M, He YJ, Borchers C, Xiong Y: **Targeting of protein ubiquitination by BTB-Cullin 3-Roc1 ubiquitin ligases.** *Nat Cell Biol* 2003, **5:**1001–1007.
11. Xu L, Wei Y, Reboul J, Vaglio P, Shin TH, Vidal M, Elledge SJ, Harper JW: **BTB proteins are substrate-specific adaptors in an SCF-like modular ubiquitin ligase containing CUL-3.** *Nature* 2003, **425:**316–321.
12. Adams J, Kelso R, Cooley L: **The kelch repeat superfamily of proteins: propellers of cell function.** *Trends Cell Biol* 2000, **10:**17–24.
13. Stogios PJ, Prive GG: **The BACK domain in BTB-kelch proteins.** *Trends Biochem Sci* 2004, **29:**634–637.
14. Bomont P, Cavalier L, Blondeau F, Ben Hamida C, Belal S, Tazir M, Demir E, Topaloglu H, Korinthenberg R, Tüysüz B, Landrieu P, Hentati F, Koenig M: **The gene encoding gigaxonin, a new member of the cytoskeletal BTB/kelch repeat family, is mutated in giant axonal neuropathy.** *Nat Genet* 2000, **26:**370–374.
15. Liang XQ, Avraham HK, Jiang S, Avraham S: **Genetic alterations of the NRP/B gene are associated with human brain tumors.** *Oncogene* 2004, **23:**5890–5900.
16. Yang Y, Allen E, Ding J, Wang W: **Giant axonal neuropathy.** *Cell Mol Life Sci: CMLS* 2007, **64:**601–609.
17. Shibata T, Kokubu A, Gotoh M, Ojima H, Ohta T, Yamamoto M, Hirohashi S: **Genetic alteration of Keap1 confers constitutive Nrf2 activation and resistance to chemotherapy in gallbladder cancer.** *Gastroenterology* 2008, **135:**1358–1368. 1368 e1351-1354.
18. Friedman JS, Ray JW, Waseem N, Johnson K, Brooks MJ, Hugosson T, Breuer D, Branham KE, Krauth DS, Bowne SJ, Sullivan LS, Ponjavic V, Gränse L, Khanna R, Trager EH, Gieser LM, Hughbanks-Wheaton D, Cojocaru RI, Ghiasvand NM, Chakarova CF, Abrahamson M, Göring HH, Webster AR, Birch DG, Abecasis GR, Fann Y, Bhattacharya SS, Daiger SP, Heckenlively JR, Andréasson S, *et al*: **Mutations in a BTB-Kelch protein, KLHL7, cause autosomal-dominant retinitis pigmentosa.** *Am J Hum Genet* 2009, **84:**792–800.
19. Louis-Dit-Picard H, Barc J, Trujillano D, Miserey-Lenkei S, Bouatia-Naji N, Pylypenko O, Beaurain G, Bonnefond A, Sand O, Simian C, Vidal-Petiot E, Soukaseum C, Mandet C, Broux F, Chabre O, Delahousse M, Esnault V, Fiquet B, Houillier P, Bagnis CI, Koenig J, Konrad M, Landais P, Mourani C, Niaudet P, Probst V, Thauvin C, Unwin RJ, Soroka SD, Ehret G, *et al*: **KLHL3 mutations cause familial hyperkalemic hypertension by impairing ion transport in the distal nephron.** *Nat Genet* 2012, **44:**456–460. S451-453.
20. **MyHits.** [http://myhits.isb-sib.ch]
21. **National Center for Biotechnology Information (NCBI).** [http://www.ncbi.nlm.nih.gov/protein]
22. **European Bioinformatics Institute (EBI).** [http:/www.ebi.ac.uk/Tools/msa/clustalo]
23. **Bioinformatics Services.** [http://www.ebi.ac.uk/Tools/phylogeny/clustalw2_phylogeny]
24. Itoh K, Chiba T, Takahashi S, Ishii T, Igarashi K, Katoh Y, Oyake T, Hayashi N, Satoh K, Hatayama I, Yamamoto M, Nabeshima Y: **An Nrf2/small Maf heterodimer mediates the induction of phase II detoxifying enzyme genes through antioxidant response elements.** *Biochem Biophys Res Commun* 1997, **236:**313–322.
25. Itoh K, Wakabayashi N, Katoh Y, Ishii T, Igarashi K, Engel JD, Yamamoto M: **Keap1 represses nuclear activation of antioxidant responsive elements by Nrf2 through binding to the amino-terminal Neh2 domain.** *Genes Dev* 1999, **13:**76–86.
26. Motohashi H, Yamamoto M: **Carcinogenesis and transcriptional regulation through Maf recognition elements.** *Cancer Sci* 2007, **98:**135–139.
27. Kobayashi M, Itoh K, Suzuki T, Osanai H, Nishikawa K, Katoh Y, Takagi Y, Yamamoto M: **Identification of the interactive interface and phylogenic conservation of the Nrf2-Keap1 system.** *Genes Cells* 2002, **7:**807–820.
28. Kobayashi A, Kang MI, Okawa H, Ohtsuji M, Zenke Y, Chiba T, Igarashi K, Yamamoto M: **Oxidative stress sensor Keap1 functions as an adaptor for Cul3-based E3 ligase to regulate proteasomal degradation of Nrf2.** *Mol Cell Biol* 2004, **24:**7130–7139.
29. Furukawa M, Xiong Y: **BTB protein Keap1 targets antioxidant transcription factor Nrf2 for ubiquitination by the Cullin 3-Roc1 ligase.** *Mol Cell Biol* 2005, **25:**162–171.
30. McMahon M, Itoh K, Yamamoto M, Hayes JD: **Keap1-dependent proteasomal degradation of transcription factor Nrf2 contributes to the negative regulation of antioxidant response element-driven gene expression.** *J Biol Chem* 2003, **278:**21592–21600.
31. Watai Y, Kobayashi A, Nagase H, Mizukami M, McEvoy J, Singer JD, Itoh K, Yamamoto M: **Subcellular localization and cytoplasmic complex status of endogenous Keap1.** *Genes Cells* 2007, **12:**1163–1178.
32. Lo SC, Hannink M: **PGAM5, a Bcl-XL-interacting protein, is a novel substrate for the redox-regulated Keap1-dependent ubiquitin ligase complex.** *J Biol Chem* 2006, **281:**37893–37903.
33. Mitsuishi Y, Motohashi H, Yamamoto M: **The Keap1-Nrf2 system in cancers: stress response and anabolic metabolism.** *Frontiers in oncology* 2012, **2:**200.
34. Padmanabhan B, Tong KI, Ohta T, Nakamura Y, Scharlock M, Ohtsuji M, Kang MI, Kobayashi A, Yokoyama S, Yamamoto M: **Structural basis for defects of Keap1 activity provoked by its point mutations in lung cancer.** *Mol Cell* 2006, **21:**689–700.
35. Singh A, Misra V, Thimmulappa RK, Lee H, Ames S, Hoque MO, Herman JG, Baylin SB, Sidransky D, Gabrielson E, Brock MV, Biswal S: **Dysfunctional KEAP1-NRF2 interaction in non-small-cell lung cancer.** *PLoS Med* 2006, **3:**e420.
36. Soltysik-Espanola M, Rogers RA, Jiang S, Kim TA, Gaedigk R, White RA, Avraham H, Avraham S: **Characterization of Mayven, a novel actin-binding protein predominantly expressed in brain.** *Mol Biol Cell* 1999, **10:**2361–2375.
37. Williams SK, Spence HJ, Rodgers RR, Ozanne BW, Fitzgerald U, Barnett SC: **Role of Mayven, a kelch-related protein in oligodendrocyte process formation.** *J Neurosci Res* 2005, **81:**622–631.
38. Jiang S, Avraham HK, Park SY, Kim TA, Bu X, Seng S, Avraham S: **Process elongation of oligodendrocytes is promoted by the Kelch-related actin-binding protein Mayven.** *J Neurochem* 2005, **92:**1191–1203.
39. Montague P, Kennedy PG, Barnett SC: **Subcellular localization of Mayven following expression of wild type and mutant EGFP tagged cDNAs.** *BMC Neurosci* 2010, **11:**63.
40. Korutla L, Wang P, Jackson TG, Mackler SA: **NAC1, a POZ/BTB protein that functions as a corepressor.** *Neurochem Int* 2009, **54:**245–252.
41. Tseng LA, Bixby JL: **Interaction of an intracellular pentraxin with a BTB-Kelch protein is associated with ubiquitylation, aggregation and neuronal apoptosis.** *Mol Cell Neurosci* 2011, **47:**254–264.
42. Hugosson T, Friedman JS, Ponjavic V, Abrahamson M, Swaroop A, Andréasson S: **Phenotype associated with mutation in the recently identified autosomal dominant retinitis pigmentosa KLHL7 gene.** *Arch Ophthalmol* 2010, **128:**772–778.
43. Wen Y, Locke KG, Klein M, Bowne SJ, Sullivan LS, Ray JW, Daiger SP, Birch DG, Hughbanks-Wheaton DK: **Phenotypic characterization of 3 families with autosomal dominant retinitis pigmentosa due to mutations in KLHL7.** *Arch Ophthalmol* 2011, **129:**1475–1482.
44. Kigoshi Y, Tsuruta F, Chiba T: **Ubiquitin ligase activity of Cul3-KLHL7 protein is attenuated by autosomal dominant retinitis pigmentosa causative mutation.** *J Biol Chem* 2011, **286:**33613–33621.
45. Uchida K, Akita Y, Matsuo K, Fujiwara S, Nakagawa A, Kazaoka Y, Hachiya H, Naganawa Y, Oh-Iwa I, Ohura K, Saga S, Kawai T, Matsumoto Y, Shimozato K, Kozaki K: **Identification of specific autoantigens in Sjogren's syndrome by SEREX.** *Immunology* 2005, **116:**53–63.
46. Cirak S, von Deimling F, Sachdev S, Errington WJ, Herrmann R, Bönnemann C, Brockmann K, Hinderlich S, Lindner TH, Steinbrecher A, Hoffmann K, Privé GG, Hannink M, Nürnberg P, Voit T: **Kelch-like homologue 9 mutation is associated with an early onset autosomal dominant distal myopathy.** *Brain* 2010, **133:**2123–2135.
47. Xu M, Da YW, Liu L, Wang F, Jia JP: **Giant axonal neuropathy caused by a novel compound heterozygous mutation in the gigaxonin gene.** *J Child Neurol* 2012. doi:10.1177/0883073812467688.

48. Kroll J, Shi X, Caprioli A, Liu HH, Waskow C, Lin KM, Miyazaki T, Rodewald HR, Sato TN: **The BTB-kelch protein KLHL6 is involved in B-lymphocyte antigen receptor signaling and germinal center formation.** *Mol Cell Biol* 2005, **25:**8531–8540.
49. Puente XS, Pinyol M, Quesada V, Conde L, Ordóñez GR, Villamor N, Escaramis G, Jares P, Beà S, González-Díaz M, Bassaganyas L, Baumann T, Juan M, López-Guerra M, Colomer D, Tubío JM, López C, Navarro A, Tornador C, Aymerich M, Rozman M, Hernández JM, Puente DA, Freije JM, Velasco G, Gutiérrez-Fernández A, Costa D, Carrió A, Guijarro S, Enjuanes A, *et al*: **Whole-genome sequencing identifies recurrent mutations in chronic lymphocytic leukaemia.** *Nature* 2011, **475:**101–105.
50. Ohta T, Iijima K, Miyamoto M, Nakahara I, Tanaka H, Ohtsuji M, Suzuki T, Kobayashi A, Yokota J, Sakiyama T, Shibata T, Yamamoto M, Hirohashi S: **Loss of Keap1 function activates Nrf2 and provides advantages for lung cancer cell growth.** *Cancer Res* 2008, **68:**1303–1309.
51. Yuan WC, Lee YR, Huang SF, Lin YM, Chen TY, Chung HC, Tsai CH, Chen HY, Chiang CT, Lai CK, Lu LT, Chen CH, Gu DL, Pu YS, Jou YS, Lu KP, Hsiao PW, Shih HM, Chen RH: **A Cullin3-KLHL20 Ubiquitin ligase-dependent pathway targets PML to potentiate HIF-1 signaling and prostate cancer progression.** *Cancer Cell* 2011, **20:**214–228.
52. Tian H, Zhang B, Di J, Jiang G, Chen F, Li H, Li L, Pei D, Zheng J: **Keap1: one stone kills three birds Nrf2, IKKbeta and Bcl-2/Bcl-xL.** *Cancer Lett* 2012, **325:**26–34.

16

An emerging role for microRNAs in NF1 tumorigenesis

Ashni Sedani, David N Cooper and Meena Upadhyaya*

Abstract

MicroRNAs (miRNAs) are a class of non-coding RNA, which have recently been shown to have a wide variety of regulatory functions in relation to gene expression. Since their identification nearly 20 years ago, miRNAs have been found to play an important role in cancer, including in neurofibromatosis type 1 (NF1)-associated tumours. NF1 is the most commonly inherited tumour predisposition syndrome and can lead to malignancy via the development of malignant peripheral nerve sheath tumours (MPNSTs). Although the mechanisms by which benign neurofibromas develop into MPNSTs still remain to be elucidated, it is becoming increasingly clear that miRNAs play a key role in this process and have the potential to be used as both diagnostic and prognostic markers of tumorigenesis.

Keywords: MicroRNAs, Neurofibromatosis type 1, Malignant peripheral nerve sheath tumours, Tumorigenesis

Introduction

miRNAs constitute a category of small RNAs, ranging between 19 and 25 nucleotides in length, which are generated from endogenous hairpin-shaped transcripts. They function predominantly as post-transcriptional regulators of gene expression by hybridizing to the 3′ untranslated regions (3′UTRs) of target mRNA molecules [1,2], leading to translational repression or cleavage of the target mRNA [3]. The first described miRNA, known as *lin-4*, was discovered in *Caenorhabditis elegans* by Lee et al. in 1993 [4]. This was later followed by the discovery of *let-7* [5], which was found to be highly conserved across many different species [6], indicating the widespread existence of miRNAs in eukaryotes. More than 1,500 human miRNA sequences have been reported in the human genome to date (miRBase; http://www.mirbase.org/), of which 50% have been found to occur within clusters, targeting either the same or different genes within the same biological pathway [7]. It has become apparent that miRNAs regulate the expression of at least 30% of all protein-coding genes in mammalian genomes [8], underlining their likely role in human genetic disease. Novel techniques developed for the identification of miRNAs have been instrumental in the rapid progress made by miRNA research. miRNAs play an important role in the development and progression of cancer. With an ever-increasing number of studies focusing on the roles of miRNAs in cancer, whether operating as oncogenes or tumour suppressor genes, our understanding of the way in which miRNAs function is steadily improving, and hence the number of potential therapeutic applications for miRNAs should also increase.

In this review, the structure, function and biogenesis of miRNA molecules are discussed in reference to the recent developments that focus upon the role of miRNAs in relation to neurofibromatosis type 1.

miRNA biogenesis, export and function

The process of miRNA biogenesis involves miRNA transcription, the transport of the miRNAs to the cytoplasm and subsequent maturation. miRNA biogenesis has been reviewed in detail by Ladomery et al. [9] and will not be specifically discussed here. However, the basic process has been summarised in Figure 1.

The mechanism by which mature miRNAs regulate gene expression depends upon the level of complementarity that exists between the miRNA and its target mRNA [17]. Gene silencing can be effected either by mRNA degradation or by inhibiting the mRNA from being translated. It has been shown that if there is complete complementarity between the miRNA and

* Correspondence: upadhyaya@cardiff.ac.uk
Institute of Medical Genetics, School of Medicine, Cardiff University, Heath Park, Cardiff CF14 4XN, UK

target mRNA sequence, then Argonaute 2, a member of the Argonaute protein family, can carry out strand selection and separation causing an RNA-induced silencing complex (RISC) to bind to its mRNA target, leading to mRNA degradation which in turn impacts upon translation [18]. If, however, the complementarity is imperfect, as seen in most cases, translational repression ensues [19]. Therefore, the main function of miRNAs appears to be in the context of gene regulation via mRNA degradation. Rarely, miRNAs can also bring about histone modification and DNA methylation of gene promoter regions, thereby indirectly altering the expression of target genes [20,21].

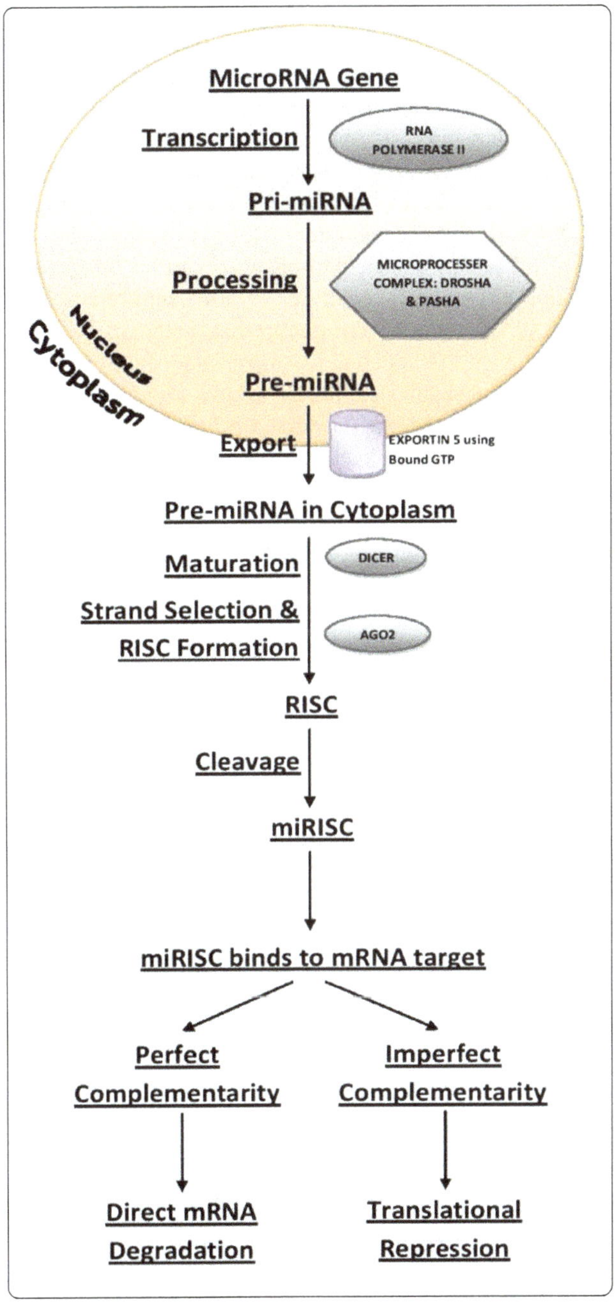

Figure 1 The flowchart highlights the processes involved in the following miRNA biogenesis: (1) The process begins inside the nucleus, where RNA polymerase II or III initiates the transcription of miRNA-coding genes to produce 'pri-microRNA's [10,11]. (2) A microprocessor complex comprising both Drosha, an RNase III class enzyme, and Pasha, identifies and cleaves pre-microRNAs generating pre-microRNAs [12-14]. (3) Pre-microRNA molecules are transferred to the cytoplasm through exportin-5-mediated transport, which uses GTP that is bound to the Ran protein. The function of exportin-5 is dependent upon the GTP-bound form of the Ran co-factor for specific binding to the corresponding substrates. Therefore, this process comprises the hydrolysis of Ran-GTP to Ran-GDP, via the Ran GTPase-activating protein in the cytoplasm [15,16]. (4) In the cytoplasm, Dicer acts to cleave pre-miRNA molecules and, with the action of Argonaute 2 which is required for miRNA-induced silencing, forms an RNA-induced silencing complex (RISC) leading to the creation of a miRNA-induced silencing complex (miRISC). (5) Interaction between the miRNA and its target mRNA in the miRISC can cause either translational repression or miRNA degradation depending upon the degree of complementarity.

Methodologies

miRNA expression profiles can be used both to categorize different types of cancer and to identify miRNA markers that can help in making prognostic predictions [22]. Initially, northern blotting was used to detect pre-miRNAs and mature miRNAs and to provide information about the regulation of the enzymes involved in miRNA biogenesis [23]. Real-time polymerase chain reaction (PCR) and microarray techniques have also been tailored to detect the expression of pre-miRNAs and mature miRNAs using either SYBR Green dye or TaqMan probes (Sigma-Aldrich Corporation, St. Louis, MO, USA) [24]. Further, Liu et al. in 2004 [25] used oligonucleotide microchips to identify distinct miRNA expression patterns in breast cancer and B cell chronic lymphocytic leukaemia. Nevertheless, miRNA microarray techniques are constantly being improved; thus, Neely et al. in 2006 [26] developed modified oligonucleotide arrays where probes for each miRNA were designed and labelled with different fluorophores whereas Lu et al. in 2005 [27] used a flow cytometry-based method analysis to demonstrate expression of miRNAs from a range of different samples. Both methods allowed the quantification of miRNA expression, thereby making cancer diagnosis through miRNA analysis more specific and accurate. The advantage of using miRNAs as markers instead of mRNAs lies in their ability to aid the classification of poorly differentiated cancers, as evidenced by the study by Rosenfeld et al. in 2008 [28], suggesting that miRNAs can be used to correctly identify the tumour tissue of origin.

The potential role of miRNAs in pathology has been studied by looking not only at their single nucleotide polymorphisms (SNPs) but also at their copy number variation (CNV). Functional polymorphisms in the 3′UTRs of miRNA genes have been reported to be associated with cancer by virtue of their altering gene expression. SNPs may occur in miRNA biogenesis pathway genes, primary miRNAs, pre-miRNAs or mature miRNA sequences and have the potential to affect the efficiency of miRNA binding to their target sites or alternatively can create or disrupt miRNA binding sites [29]. In a recent study, Gong et al. [30] identified 48 SNPs in human miRNA seed regions and a large number of SNPs in 3′UTRs with the potential to either disturb or create miRNA target interactions. They confirmed the loss-of-function and gain-of-function SNPs by luciferase assay.

Zhang et al. in 2006 [31] found that a large proportion of loci containing miRNA genes exhibited somatic copy number alterations and, amongst the three cancer types, they identified 41 miRNAs with copy number changes. These miRNA copy number changes also correlated with the levels of miRNA expression in these cancers. High frequency copy number changes were also noted in the genes encoding Dicer (*DICER1*) and Argonaute 2 (*EIF2C2*), both of which are required for miRNA biogenesis. These findings are compatible with the view that somatic miRNA copy number changes are common in cancer and could potentially account for at least a proportion of the miRNA deregulation found in many tumour types. Using bioinformatic tools, Marcinkowska et al. in 2011 [32] have demonstrated that miRNA loci are under-represented in highly polymorphic and well-validated CNV regions. Thus, CNV-miRNAs represent functional variants of potential importance for genotype/phenotype association studies.

miRNAs in neurofibromatosis type 1

Neurofibromatosis type 1 (NF1), a familial tumour predisposition syndrome, is characterised by the growth of benign and malignant tumours involving the peripheral and central nervous system. NF1 results from inactivating germline mutations of the *NF1* gene located at 17q11.2 [33]. Most NF1 patients develop multiple benign cutaneous neurofibromas, with approximately 30% to 50% of patients also developing larger plexiform neurofibromas. About 10% of patients eventually develop malignant peripheral nerve sheath tumours (MPNSTs), which are aggressive tumours that pose significant diagnostic and therapeutic challenges. Half of all MPNSTs diagnosed occur in association with NF1, with affected patients exhibiting a poor prognosis. With no effective treatment available, radical surgery and chemo and radiotherapy are required to reduce tumour recurrence and metastasis and prolong patient survival.

The process of MPNST pathogenesis is poorly understood owing to its complex histopathology and the underlying molecular mechanisms. Biallelic *NF1* gene inactivation is essential for tumour development. However, it is now known that additional molecular changes and the tumour micro-environment are associated with the progression of this type of tumour. There is currently no defined molecular signature for MPNST development. Constitutive activation of several critical cell signalling cascades also occurs in MPNSTs. Multidisciplinary collaborative efforts are clearly essential to fully decipher both the complex molecular basis of MPNST development and to define potential therapeutic targets.

A general characteristic of cancer cells is uncontrolled growth and, in many cases, miRNAs can either promote or suppress this growth. Previous investigations have shown that miRNAs have key functions in the development of cancer, in relation to a range of different cellular processes including cell differentiation, developmental control, neural development, cell proliferation, apoptosis [34,35] and organ development [3]. Thus, the role of a given miRNA in cancer pathogenesis can be categorised as being either of oncogene or tumour suppressor gene nature. Moreover, it is thought that >50% of miRNA-coding genes are located in cancer-associated genomic regions or in fragile sites [36]. It is now known that miRNAs are associated with a range of different cancers, including chronic leukaemias, acute leukaemias and myelodysplastic syndromes, lymphomas, multiple myeloma, hepatocellular carcinoma, breast, lung and colon cancer, amongst others.

Several research groups have studied the role of miRNA in NF1-associated malignancy. Here we focus on miRNAs miR-29c, miR-34a, miR-214, miR-10b, miR204 and miR-21 which have previously been directly implicated in NF1 tumorigenesis (summarized in Table 1).

miR-34a

One of the earliest studies of miRNAs in NF1 was carried out by Subramanian et al. [37]. Their genome-wide

Table 1 Functionally characterised miRNAs identified in NF1-MPNSTs

miRNA	Change in expression in MPNSTs	Tumour suppressor or oncogene role	Reference
miR-34a	Down-regulated	Tumour suppressor	[37]
miR-214	Over-expressed	Oncogene	[37]
miR-10b	Over-expressed	Oncogene	[37,38]
miR-29c	Down-regulated	Tumour suppressor	[39]
miR204	Down-regulated	Tumour suppressor	[40]
miRNA-21	Over-expressed	Oncogene	[41]

transcriptome analyses revealed that the development of malignancy from neurofibroma to MPNST correlates with the loss of expression of a number of genes rather than an increase in expression. This subsequently led to miRNA expression profiling which demonstrated the down-regulation of miR-34a in most MPNSTs as compared to neurofibromas. This loss of miR-34a could contribute to the development of malignancy. miR-34 is known to be a direct target of p53 in a variety of neoplasms including colorectal carcinoma and neuroblastoma in which lower levels of this miRNA are associated with the suppression of apoptosis. Forced expression of miR-34a in MPNST cell lines that are deficient in miR-34a leads to increased apoptosis whereas the forced expression of p53 in the same cell line results in a similar effect, indicating that the expression of p53 results in apoptosis through a mechanism involving miR-34a. The study of Subramanian et al. in 2010 also revealed an increase in the expression levels of a further nine miRNAs, following induced expression of p53 in MPNSTs. Interestingly, six of these (including miR-638, miR-373, miR-492, miR-126, miR-140 and miR-491), have been shown to be involved in promoting tumorigenic processes such as invasion, proliferation and metastasis.

Using a systems biology approach, Lee et al. [42] identified a regulatory network which involved the E2F family: E2F7/E2F8 in several cell cycle-related gene modules. miR-34a over-expression was found to lead to increased activity of E2F7/E2F8 transcription factors and cell cycle genes. These transcription factors are disproportionately associated with DNA damage repair, cell growth and development [42,43], and the altered expression levels of this family of transcription factors has been noted in cancerous cells [44], indicating that miR-34a could be a target for therapeutic intervention. As E2F transcription factors are involved in transcriptional regulation as well as in DNA repair and cell proliferation, it is possible that an alteration in the expression of activators and suppressors of E2F7 and E2F8 transcription may play a role in the development of MPNSTs. However, recent data by Presneau et al. [39] failed to confirm the work by Subramanian et al. [37] regarding miR-34a. This was deemed to be due either to differences in the methodologies used or to the use of different groups of patients based on differences in NF1 diagnostic criteria. Recent reports indicate that miR-34a has also been shown to act as a tumour suppressor through its dysregulation in a number of other carcinomas including glioblastoma multiforme tumours [45], breast cancer [46], head and neck squamous cell carcinoma [47] and osteosarcoma [48], suggesting that it could represent a significant gene target in cancer therapeutics.

miR-214

Subramanian et al. [37] identified miR-214 as having the highest expression level of all miRNAs screened in their study of NF1-MPNSTs. miR-214 had previously been shown to be expressed at an increased level in the blood of breast and ovarian cancer patients, indicating that it could be used as an indicator of malignancy [49,50]. Yang et al. [50] proposed that miR-214 induces cell survival and cisplatin resistance through targeting the 3′UTR of the *PTEN* gene, which leads to down-regulation of the PTEN protein and the activation of the Akt pathway, thereby promoting cell survival. More recently, Peng et al. [51] found that miR-214 can inhibit cancer cell proliferation and migration by targeting *GALNT7.* This is supported by data from Shih et al. [52], who showed that miR-214 down-regulation can contribute to tumour angiogenesis and is associated with increased tumour recurrence and a poor prognosis. In their study, Subramanian et al. [37] also identified a metastasis-promoting factor, *TWIST1*, as promoting expression of miR-214. *TWIST1* had previously been noted to increase metastasis in a number of different carcinomas, but its exact role in NF1 tumorigenesis has not yet been elucidated. Taken together with the above data, it is suggested that *TWIST1* may regulate miR-214 expression thereby contributing to tumorigenesis [53].

miR-10b

By inhibiting the expression of miR-10b in NF1-MPNSTs, Subramanian et al. [37] demonstrated decreased cell proliferation and migration, indicating an important function for miR-10b in the transformation of benign NF1-associated neurofibromas to MPNSTs. These workers also showed that the expression of miR-10b is considerably higher in NF1-MPNST cell lines, NF1-MPNST tumour tissues and primary Schwann cells by comparison with benign neurofibromas. This suggests that miR-10b could act as a biomarker to differentiate between NF1-MPNSTs and neurofibromas. miR-10b belongs to the miR-10 cluster of miRNAs and is highly conserved between different species. Its location within the Hox gene clusters suggests that it could share the same mechanisms of regulation as the Hox genes [54]. Supporting this notion that over-expressed miRNAs of the miR-10 family may play a role in cancer, miR-10b has also been found to be overexpressed in B cell chronic lymphocytic leukaemia [36] as well as in acute myeloid leukaemias associated with mutations in the *NPM1* gene [55].

miR-10b expression has also been shown as enhanced by increased expression of *TWIST1* in MPNST cells [56]. Chai et al. [38] have suggested that it is the increased expression of *TWIST1* that may cause increased expression of miR-10b in the MPNSTs of NF1 patients. In their study, which compared MPNST cell lines from NF1 patients with those from sporadic tumours, Chai et al. [38] identified miR-10b, miR-155 and miR-335 as being over-expressed and Let-7a and Let-7b as being under-expressed in the NF1-MPNST cell lines. Further investigation showed that miR-10b reduced cell migration, invasion and proliferation. While inhibiting miR-155 did not correct the abnormal growth behaviour of NF1 MPNST cells, inhibiting miR-335 or enhancing let-7a expression partially corrected some abnormal growth properties of these tumour cells. These findings suggest that changes in miR-155 may represent a consequence of NF1 MPNST tumour formation, while changes in miR-335 and let-7 expression may contribute to progression of NF1 MPNSTs. These speculations are supported by the observation that *RAS* and *tenascin C* are deregulated in NF1 MPNSTs. Subsequently, these authors went on to demonstrate that miR-10b targets the *NF1* mRNA 3′UTR, thereby repressing the expression of neurofibromin protein. Therefore, it is suggested that miR-10b could specifically target neurofibromin to control NF1 tumorigenesis and progression. Irrespective of whether or neurofibromin is functional, as long as there is expression of the *NF1* mRNA, it is possible for the miR-10b to target its 3′UTR to suppress expression of neurofibromin protein. Chai et al. [38] also suggested that miR-10b could target other genes, and co-operate with other miRNAs such as miR-335 and let-7, to promote NF1 tumorigenesis and progression.

miR-29c

Presneau et al. [39] aimed to identify a molecular target to help discriminate between neurofibromas and MPNSTs. In their study of ten matched pairs of samples of MPNSTs and neurofibromas from NF1 patients, Presneau et al. [39] showed miR-210 to have been upregulated, and a series of miRNAs to have been down-regulated (miR-30e, miR-30c, miR-340, miR-139-5p, miR-29c and Let-7g) in MPNSTs. Of these miR-29c was the most down-regulated; the gene targets of miR-29c include *COL1A1*, *COL21A1*, *COL5A2* and *TDG*, all of which were down-regulated in MPNSTs. This was confirmed using synthetic oligonucleotide mimics. Further assays showed increased migration and invasion of MPNST cells following treatment with a miR-29c mimic. Presneau et al. [39] postulated that the decreased expression levels of miR-29c are mediated by the activation of a hepatocyte growth factor receptor, *cMET*, which has been shown to be activated in MPNSTs. This hypothesis is supported by the findings of Kwiecinski et al. [57] who demonstrated that hepatocyte growth factor receptor can inhibit collagen synthesis by activating miR-29a and miR-29b. Together, these data suggest that miR-29c is regulated by the action of *cMET* which, when activated, can stimulate miR-29 to control cell migration and invasion. Thus, miR-29c can act as a tumour suppressor and could potentially be used as a means to distinguish malignant from benign tumours. This suggestion has been borne out by findings in colorectal cancer, where analysis of mRNA expression profiles has indicated that miR-29c can predict the recurrence of colorectal cancer [58], and in hepatitis B virus-related hepatocellular carcinoma, where miR29c inhibits cell proliferation and promotes apoptosis [59].

miR-204

Recently, Gong et al. [40] reported that miR-204 contributes to the growth of MPNSTs, particularly in NF1. They postulated that this miRNA plays an important role in the carcinogenic process as it is found in cancer-associated regions of the genome and has previously been shown to be subject to high-frequency loss of heterozygosity in tumours [60]. miR-204 has also been found to act as a tumour suppressor gene in various other tumours including breast, kidney and prostate cancers [61]. This study demonstrated that the expression of miR-204 is down-regulated in tissue, which is derived from both NF1- and non-NF1-related tumours. By inducing the expression of miR-204 in MPNSTs of both NF1 and non-NF1 origin, the abnormal cellular characteristics were reversed and cell proliferation was reduced. Specifically in an NF1-related tumour cell line, induced expression of miR-204 resulted in decreased progression of malignancy and tumour development. Further bioinformatic analysis revealed that miR-204 targets *HMGA2*, a gene that regulates RAS signalling, suggesting that miR-204 may also contribute indirectly to the development of malignancy. It was also found that *HMGA2* expression is inhibited by miR-204, revealing an alternative pathway for tumour progression. It is still not clear whether miR-204 alone is sufficient to promote carcinogenesis in MPNSTs, as earlier studies have indicated that p53 inactivation and subsequent loss of expression of miR-34a may contribute to MPNST development [37]. Although these results have only been confirmed *in vitro*, miR-204 could potentially act as a biomarker for cancer diagnosis as well as an effective target for the development of therapeutic treatment.

miR-21

In a recent study, Itani et al. [41] analysed a panel of 12 MPNSTs, 11 neurofibromas, five normal nerves and three MPNST cell lines by mRNA expression profiling. The expression of miR-21 was significantly higher in MPNSTs than in the neurofibromas or MPNST cell lines. Transfection of miR-21 inhibitor significantly increased caspase activity ($p < 0.001$) and suppressed cell growth ($p < 0.05$) while upregulating the level of PDCD4 protein. Hence, these results indicate that miR-21 is likely to play an important role in MPNST progression through its target *PDCD4*.

NF1 microdeletions

It has been estimated that 5% of NF1 patients possess a germline 1.4-Mb microdeletion [62]. This results from the unequal recombination between two homologous NF1 low copy-number repeats [63]. NF1-microdeleted patients have an increased risk of developing MPNSTs [64]. They also appear to exhibit a more severe clinical phenotype in comparison to individuals with intragenic *NF1* mutations [65]. Analysis of the NF1 microdeleted region reveals that it contains a minimum of 16 protein coding genes, four pseudogenes and two microRNAs [66]. A recent study by Pasmant et al. [67] looked at the two miRNAs located within the 1.4-Mb microdeleted region in a set of MPNSTs and benign neurofibromas of NF1 microdeleted patients. They found that the two miRNA genes (*MIR3652* and *MIR193A* at 17q11.2 encoding miR-365-2 and miR-193a, respectively) displayed no differences in the expression between the tumour types, despite miR-193a having been previously categorized as a tumour suppressor in oral squamous cell carcinoma [68] and despite miR-365-2 having been identified as having an anti-proliferative role in colon cancer [69]. Further study will be required to assess the possible role of these two miRNAs in NF1 tumorigenesis.

NF1-phaeochromocytomas

Tömböl et al. [70] analysed the expression pattern of miRNAs in patients with NF1-associated pheochromocytomas by real-time quantitative reverse-transcription PCR. The results of their study revealed 16 differentially expressed miRNAs; their pathway analysis suggested that Notch- and G-protein-coupled receptor signalling may be involved in tumour recurrence. These authors also demonstrated the successful use of formalin-fixed paraffin-embedded samples for the analysis of miRNAs in phaeochromocytomas.

Epigenetic regulation of microRNAs in cancer

DNA methylation in the 5′ regulatory regions of genes is a major epigenetic mechanism. The role of aberrant DNA hypermethylation in the regulation of miRNA expression in human cancer has also been explored [71]. This study identified 122 miRNAs which were reported to be epigenetically regulated in 23 cancer types. Human oncomirs (miRNAs) with a role in cancer are designated as oncogenic miRNAs or oncomirs. High methylation levels compared to the protein-coding genes and at least half of the epigenetically regulated miRNAs were involved with different cancer types.

Both DNA methylation and mRNA regulation can suppress gene expression and their corresponding gene product. Su et al. [72] demonstrated that miRNAs tend to target genes with a low level of DNA methylation level in their promoter regions. They also found that miRNA target sites were significantly enriched in genes located in differentially methylated regions or partially methylated domains and that cancer genes tend to be characterized by a low level of methylation and more miRNA target sites.

miRNAs as prognostic and diagnostic biomarkers

Dysregulation of miRNAs is fundamental to the pathogenesis of many cancers. miRNAs that regulate the expression of tumour suppressor genes and oncogenes are candidates for use in targeted therapies [73]. An improved understanding of the underlying molecular mechanisms is still required for many cancers so as to make possible the development of effective targeted therapies. Krutzfeldt et al. [74] created chemically modified antagomirs, molecules which are complementary to miRNAs and which provide a useful way of silencing specific miRNAs *in vivo*. Just as one miRNA may regulate multiple targets, one target may also be regulated by a number of different miRNAs. Hence, specificity is an important factor to consider in designing a therapeutic approach.

miRNAs are increasingly being identified as useful diagnostic and prognostic markers. One example of this is in hepatocellular carcinoma (HCC) in which it has been shown that low levels of miR-26 can be indicative of a poor prognosis [75]. These patients have also been shown to benefit from a specific type of interferon-α therapy, showing that miR-26 can be used to identify HCC patients who would be more likely to respond well to this type of treatment. miRNAs can also be shown to overcome drug resistance when targeted, in chemo-resistance [76] and resistance to anti-oestrogenic therapies [77,78], demonstrating the range of different treatment methods to which miRNAs can contribute. miRNA delivery may be used to counteract carcinogenesis. miRNAs are reliable biomarkers for testing the efficiency of chemoprevention and may be used to counteract carcinogenesis [79].

As well as individual miRNAs being able to act as biomarkers and therapeutic targets, Han et al. [80], have shown that the three genes involved in miRNA biogenesis, namely *DICER1*, *DROSHA* and *XPO5* (exportin 5), have also been shown to have therapeutic potential, at least in the case of bladder urothelial carcinoma. These genes are vital for miRNA development, and their silencing results in the inhibition of cell proliferation and apoptosis. Han et al. [80] showed that all three genes were up-regulated and had higher expression in high-grade carcinomas than low-grade carcinomas. These differential expression patterns indicate that *DICER1*, *DROSHA* and *XPO5* could play active roles in carcinogenesis.

The use of miRNAs as useful biomarkers of tumorigenesis is supported by the finding that they are secreted into bodily fluids [81] and, hence, are circulating around the body so that they can be easily and accurately observed by means of microarray and quantitative PCR methods, allowing their detection to be both sensitive and specific [82]. There are already clinical diagnostic tests available that use miRNAs as biomarkers, such as the ProOnc TumorSource Dx, a proprietary test offered by Prometheus Labs (San Diego, CA, USA) (http://www.prometheuslabs.com), that determines the expression levels of 48 different miRNA biomarkers in a tissue sample, from which the results are used to determine the tissue of origin of metastatic cancer.

Conclusions

The discovery of miRNAs nearly 20 years ago introduced us to a new regulatory mechanism enabling a better understanding of the molecular pathogenesis of cancers. Dysregulation of miRNAs is fundamental to the pathogenesis of many cancers. miRNAs have the potential to target as many as several hundred genes simultaneously making them attractive prognostic biomarkers and therapeutic targets in cancer. miRNAs are not only involved in tumour progression, but also play a role in cancer invasion, metastasis, epigenetic alterations, chemo-resistance and radio-resistance. Although research on the role of miRNAs in NF1 tumorigenesis is still in its infancy, the experimental data obtained so far indicate that a number of miRNAs may be involved in NF1 tumorigenesis, including miR-29c, miR-34a, miR-214, miR-10b, miR-204 and miR-21. However, we lack an understanding of how different miRNAs identified in NF1 tumours might interact with neurofibromin and other tumour-associated proteins and whether these miRNAs can be linked to specific cancer signalling pathways. miRNAs involved in regulating the expression of oncogenes and tumour suppressor genes are candidates for targeted therapy for NF1 tumours. Therefore, it is hoped that the study of these small RNAs will eventually make a significant difference in treating NF1, at least to delay, if not entirely eliminate, the onset of tumorigenesis. The identification not only of differentially expressed microRNAs in tumours but also their target genes is providing new avenues for therapeutic approaches. As with any new therapeutic approach, there are of course many obstacles to be overcome before miRNAs can be used in clinical practise. However, it appears to present a very promising therapeutic avenue.

Competing interests
The authors declare that they have no competing interests.

Authors' contributions
AS contributed to the compilation of the first draft, DNC and MU improved the manuscript. All authors read and approved the final manuscript.

References

1. Ambros V: **The functions of animal microRNAs.** *Nature* 2001, **431**:350–355.
2. Bartel DP: **MicroRNAs: genomics, biogenesis, mechanism and function.** *Cell* 2004, **116**:281–297.
3. Lai EC: **MicroRNAs are complementary to 3′UTR sequence motifs that mediate negative post-transcriptional regulation.** *Nat Genet* 2002, **30**:363–364.
4. Lee RC, Feinbaum RL, Ambros V: **The C. elegans heterochronic gene lin-4 encodes small RNAs with antisense complementarity to lin-14.** *Cell* 1993, **75**:843–854.
5. Reinhart BJ, Slack FJ, Basson M, Pasquinelli AE, Bettinger JC, Rougvie AE, Horvitz HR, Ruvkun G: **The 21-nucleotide let-7 RNA regulates developmental timing in *Caenorhabtidis elegans*.** *Nature* 2000, **403**:901–906.
6. Pasquinelli AE, Reinhart BJ, Slack FJ, Martindale MQ, Kuroda MI, Maller B, Hayward DC, Ball EE, Degnan B, Muller P, Spring J, Srinivasan A, Fishman M, Finnerty J, Corbo J, Levine M, Leahy P, Davidson E, Ruvkun G: **Conservation of the sequence and temporal expression of Let-7 heterochronic regulatory RNA.** *Nature* 2000, **408**:86–89.
7. Yu J, Wang F, Yang GH, Wang FL, Ma YN, Du ZW, Zhang JW: **Human microRNA clusters: genomic organization and expression profile in leukemia cell lines.** *Biochem Biophys Res Commun* 2006, **13**:59–68.
8. Sayed D, Abdellatif M: **MicroRNAs in development and disease.** *Physiol Rev* 2011, **91**:827–887.
9. Ladomery MR, Maddocks DG, Wilson ID: **MicroRNAs: their discovery, biogenesis, function and potential use as biomarkers in non-invasive prenatal diagnostics.** *Int J Mol Epidemiol Genet* 2011, **2**:253–260.
10. Lee Y, Jeon K, Lee JT, Kim S, Kim VN: **MicroRNA maturation: stepwise processing and subcellular localisation.** *EMBO J* 2002, **23**:4051–4060.
11. Zeng Y, Yi R, Cullen BR: **Recognition and cleavage of primary microRNA precursors by the nuclear processing enzyme Drosha.** *EMBO J* 2005, **24**:138–148.
12. Denli AM, Tops BBJ, Plasterk RHA, Ketting RF, Hannon GJ: **Processing of primary microRNAs by the microprocessor complex.** *Nature* 2004, **432**:231–235.
13. Gregory RI, Yan KP, Amuthan G, Chendrimada T, Doratotaj B, Cooch N, Shiekhatter R: **The microprocessor complex mediates the genesis of microRNAs.** *Nature* 2004, **432**:235–240.
14. Landthaler M, Yalcin A, Tuschl T: **The human DiGeorge syndrome critical region gene 8 and its D. melanogaster homolog are required for miRNA biogenesis.** *Curr Biol* 2004, **14**:2162–2167.
15. Yi R, Qin Y, Macara IG, Cullen BR: **Exportin-5 mediates the nuclear export of pre-microRNAs and short hairpin RNAs.** *Genes Dev* 2003, **17**:3011–3016.
16. Lund E, Guttinger S, Calado A, Dahlberg JE, Kutay U: **Nuclear export of microRNA precursors.** *Science* 2004, **303**:95–98.
17. Hwang HW, Mendell JT: **MicroRNAs in cell proliferation, cell death and tumourigenesis.** *Br J Cancer* 2006, **94**:776–780.
18. Matranga C, Tomari Y, Shin C, Bartel DP, Zamore PD: **Passenger-strand cleavage facilitates assembly of siRNA into Ago2-containing RNAi enzyme complexes.** *Cell* 2005, **123**:607–620.
19. Winter J, Jung S, Keller S, Gregory RI, Diederichs S: **Many roads to maturity: microRNA biogenesis pathways and their regulation.** *Nat Cell Biol* 2009, **11**:228–234.
20. Tan G, Shi Y, Wu ZH: **MicroRNA-22 promotes cell survival upon UV radiation by repressing PTEN.** *Biochem Biophys Res Commun* 2012, **2012** (417):546–551.
21. Hawkins PG, Morris KV: **RNA and transcriptional modification of gene expression.** *Cell Cycle* 2008, **7**:602–607.
22. Esquela-Kerscher A, Slack FJ: **Oncomirs-microRNAs with a role in cancer.** *Nat Rev Cancer* 2006, **6**:259–269.

23. Hammond SM: **MicroRNA detection comes of age.** *Nat Methods* 2006, **3**:12–13.
24. Chen C, Ridzon DA, Broomer AJ, Zhou Z, Lee DH, Nguyen JT, Barbisin M, Xu NL, Mahuvakar VR, Andersen MR, Lao KQ, Livak KJ, Guegler KJ: **Real-time quantification of microRNAs by stem-loop RT-PCR.** *Nucleic Acids Res* 2005, **33**:e179.
25. Liu CG, Calin GA, Meloon B, Gamliel N, Sevignani C, Ferracin M, Dumitru CD, Shimizu M, Zupo S, Dono M, Alder H, Bullrich F, Negrini M, Croce CM: **An oligonucleotide microchip for genome-wide microRNA profiling in human and mouse tissues.** *Proc Nat Acad Sci USA* 2004, **101**:9740–9744.
26. Neely LA, Patel S, Garver J, Gallo M, Hackett M, McLaughlin S, Nadel M, Harris J, Gullans S, Rooke J: **A single-molecule method for the quantitation of microRNA gene expression.** *Nat Methods* 2006, **3**:41–46.
27. Lu J, Getz G, Miska EA, Alvarez-Saavedra E, Lamb J, Peck D, Sweet-Cordero A, Ebert BL, Mak RH, Ferrando AA, Downing JR, Jacks T, Horvitz HR, Golub TR: **MicroRNA expression profiles classify human cancers.** *Nature* 2005, **435**:834–838.
28. Rosenfeld N, Aharonov R, Meiri E, Rosenwald S, Spector Y, Zepeniuk M, Benjamin H, Shabes N, Tabak S, Levy A, Lebanony D, Goren Y, Silberschein E, Targan N, Ben-Ari A, Gilad S, Sion-Vardy N, Tobar A, Feinmesser M, Kharenko O, Nativ O, Nass D, Perelman M, Yosepovich A, Shalmon B, Polak-Charcon S, Fridman E, Avniel A, Bentwich I, *et al*: **MicroRNAs accurately identify cancer tissue origin.** *Nat Biotechnol* 2008, **26**:462–469.
29. Slaby O, Bienertova-Vasku J, Svoboda M, Vyzula R: **Genetic polymorphisms and microRNAs: new direction in molecular epidemiology of solid cancer.** *J Cell Mol Med* 2012, **16**:8–21.
30. Gong J, Tong Y, Zhang HM, Wang K, Hu T, Shan G, Sun J, Guo AY: **Genome-wide identification of SNPs in microRNA genes and the SNP effects on microRNA target binding and biogenesis.** *Hum Mutat* 2012, **33**:254–263.
31. Zhang L, Huang J, Yang N, Greshock J, Megraw MS, Giannakakis A, Liang S, Naylor TL, Barchetti A, Ward MR, Yao G, Medina A, O'brien-Jenkins A, Katsaros D, Hatzigeorgiou A, Gimotty PA, Weber BL, Coukos G: **microRNAs exhibit high frequency genomic alterations in human cancer.** *Proc Natl Acad Sci USA* 2006, **103**:9136–9141.
32. Marcinkowska M, Szymanski M, Krzyzosiak WJ, Kozlowski P: **Copy number variation of microRNA genes in the human genome.** *BMC Genomics* 2011, **12**:183.
33. Upadhyaya M: **Genetic basis of tumorigenesis in NF1 malignant peripheral nerve sheath tumors.** *Front Biosci* 2011, **16**:937–951.
34. Cheng AM, Byrom MW, Shelton J, Ford LP: **Antisense inhibition of human miRNAs and indications for involvement of miRNA in cell growth and apoptosis.** *Nucleic Acids Res* 2005, **33**:1290–1297.
35. Cimmino A, Calin GA, Fabri M, Iorio MV, Ferracin M, Shimizu M, Wojcik SE, Aqelin RI, Zupo S, Dono M, Rassenti L, Alder H, Volinia S, Liu CG, Kipps TJ, Negrini M, Croce CM: **miR-15 and miR-16 induce apoptosis by targeting BCL2.** *Proc Natl Acad Sci USA* 2005, **102**:13944–13949.
36. Calin GA, Sevignani C, Dumitru CD, Hyslop T, Noch E, Yendamuri S, Shimizu M, Rattan S, Bullrich F, Negrini M, Croce CM: **Human microRNA genes are frequently located at fragile sites and genomic regions involved in cancers.** *Proc Natl Acad Sci USA* 2004, **101**:2999–3004.
37. Subramanian S, Thayanithy V, West RB, Lee CH, Beck AH, Zhu S, Downs-Kelly E, Montgomery K, Goldblum JR, Hogendoorn PC, Corless CL, Oliveira AM, Dry SM, Nielsen TO, Rubin BP, Fletcher JA, Fletcher CD, van de Rijn M: **Genome-wide transcriptome analyses reveal p53 inactivation mediated loss of miR-34a expression in malignant peripheral nerve sheath tumours.** *J Pathol* 2010, **220**:58–70.
38. Chai G, Liu N, Ma J, Li H, Oblinger JL, Prahalad AK, Gong M, Chang LS, Wallace M, Muir D, Guha A, Phipps RJ, Hock JM, Yu X: **MicroRNA-10b regulates tumourigenesis in neurofibromatosis type 1.** *Cancer Sci* 2010, **101**:1997–2004.
39. Presneau N, Eskandarpour MS, Henderson S, Halai D, Tirabosco R, Flanagan AM: **Micro-RNA profiling of peripheral nerve sheath tumours identifies miR-29c as a tumour suppressor gene involved in tumour progression.** *Br J Cancer* 2012, doi:10.1038/bjc.2012.518.
40. Gong M, Ma J, Li M, Zhou M, Hock JM, Yu X: **MicroRNA-204 critically regulates carcinogenesis in malignant peripheral nerve sheath tumors.** *Neuro Oncol* 2012, **14**:1007–1017.
41. Itani S, Kunisada T, Morimoto Y, Yoshida A, Sasaki T, Ito S, Ouchida M, Sugihara S, Shimizu K, Ozaki T: **MicroRNA-21 correlates with tumorigenesis in malignant peripheral nerve sheath tumor (MPNST) via programmed cell death protein 4 (PDCD4).** *J Cancer Res Clin Oncol* 2012, **138**:1501–1509.
42. Lee Ming J, Choji H, Galas DJ, Wang K: **The systems biology of neurofibromatosis type 1 - critical roles for microRNA.** *Exp Neurol* 2012, **235**:464–464.
43. Lammens T, Li J, Leone G, De Veylder L: **Atypical E2Fs: new players in the E2F transcription factor family.** *Trends Cell Biol* 2009, **19**:111–118.
44. Reimer D, Sadr S, Wiedemair A, Stadlmann S, Concin N, Hofstetter G, Müller-Holzner E, Marth C, Zeimet AG: **Clinical relevance of E2F family members in ovarian cancer - an evaluation in a training set of 77 patients.** *Clin Cancer Res* 2007, **13**:144–151.
45. Yin D, Ogawa S, Kawamata N, Leiter A, Ham M, Li D, Doan NB, Said JW, Black KL, Koeffler PH: **miR-34a functions as a tumor suppressor modulating EGFR in glioblastoma multiforme.** *Oncogene* 2012, **10**:1038.
46. Li L, Yuan L, Luo J, Gao J, Guo J, Xie X: **MiR-34a inhibits proliferation and migration of breast cancer hrough down-regulation of Bcl-2 and SIRT1.** *Clin Exp Med* 2012, doi:10.1007/s10238-012-0186-5.
47. Kumar B, Yadav A, Lang J, Teknos TN, Kumar P: **Dysregulation of microRNA-34a expression in head and neck squamous cell carcinoma promotes tumor growth and tumor angiogenesis.** *PLoS One* 2012, **7**:e37601.
48. Yan K, Gao J, Yang T, Ma Q, Qiu X, Fan Q, Ma B: **MicroRNA-34a inhibits the proliferation and metastasis of osteosarcoma cells both *in vitro* and *in vivo*.** *PLoS One* 2012, **7**:e33778.
49. Schwarzenbach H, Milde-Langosch K, Steinbach B, Müller V, Pantel K: **Diagnostic potential of PTEN-targeting miR-214 in the blood of breast cancer patients.** *Breast Cancer Res Treat* 2012, **134**:933–941.
50. Yang H, Kong W, He L, Zhao JJ, O'Donnell JD, Wang J, Wenham RM, Coppola D, Kruk PA, Nicosia SV, Cheng JQ: **MicroRNA expression profiling in human ovarian cancer: miR-214 induces cell survival and cisplatin resistance by targeting PTEN.** *Cancer Res* 2008, **68**:425–433.
51. Peng RQ, Wan HY, Li HF, Liu M, Li X, Tang H: **MicroRNA-214 suppresses growth and invasiveness of cervical cancer cells by targeting UDP-*N*-acetyl-α-D-galactosamine:polypeptide *N*-acetylgalactosaminyltransferase 7.** *J Biol Chem* 2012, **287**:14301–14309.
52. Shih TC, Tien YJ, Wen CJ, Yeh TS, Yu MC, Huang CH, Lee YS, Yen TC, Hsieh SY: **MicroRNA-214 downregulation contributes to tumor angiogenesis via inducing secretion of hepatoma-derived growth factor in human hepatoma.** *J Hepatol* 2012, **57**:584–591.
53. Lee YB, Bantounas I, Lee DY, Phylactou L, Caldwell MA, Uney JB: **Twist-1 regulates the miR-199a/214 cluster during development.** *Nucleic Acids Res* 2009, **1**:123–128.
54. Tanzer A, Amemiya CT, Kim CB, Stadler PF: **Evolution of microRNAs located within Hox gene clusters.** *J Exp Zool B Mol Dev Evol* 2005, **304**:75–85.
55. Garzon R, Garofalo M, Martelli MP, Briesewitz R, Wang L, Fernandez-Cymering C, Volinia S, Liu CG, Schnittger S, Haferlach T, Liso A, Diverio D, Mancini M, Meloni G, Foa R, Martelli MF, Mecucci C, Croce CM, Falini B: **Distinctive microRNA signature of acute myeloid leukemia bearing cytoplasmic mutated nucleophosmin.** *Proc Natl Acad Sci USA* 2008, **105**:3945–3950.
56. Ma L, Teruya-Feldstein J, Weinberg RA: **Tumour invasion and metastasis initiated by microRNA-10b in breast cancer.** *Nature* 2007, **449**:682–688.
57. Kwiecinski M, Noetel A, Elfimova N, Trebicka J, Schievenbusch S, Strack I, Molnar L, von Brandenstein M, Töx U, Nischt R, Coutelle O, Dienes HP, Odenthal M: **Hepatocyte growth factor (HGF) inhibits collagen I and IV synthesis in hepatic stellate cells by miRNA-29 induction.** *PLoS One* 2011, **6**:e24568.
58. Kuo TY, Hsi E, Yang IP, Tsai PC, Wang JY, Juo SH: **Computational analysis of mRNA expression profiles identifies microRNA-29a/c as predictor of colorectal cancer early recurrence.** *PLoS One* 2012, **7**:e31587.
59. Wang CM, Wang Y, Fan CG, Xu FF, Sun WS, Liu YG, Jia JH: **miR-29c targets TNFAIP3, inhibits cell proliferation and induces apoptosis in hepatitis B virus-related hepatocellular carcinoma.** *Biochem Biophys Res Commun* 2011, **411**:586–592.
60. Bauer VL, Braselmann H, Henke M, Mattern D, Walch A, Unger K, Baudis M, Lassmann S, Huber R, Wienberg J, Werner M, Zitzelsberger HF: **Chromosomal changes characterize head and neck cancer with poor prognosis.** *J Mol Med* 2008, **86**:1353–1365.
61. Wang FE, Zhang C, Maminishkis A, Dong L, Zhi C, Li R, Zhao J, Majerciak V, Gaur AB, Chen S, Miller SS: **MicroRNA-204/211 alters epithelial physiology.** *FASEB J* 2010, **24**:1552–1571.

62. Kluwe L, Siebert R, Gesk S, Friedrich RE, Tinschert S, Kehrer-Sawatzki H, Mautner VF: **Screening 500 unselected neurofibromatosis 1 patients for deletions of the *NF1* gene.** *Hum Mutat* 2004, **23:**111–116.
63. Dorschner MO, Sybert VP, Weaver M, Pletcher BA, Stephens K: **NF1 microdeletion breakpoints are clustered at flanking repetitive sequences.** *Hum Mol Genet* 2000, **9:**35–46.
64. De Raedt T, Brems H, Lopez-Correa C, Vermeesch JR, Marynen P, Legius E: **Genomic organization and evolution of the NF1 microdeletion region.** *Genomics* 2004, **84:**346–360.
65. Upadhyaya M, Ruggieri M, Maynard J, Osborn M, Hartog C, Mudd S, Penttinen M, Cordeiro I, Ponder M, Ponder BAJ, Krawczak M, Cooper DN: **Gross deletions of the neurofibromatosis type 1 (*NF1*) gene are predominantly of maternal origin and commonly associated with a learning disability, dysmorphic features and developmental delay.** *Hum Genet* 1998, **102:**591–597.
66. Jenne DE, Tinschert S, Dorschner MO, Hameister H, Stephens K, Kehrer-Sawatzki H: **Complete physical map and gene content of the human NF1 tumour suppressor region in human and mouse.** *Genes Chrom Cancer* 2003, **37:**111–120.
67. Pasmant E, Masliah-Planchon J, Lévy P, Laurendeau I, Ortonne N, Parfait B, Valeyrie-Allanore L, Leroy K, Wolkenstein P, Vidaud M, Vidaud D, Bièche I: **Identification of genes potentially involved in the increased risk of malignancy in NF1-microdeleted patients.** *Mol Med* 2011, **17:**79–87.
68. Kozaki K, Imoto I, Mogi S, Omura K, Inazawa J: **Exploration of tumour-suppressive microRNAs silenced by DNA hypermethylation in oral cancer.** *Cancer Res* 2008, **68:**2094–2105.
69. Nie J, Liu L, Zheng W, Chen L, Wu X, Xu Y, Du X, Han W: **microRNA-365, down-regulated in colon cancer, inhibits cell cycle progression and promotes apoptosis of colon cancer cells by probably targeting cyclin D1 and Bcl-2.** *Carcinogenesis* 2012, **33:**220–225.
70. Tömböl Z, Eder K, Kovács A, Szabó PM, Kulka J, Likó I, Zalatnai A, Rácz G, Tóth M, Patócs A, Falus A, Rácz K, Igaz P: **MicroRNA expression profiling in benign (sporadic and hereditary) and recurring adrenal pheochromocytomas.** *Mod Pathol* 2010, **23:**1583–1595.
71. Kunej T, Godnic I, Ferdin J, Horvat S, Dovc P, Calin GA: **Epigenetic regulation of microRNAs in cancer: an integrated review of literature.** *Mutat Res* 2011, **717:**77–84.
72. Su Z, Xia J, Zhao Z: **Functional complementation between transcriptional methylation regulation and post-transcriptional microRNA regulation in the human genome.** *BMC Genomics* 2011, **5:**S15.
73. Nana-Sinkam SP, Croce CM: **MicroRNAs as therapeutic targets in cancer.** *Transl Res* 2011, **157:**216–225.
74. Krutzfeldt J, Rajewsky N, Braich R, Rajeev KG, Tuschl T, Manoharan M, Stoffel M: **Silencing of microRNAs *in vivo* with 'antagomirs'.** *Nature* 2005, **438:**685–689.
75. Ji J, Shi J, Budhu A, Yu Z, Forgues M, Roessler S, Ambs S, Chen Y, Meltzer PS, Croce CM, Qin LX, Man K, Lo CM, Lee J, Ng IO, Fan J, Tang ZY, Sun HC, Wang XW: **MicroRNA expression, survival, and response to interferon in liver cancer.** *N Engl J Med* 2009, **361:**1437–1447.
76. Meng F, Henson R, Lang M, Wehbe H, Maheshwari S, Mendell JT, Jiang J, Schmittgen TD, Patel T: **Involvement of human micro-RNA in growth and response to chemotherapy in human cholangiocarcinoma cell lines.** *Gastroenterology* 2006, **2006**(130):2113–2129.
77. Miller TE, Ghoshal K, Ramaswamy B, Roy S, Datta J, Shapiro CL, Jacob S, Majumder S: **MicroRNA-221/222 confers tamoxifen resistance in breast cancer by targeting p27Kip1.** *J Biol Chem* 2008, **283:**29897–29903.
78. Zhao JJ, Lin J, Yang H, Kong W, He L, Ma X, Coppola D, Cheng JQ: **MicroRNA-221/222 negatively regulates estrogen receptor alpha and is associated with tamoxifen resistance in breast cancer.** *J Biol Chem* 2008, **283:**31079–31086.
79. Izzotti A: **Molecular medicine and the development of cancer chemopreventive agents.** *Ann N Y Acad Sci* 2012, **1259:**26–32.
80. Han Y, Liu Y, Gui Y, Cai Z: **Inducing cell proliferation inhibition and apoptosis via silencing Dicer, Drosha, and Exportin 5 in urothelial carcinoma of the bladder.** *J Surg Oncol* 2012, doi:10.1002/jso.23214. Epub ahead of print.
81. Steer CJ, Subramanian S: **Circulating microRNAs as biomarkers: a new frontier in diagnostics.** *Liver Transpl* 2012, **18:**265–269.
82. Ajit SK: **Circulating microRNAs as biomarkers, therapeutic targets, and signaling molecules.** *Sensors (Basel)* 2012, **12:**3359–3369.

17

Gene selection and cancer type classification of diffuse large-B-cell lymphoma using a bivariate mixture model for two-species data

Yuhua Su[1*], Dahlia Nielsen[2], Lei Zhu[3], Kristy Richards[4], Steven Suter[5], Matthew Breen[6], Alison Motsinger-Reif[7] and Jason Osborne[7]

Abstract

A bivariate mixture model utilizing information across two species was proposed to solve the fundamental problem of identifying differentially expressed genes in microarray experiments. The model utility was illustrated using a dog and human lymphoma data set prepared by a group of scientists in the College of Veterinary Medicine at North Carolina State University. A small number of genes were identified as being differentially expressed in both species and the human genes in this cluster serve as a good predictor for classifying diffuse large-B-cell lymphoma (DLBCL) patients into two subgroups, the germinal center B-cell-like diffuse large B-cell lymphoma and the activated B-cell-like diffuse large B-cell lymphoma. The number of human genes that were observed to be significantly differentially expressed (21) from the two-species analysis was very small compared to the number of human genes (190) identified with only one-species analysis (human data). The genes may be clinically relevant/important, as this small set achieved low misclassification rates of DLBCL subtypes. Additionally, the two subgroups defined by this cluster of human genes had significantly different survival functions, indicating that the stratification based on gene-expression profiling using the proposed mixture model provided improved insight into the clinical differences between the two cancer subtypes.

Keywords: Mixture models, Gene expression, Homology, Lymphoma

Introduction

Diffuse large-B-cell lymphoma (DLBCL), the most common type of non-Hodgkin lymphoma in adults, accounts for 30% to 40% of newly diagnosed lymphomas and has an annual incidence in America of more than 25,000 cases. Combination chemotherapy has transformed DLBCL from a fatal disease into one that is often curable, but only approximately 50% of all patients are cured [1,2]. This suggests that DLBCL actually comprises several subgroups that differ in responsiveness to chemotherapy. The attempts to define subgroups of DLBCL have often failed due to diagnostic discrepancies. Clinically, the International Prognostic Index (IPI) [3] has been developed for use in the design of future therapeutic trials in patients with aggressive non-Hodgkin lymphoma and in the selection of appropriate therapeutic approaches for individual patients. However, IPI has not been used successfully to predict outcomes in DLBCLs so that patients can be stratified correctly for therapeutic trials. This may be attributed to the fact that the clinical factors of IPI (age, tumor stage, serum lactate dehydrogenase concentration, performance status, and number of extranodal disease sites) neither provide molecular insight into the heterogeneity of DLBCL nor identify specific therapeutic targets [4,5].

Recent developments in microarray technology allow researchers to accurately and precisely measure gene expression patterns in lymphomas which provides the opportunity to revolutionize the way these tumors are grouped and treated. In other words, studying gene expression profiles in lymphomas may provide the opportunity to identify pathways on which the tumor depends and to target the pathways for the development of new drugs. Indeed, gene-expression profiling studies have distinguished three molecular subtypes of DLBCL:

*Correspondence: yhsejo@gmail.com
[1]Dr. Su's Statistics, Department of Human Nutrition, Food, and Animal Sciences, University of Hawaii at Manoa, Honolulu, HI 96822, USA
Full list of author information is available at the end of the article

germinal-center B-cell-like (GCB) DLBCL, activated B-cell-like (ABC) DLBCL, and primary mediastinal B-cell lymphoma (PMBL) [2,5-8].

The first attempt at examining gene expression profiling to identify distinct B-cell malignancies was made by Alizadeh et al. [9]. A hierarchical clustering algorithm [10] was used to group genes on the basis of similarity of their expression over all subjects. Subjects were also grouped based on the similarities in gene expression using the same clustering method. Two distinct subgroups of DLBCL were found based on the gene expression analysis: GCB DLBCL and ABC DLBCL. Alizadeh et al. [9] discovered that almost all genes that defined GCB DLBCL were highly expressed in normal germinal center B cells and, by contrast, most genes that defined ABC DLBCL were not expressed in normal germinal center B cells. In addition, there was a substantial and significant difference in the average five-year survival rate between patients with GCB DLBCL and ABC DLBCL.

Inspired by the work of Alizadeh [9], Rosenwald et al. [5] found that most of the genes with expression patterns that correlated with survival of the DLBCL subgroups fell within four gene-expression signatures. *A gene-expression signature is a group of genes expressed in a specific cell lineage or stage of differentiation or during a particular biologic response* and *hence genes within the same gene-expression signature are probably associated with similar biologic aspects of tumor* [5]. The authors in [5] then developed a molecular predictor consisting of 17 genes for the likelihood of survival after chemotherapy according to gene expression profiles of lymphomas. Shipp et al. [4] adopted the weighted-voting algorithm [11] to develop an outcome predictor with 13 genes and were able to classify two categories of DLBCL patients with very different five-year overall survival rates. Note that there is no overlap among the genes in the models derived in [4] and [5].

Wright et al. [8] formulated a DLBCL subgroup predictor based on Bayes' rule, applied this method to the DLBCL gene expression data in [5], and constructed a 27-gene DLBCL subgroup predictor. Next, a new predictor including 14 genes among the previous predictor was constructed and applied to another set of gene expression data from DLBCLs [4]. Wright et al. [8] also demonstrated that the proposed algorithm can define cancer subgroups based on gene expression differences regardless of the DNA microarray platforms and could be used clinically to provide diagnostic information as the resulting survival rates were significantly different for the identified GCB and ABC DLBCL subgroups.

A panel of 36 genes whose expression predicts survival in DLBCL was identified by Lossos et al. [1] through literature review. They [1] selected 6 out of the 36 genes by ranking them on the basis of their predictive power for DLBCL survival obtained by univariate analysis. A 6-gene multivariate Cox proportional-hazards regression model for prediction of survival in DLBCL was constructed and applied to the data from [4] and [5]. Lossos et al. [1] concluded that the measurement of the expression of the six genes was sufficient to predict overall survival in DLBCL after stratifying patients into different risk groups based on their IPI score.

More recently, Blenk et al. [12] analyzed an enlarged data set (original data were generated by [5]) to confirm that there are clear expression differences between ABC and GCB DLBCL. To detect differentially expressed genes, they [12] used *limma* in [13] and further determined 50 best separating genes for class discovery. An optimal classifier with only 18 genes for distinguishing DLBCL subgroups was conducted. In addition, an optimal molecular survival predictor with only six genes was obtained. However, there was no overlap among the genes used in the classifier and the survival predictor established in [12].

Models introduced in [1,4,5,8,9,12] can be used to distinguish the subgroups in DLBCL and identify rational targets for research into treatment intervention. Moreover, the predictor identified by each study involved only a small number of genes and thus the needed DNA microarrays may be easily developed for clinical prediction. Nonetheless, genes seldom overlap in these models. Blenk et al. [12] showed that 6 of the 18 genes used in the optimal classifier were found again after analyzing another data set from [4]. However, none of these genes were identified in a subsequent investigation of survival [12].

Due to technical differences, the composition of the microarrays used, and the different algorithms used for constructing predictive models, it remains unclear which method and which model best captures the molecular and clinical heterogeneity of diffuse large-B-cell lymphoma. Therefore, the goal in this research was to give an example of how bivariate data can be used for clinical research.

Methods

Let $X_{a_{ij}}$ and $X_{h_{il}}$ denote gene expression measurements from the ith orthologous gene pair [14] for the jth animal and the lth human. The following independent linear models describe the association between gene expression and treatment (cancer type):

$$X_{a_{ij}} = \beta_{0a_i} + \beta_{1a_i} T_{a_j} + e_{a_{ij}}, \quad (1)$$
$$X_{h_{il}} = \beta_{0h_i} + \beta_{1h_i} T_{h_l} + e_{h_{il}}, \quad (2)$$

where T_{a_j} and T_{h_l} are $\{0,1\}$ treatment indicators, and $e_{a_{ij}}$ and $e_{h_{il}}$ are independent $N(0,\sigma_a^2)$ and $N(0,\sigma_h^2)$ random variables. The σ_a^2 and σ_h^2 are variances for $e_{a_{ij}}$ and $e_{h_{il}}$, respectively. A given gene can be classified as non-differentially expressed (NDE, showing no signs of treatment effects), positively differentially expressed (pDE, showing positive treatment effects), or negatively differentially expressed (nDE, showing negative treatment effects). Furthermore, we assume dependency between differentially expressed orthologs. Therefore, for a human and animal gene pair, there are nine possibilities for categorizing this pair of genes, illustrated in Table 1.

The following two-species nine-component bivariate normal mixture model in [15,16] is proposed to simultaneously model the vectors of the estimated treatment effects $(\hat{\beta}_{1a_i}, \hat{\beta}_{1h_i})^T$ obtained from Equations 1 and 2:

$$\begin{aligned}\begin{pmatrix}\hat{\beta}_{1a_i}\\ \hat{\beta}_{1h_i}\end{pmatrix} &\sim \pi_0 N\left(\begin{pmatrix}0\\0\end{pmatrix}, \begin{pmatrix}\sigma_{a0}^2 & 0\\ 0 & \sigma_{h0}^2\end{pmatrix}\right)\\ &+\pi_1 N\left(\begin{pmatrix}\mu_{a1}\\ \mu_{h1}\end{pmatrix}, \begin{pmatrix}\sigma_{a1}^2 & \rho_1\sigma_{a1}\sigma_{h1}\\ \rho_1\sigma_{a1}\sigma_{h1} & \sigma_{h1}^2\end{pmatrix}\right)\\ &+\pi_2 N\left(\begin{pmatrix}\mu_{a2}\\ \mu_{h2}\end{pmatrix}, \begin{pmatrix}\sigma_{a2}^2 & \rho_2\sigma_{a2}\sigma_{h2}\\ \rho_2\sigma_{a2}\sigma_{h2} & \sigma_{h2}^2\end{pmatrix}\right)\\ &+\pi_3 N\left(\begin{pmatrix}\mu_{a3}\\ \mu_{h3}\end{pmatrix}, \begin{pmatrix}\sigma_{a3}^2 & \rho_3\sigma_{a3}\sigma_{h3}\\ \rho_3\sigma_{a3}\sigma_{h3} & \sigma_{h3}^2\end{pmatrix}\right)\\ &+\pi_4 N\left(\begin{pmatrix}\mu_{a4}\\ \mu_{h4}\end{pmatrix}, \begin{pmatrix}\sigma_{a4}^2 & \rho_4\sigma_{a4}\sigma_{h4}\\ \rho_4\sigma_{a4}\sigma_{h4} & \sigma_{h4}^2\end{pmatrix}\right)\\ &+\pi_5 N\left(\begin{pmatrix}0\\ \mu_{h5}\end{pmatrix}, \begin{pmatrix}\sigma_{a5}^2 & 0\\ 0 & \sigma_{h5}^2\end{pmatrix}\right)\\ &+\pi_6 N\left(\begin{pmatrix}0\\ \mu_{h6}\end{pmatrix}, \begin{pmatrix}\sigma_{a6}^2 & 0\\ 0 & \sigma_{h6}^2\end{pmatrix}\right)\\ &+\pi_7 N\left(\begin{pmatrix}\mu_{a7}\\ 0\end{pmatrix}, \begin{pmatrix}\sigma_{a7}^2 & 0\\ 0 & \sigma_{h7}^2\end{pmatrix}\right)\\ &+\pi_8 N\left(\begin{pmatrix}\mu_{a8}\\ 0\end{pmatrix}, \begin{pmatrix}\sigma_{a8}^2 & 0\\ 0 & \sigma_{h8}^2\end{pmatrix}\right),\end{aligned} \tag{3}$$

where π_k , $k = 0, \ldots, 8$ denote the mixing weights (the probability that an observation belongs to the kth component). Note that $\sum_{k=0}^{8} \pi_k = 1$ and $\pi_k \geq 0$. $(\mu_{ak}, \mu_{hk})^T$ and $(\sigma_{ak}^2, \sigma_{hk}^2)^T$ are the vectors of the means and variances, respectively, for each species in each mixture component. ρ_k denotes the correlation between orthologs under the kth category. To accommodate the possible patterns of

Table 1 Possible categories of $(\beta_{1a_i}, \beta_{1h_i})^T$

Category	$(\beta_{1a_i}, \beta_{1h_i})$	$(\mu_{\beta_{1a_i}}, \mu_{\beta_{1h_i}})$	Corr$(\beta_{1a_i}, \beta_{1h_i})$
0	(NDE,NDE)	(0, 0)	0
1	(pDE,pDE)	(+, +)	ρ_1
2	(nDE,nDE)	(−, −)	ρ_2
3	(pDE,nDE)	(+, −)	ρ_3
4	(nDE,pDE)	(−, +)	ρ_4
5	(NDE,pDE)	(0, +)	0
6	(NDE,nDE)	(0, −)	0
7	(pDE,NDE)	(+, 0)	0
8	(nDE,NDE)	(−, 0)	0

the gene expression for animal and human due to treatment intervention (different cancer types), the following constraints are imposed: $\mu_{a1} \geq 0$, $\mu_{h1} \geq 0$, $\mu_{a2} \leq 0$, $\mu_{h2} \leq 0$, $\mu_{a3} \geq 0$, $\mu_{h3} \leq 0$, $\mu_{a4} \leq 0$, $\mu_{h4} \geq 0$, $\mu_{h5} \geq 0$, $\mu_{h6} \leq 0$, $\mu_{a7} \geq 0$, and $\mu_{a8} \leq 0$; $\rho_0 = 0$, $\rho_5 = 0$, $\rho_6 = 0$, $\rho_7 = 0$, and $\rho_8 = 0$.

Gene membership is determined according to the maximum posterior probability that an observation $(\hat{\beta}_{1a_i}, \hat{\beta}_{1h_i})^T$ comes from the kth component of the mixture.

A parametric bootstrap method in [17,18] to estimate the standard errors for the estimated parameters is provided. Bootstrapping is the practice of estimating properties of an estimator by measuring those properties when sampling from an approximating distribution. The basis of the bootstrap methodology is simple. In the parametric bootstrap setting, consider F to be a member of some prescribed parametric family and obtain $\widehat{F}_n$ by estimating the family parameters, in this case, $(\pi_k, \mu_{ak}, \mu_{hk}, \Sigma_k)^T$, $k = 0, \ldots, 8$, from the data. In each iteration, by generating an *iid* random sequence, called a 'resample' from the distribution $\widehat{F}_n$, new estimates of the parameters are obtained and the sampling properties (such as the mean, standard deviation, bias, and shape) can be evaluated.

The procedure of the parametric bootstrap resampling method to obtain the estimated standard errors of the estimated parameters for the nine-component mixture model is described as follows:

1. $\widehat{F}_n$ is formed by substituting the estimates of $(\mu_{ak}, \mu_{hk})^T$ and Σ_k into the 9-component mixture model (3).
2. The numbers of genes in category 0 through category 8 $(n_0, n_1, \ldots, n_8)$ are drawn from a multinomial distribution with parameters n and $\mathbf{p}$. n is the number of trials for each multinomial random variable. In this study, it is equal to the number of orthologs in two-species data. $\mathbf{p}$ is the vector of event probabilities for each trial. In this study, $\mathbf{p}$ is the vector of the mixing weights estimated from the data. The new mixing weights are then calculated for the bootstrap resampling and plugged into the nine-component mixture model (Equation 3) to form $\widehat{F}_n$.
3. Bootstrap samples $(\hat{\beta}^*_{1a_i}, \hat{\beta}^*_{1h_i})^T$ of size n are drawn from $\widehat{F}_n$ formed above.
4. For each bootstrap resampling, obtain the numerically approximated maximum likelihood estimates for the parameters in the nine-component mixture using the expectation-maximization (EM) algorithm.
5. Repeat steps 1 to 4 B times independently. B is the number of bootstrap replications. Calculate the

empirical standard deviation of a series of bootstrap replications of $\hat{\theta}$ accordingly. $\hat{\theta}$ is the estimator of θ , the parameter of interest. Since the standard error of the mean ($s/\sqrt{n}$, sample standard deviation divided by the squared root of the size of the sample) is the estimate of the true standard deviation of the sample mean ($\sigma/\sqrt{n}$, standard deviation for the population divided by the squared root of the size of the sample), essentially, the standard deviation of the bootstrap estimator obtained here is an estimation of the standard error of the mean for the parameter of interest. The bootstrap standard error $\widehat{SE}_B$ of $\hat{\theta}$ is calculated as follows:

$$\widehat{SE}(\hat{\theta})_B = \sqrt{\frac{1}{B-1}\sum_{b=1}^{B}(\hat{\theta}_b^* - \bar{\hat{\theta}}^*)^2},$$

where $\hat{\theta}_b^*$ is the estimator of θ calculated from the bth bootstrap resample $(b = 1, \ldots, B)$, $\bar{\hat{\theta}}^* = \sum_{b=1}^{B} \hat{\theta}_b^*/B$; B is the total number of resamples (each of size n) collected from the empirical estimate of F.

Data sources

In order to improve treatments for non-Hodgkin lymphoma in human and canine patients, researchers from North Carolina State University's College of Veterinary Medicine and the University of North Carolina at Chapel Hill Lineberger Comprehensive Cancer Center conducted research to study tissue samples from human and canine non-Hodgkin lymphoma patients, with the hope of creating a genomic profile of non-Hodgkin lymphoma that would give oncologists and veterinarians greater insight into the disease's biology and obtain the information that could lead to a clinical benefit for both species. The study protocol was approved by the Institutional Animal Care and Use Committee of North Carolina State University.

The team recruited dogs diagnosed with lymphoma to collect tissue samples for study. The dog data were measured at the probe set level on Affymetrix Canine Genome 2.0 array (Canine_2, Affymetrix Inc., Santa Clara, CA, USA), with a total number of probe sets equal to 43,035. Forty-eight dogs with one of the following diagnostic results were recruited: B-cell lymphoma (27 dogs), T-cell lymphoma (10 dogs), B-cell acute lymphoblastic leukemia (1 dog), T-cell acute lymphoblastic leukemia (4 dogs), and normal (6 dogs). Among the 27 dogs with B-cell lymphoma, 14 of them were diagnosed histopathologically with DLBCL. The 14 DLBCL patients could be further divided into two subgroups: 5 ABC DLBCL patients and 9 GCB DLBCL patients. For the purpose of this research, only data for the 14 dogs with DLBCLs were used. The dog microarray gene expression data were LOESS normalized by JMP Genomics 4.0 (Cary, NC, USA).

Corresponding data for human patients with lymphoma were extracted from the Gene Expression Omnibus (GEO) database [19]. Data for 460 lymphoma patients were retrieved from two series with GEO accession number: GSE10846 [7] and GSE11318 [6]. The human data were measured at the probe set level on Affymetrix Human Genome U133 2.0 array (HG-U133_Plus_2), with a total number of probe sets equal to 54,675. The human microarray gene expression data were also LOESS normalized by JMP Genomics 4.0. Based on the gene expression, two distinct subgroups were identified after principle component analysis. This implied that there may be a strong batch effect among the samples. Hence, only samples from one of these two subgroups were included in the data analysis. This resulted in 219 human subjects consisting of 31 PMBL, 78 ABC DLBCLs, 80 GCB DLBCLs, and 29 unclassified DLBCLs (distinguishing between subgroups of DLBCL is through gene-expression profiling [6,7]). To make the animal and human data comparable, only data for ABC and GCB DLBCLs with corresponding survival information were used. This resulted in a final dataset with 77 ABC DLBCL patients and 79 GCB DLBCL patients.

After averaging probe sets across a gene to obtain a gene-level transcript value, the orthologous information from HomoloGene release 64 at website ftp://ftp.ncbi.nih.gov/pub/HomoloGene/build64/ was applied to acquire the mappings between dog and human. This led to a total of 6,566 pairs of dog and human orthologs.

Data analysis

We recall that the objective of the data analysis was to identify rational targets (genes) for treatment intervention simultaneously for both dog and human lymphoma patients with the hope of giving researchers greater insight into the disease's biology. Furthermore, it was also of interest to verify if the targeted genes can serve as a good predictor to clinically distinguish subgroups of DLBCL in humans. Because the samples in humans that were used to estimate the distribution of the bivariate mixture model were also used to build the classification function, there was a possibility of over-fitting, resulting in a model that would indicate an over-optimistic separation between the subgroups than would be found in independent data. To avoid the biased classification result, a leave-one-out-cross-validation (LOOCV) procedure [20] was introduced as the following steps:

1. Use all 14 observations for dogs and obtain the estimated coefficients of cancer type effect on gene

expression $\hat{\beta}_{1a_i}, i = 1, \ldots, 6,566$. Omit one observation from the 156 human observations and obtain the estimated coefficients of cancer type effect $\hat{\beta}_{1h_i}$.

2. Use all $(\hat{\beta}_{1a_i}, \hat{\beta}_{1h_i})^T$ to construct the nine-component bivariate normal mixture model. Identify gene membership accordingly.
3. Use genes classified into categories (1, 2, 3, and 4) (differentially expressed in both species) to develop a classification rule based on the remaining 155 human observations. Develop another classification rule based on genes classified into categories (1, 2, 3, 4, 5, and 6) (differentially expressed in human).
4. For the purpose of comparison, identify differentially expressed human genes by performing a single species analysis for human only. Choose genes based on the p values of the t statistics after adjusting for multiple comparison by controlling the false discovery rate (FDR) [21] at levels 0.01 and 0.00001.
5. Classify the holdout human observation using the classification rules constructed in steps 3 and 4.
6. Repeat steps 1, 2, 3, 4 and 5 until every one of the human observations is classified.

The classification rule was established through the M-dimensional centroid obtained from the k-means [22] clustering process applied to the training set. M was the number of genes retained for performing cancer type classification. k was equal to 2 as there were two types of cancer. SAS PROC FASTCLUS [23] was used to carry out the k-means clustering.

Since k-means does the clustering, and not the classification, the class of each cluster has to be determined for the classification rule before it can be used to classify future observations. Table 2 demonstrates the results of the k-means clustering.

Clusters were designated so that the minimum misclassification rate was achieved. Therefore,

$$\begin{cases} \text{if} \quad n_{12} + n_{21} < n_{22} + n_{11} \\ \Rightarrow \text{cluster 1 = "ABC DLBCL" and cluster 2 = "GCB DLBCL"}, \\ \text{if} \quad n_{12} + n_{21} > n_{22} + n_{11} \\ \Rightarrow \text{cluster 1 = "GCB DLBCL" and cluster 2 = "ABC DLBCL"}, \\ \text{if} \quad n_{12} + n_{21} = n_{11} + n_{22} \\ \Rightarrow \text{randomly assign cluster labels.} \end{cases}$$

Table 2 The k-means clustering results

	Cluster 1	Cluster 2
ABC DLBCL	n_{11}	n_{12}
GCB DLBCL	n_{21}	n_{22}

The classification rule established at the lth LOOCV procedure was then

$$\begin{cases} \text{if} \sum_{m=1}^{M_l} (x_{h_{ml}} - \mu_{l,1m}^{\text{centroid}})^2 < \sum_{m=1}^{M_l} (x_{h_{ml}} - \mu_{l,2m}^{\text{centroid}})^2 \\ \Rightarrow \text{classify the } l\text{th human subject into cluster 1,} \\ \text{else} \Rightarrow \text{classify the } l^{\text{th}} \text{ human subject into cluster 2.} \end{cases}$$

M_l was the total number of genes retained at the lth LOOCV procedure for cancer type classification. $l = 1, \ldots, 156$, as there were 156 human DLBCL patients. $x_{h_{ml}}$ was the mth gene expression for the lth hold-out human subject. For the lth LOOCV procedure, $\mu_{l,1m}^{\text{centroid}}$ and $\mu_{l,2m}^{\text{centroid}}$ were the mth centroid means $(m = 1, \ldots, M_l)$ calculated from the k-means $(k = 2)$ algorithm for cluster 1 and cluster 2, respectively.

Results

Parameter estimation

The maximum likelihood estimates of the parameters in the nine-component bivariate normal mixture model computed using the EM algorithm [24] are given in Table 3. The estimated mixture weight for category 0 was $\hat{\pi}_0 = 0.823$ indicating approximately 5,404 $(6,566 \times 0.823)$ pairs of uninteresting dog and human orthologs. $(\mu_a, \mu_h)^T$ denotes the mean vector of each mixture component. Most of the estimated mean vectors were slightly larger in categories 1 through 4 than those in categories 5 through 8. It appeared that the magnitude of the estimated difference of expression in genes related to lymphoma in both species tended to be larger than in genes where differential expression was exhibited in only one species.

Gene selection and cancer type classification

For the 156 LOOCV instances, the proposed mixture model determined 21 (14 genes appearing in the intersection of all hold-outs) human genes in categories (1, 2, 3, and 4) and 279 (185 genes appearing in the intersection of all hold-outs) human genes in categories (1, 2, 3, 4, 5, and 6). While analyzing the human data alone and controlling the FDR at levels 0.01 and 0.00001, 935 (706 genes appearing in the intersection of all hold-outs) and 190 (139 genes appearing in the intersection of all hold-outs) genes were identified as differentially expressed, respectively. Figure 1 shows the scatter plots of $(\hat{\beta}_{1a}, \hat{\beta}_{1h})^T$ for all orthologs and the 21 pairs of orthologs in categories (1, 2, 3, and 4); i.e., the genes in this group showed evidence of distinguishing the two types of cancer for both species. Clearly, most of the pairs scattered around the $(0, 0)$ origin, indicating that these genes (for both species) did not have potential for serving as markers that could distinguish the two subgroups of DLBCL.

After identifying human genes that showed signs of discriminating between ABC DLBCL and GCB DLBCL and

Table 3 Summary of parameter estimates for the bivariate mixture model averaged over the 156 LOOCV outcomes

Category	Parameter					
	π_k	μ_{ak}	μ_{hk}	σ^2_{ak}	$\rho_k\sigma_{ak}\sigma_{hk}$	σ^2_{hk}
0	0.823(0.077)	NE	NE	0.013(0.001)	NE	0.012(0.001)
1	0.001(0.005)	0.341(0.081)	0.022(0.130)	0.004(0.010)	0.001(0.017)	0.022(0.060)
2	0.001(0.001)	-0.602(0.243)	-0.831(0.193)	0.199(0.082)	-0.128(0.048)	0.089(0.036)
3	0.001(0.004)	0.495(0.195)	-0.564(0.244)	0.042(0.078)	-0.042(0.041)	0.119(0.074)
4	0.000(0.003)	-1.131(0.422)	0.758(0.305)	0.000(0.028)	0.000(0.015)	0.000(0.050)
5	0.020(0.008)	NE	0.492(0.121)	0.020(0.021)	NE	0.058(0.049)
6	0.011(0.004)	NE	-0.517(0.136)	0.034(0.093)	NE	0.040(0.044)
7	0.130(0.077)	0.331(0.038)	NE	0.018(0.009)	NE	0.025(0.001)
8	0.012(0.008)	-0.478(0.339)	NE	0.011(0.051)	NE	0.042(0.054)

Numbers in parentheses are the bootstrap standard errors; $B = 5,000$ (the number of bootstrap replications); *NE* not estimated.

based either on two-species analysis (the nine-component bivariate mixture model) or on single-species (human only) analysis, the next step in the LOOCV procedure was to classify the hold-out human subject according to a classification rule established using the same set of genes. Table 4 summarizes the classification results over the 156 LOOCV instances under the four different gene selection criteria. It was interesting to see that using human genes from categories (1, 2, 3, and 4), categories (1, 2, 3, 4, 5, and 6) (two-species analysis), and the genes selected by controlling FDR at 0.00001 (single-species analysis) gave a very similar number of misclassifications, 17, 16, and 19, respectively. Nonetheless, choosing FDR = 0.01, the gene list was largely expanded. The enlarged gene

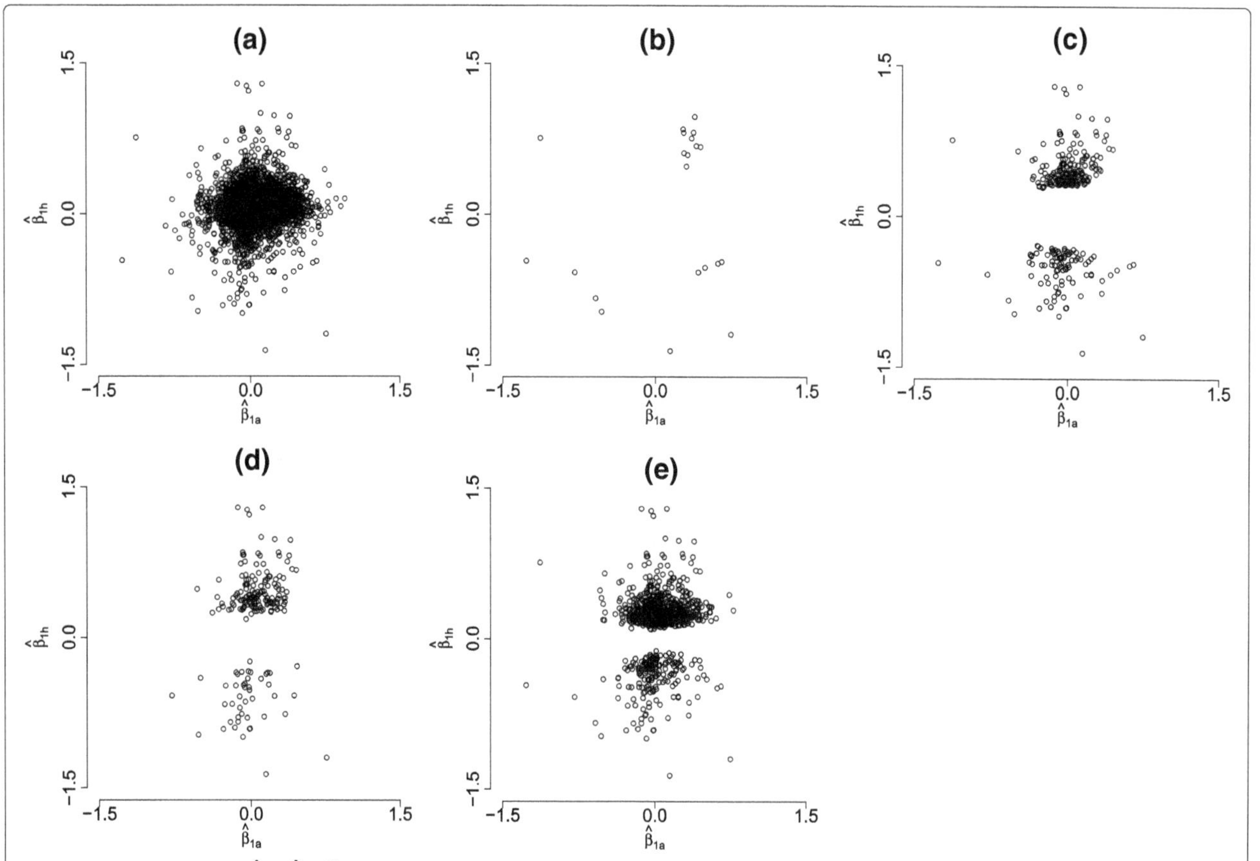

Figure 1 Scatter plots of $(\hat{\beta}_{1a}, \hat{\beta}_{1h})^T$. (**a**) all orthologs, (**b**) orthologs differentially expressed in both species (categories (1, 2, 3, and 4)), (**c**) orthologs for which the corresponding human genes are differentially expressed (categories (1, 2, 3, 4, 5, and 6)), (**d**) orthologs identified by analyzing the human data alone and controlling FDR at 0.00001, and (**e**) orthologs identified by analyzing the human data alone and controlling FDR at 0.01.

Table 4 Misclassification tables using different criteria

	Categories (1, 2, 3, and 4)		Categories (1, 2, 3, 4, 5, and 6)		FDR = 0.00001		FDR = 0.01	
Model prediction/subgroup	ABC	GCB	ABC	GCB	ABC	GCB	ABC	GCB
ABC DLBCL	72	5	64	13	58	19	0	77
GCB DLBCL	12	67	3	76	0	79	2	77

list resulted in a very poor classification result: 79 subjects were misclassified, among whom the entire group of ABC DLBCLs were misclassified as GCB DLBCLs. Misclassification rates were 0.109, 0.103, 0.122, and 0.506, accordingly. It was reasonable to conclude that the classification results based on two-species (dog and human) data, in general, may outperform those based on only single-species (human) data.

Prognostic DLBCL sub-categories defined by gene expression profiles

Does the taxonomy of DLBCL derived from gene expression patterns define clinically distinct subgroups of patients? To confirm that these two DLBCL subgroups defined by gene expression (the 21 genes in categories (1, 2, 3, and 4)) were both biologically and clinically distinct so that the mixture model approach could form the basis of a robust diagnostic test that may prove useful in assessing the results of therapeutic trials in DLBCL, overall survival and subgroup survival based on two types of gene-expression profiling, in [6] and [7] and the proposed mixture model approach, were plotted.

Figure 2 shows the nonparametric Kaplan-Meier survival probability estimates [25] for patients with DLBCL under two situations, unstratified and stratified, by gene-expression profiling. Treating the DLBCL patients regardless of the biological difference between the subgroups gave a 5-year survival rate of 45%. The 5-year survival rates after stratifying the patients according to the gene-expression profiling performed in [6] and [7] were 31% for ABC DLBCL and 59% for GCB DLBCL as compared with the rates of 29% for ABC DLBCL and 64% for GCB DLBCL if patients were stratified by the gene-expression profiling results based on the proposed nine-component mixture model. Under both types of stratification, ABC and GCB DLBCL were associated with statistically significant differences in overall survival ($p < 0.0001$). A log-rank test [26] was used to test the hypothesis of equal survival functions. The molecular dissection of DLBCL by gene-expression profiling using the proposed nine-component mixture model apparently identified different features of these patients that influence their survival.

As determined by gene-expression profiling performed in [6] and [7], among the 156 patients, there were 77 ABC DLBCLs and 79 GCB DLBCLs. Conversely, the stratification stated by the gene-expression profiling using the proposed nine-component mixture model gave a result of 84 ABC DLBCLs and 72 GCB DLBCLs. More specifically, five of the ABC DLBCLs had been classified as GCB DLBCLs, and 12 of the GCB DLBCLs had been categorized as ABC DLBCLs. However, the difference between the median survival time (years) of the subgroups stratified by gene-expression profiling performed in [6] and [7] was smaller than that of the subgroups stratified by gene expression profiling using the proposed nine-component mixture model (8.76 vs. 9.31). This may imply

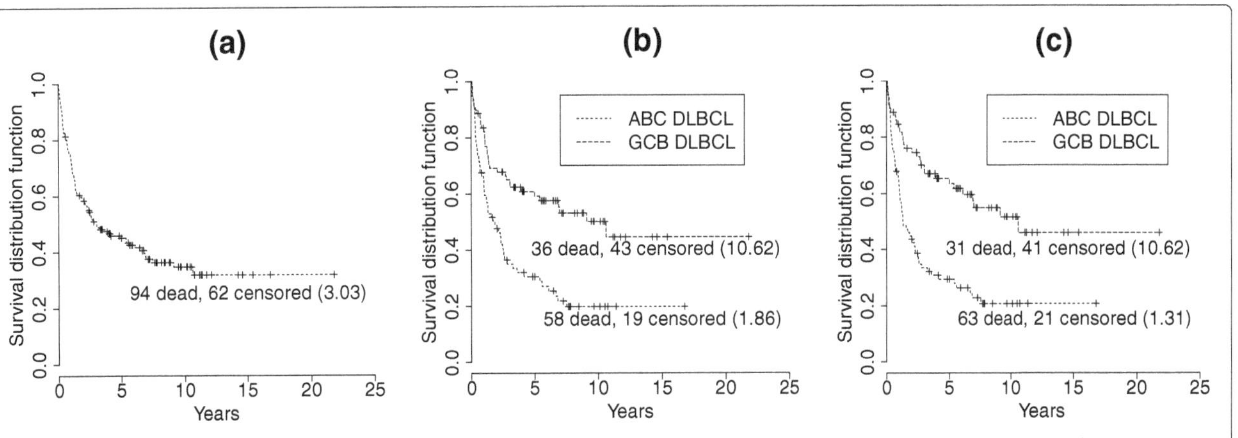

Figure 2 Kaplan-Meier survival probability estimates for the dog and human lymphoma study. (**a**) No stratification, (**b**) stratification based on the results of gene-expression profiling performed in [6] and [7], and (**c**) stratification based on the gene-expression profiling resulted from the proposed nine-component mixture model. Numbers in parentheses are medians.

that the stratification based on the gene expression profiling using the proposed nine-component mixture model provided better insight for the clinical difference between ABC and GCB DLBCL. These results suggested that the microarray-based outcome predictor not only reflected the clinical difference between the two DLBCL subgroups, but also provided a possible strategy of investigation for further individualization of patient treatment.

Justification of the 21 selected human genes

To validate the relevance between specific genes and phenotypes, a careful search of the literature was undertaken using Entrez Gene [27]. Some of these 21 genes (the genes in Table 5 with Entrez ID highlighted in italics) were identified by this search as potentially associated with the development of DLBCL. A brief summary of the relationship between these candidate genes and the development of DLBCL is given as follows:

1. *CD39* [Entrez Gene:953] is a B lymphocyte activation marker and has powerful functions in the immune system [28].
2. The expression pattern of *JAW1* [Entrez Gene:4033], a lymphoid-restricted protein, suggested that this protein may have a role in the developmentally regulated trafficking of the antigen receptors in B cells and may influence lymphoid development [29]. Tedoldi et al. [30] pointed out that high levels of *Jaw1* mRNA were found in germinal center B-cells and in diffuse large B-cell lymphomas of germinal center subtype.
3. The importance of *LMO2* [Entrez Gene:4005], though its function in germinal center cells is unknown, as a candidate marker involved in the development of DLBCL has been discussed in several papers. Natkunam et al. [31] studied *LMO2* at the protein level and confirmed that *LMO2* is expressed specifically in germinal center B cells, which is fully in keeping with gene-expression profiling studies that showed high levels of *LMO2* mRNA in germinal center B cells. They in [31] also observed that among DLBCLs, *LMO2* tended to be expressed in cases assigned by phenotyping to the GCB categories and can therefore be added to the panel of markers that pathologists may use to subcategorize lymphomas. Morton et al. [32] claimed that *LMO2* is one of the candidate genes involved in lymphocyte development and is highly expressed in germinal center lymphocytes. Durnick et al. [33] studied the relationship between *LMO2* expression and *t(14;18)/IGH-BCL2*, a specific marker of lymphomas of germinal center origin and has been specifically associated with the GCB subgroup of DLBCL as determined by gene expression profiling but not in the ABC cases. There was a statistically significant association between *IGH-BCL2* fusion and *LMO2* protein expression and hence *LMO2* was suggested as a potential marker for the GCB phenotype. A similar conclusion has also been reached by [1].
4. Germinal center B lymphocytes prominently express at least two regulators of G-protein signaling (RGS) proteins, *RGS1* and *RGS13* [Entrez Gene:6003]. RGS is a family of proteins acting to limit and modulate heterotrimeric G-protein signaling. Han et al. [34] discovered that RGS1 and RGS13 act together to regulate chemokine receptor signaling in human germinal center B lymphocytes. The results provide some insight toward finding methods to reduce or eliminate an organism's negative reaction to a treatment stimulus.
5. The importance of the transcription factor *FOXP1* [Entrez Gene:27086] as marker for the activated B-cell-like signature has been well-established [5,9]. Banham et al. [35] investigated the prognostic importance of FOXP1 protein expression in DLBCL and found that the overall empirical survival curves for the two subgroups based on the expression of *FOXP1* are significantly different. Goatly et al. [36] made an attempt to discover the underlying molecular mechanism of *FOXP1* expression in lymphoma development by investigating the *FOXP1* translocation, copy number change, and protein expression in mucosa-associated lymphoid tissue lymphoma and DLBCL. Korac and Dominis [37] explored the association between *FOXP1, BCL2,* and *BCL6* gene expression in diffuse large B-cell lymphoma tumor cells. *FOXP1* protein was detected in 28 patients; genetic abnormalities involving the *FOXP1* locus were found in 19 patients, and both were present in 13 patients, among the samples of lymph nodes from 53 patients with newly diagnosed DLBCL. *FOXP1* genetic abnormalities have been found to be associated with both *BCL2* and *BCL6* expression. Though it has been discovered that *BCL2* and *BCL6* proteins have an impact on diffuse large B-cell lymphoma development and outcome, they may not be good prognostic markers. *FOXP1* has played a role in the development of DLBCL. The identified association among *FOXP1, BCL2,* and *BCL6* indicates the possibilities of uncovering the development process in diffuse large B-cell lymphoma tumor cells. In addition, Nyman et al. [38] used *FOXP1* and *MUM1/IRF4* as activated B-cell-like markers to distinguish patients between the activated B-cell-like and other diffuse large B-cell lymphoma subtypes. Most recently, six common prognostic biomarkers, including *FOXP1,* were used to conclusively decide the cut-off values calculated by receiver operating

Table 5 Summary of the gene-specific information (retrieved from Entrez Gene, an NCBI's database for gene-specific information)

Entrez Gene ID	Category	Dog ortholog	Frequency[a]	Symbol	Official full name
953	1	486810	156	CD39; ATPDase; FLJ40921; FLJ40959; NTPDase-1; DKFZp686D194; DKFZp686I093; ENTPD1	Ectonucleoside triphosphate diphosphohydrolase 1
1278	2	403824	156	OI4; COL1A2	Collagen, type I, alpha 2
2530	1	448804	156	MGC26465; FUT8	Fucosyltransferase 8 (alpha (1,6) fucosyltransferase)
4005	2	609006	156	TTG2; RBTN2; RHOM2; RBTNL1; LMO2	LIM domain only 2 (rhombotin-like 1)
4033	3	486631	156	JAW1; LRMP	Lymphoid-restricted membrane protein
5919	2	475532	156	TIG2; HP10433; RARRES2	Retinoic acid receptor responder (tazarotene induced) 2
6003	3	612789	124	MGC17173; RGS13	Regulator of G-protein signaling 13
6856	3	475889	154	SYPL; H-SP1; SYPL1	Synaptophysin-like 1
6925	1	403949	156	E2-2; ITF2; PTHS; SEF2; SEF2-1; SEF2-1A; SEF2-1B; bHLHb19; MGC149723; MGC149724; TCF4	Transcription factor 4
7037	1	403703	11	TFR; CD71; TFR1; TRFR; TFRC	Transferrin receptor (p90, CD71)
9435	1	485701	156	C6ST; GST2; GST-2; Gn6ST-1; CHST2	Carbohydrate (*N*-acetylglucosamine-6-*O*) sulfotransferase 2
9760	2	486964	156	TOX1; KIAA0808; TOX	Thymocyte selection-associated high mobility group box
10447	3	612336	154	ILEI; GS3786; FAM3C	Family with sequence similarity 3, member C
23075	3	485385	4	HSPC321; SWAP-70; FLJ39540; KIAA0640; SWAP70	SWAP switching B-cell complex 70kDa subunit
25816	1	481428	156	GG2-1; SCCS2; SCC-S2; MDC-3.13; TNFAIP8	Tumor necrosis factor, alpha-induced protein 8
27086	1	484692	156	QRF1; 12CC4; hFKH1B; HSPC215; FLJ23741; MGC12942; MGC88572; MGC99551; FOXP1	Forkhead box P1
56941	2	484628	156	DC12; MGC111075; C3orf37	Chromosome 3 open reading frame 37
81552	1	608562	145	ECOP; GASP; FLJ20532; DKFZp564K0822, VOPP1	Vesicular, overexpressed in cancer, prosurvival protein 1
81641	1	479002	116	Apm; Apn; KZP; AP-M; AP-N; Lap1; rAPN; Anpep	Alanyl (membrane) aminopeptidase
121355	4	477590	156	FAM112B; FLJ32942; GTSF1	Gametocyte specific factor 1
219972	1	475960	156	MPG1; MGC132657; MGC138435; MPEG1	Macrophage expressed 1

For the 21 human genes in categories (1, 2, 3, and 4) determined by the bivariate mixture model.
Genes in *italics* were identified by this search as potentially associated with the development of DLBCL.
[a]number of times the corresponding gene was found in the classification gene set for the 156 LOOCV instances.

curves to predict survival for DLBCL patients [39]. All these results suggested that FOXP1 expression may be important in DLBCL pathogenesis.

Among the 21 selected genes, five (from categories 1, 2, and 3) have been carefully examined to explore their association with the development of lymphoma. From the mixture model assumption, genes in the same category should react to the stimulus (drug treatment, cancer type, etc.) in a similar manner. Hence, the implications of these 21 genes (some of them may not have been studied scrupulously) in lymphoma may provide timely and important insight on guiding future investigations of their roles in both B-cell biology and lymphoma development.

Conclusions

Since the development of high throughput gene expression technology, the important and difficult task of searching for genes that exhibit differences across species (cancer types or treatment groups in drug trials) has been the focus of much research. Simultaneously analyzing gene expression across two species takes into account the biological similarity between different organisms while identifying genes that could be potential prognostic markers and increase the power to detect differences. Identification of the relevant genes and a better understanding of the associated molecular pathways may open new possibilities in cancer diagnosis and treatment. Furthermore, it may become a practical assay for newly diagnosed patients to optimize their clinical management.

In this case study, the application of the proposed nine-component mixture model successfully reduced the quantities of variables (genes) needed to be investigated for the study of two types of DLBCL in humans. The dimension of variables decreased from 6,566 to 21, a cluster of genes that were identified as being differentially expressed in both species. On the other hand, an analysis of data from one species that selected genes using a specified FDR led to a much longer list of differentially expressed human genes (935 genes with FDR = 0.01 and 190 with FDR = 0.00001). Furthermore, the misclassification rate for human cancer type classification using clustering with gene expression from these 21 genes identified by the bivariate mixture model was remarkably low. The survivorship of the patients stratified according to this clustering was very different across the two types of cancer, indicating that the stratification based on gene-expression profiling using the proposed nine-component mixture model provided better insight for the clinical differences between the two types of cancer.

While validating the relevance of the identified human genes through NCBI's database, literature, if any, for the corresponding dog orthologs were also searched. Far less research about DLBCL has been conducted for canines. As the model assumption is based on the biological mechanism behind humans and animals, the promising DLBCL classification results based on the human genes may be extended to dogs. Furthermore, currently, direct experiments on humans are not practical. This research provides the possibility for scientists to conduct observational or experimental research on modeling organisms as the first step to understand phenotypes, and then extend the findings to humans for further investigation.

Abbreviations

DLBCL, diffuse large-B-cell lymphoma; GCB DLBCL, germinal-center B-cell-like diffuse large-B-cell lymphoma; ABC DLBCL, activated B-cell-like diffuse large-B-cell lymphoma.

Competing interests

The authors declare that they have no competing interests.

Authors' contributions

All authors read and approved the final manuscript.

Acknowledgements

The authors thank Dr. Steven Suter, professor of clinical sciences and Dr. Matthew Breen from the College of Veterinary Medicine, North Carolina State University for the access to the dog lymphoma expression data.

Author details

[1] Dr. Su's Statistics, Department of Human Nutrition, Food, and Animal Sciences, University of Hawaii at Manoa, Honolulu, HI 96822, USA. [2] Bioinformatics Research Center, North Carolina State University, Raleigh, NC 27695, USA. [3] Biomarker and Predictive Analytics, GlaxoSmithKline, 5 Moore Drive, Research Triangle Park, NC 27709, USA. [4] Department of Genetic, University of North Carolina, Chapel Hill, NC 27599, USA. [5] Department of Clinical Sciences, Center for Comparative Medicine & Translational Research, North Carolina State University, Raleigh, NC 27695, USA. [6] Department of Molecular Biomedical Sciences, College of Veterinary Medicine, North Carolina State University, Raleigh, NC 27695, USA. [7] Department of Statistics, North Carolina State University, Raleigh, NC 27695, USA.

References

1. Lossos I, Czerwinski DK, Alizadeh AA, Wechser MA, Tibshirani R, Botstein D, Levy R: **Prediction of survival in diffuse large-B-cell lymphoma based on the expression of six genes.** *N Engl J Med* 2004, **350:**1828–1837.
2. Lenz G, Staudt L: **Aggressive lymphomas.** *N Engl J Med* 2010, **362:**1417–1429.
3. The International Non-Hodgkin's Lymphoma Prognostic Factors Project: **A predictive model for aggressive non-Hodgkin's lymphoma.** *N Engl J Med* 1993, **329:**987–992.
4. Shipp MA, Ross KN, Tamayo P, Weng AP, Kutok JL, Aguiar RC, Gaasenbeek M, Angelo M, Reich M, Pinkus GS, Ray TS, Koval MA, Last KW, Norton A, Lister TA, Mesirov J, Neuberg DS, Lander ES, Aster JC, Golub TR: **Diffuse large B-cell lymphoma outcome prediction by gene-expression profiling and supervised machine learning.** *Nat Med* 2002, **8:**68–74.
5. Rosenwald A, Wright G, Chan WC, Connors JM, Campo E, Fisher RI, Gascoyne RD, Muller-Hermelink HK, Smeland EB, Giltnane JM, Hurt EM, Zhao H, Averett L, Yang L, Wilson WH, Jaffe ES, Simon R, Klausner RD, Powell J, Duffey PL, Longo DL, Greiner TC, Weisenburger DD, Sanger WG, Dave BJ, Lynch JC, Vose J, Armitage JO, Montserrat E, Lpez-Guillermo A, et al.: **The use of molecular profiling to predict survival after chemotherapy for diffuse large-B-cell lymphoma.** *N Engl J Med*, **346:**1937–1947.
6. Lenz G, Wright GW, Emre NC, Kohlhammer H, Dave SS, Davis RE, Carty S, Lam LT, Shaffer AL, Xiao W, Powell J, Rosenwald A, Ott G, Muller-Hermelink HK, Gascoyne RD, Connors JM, Campo E, Jaffe ES, Delabie J, Smeland EB, Rimsza LM, Fisher RI, Weisenburger DD, Chan WC, Staudt LM: **Molecular**

subtypes of diffuse large B-cell lymphoma arise by distinct genetic pathways. *Proc Nat Acad Sci USA* 2008, **105:**13520–13525.

7. Lenz G, Wright G, Dave SS, Xiao W, Powell J, Zhao H, Xu W, Tan B, Goldschmidt N, Iqbal J, Vose J, Bast M, Fu K, Weisenburger DD, Greiner TC, Armitage JO, Kyle A, May L, Gascoyne RD, Connors JM, Troen G, Holte H, Kvaloy S, Dierickx D, Verhoef G, Delabie J, Smeland EB, Jares P, Martinez A, Lopez-Guillermo A, et al.: **Stromal gene signatures in large-B-cell lymphomas.** *N Engl J Med* 2008, **359:**2314–2323.
8. Wright G, Tan B, Rosenwald A, Hurt EH, Wiestner A, Staudt LM: **A gene expression-based method to diagnose clinically distinct subgroups of diffuse large B-cell lymphoma.** *Proc Nat Acad Sci USA* 2003, **100:**9991–9996.
9. Alizadeh AA, Eisen MB, Davis RE, Ma C, Lossos IS, Rosenwald A, Boldrick JC, Sabet H, Tran T, Yu X, Powell JI, Yang L, Marti GE, Moore T, Hudson JJr, Lu L, Lewis DB, Tibshirani R, Sherlock G, Chan WC, Greiner TC, Weisenburger DD, Armitage JO, Warnke R, Levy R, Wilson W, Grever MR, Byrd JC, Botstein D, Brown PO, Staudt LM, et al.: **Distinct types of diffuse large B-cell lymphoma identified by gene expression profiling.** *Nature* 2000, **403:**503–511.
10. Eisen M, Spellman PT, Brown PO, Botstein D: **Cluster analysis and display of genome-wide expression patterns.** *Proc Nat Acad Sci USA* 1998, **95:**14863–14868.
11. Golub T, Slonim DK, Tamayo P, Huard C, Gaasenbeek M, Mesirov JP, Coller H, Loh ML, Downing JR, Caligiuri MA, Bloomfield CD, Lander ES: **Molecular classification of cancer: class discovery and class prediction by gene expression monitoring.** *Science* 1999, **286:**531–537.
12. Blenk S, Engelmann J, Weniger M, Schultz J, Dittrich M, Rosenwald A, Mller-Hermelink HK, Mller T, Dandekar T: **Germinal center B cell-like (GCB) and activated B cell-like (ABC) type diffuse large B cell lymphoma (DLBCL): analysis of molecular predictors, signatures, cell cycle state and patient survival.** *Cancer Inform* 2007, **3:**399–420.
13. Smyth G: **Linear models and empirical Bayes methods for assessing differential expression in microarray experiments.** *Stat Appl Genet Mol Biol* 2004, **3:**3.
14. Sonnhammer E, Koonin E: **Orthology, paralogy and proposed classification for paralog subtypes.** *TIG* 2002, **18:**619–620.
15. McLachlan G, Basford K: *Mixture models: inference and applications to clustering*. New York: Marcel Dekker; 1988.
16. McLachlan G, Peel D: *Finite mixture models*. New York: Wiley; 2000.
17. Efron B: **Bootstrap methods: another look at the jackknife.** *Ann Stat* 1979, **7:**1–26.
18. Efron B: **Better bootstrap confidence intervals.** *J Am Stat Assoc* 1987, **82:**171–185.
19. Barrett T, Troup DB, Wilhite SE, Ledoux P, Rudnev D, Evangelista C, Kim IF, Soboleva A, Tomashevsky M, Marshall KA, Phillippy KH, Sherman PM, Muertter RN, Edgar R: **NCBI GEO: archive for high-throughput functional genomic data.** *Nucl Acids Res* 2009, **37:**D885—D890.
20. Lachenbruch P, Mickey M: **Estimation of error rates in discriminant analysis.** *Technometrics* 1968, **10:**1–11.
21. Benjamini Y, Hochberg Y: **Controlling the false discovery rate: a practical and powerful approach to multiple testing.** *J Roy Statist Soc Ser B* 1995, **57:**289–300.
22. MacQueen J: **Some methods for classification and analysis of multivariate observations.** In *Proceedings of Fifth Berkeley Symposium on Math Statistics and Probability. Statistics*. Berkeley: 1965 June 21-July 18, Statistical Laboratory of the University of California; 1965**1:**281–297 .
23. SAS: **SAS onlineDoc® 9.1.3.** (2002-2008) Available at http://support.sas.com/onlinedoc/913.
24. Dempster A, Laird N, Rubin D: **Maximum likelihood from incomplete data via the EM algorithm.** *J Roy Statist Soc Ser B* 1977, **39:**1–38.
25. Kaplan E, Meier P: **Nonparametric estimation from incomplete observations.** *J Am Stat Assoc* 1958, **53:**457–481.
26. Mantel N: **Evaluation of survival data and two new rank order statistics arising in its consideration.** *Cancer Chemother Rep* 1966, **50:**163–170.
27. Maglott D, Ostell J, Pruitt KD, Tatusova T: **Entrez Gene: gene-centered information at NCBI.** *Nucl Acids Res* 2007, **35:**D26—D31.
28. Spanevello R, Mazzanti CM, Schmatz R, Thom G, Bagatini M, Correa M, Rosa C, Stefanello N, Bell LP, Moretto MB, Oliveira L, Morsch VM, Schetinger MR: **The activity and expression of NTPDase is altered in lymphocytes of multiple sclerosis patients.** *Clin Chim Acta* 2009, **411:**210–214.
29. Behrens T, Kearns GM, Rivard JJ, Bernstein HD, Yewdell JW, Staudt LM: **Carboxyl-terminal targeting and novel post-translational processing of JAW1, a lymphoid protein of the endoplasmic reticulum.** *J Biol Chem* 1996, **271:**23528–23534.
30. Tedoldi S, Paterson JC, Cordell J, Tan SY, Jones M, Manek S, Dei Tos, A P, Roberton H, Masir N, Natkunam Y, Pileri SA, Facchetti F, Hansmann ML, Mason DY, Marafioti T: **Jaw1/LRMP, a germinal centre-associated marker for the immunohistological study of B-cell lymphomas.** *J Pathol* 2006, **209:**454–463.
31. Natkunam Y, Zhao S, Mason DY, Chen J, Taidi B, Jones M, Hammer AS, Hamilton Dutoit, S, Lossos IS, Levy R: **The oncoprotein LMO2 is expressed in normal germinal-center B cells and in human B-cell lymphomas.** *Blood* 2007, **109:**1636–1642.
32. Morton LM, Purdue MP, Zheng T, Wang SS, Armstrong B, Zhang Y, Menashe I, Chatterjee N, Davis S, Lan Q, Vajdic CM, Severson RK, Holford TR, Kricker A, Cerhan JR, Leaderer B, Grulich A, Yeager M, Cozen W, Hoar Zahm, S, Chanock SJ, Rothman N, Hartge P: **Risk of non-Hodgkin lymphoma associated with germline variation in genes that regulate the cell cycle, apoptosis, and lymphocyte development.** *Cancer Epidemiol Biomarkers Prev* 2009, **18:**1259–1270.
33. Durnick D, Law ME, Maurer MJ, Natkunam Y, Levy R, Lossos IS, Kurtin PJ, McPhail ED: **Expression of LMO2 is associated with t(14;18)/IGH-BCL2 fusion but not BCL6 translocations in diffuse large B-cell lymphoma.** *Am J Clin Path* 2010, **134:**278–281.
34. Han J, Huang NN, Kim DU, Kehrl JH: **RGS1 and RGS13 mRNA silencing in a human B lymphoma line enhances responsiveness to chemoattractants and impairs desensitization.** *J Leukoc Biol* 2006, **79:**1357–1367.
35. Banham A, Connors JM, Brown PJ, Cordell JL, Ott G, Sreenivasan G, Farinha P, Horsman DE, Gascoyne RD: **Expression of the FOXP1 transcription factor is strongly associated with inferior survival in patients with diffuse large B-cell lymphoma.** *Clin Cancer Res* 2005, **11:**1065–1072.
36. Goatly A, Bacon CM, Nakamura S, Ye H, Kim I, Brown PJ, Ruskon-Fourmestraux A, Cervera P, Streubel B, Banham AH, Du MQ: **FOXP1 abnormalities in lymphoma: translocation breakpoint mapping reveals insights into deregulated transcriptional control.** *Mod Pathol* 2008, **21:**902–911.
37. Korac P, Dominis, M: **Prognostic markers and gene abnormalities in subgroups of diffuse large B-cell lymphoma: single center experience.** *Clin Sci* 2008, **49:**618–624.
38. Nyman H, Jerkeman M, Karjalainen-Lindsberg ML, Banham AH, Leppä S: **Prognostic impact of activated B-cell focused classification in diffuse large B-cell lymphoma patients treated with R-CHOP.** *Mod Pathol* 2009, **22:**1094–1101.
39. Tzankov A, Zlobec I, Went P, Robl H, Hoeller S, Dirnhofer S: **Prognostic immunophenotypic biomarker studies in diffuse large B cell lymphoma with special emphasis on rational determination of cut-off scores.** *Leuk Lymphoma* 2010, **21:**902–911.

18

Molecular heterogeneity in malignant peripheral nerve sheath tumors associated with neurofibromatosis type 1

Laura Thomas[1], Victor-Felix Mautner[2], David N Cooper[1] and Meena Upadhyaya[1*]

Abstract

Neurofibromatosis type-1 (NF1), resulting from *NF1* gene loss of function, is characterized by an increased risk of developing benign and malignant peripheral nerve sheath tumors (MPNSTs). Whereas the cellular heterogeneity of NF1-associated tumors has been well studied, the molecular heterogeneity of MPNSTs is still poorly understood. Mutational heterogeneity within these malignant tumors greatly complicates the study of the underlying mechanisms of tumorigenesis. We have explored this molecular heterogeneity by performing loss of heterozygosity (LOH) analysis of the *NF1*, *TP53*, *RB1*, *PTEN*, and *CDKN2A* genes on sections of 10 MPNSTs derived from 10 unrelated NF1 patients. LOH data for the *TP53* gene was found to correlate with the results of p53 immunohistochemical analysis in the same tumor sections. Further, approximately 70% of MPNSTs were found to display intra-tumoral molecular heterogeneity as evidenced by differences in the level of LOH between different sections of the same tumor samples. This study constitutes the first systematic analysis of molecular heterogeneity within MPNSTs derived from NF1 patients. Appreciation of the existence of molecular heterogeneity in NF1-associated tumors is important not only for optimizing somatic mutation detection, but also for understanding the mechanisms of NF1 tumorigenesis, a prerequisite for the development of specifically targeted cancer therapeutics.

Keywords: Neurofibromatosis type 1, Malignant peripheral nerve sheath tumors, Molecular heterogeneity, *TP53*

Introduction

Neurofibromatosis type 1 (NF1) (MIM 162200) is an autosomal dominant disorder affecting approximately 1 in 4,000 people worldwide [1]. NF1 is characterized by variable clinical features including benign cutaneous neurofibromas and plexiform neurofibromas in addition to pigmentary abnormalities comprising *café-au-lait* macules, Lisch nodules of the iris, and axillary and inguinal freckling. Learning difficulties and orthopedic problems also occur in up to 50% of individuals with NF1 [2]. Malignant complications are a less frequent but potentially much more serious manifestation of NF1. These often lead to premature death in individuals with NF1 and include malignant peripheral nerve sheath tumors (MPNSTs) which occur in approximately 10% to 15% of patients [3], pheochromocytomas, brain tumors, optic gliomas, gastrointestinal stromal tumors, and breast carcinomas [4].

The *NF1* gene, located at 17q11.2, encodes neurofibromin, a 2818 amino acid protein which is expressed at a high level in the brain and central nervous system [4]. Neurofibromin is a highly conserved RAS-GAP which negatively regulates Ras signaling [5-7] and the multiple downstream effectors activated by Ras, such as the PI3K and the MAPK (mitogen-activated kinase) signaling cascades that are involved in regulating cell proliferation, DNA synthesis, and apoptosis. The loss of neurofibromin function due to *NF1* gene inactivation therefore results in the constitutive activation of many of these down-regulated systems leading to increased cell proliferation and an increased likelihood of tumorigenesis.

In line with the tumor suppressor role of the *NF1* gene, mutational inactivation of both NF1 alleles is required to change the phenotype of the cell: a first (inherited) mutation in one *NF1* allele is followed by the somatic loss of the remaining wild-type *NF1* allele via a

* Correspondence: upadhyaya@cardiff.ac.uk
[1]Institute of Medical Genetics, School of Medicine, Cardiff University, Cardiff CF14 4XN, UK

number of different mutational mechanisms. Loss of heterozygosity (LOH), for example, represents a common form of loss of function of the wild-type *NF1* allele in somatic cells such as Schwann cells which form neurofibromas, owing to the presence of an inherited *NF1* gene lesion on the other allele. [8,9] LOH is known to be caused by a number of mechanisms including deletions of genetic material and the loss of a whole chromosome by nondisjunction with or without reduplication. However, mitotic recombination has been demonstrated to be the most common event accounting for LOH in NF1-associated tumors [9].

In addition to *NF1* gene mutations, a number of other loci are also known to be involved in the process of NF1 tumorigenesis. Thus, additional somatic mutations have been identified in NF1-associated MPNSTs that affect several genes encoding proteins involved in cell cycle regulation: *TP53, RB1, CDKN2A* [10-17], and *PTEN* [18]. Alterations in *TP53* and *RB1* have also been identified in plexiform neurofibromas [19] and more recently in cutaneous neurofibromas from patients with a high tumor burden [20]. These genetic alterations act so as to promote cellular proliferation as a consequence of *CDKN2A* loss and to bring about abnormal cell cycle arrest mediated by DNA damage and aberrant apoptosis as a consequence of the loss of *TP53* and *RB1*.

Tumor heterogeneity is a notoriously challenging aspect of cancer biology, responsible for introducing very significant complexity into both the study of the underlying mechanisms of tumor development and the therapeutic context [21-23]. Tumor heterogeneity has been modeled using a number of different biomarkers to identify the extent of heterogeneity at the cellular, molecular, and genome architectural levels [24,25]. Cellular heterogeneity is a well-established feature of NF1-associated tumors, particularly in benign cutaneous neurofibromas in which only the Schwann cells harbor *NF1* mutations, although the tumors also contain fibroblasts, mast cells, perineural cells, and axons [26]. The tumor microenvironment is also known to impact upon the development of NF1-associated tumors, with mast cells a likely contributor to neurofibroma development [27]. As with benign neurofibromas, malignant NF1-associated tumors are known to be heterogeneous in nature, invariably containing diverse subpopulations of tumor cells, including benign and malignant cells, fibroblasts, and infiltrating inflammatory cells [26]. At the molecular level, malignant tumors are recognized as being highly heterogeneous in terms of both their accumulated genetic mutations and their phenotypic [*CDKN2A, TP53, RB1*] expression profiles [13,15,16].

Analysis of molecular and cellular heterogeneity using a variety of methods promises to generate important new insights into tumor biology as well as the underlying processes of tumorigenesis. This is the first study to comprehensively determine the level of molecular heterogeneity in a panel of MPNSTs derived from patients with NF1. It is hoped that this will provide further understanding of the molecular heterogeneity of malignant tumors in the context of the underlying background cellular and genome architectural heterogeneity. Furthermore, such studies may allow both therapeutic sensitivities and the efficacy of potential drug treatments to be comprehensively evaluated.

Materials and methods

Patients

Ten unrelated patients, all exhibiting the NIH diagnostic criteria for NF1 (reviewed by Upadhyaya [1]) were analyzed in this study. Germline mutations have been detected in 7 of the 10 patients (Table 1); however, full clinical details were not available from all patients. A total of 10 MPNSTs derived from these patients were carefully and individually macrodissected to yield clean sections which were in turn further subdivided. The number and size of the various sections and subsections were mainly dependent upon the size of the original tumor (Table 1 and Additional file 1: Supplementary Figure S1). DNA was extracted from all sections of tumor samples and corresponding constitutional (blood) samples by means of the phenol/chloroform extraction method [28]. This study obtained approval from the appropriate institutional review boards. All patients involved provided their informed consent.

LOH analysis

LOH analysis was performed on all sections derived from the 10 MPNSTs and their corresponding lymphocyte DNA samples with a panel of fluorescently tagged microsatellite markers located within the five genes investigated: *NF1* (*D17S799, J1J2, IVS27, EV120, IVS38, 3'NF1-1, D17S798, D17S250*, and *D17S1822*) [28], *TP53* (D17S796, *TP53 Inv, TP53 c.72, TP53 Exon 6, D17S938*, and *D17S804*) [29,30], *RB1* (*D13S118, D13S153, D13S917, RB1.2, RB1.26*, and *D13S119*) [31,32], *CDKN2A* (*D9S1751, D9S942, D9S304*, and *D9S748*) [33,34], and *PTEN* (*D10S2491, D10S215*, exon 3, and exon 8) [35]. Molecular heterogeneity was assessed by noting differences in the level of LOH between different sections of the same tumor sample.

Markers were analyzed by means of an ABI 3100 genetic analyzer using Genotyper and Genescan software (Applied Biosystems, Warrington, UK) [28]. Allele loss in a tumor was scored if the area under one allelic peak in the tumor section was reduced relative to the other allele, after correction of the relative peak areas against the corresponding lymphocyte DNA sample. For LOH to be confirmed, at least two adjacent markers were

Table 1 Analysis of molecular heterogeneity with respect to *NF1*, *TP53*, *RB1*, *CDKN2A*, and *PTEN* in 10 MPNSTs

Tumor	Tumor number	Tumor section	Tumor subsection	*NF1*	*TP53*	*RB1*	*PTEN*	*CDKN2A*
1	T196.22	A	1	LOH	LOH	LOH	LOH	LOH
			2	LOH	LOH	LOH	LOH	LOH
			3	LOH	LOH	50% LOH	LOH	LOH
			4	1 2	1 2	1 2	1 2	1 2
			5	LOH	LOH	50% LOH	LOH	LOH
			6	LOH	LOH	LOH	LOH	LOH
			7	LOH	LOH	LOH	LOH	LOH
			8	LOH	LOH	50% LOH	50% LOH	LOH
			9	1 2	LOH	1 2	LOH	LOH
			10	1 2	LOH	1 2	LOH	LOH
		B	1	LOH	50% LOH	50% LOH	50% LOH	1 2
			2	LOH	50% LOH	50% LOH	50% LOH	1 2
			3	LOH	50% LOH	50% LOH	50% LOH	1 2
			4	LOH	50% LOH	50% LOH	50% LOH	1 2
			5	50% LOH	50% LOH	50% LOH	50% LOH	1 2
			6	LOH	50% LOH	50% LOH	50% LOH	1 2
			7	LOH	50% LOH	50% LOH	50% LOH	1 2
			8	LOH	50% LOH	50% LOH	50% LOH	1 2
			9	LOH	50% LOH	50% LOH	50% LOH	1 2
			10	LOH	50% LOH	50% LOH	50% LOH	1 2
		C	1	LOH	LOH	50% LOH	LOH	1 2
			2	LOH	LOH	50% LOH	LOH	1 2
			3	LOH	LOH	50% LOH	LOH	1 2
			4	LOH	LOH	50% LOH	LOH	1 2
			5	1 2	LOH	1 2	50% LOH	50% LOH
			6	LOH	LOH	50% LOH	LOH	50% LOH
			7	LOH	LOH	50% LOH	LOH	50% LOH
			8	LOH	LOH	50% LOH	LOH	50% LOH
			9	LOH	LOH	50% LOH	LOH	50% LOH
			10	LOH	LOH	50% LOH	LOH	50% LOH
		D	1	LOH	LOH	50% LOH	LOH	50% LOH
			2	LOH	LOH	50% LOH	50% LOH	1 2
			3	LOH	LOH	50% LOH	LOH	LOH
			4	LOH	LOH	50% LOH	LOH	LOH
			5	LOH	LOH	50% LOH	LOH	LOH
			6	LOH	LOH	50% LOH	LOH	LOH
			7	LOH	LOH	50% LOH	LOH	LOH
			8	LOH	LOH	50% LOH	LOH	LOH
			9	LOH	LOH	50% LOH	LOH	LOH
			10	LOH	LOH	50% LOH	LOH	LOH
		E	1	LOH	1 2	1 2	1 2	1 2
			2	LOH	1 2	1 2	50% LOH	1 2
			3	50% LOH	1 2	1 2	1 2	1 2
			4	LOH	1 2	1 2	50% LOH	1 2
			5	1 2	1 2	1 2	0%	1 2
			6	50% LOH	1 2	1 2	50% LOH	1 2
			7	50% LOH	1 2	1 2	0%	1 2

Table 1 Analysis of molecular heterogeneity with respect to *NF1*, *TP53*, *RB1*, *CDKN2A*, and *PTEN* in 10 MPNSTs *(Continued)*

			8	LOH	1 2	1 2	1 2	1 2
			9	LOH	1 2	1 2	1 2	1 2
			10	LOH	1 2	1 2	1 2	1 2
2	T516	A	1	LOH	50% LOH	1 2	1 2	1 2
			2	1 2	50% LOH	1 2	1 2	1 2
		B	1	50% LOH	50% LOH	1 2	1 2	1 2
			2	50% LOH	50% LOH	1 2	1 2	1 2
		C	1	1 2	1 2	1 2	1 2	1 2
			2	1 2	1 2	1 2	1 2	1 2
3	T517	A	1	LOH	50% LOH	1 2	1 2	1 2
			2	LOH	50% LOH	1 2	1 2	1 2
		B	1	LOH	50% LOH	1 2	1 2	1 2
			2	1 2	1 2	50% LOH	1 2	1 2
4	T518	A	1	1 2	50% LOH	50% LOH	1 2	1 2
			2	LOH	1 2	50% LOH	1 2	50% LOH
		B	1	LOH	50% LOH	1 2	1 2	1 2
			2	1 2	1 2	1 2	1 2	1 2
		C	1	1 2	1 2	1 2	1 2	1 2
			2	1 2	1 2	1 2	1 2	1 2
5	T519	A	1	1 2	50% LOH	50% LOH	1 2	1 2
			2	50% LOH	50% LOH	50% LOH	1 2	1 2
		B	1	50% LOH	50% LOH	1 2	1 2	1 2
			2	50% LOH	50% LOH	50% LOH	1 2	1 2
6	T521	A	1	LOH	1 2	1 2	1 2	1 2
			2	LOH	1 2	1 2	1 2	1 2
		B	1	LOH	1 2	1 2	1 2	1 2
			2	LOH	1 2	1 2	1 2	1 2
7	T522	A	1	LOH	1 2	1 2	1 2	1 2
			2	LOH	1 2	1 2	1 2	1 2
8	T523	A	1	LOH	1 2	1 2	1 2	1 2
			2	LOH	1 2	1 2	LOH	1 2
9	T524	A	1	LOH	1 2	1 2	1 2	LOH
			2	LOH	1 2	1 2	1 2	LOH
10	T525	A	1	LOH	1 2	1 2	1 2	1 2
			2	LOH	1 2	1 2	1 2	1 2
		B	1	LOH	1 2	1 2	1 2	LOH
			2	LOH	1 2	1 2	1 2	LOH

LOH denotes samples in which approximately 100% LOH of the second allele has occurred; 50% LOH denotes samples in which approximately 50% of the second allele was lost; 1 2 denotes samples in which the marker was clearly present in the heterozygous state, denoting the absence of LOH. The results represent the summed data for all markers analyzed at each genetic loci (*NF1*, *TP53*, *RB1*, *CDKN2A* and *PTEN*).

required to exhibit a reduced signal by at least 50%. Samples were deemed to display LOH when complete (approximately 100%) loss of the second allele was evident. Samples exhibiting between approximately 50% and 99% loss of the second allele were termed '50% LOH', whereas a marker which demonstrated no LOH (approximately 0% to 49%) was simply classed as heterozygous ('1 2').

p53 Immunohistochemical analysis

Immunohistochemical (IHC) analysis of p53 was performed on five sections derived from five MPNSTs (T196.22, T516, T517, T518, and T519) which were found by LOH analysis to exhibit molecular heterogeneity with respect to the *TP53* gene (Table 1). Immunohistochemistry was performed using a standard protocol [9]. Briefly, 5-μm-thick slides were cut from blocks of formalin-fixed paraffin-embedded MPNST tissue using a microtome (Leica Microsystems, Wetzlar, Germany). Deparaffination was completed in ethanol and xylene prior to antigen recovery which was performed using boiling citrate buffer. Endogenous peroxidase was blocked with 3% hydrogen peroxide, while goat serum (Vector Labs, Peterborough, UK) was used in the blocking step. A 100-μl pre-diluted mouse anti-p53 monoclonal primary antibody (Launch Diagnostics, Kent, UK) was used as supplied and added to each slide and incubated at 4 °C overnight. Each slide was then incubated with 100 μl secondary antibody (Vector Labs) for 30 min and subsequently with 100 μl ABC peroxidase (Vector Labs) for 30 min. DAB (Vector Labs) was added to each slide to allow the color to develop. Slides were dehydrated and mounted with DPX (VWR).

Results

LOH analysis

Varying sizes of 10 MPNST tumors, derived from 10 different individuals, were independently sectioned, and the LOH of five genes (*NF1*, *TP53*, *RB1*, *CDKN2A*, and *PTEN*) was analyzed for each section. Germline mutations were detected in 7 of the 10 patients. Although this is a relatively small sample, the germline mutation does not appear to correlate with the level of molecular heterogeneity. LOH of the *NF1* gene was identified in all 10 tumors. In addition, LOH was noted for the *TP53* gene (five tumors: T196.22, T516, T517, T518, and T519), the *RB1* gene (four tumors: T196.22, T517, T518, and T519), the *CDKN2A* gene (four tumors: T196.22, T518, T524, and T525), and the *PTEN* gene (two tumors: T196.22 and T523) (Table 1, Figure 1, and Additional file 2: Supplementary Table S1). In only 2 of the 10 tumors (T521 and T522) was LOH not found in at least one of the four loci other than *NF1* (i.e. *TP53*, *RB1*, *CDKN2A* or *PTEN*). Further, 7 of the 10 tumors (70%) were found to exhibit intra-tumoral molecular heterogeneity with respect to at least one gene, as defined by a varying level of LOH within the same tumor (T196.22, T516, T517, T518, T519, T523, T525; i.e., between the subsections). Additional cytogenetic analysis was not available to confirm the LOH identified.

Some of the larger tumors (e.g., T521) were found to exhibit no molecular heterogeneity, whereas some smaller tumors (e.g., T523) displayed molecular heterogeneity albeit only with respect to a specific gene. Additionally, five of the tumors analyzed in this study were known to be high grade (T196.22, T517, T519, T522, and T525). Four of these high grade tumors in our cohort exhibited molecular heterogeneity (*viz.* T196.22, T517, T519, and T525), whereas such heterogeneity was absent in the remaining sample graded as high (T522). For the remaining samples, details on the grade of tumor were unknown. The extent of LOH in the *NF1* gene was also found to vary between sections of the same tumor. Thus, some sections displayed LOH over the entire *NF1* gene and surrounding regions, whereas other sections of the same tumor only exhibited LOH within a portion of the *NF1* gene. Details of the extent of LOH in each tumor are given in Additional file 2: Supplementary Table S1.

p53 Immunohistochemical analysis

IHC analysis of the tissue distribution of p53 was found to correlate broadly with the results of the LOH analysis (Figure 2). Thus, different sections of the five MPNST tumors analyzed were found to display differences in staining for p53 that closely matched the presence or absence of LOH for the *TP53* gene (Table 1). For example, sections A, C, and D of T196.22 displayed complete LOH of the *TP53* gene in the majority of MPNST sections, and this was reflected in higher p53 expression as seen by IHC in these samples (Figure 2B,C). Conversely, section E (T196.22) showed no p53 expression by IHC peroxidase staining, and this section was found not to display any LOH (Figure 2D). Additionally, section B (T196.22) showed lower levels of staining (Figure 2B) than that of T196.22 section C (Figure 2C) but more than that of T196.22 section E (Figure 2D). These results correlate with those of the LOH analysis in which section T196.22 section B was found to have 50% LOH, but section T196.22 section C had 100% LOH and section E (T196.22) had no LOH. p53 Positivity by IHC has previously been reported in 60% of MPNSTs, whereas neurofibromas are p53 immunonegative [36].

Discussion

Cellular heterogeneity is a well-known complication in the analyses of NF1-associated tumors. By contrast, heterogeneity at the molecular level in NF1-associated tumors has scarcely been addressed. In this study, we set out to determine the extent of molecular heterogeneity within and between 10 MPNSTs, derived from 10 unrelated NF1 patients, by determining the differences in the levels of LOH at the *NF1*, *TP53*, *RB1*, *CDKN2A*, and *PTEN* gene loci. The results of this study indicated that 70% of the MPNST tumors studied exhibit molecular heterogeneity between sections of the same tumor sample. This heterogeneity was especially evident in the case of those sections from the same tumor which were anatomically adjacent to each other prior to dissection but which had nevertheless been found to differ with respect to the degree of LOH. Indeed, some sections were found to be entirely devoid of LOH for all five gene loci analyzed but were located beside sections exhibiting complete LOH for one or more of these genes (e.g., T196.22 section A4). Prior to dissection, in a number of the MPNST tumor sections under study, there were clearly

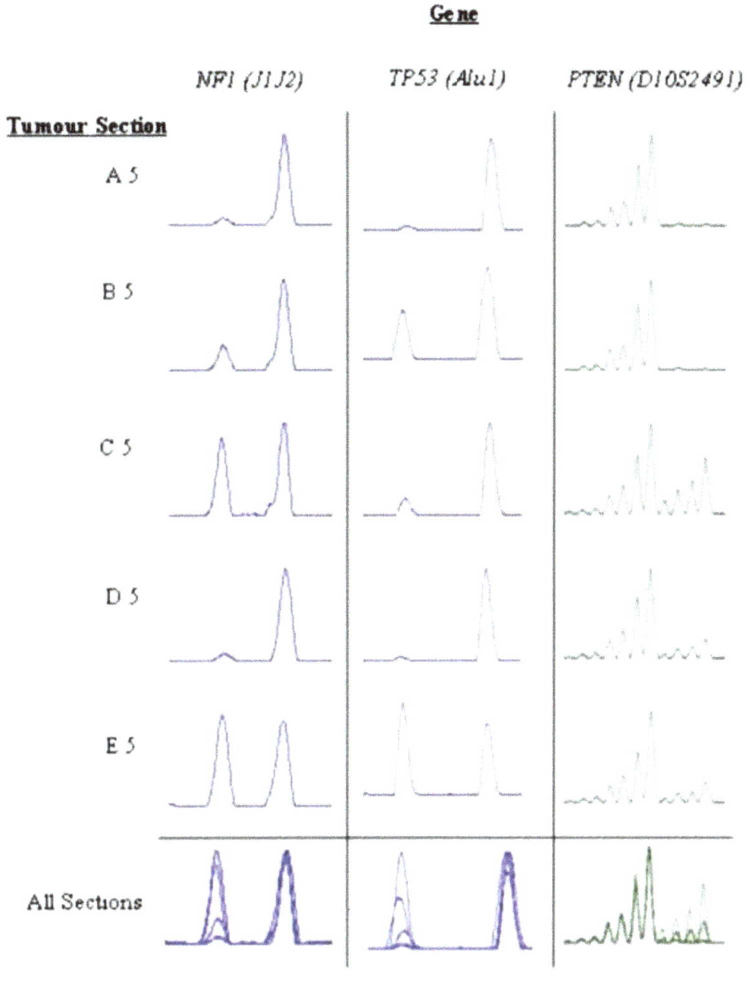

Figure 1 LOH patterns in *NF1*, *TP53*, and *PTEN* within sections A to E derived from T196.22. *All sections* represents the overlaid LOH results from all five sections (**A** to **E**) illustrating the different levels of gene-specific LOH observed within a single tumor. The results presented are representative of LOH at each genetic loci and are derived from individual markers analyzed at each of these loci (*NF1 - J1J2*, *TP53 - Alu1*, and *PTEN - D10S2491*).

defined centrally located tumor portions (T196.22 subsection 5 A to E, T516 section B, T518 section B). These areas corresponded to the sections in which different levels of LOH and subsequently *TP53* staining were identified (T196.22 section B5, T196.22 section C5, T196.22 section E5; Figure 2).

The observation that *TP53* LOH correlates directly with the p53 expression, as demonstrated here, has been observed in previous studies [37,38]. However, the precise relationship between *TP53* LOH and p53 protein expression remains unclear since some studies have identified p53 expression in tumors which have no *TP53* LOH. This may be explicable in terms of the presence of two *TP53* alleles, one mutant and the other wild-type in a given cell type, resulting in the production of both wild-type and mutant p53 protein. As a consequence, p53 may be detected by IHC even in the absence of p53 function. This suggests that in the context of evaluating tumor heterogeneity, IHC analysis is unlikely to be as reliable as the other molecular genotyping methods. IHC analysis could therefore be replaced by more accurate methods including AQUA [39,40] and tissue analysis with multiplex quantum dots (QD) [25] to yield a digital map of molecular and cellular heterogeneity to improve the sensitivity of detection and the prediction of a therapeutic response.

p53 is associated with malignant transformation in NF1-associated tumors [18] and LOH of the *TP53* gene was identified in 5 of the 10 tumors under study (Table 1, Additional file 2: Supplementary Table S1). *TP53* has also been found to manifest in intra-tumoral molecular heterogeneity with respect to its mutation in other tumor types, including breast cancer [41,42]. In pancreatic cancer, molecular heterogeneity is evident in cells with different capacities for initiating metastasis [43] suggesting that molecular heterogeneity may well prove to be

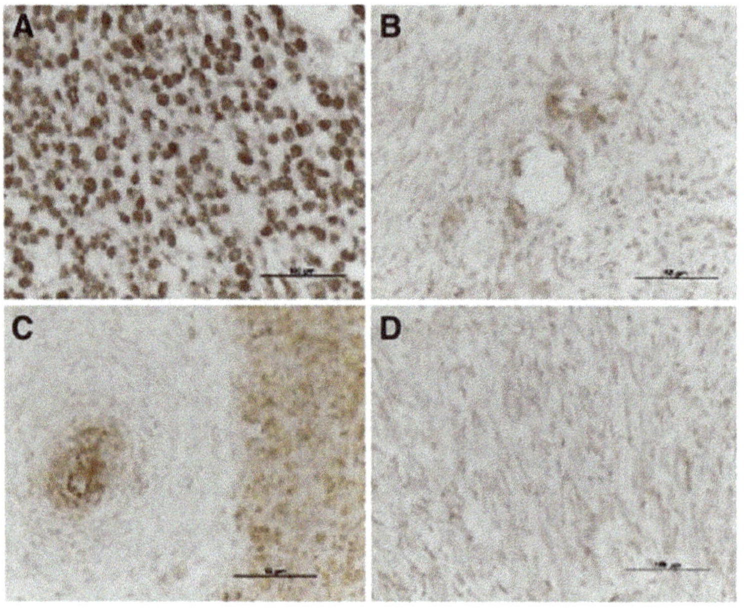

Figure 2 Immunohistochemical analysis of p53 on section 5 B,C and E (T196.22). (**A**) Positive control; breast carcinoma localized positive stain for p53. (**B**) T196.22,B5; slight localized positive p53 staining in a few cells. (**C**) T196.22,C5; localized positive and negative staining for p53. (**D**) T196.22,E5; Lack of p53 immunohistochemical staining.

the rule rather than the exception. If the molecular heterogeneity identified in this set of tumors was to emerge as relevant to MPNST development, we may have to revise our view not only of MPNST tumor biology, but also of the basic processes underlying MPNST tumorigenesis.

It might be assumed that, owing to the large size of some of the MPNST tumors, they would be divisible into a larger number of sections thereby allowing molecular heterogeneity to be assessed more clearly. However, the size of the tumor was not found to correlate with the level of molecular heterogeneity detected. It is, however, possible that intra-tumoral molecular heterogeneity could be related in some way to the grade of tumor, at least for those tumor samples analyzed here. A larger study is clearly warranted in order to determine whether these results could be replicated in a larger set of NF1-associated MPNSTs.

The pathological diagnosis of an MPNST is usually held to represent the 'gold standard' for the purposes of analysis and currently relies on the examination of not just one but a number of different sections. The results of this study, and from other previous studies on solid tumors [44-46], are broadly illustrative of the importance of careful dissection in the analysis of large tumors and suggest that in the interest of diagnostic accuracy, molecular analysis should be performed on several tumor sections alongside a pathological diagnosis. The clear implication for those studies that involve microarray analysis is that replicates across several sections would be advisable.

The results of this study therefore have important implications for molecular studies of NF1-associated tumor specimens. For example, although molecular techniques currently employed in mutation detection in large solid tumors are adequate for identifying and characterizing the underlying molecular and genetic aberrations, the potential for molecular heterogeneity means that a single dissected piece of tumor should not be assumed to be representative of the tumor as a whole; as a consequence, some somatic mutations may well be missed.

Although MPNSTs only develop in approximately 15% of NF1 patients, they represent a frequent cause of lethal progression of the NF1 phenotype. The prognosis for individuals diagnosed with an MPNST is usually very poor; 5-year survival rates in patients with advanced non-resectable and/or metastatic MPNSTs that have exhibited a limited response to chemotherapy are in the order of 20% to 50%, while 10-year survival rates are as low as 7.5% [47]. Treatment options for MPNSTs are currently rather limited, and complete surgical excision with clear margins is the recommended therapy for MPNSTs. A larger study is required in order to determine the full extent of molecular heterogeneity within MPNSTs in NF1 patients. However, such a study will be laborious and time-consuming to set up especially as MPNSTs are quite rare.

Genomic instability and high intra-tumoral genetic heterogeneity may synergize so as to accelerate the evolutionary processes within the tumor leading to the development of resistance to cytotoxic and targeted anticancer drugs. Improvements clearly need to be made to the treatment regimes for patients with MPNSTs. The results from this study indicate that while drugs can be developed *in vitro* and in *vivo* animal studies that would be capable of targeting the genes involved in the genesis of MPNSTs, the efficacy of these drugs is likely to be somewhat limited unless the cellular, molecular, and architectural heterogeneity of the tumor are considered alongside the tumor microenvironment.

This study represents the first systematic analysis of molecular heterogeneity in MPNSTs associated with NF1. The molecular heterogeneity evident at a number of different gene loci indicates that there is an urgent need not only for the integration of molecular and morphological biomarkers in cancer diagnosis, but also for the development of specific treatments for NF1-associated MPNSTs.

Competing interests

The authors declare that they have no competing interests.

Authors' contributions

LT performed the laboratory work and contributed to writing; V-FM provided the tumors; DNC contributed to writing; and MU conceived this study and provided overall directions. All authors read and approved the final manuscript.

Acknowledgments

We are grateful to all the patients who have participated in this study. We thank Cancer Research UK for the financial support. We would also like to thank David Viskochil for his comments on this manuscript in addition to Mark Aldred for his contributions to the immunohistochemical analysis.

Author details

[1]Institute of Medical Genetics, School of Medicine, Cardiff University, Cardiff CF14 4XN, UK. [2]Department of Maxillofacial Surgery, University Medical Centre Hamburg-Eppendorf, Hamburg D-20246, Germany.

References

1. Upadhyaya M: **Neurofibromatosis type 1: diagnosis and recent advances.** *Expert Opin Med Diagn* 2010, **4**:307–322.
2. Ferner RE: **The neurofibromatoses.** *Pract Neurol* 2010, **10**:82–93.
3. Upadhyaya M: **Genetic basis of tumorigenesis in NF1 malignant peripheral nerve sheath tumors.** *Front Biosci* 2011, **16**:937–951.
4. Jett K, Friedman JM: **Clinical and genetic aspects of neurofibromatosis 1.** *Genet Med* 2010, **12**:1–11.
5. Upadhyaya M: ***Neurofibromatoses (Monographs in Human Genetics).*** In *NF1 gene structure and NF1 genotype/phenotype correlations.* Edited by Kaufmann D. Switzerland: S Karger AG; 2008:46–62.
6. Cichowski K, Jacks T: ***NF1* tumor suppressor gene function: narrowing the GAP.** *Cell* 2001, **104**:593–604.
7. Arun D, Gutmann DH: **Recent advances in neurofibromatosis type 1.** *Curr Opin Neurol* 2004, **17**:101–105.
8. Thomas L, Spurlock G, Eudall C, Thomas NS, Mort M, Hamby SE, Chuzhanova N, Brems H, Legius E, Cooper DN, Upadhyaya M: **Exploring the somatic NF1 mutational spectrum associated with NF1 cutaneous neurofibromas.** *Eur J Hum Genet* 2012, **20**(4):411–419.
9. Garcia-Linares C, Fernández-Rodríguez J, Terribas E, Mercadé J, Pros E, Benito L, Benavente Y, Capellà G, Ravella A, Blanco I, Kehrer-Sawatzki H, Lázaro C, Serra E: **Dissecting loss of heterozygosity (LOH) in neurofibromatosis type 1-associated neurofibromas: Importance of copy neutral LOH.** *Hum Mutat* 2011, **32**(1):78–90.
10. Gottfried ON, Viskochil DH, Fults DW, Couldwell WT: **Molecular, genetic, and cellular pathogenesis of neurofibromas and surgical implications.** *Neurosurgery* 2006, **58**:1–16.
11. Brekke HR, Ribeiro FR, Kolberg M, Agesen TH, Lind GE, Eknaes M, Hall KS, Bjerkehagen B, van den Berg E, Teixeira MR, Mandahl N, Smeland S, Mertens F, Skotheim RI, Lothe RA: **Genomic changes in chromosomes 10, 16, and X in malignant peripheral nerve sheath tumors identify a high-risk patient group.** *J Clin Oncol* 2010, **28**:1573–1582.
12. Kourea HP, Orlow I, Scheithauer BW, Cordon-Cardo C, Woodruff JM: **Deletions of the INK4A gene occur in malignant peripheral nerve sheath tumors but not in neurofibromas.** *Am J Pathol* 1999, **155**:1855–1860.
13. Nielsen GP, Stemmer-Rachamimov AO, Ino Y, Moller MB, Rosenberg AE, Louis DN: **Malignant transformation of neurofibromas in neurofibromatosis 1 is associated with *CDKN2A*/p16 inactivation.** *Am J Pathol* 1999, **155**:1879–1884.
14. Mawrin C, Kirches E, Boltze C, Dietzmann K, Roessner A, Schneider-Stock R: **Immunohistochemical and molecular analysis of p53, RB, and PTEN in malignant peripheral nerve sheath tumors.** *Virchows Arch* 2002, **440**:610–615.
15. Mantripragada KK, Spurlock G, Kluwe L, Chuzhanova N, Ferner RE, Frayling IM, Dumanski JP, Guha A, Mautner V, Upadhyaya M: **High-resolution DNA copy number profiling of malignant peripheral nerve sheath tumors using targeted microarray-based comparative genomic hybridization.** *Clin Cancer Res* 2008, **14**:1015–1024.
16. Cichowski K, Shih TS, Schmitt E, Santiago S, Reilly K, McLaughlin ME, Bronson RT, Jacks T: **Mouse models of tumor development in neurofibromatosis type 1.** *Science* 1999, **286**:2172–2176.
17. Miller SJ, Rangwala F, Williams J, Ackerman P, Kong S, Jegga AG, Kaiser S, Aronow BJ, Frahm S, Kluwe L, Mautner V, Upadhyaya M, Muir D, Wallace M, Hagen J, Quelle DE, Watson MA, Perry A, Gutmann DH, Ratner N: **Large-scale molecular comparison of human Schwann cells to malignant peripheral nerve sheath tumor cell lines and tissues.** *Cancer Res* 2006, **66**:2584–2591.
18. Gregorian C, Nakashima J, Dry SM, Nghiemphu PL, Smith KB, Ao Y, Dang J, Lawson G, Mellinghoff IK, Mischel PS, Phelps M, Parada LF, Liu X, Sofroniew MV, Eilber FC, Wu H: **PTEN dosage is essential for neurofibroma development and malignant transformation.** *Proc Natl Acad Sci USA* 2009, **106**:19479–19484.
19. Upadhyaya M, Spurlock G, Monem B, Thomas N, Friedrich RE, Kluwe L, Mautner V: **Germline and somatic *NF1* gene mutations in plexiform neurofibromas.** *Hum Mutat* 2008, **29**:112–122.
20. Thomas L, Kluwe L, Chuzhanova N, Mautner V, Upadhyaya M: **Analysis of *NF1* somatic mutations in cutaneous neurofibromas from patients with high tumor burden.** *Neurogenetics* 2010, **11**:391–400.
21. Visvader JE: **Cells of origin in cancer.** *Nature* 2011, **469**:314–322.
22. Gibson P, Tong Y, Robinson G, Thompson MC, Currle DS, Eden C, Kranenburg TA, Hogg T, Poppleton H, Martin J, Finkelstein D, Pounds S, Weiss A, Patay Z, Scoggins M, Ogg R, Pei Y, Yang ZJ, Brun S, Lee Y, Zindy F, Lindsey JC, Taketo MM, Boop FA, Sanford RA, Gajjar A, Clifford SC, Roussel MF, McKinnon PJ, Gutmann DH, *et al*: **Subtypes of medulloblastoma have distinct developmental origins.** *Nature* 2010, **468**:1095–1099.
23. Kalamarides M, Stemmer-Rachamimov AO, Niwa-Kawakita M, Chareyre F, Taranchon E, Han ZY, Martinelli C, Lusis EA, Hegedus B, Gutmann DH, Giovannini M: **Identification of a progenitor cell of origin capable of generating diverse meningioma histological subtypes.** *Oncogene* 2011, **30**(20):2333–2344.
24. Singh DK, Ku CJ, Wichaidit C, Steininger RJ III, Wu LF, Altschuler SJ: **Patterns of basal signaling heterogeneity can distinguish cellular populations with different drug sensitivities.** *Mol Syst Biol* 2010, **6**:369.
25. Liu J, Lau SK, Varma VA, Moffitt RA, Caldwell M, Liu T, Young AN, Petros JA, Osunkoya AO, Krogstad T, Leyland-Jones B, Wang MD, Nie S: **Molecular**

mapping of tumor heterogeneity on clinical tissue specimens with multiplexed quantum dots. *ACS Nano* 2010, **4**:2755–2765.

26. Friedman J: *Gutmann DH, Maccollin M, Riccardi VM: Neurofibromatosis: Phenotype, Natural History, and Pathogenesis*. Baltimore: The Johns Hopkins University Press; 1999.
27. Le LQ, Parada LF: **Tumor microenvironment and neurofibromatosis type I: connecting the GAPs.** *Oncogene* 2007, **26**:4609–4616.
28. Upadhyaya M, Han S, Consoli C, Majounie E, Horan M, Thomas NS, Potts C, Griffiths S, Ruggieri M, von Deimling A, Cooper DN: **Characterization of the somatic mutational spectrum of the neurofibromatosis type 1 (*NF1*) gene in neurofibromatosis patients with benign and malignant tumors.** *Hum Mutat* 2004, **23**:134–146.
29. McDaniel T, Carbone D, Takahashi T, Chumakov P, Chang EH, Pirollo KF, Yin J, Huang Y, Meltzer SJ: **The *Msp*I polymorphism in intron 6 of p53 (*TP53*) detected by digestion of PCR products.** *Nucleic Acids Res* 1991, **19**:4796.
30. Hartmann A, Rösner U, Schlake G, Dietmaier W, Zaak D, Hofstaedter F, Knuechel R: **Clonality and genetic divergence in multifocal low-grade superficial urothelial carcinoma as determined by chromosome 9 and p53 deletion analysis.** *Lab Invest* 2000, **80**:709.
31. Belchis DA, Meece CA, Benko FA, Rogan PK, Williams RA, Gocke CD: **Loss of heterozygosity and microsatellite instability at the retinoblastoma locus in osteosarcomas.** *Diagn Mol Pathol* 1996, **5**:214–219.
32. Yandell DW, Dryja TP: **Detection of DNA sequence polymorphisms by enzymatic amplification and direct genomic sequencing.** *Am J Hum Genet* 1989, **45**:547–555.
33. Cairns P, Polascik TJ, Eby Y, Tokino K, Califano J, Merlo A, Mao L, Herath J, Jenkins R, Westra W, Rutter JL, Buckler A, Gabrielson E, Tockman M, Cho KR, Hedrick L, Bova GS, Isaacs W, Koch W, Schwab D, Sidransky D: **Frequency of homozygous deletion at p16/ *CDKN2* in primary human tumors.** *Nat Genet* 1995, **11**:210–212.
34. Pollock PM, Welch J, Hayward NK: **Evidence for three tumor suppressor loci on chromosome 9p involved in melanoma development.** *Cancer Res* 2001, **61**:1154–1161.
35. Li YL, Tian Z, Wu DY, Fu BY, Xin Y: **Loss of heterozygosity on 10q23.3 and mutation of tumor suppressor gene *PTEN* in gastric cancer and precancerous lesions.** *World J Gastroenterol* 2005, **11**:285–288.
36. Liapis H, Marley EF, Lin Y, Dehner LP: **p53 and Ki-67 proliferating cell nuclear antigen in benign and malignant peripheral nerve sheath tumors in children.** *Pediatr Dev Pathol* 1999, **2**:377–384.
37. Otis CN, Krebs PA, Quezado MM, Albuquerque A, Bryant B, San Juan X, Kleiner D, Sobel ME, Merino MJ: **Loss of heterozygosity in p53, *BRCA1*, and estrogen receptor genes and correlation to expression of p53 protein in ovarian epithelial tumors of different cell types and biological behaviour.** *Hum Pathol* 2002, **31**:233–238.
38. Götte K, Riedel F, Neubauer J, Schäfer C, Coy JF, Hörmann K: **The relationship between allelic imbalance on 17p, p53 mutation and p53 overexpression in head and neck cancer.** *Int J Oncol* 2001, **19**:331–336.
39. McCabe A, Dolled-Filhart M, Camp RL, Rimm DL: **Automated quantitative analysis (AQUA) of in situ protein expression, antibody concentration, and prognosis.** *J Natl Cancer Inst* 2005, **97**:1808–1815.
40. Camp RL, Chung GG, Rimm DL: **Automated subcellular localization and quantification of protein expression in tissue microarrays.** *Nat Med* 2002, **8**:1323–1327.
41. Clark SE, Warwick J, Carpenter R, Bowen RL, Duffy SW, Jones JL: **Molecular subtyping of DCIS: heterogeneity of breast cancer reflected in pre-invasive disease.** *Br J Cancer* 2011, **104**:120–127.
42. Lennington WJ, Jensen RA, Dalton LW, Page DL: **Ductal carcinoma *in situ* of the breast.** *Heterogeneity of individual lesions. Cancer* 1994, **73**:118–124.
43. Campbell PJ, Yachida S, Mudie LJ, Stephens PJ, Pleasance ED, Stebbings LA, Morsberger LA, Latimer C, McLaren S, Lin ML, McBride DJ, Varela I, Nik-Zainal SA, Leroy C, Jia M, Menzies A, Butler AP, Teague JW, Griffin CA, Burton J, Swerdlow H, Quail MA, Stratton MR, Iacobuzio-Donahue C, Futreal PA: **The patterns and dynamics of genomic instability in metastatic pancreatic cancer.** *Nature* 2010, **467**:1109–1113.
44. Alizadeh AA, Eisen MB, Davis RE, Ma C, Lossos IS, Rosenwald A, Boldrick JC, Sabet H, Tran T, Yu X, Powell JI, Yang L, Marti GE, Moore T, Hudson J Jr, Lu L, Lewis DB, Tibshirani R, Sherlock G, Chan WC, Greiner TC, Weisenburger DD, Armitage JO, Warnke R, Levy R, Wilson W, Grever MR, Byrd JC, Botstein D, Brown PO, *et al*: **Distinct types of diffuse large B-cell lymphoma identified by gene expression profiling.** *Nature* 2000, **403**:503–511.
45. Whitehall VL, Wynter CV, Walsh MD, Simms LA, Purdie D, Pandeya N, Young J, Meltzer SJ, Leggett BA, Jass JR: **Morphological and molecular heterogeneity within non microsatellite instability-high colorectal cancer.** *Cancer Res* 2002, **62**:6011–6014.
46. Stingl J, Caldas C: **Molecular heterogeneity of breast carcinomas and the cancer stem cell hypothesis.** *Nat Rev Cancer* 2007, **7**:791–799.
47. Katz D, Lazar A, Lev D: **Malignant peripheral nerve sheath tumor (MPNST): the clinical implications of cellular signalling pathways.** *Exp Rev Mol Med* 2009, **11**:e30.

19

Viral expression associated with gastrointestinal adenocarcinomas in TCGA high-throughput sequencing data

Daria Salyakina[1*] and Nicholas F Tsinoremas[1,2]

Abstract

Background: Up to 20% of cancers worldwide are thought to be associated with microbial pathogens, including bacteria and viruses. The widely used methods of viral infection detection are usually limited to a few *a priori* suspected viruses in one cancer type. To our knowledge, there have not been many broad screening approaches to address this problem more comprehensively.

Methods: In this study, we performed a comprehensive screening for viruses in nine common cancers using a multistep computational approach. Tumor transcriptome and genome sequencing data were available from The Cancer Genome Atlas (TCGA). Nine hundred fifty eight primary tumors in nine common cancers with poor prognosis were screened against a non-redundant database of virus sequences. DNA sequences from normal matched tissue specimens were used as controls to test whether each virus is associated with tumors.

Results: We identified human papilloma virus type 18 (HPV-18) and four human herpes viruses (HHV) types 4, 5, 6B, and 8, also known as EBV, CMV, roseola virus, and KSHV, in colon, rectal, and stomach adenocarcinomas. In total, 59% of screened gastrointestinal adenocarcinomas (GIA) were positive for at least one virus: 26% for EBV, 21% for CMV, 7% for HHV-6B, and 20% for HPV-18. Over 20% of tumors were co-infected with multiple viruses. Two viruses (EBV and CMV) were statistically significantly associated with colorectal cancers when compared to the matched healthy tissues from the same individuals ($p = 0.02$ and 0.03, respectively). HPV-18 was not detected in DNA, and thus, no association testing was possible. Nevertheless, HPV-18 expression patterns suggest viral integration in the host genome, consistent with the potentially oncogenic nature of HPV-18 in colorectal adenocarcinomas. The estimated counts of viral copies were below one per cell for all identified viruses and approached the detection limit.

Conclusions: Our comprehensive screening for viruses in multiple cancer types using next-generation sequencing data clearly demonstrates the presence of viral sequences in GIA. EBV, CMV, and HPV-18 are potentially causal for GIA, although their oncogenic role is yet to be established.

Keywords: Cancer, Papilloma virus, Herpes virus

Background

Viruses may be more commonly associated with malignant diseases than previously considered [1]. Reported associations do not always mean that a virus is a direct cause of the cancer; they can be the result of contamination, viral infection without causal involvement ('passenger'), and an indirect or direct causal relationship. Regardless of the causal relationship, viruses may have significant clinical implications in human cancers through contribution to dramatic changes in the microenvironment and immunosurveillance.

The main strategies to detect and type various viruses in cancers usually address individual protein biomarkers, serological tests, or DNA/RNA detection of one or a few viruses at a time. The major disadvantage of these strategies is failure to detect viruses not previously known to be associated with a particular cancer type. In this report, we introduce a new and substantially different

* Correspondence: dsalyakina@med.miami.edu
[1]Center for Computational Science, University of Miami, 1120 NW 14 St, Miami, FL 33136, USA

way of addressing this problem by utilizing next-generation sequencing (NGS) data to detect both human and non-human nucleic acids in tumor specimens. This approach does not require any prior knowledge of viruses involved and can identify all known viral genomes. NGS provides the opportunity to detect viral transcripts with high sensitivity in the host tissue at frequencies less than 1 RNA molecule in 1 million [2]. Whole genome or transcriptome tumor sequencing data provides a unique resource for the development of new and powerful methodologies to detect and characterize viruses in cancers.

'Computational subtraction' is the general concept for detecting infectious agents in the host NGS material [3]. During this procedure, human and artifact sequences are removed from the NGS data and the remaining sequences are aligned to bacterial or viral references from existing databases. A few groups have implemented computational subtraction procedures for this purpose [4,5]. To date, NGS data was successfully used for virus identification in human papilloma virus (HPV)-associated squamous cell carcinomas [6-9] and hepatitis B virus (HBV)-mediated hepatocellular carcinomas [5], while other cancer types and viruses largely remain out of the picture.

In this study, we present a comprehensive screening for viruses in NGS data of nine common cancers in 1,007 patients, using The Cancer Genome Atlas (TCGA) data. TCGA is a joint project of the National Cancer Institute (NCI) and the National Human Genome Research Institute (NHGRI). The goal of the TCGA project is to collect and systematically explore the entire spectrum of genomic changes involved in more than 20 types of human cancers. Comprehensive genomic characterization has been published for three out of nine cancers studied so far (lung squamous cell carcinoma, colon, and rectum adenocarcinoma) [10,11]. Colon and rectum adenocarcinoma were shown to belong to one cancer type based on their molecular profiles. In addition to the screening for viruses, we perform association analysis of identified viruses with tumor vs. paired non-malignant tissue from the same patients in order to determine whether the presence of a virus is significantly associated with tumors and not the normal cell types.

Results and discussion

Screening for viruses

Screening for viruses is an essential step in the continuum of research that is expected to lead to new treatment strategies in patients with virus-positive tumors. In this study, we performed the systematic screening for potentially oncogenic viruses in nine cancer types from TCGA (Table 1), most of which were not previously known to be associated with viruses or have controversial reports in this regard [12,13]. After subtraction of non-viral sequences, unaligned fragments were used in virus identification (Figure 1). Sequences of Epstein-Barr virus (EBV), cytomegalovirus (CMV), roseola virus (HHV-6B), Kaposi's sarcoma-associated human virus (KSHV), and human papilloma virus type 18 (HPV-18) were identified in transcriptomes of three gastrointestinal adenocarcinomas (GIA): stomach, rectum, and colon adenocarcinomas (STAD, READ, and COAD, respectively). In total, 83% of the viral reads mapped to the known coding regions. The remaining six cancer types (Table 1) were virus negative according to our computational pipeline. Table 2 represents a summary for the sequencing data in the GIA samples and matched controls.

Table 1 Sample size for available DNA and RNA sequencing data in primary tumors and paired control samples

Cohort	Primary tumor		Matched controls	
			Blood	Solid tissue
	RNA	DNA	DNA	DNA
AML, acute myeloid leukemia	123	nt	nt	nt
COAD, colon adenocarcinoma	194	77	56	16
KIRK, kidney renal clear carcinoma	132	nt	nt	nt
KIRP, kidney renal papillary cell carcinoma	15	nt	nt	nt
LUAD, lung adenocarcinoma	58	nt	nt	nt
LUSK, lung squamous cell carcinoma	151	nt	nt	nt
READ, rectum adenocarcinoma	71	40	35	4
STAD, stomach adenocarcinoma	57	3	0	2
UCEC, uterine corpus endometrioid carcinoma	157	nt	nt	nt

Control samples were derived from either whole blood or adjacent normal tissue (not both) from the same patient. nt, not tested.

Viruses in gastrointestinal adenocarcinomas

EBV, CMV, and HHV-6B were detected in all three GIA, while HPV-18 was detected in colorectal cancers only. In total, 189 (58.7%) GIA samples were infected with at least one virus: 83 (25.8%) with EBV, 67 (20.8%) with CMV, 22 (6.8%) with HHV-6B, and 64 (19.8%) with HPV-18 (Figure 2). One STAD RNA sample was KSHV positive with 115 sequence reads mapping to 3,280 bases of the viral genome (Additional file 1: Table S1). During the review of this paper, another group published a very similar study including 3,775 tumors from TCGA [14]. However, in their computational pipeline, Khoury with colleagues did not detect any viral sequences in 138 COAD and 66 READ samples. In addition, they only reported four EBV-positive samples in the STAD. Khoury et al. used a different sequence aligner (MOSAIK) and more stringent cutoff for the viral gene expression detection. Although no explicit cutoff is stated in the paper

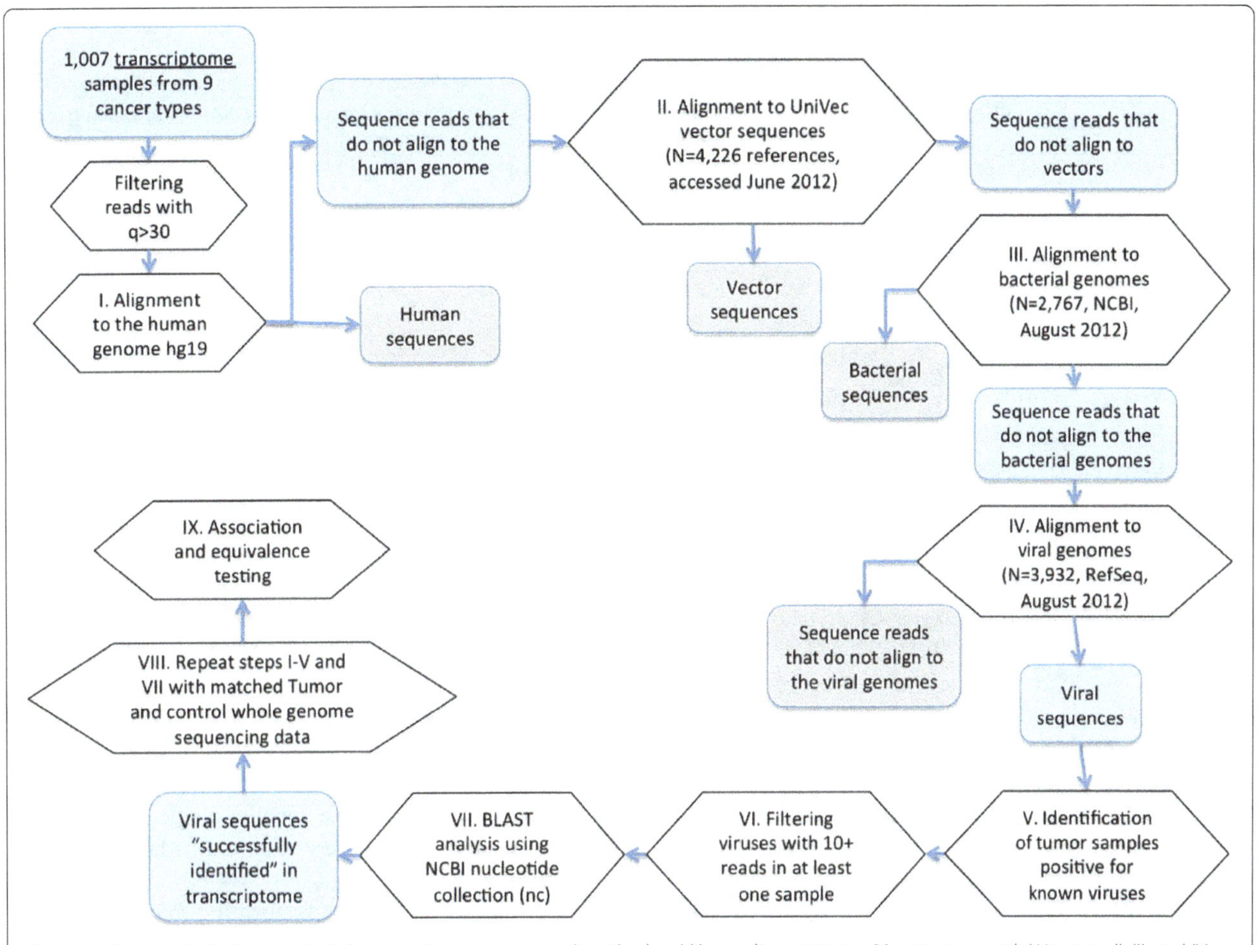

Figure 1 Data analysis flowchart. Before step I, sequencing reads with phred-like quality scores $q < 30$ were removed. N in steps II, III, and IV reflects the number of reference sequences from corresponding databases. For the alignment in steps II, III, and IV, we combined reference fasta files into 'supergenomes' including vector sequences, bacterial genomes, and viral genomes, respectively. Each individual reference sequence in the 'supergenome' was treated as a chromosome. All supergenome reference files were indexed before alignment steps.

[14], the VirusSeq pipeline [5] implemented in their study uses 1,000 reads as a cutoff for virus detection. In our case, the number of identified reads was far below 1,000 for all transcriptomes, except two EBV-positive STAD tumors. The probable reason for using such a high cutoff in VirusSeq pipeline is the high number of false-positive results due to the homology of the contaminating vector and bacterial sequences. In our pipeline, adding steps II and III, in which these sequences are subtracted, alleviates this problem, reducing the number of unaligned RNA-seq reads by 19% on average before aligning to the virus reference. In our experience, these two steps are essential since they eliminate false-positive findings and increase specificity of the method. We included here 57 STAD samples, not 71 as in [14]. To our knowledge, 14 additional patients reported in [14] have withdrawn their consent to participate in TCGA study (as of November 1, 2012).

All viruses identified in GIA are ubiquitous in human population. The first encounter with EBV, CMV, and HHV-6B infection usually happens in early childhood and results in latent lifelong infection with a prevalence of over 90% in adults [15-21]. Similarly, KSHV infects 7.2% and 49% of the population depending on the geographical region [22-24]. At the same time, HPV is the most common sexually transmitted infection with a lifelong prevalence of 71%, although unlike herpes virus infections, about 90% of HPV infection is cleared within 2 years without any consequences [25].

EBV, HPV-18, KSHV, and CMV have been linked to multiple cancers and potentially are oncogenic in GIA. EBV has been accepted as an infective agent of gastric and colorectal carcinomas. Nearly 10% of all gastric cancers [26-30] and up to 30% of colorectal carcinomas [31-35] have been found to be EBV-infected monoclonal epithelial cells. In TCGA, 45.6% of STAD, 22.6% of COAD, and 31% of READ samples were EBV positive [36,37] (Figure 2). Multiple studies have also shown significant association of high-risk HPV types with colorectal cancers with infection rate of up to 84% [38-41]. The

Table 2 Total number of next-generation sequencing reads/fragments available for gastrointestinal cancers organized by cancer and tissue type

Cohort	Statistics	Primary tumor	Primary tumor		Blood		Solid tissue	
		RNA	DNA	Human genome coverage[a]	DNA	Human genome coverage[a]	DNA	Human genome coverage[a]
COAD	Min	5,244,743	60,872,080	0.47	64,637,478	0.50	148,341,394	1.18
	Mean	26,127,635	205,217,167	1.63	182,959,915	1.45	224,838,391	1.77
	Median	27,424,762	196,408,988	1.57	193,657,350	1.49	196,072,876	1.57
	Max	64,021,517	1,162,469,344	9.43	354,790,740	2.85	429,443,164	3.36
READ	Min	19,665,974	89,943,982	0.70	90,122,736	0.70	95,061,666	0.75
	Mean	26,782,703	225,818,442	1.79	214,787,544	1.71	150,549,985	1.19
	Median	27,121,702	227,226,239	1.81	224,045,358	1.80	159,027,517	1.26
	Max	33,338,326	461,153,444	3.68	367,295,986	2.93	189,083,240	1.47
STAD	Min	127,157,036	259,701,502	2.08	NA	NA	418,702,808	3.34
	Mean	155,138,810	300,668,630	2.40	NA	NA	448,318,606	3.58
	Median	155,490,548	280,015,346	2.23	NA	NA	448,318,606	3.58
	Max	193,445,130	362,289,042	2.88	NA	NA	477,934,404	3.82

Paired reads are counted as two single fragments. COAD, colon adenocarcinoma; READ, rectum adenocarcinoma; STAD, stomach adenocarcinoma; NA, no data available. [a]Average coverage was calculated as the number of reads multiplied by the average read length (51 nt) and divided by the corresponding genome length, divided by two for diploid genome.

detected frequency of HPV-18 in TCGA was substantially lower: 31% in COAD and 0.4% in READ. Differences in frequencies between previously reported and our studies can result from multiple factors, such as varying sensitivity of detection methods used as well as population demographics. For instance, EBV positivity in STAD has been reported to be higher in males, young subjects, non-antral subsites, diffuse-type histology, and in studies from the Americas [27]. Given the sample size of the STAD cohort and the number of viruses, no epidemiological analyses were done. COAD and READ combined provided a sufficient sample size for association testing with clinical and demographic variables (Additional file 1: Tables S2–S12). No association with gender, age at initial diagnosis, histological type or 'M' and 'N' staging was found. Nominal p values are shown in Table 3. After correction for multiple testing, the only association of HPV-18 infection with anatomic subdivision was statistically significant. HPV-18 was predominantly associated with tumors located in the cecum and ascending colon. No large epidemiological studies for HPV-associated COAD are available thus far to compare these results to.

CMV is also capable of transforming mammalian cells through various pathways [42] and has been linked to colorectal cancer, although available evidence is scarce [43]. KSHV causes Kaposi's sarcoma [44] and, to our knowledge, has not yet been associated with gastric adenocarcinomas. This may be a special case of STAD that needs further investigation.

Co-infection with multiple viruses

A substantial proportion of GIA was co-infected with multiple viruses: 46 (23%) COAD, 11 (19.3%) STAD, and

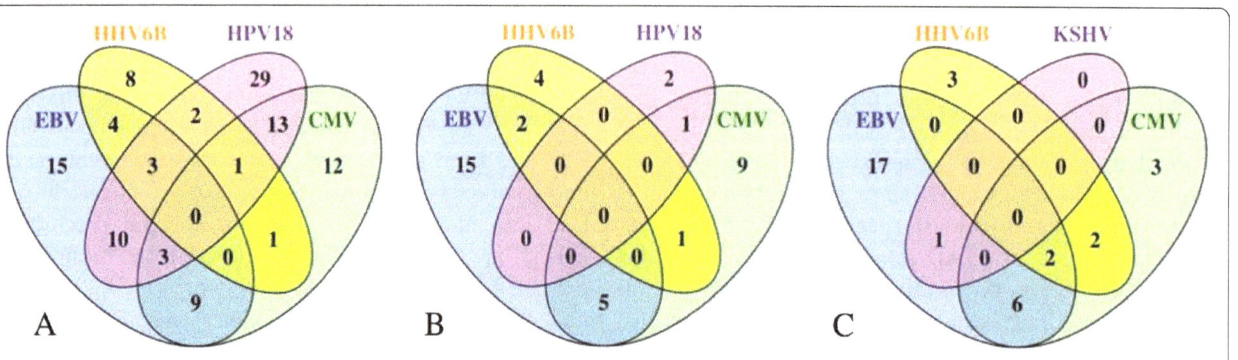

Figure 2 Counts of tumors with viral co-infection. (A) In the COAD, **(B)** in the READ, and **(C)** in the STAD. Tumors were considered virus positive when viral sequences were identified in the tumor transcriptome or genome.

Table 3 Nominal *p* values for association testing of virus with clinical and demographic phenotypes

Phenotype	HPV-18	EBV	CMV	HHV-6B
Gender	1.00	1.00	1.00	0.54
Age at initial diagnosis	0.22	0.51	0.07	0.26
Anatomic subdivision	5.0E − 05*	0.23	0.06	0.02
Histological type	0.39	0.52	0.82	0.55
History of colon polyps	3.0E − 03	0.77	0.22	0.83
Pathologic M	0.84	0.32	0.21	1.00
Pathologic N	0.59	0.11	0.58	0.13
Pathologic T	0.33	0.03	0.09	0.48
Stage	0.89	0.01	0.12	0.64

*p value is significant after Bonferroni correction at $\alpha = 0.05$.

9 (12.7%) READ. Figure 2 shows how many tumors were co-infected. These multiple viruses may either co-exist in the same cancer cells or populate different cell types that compose or infiltrate the tumor. Szostek et al. suggests that co-infection with HHVs, especially CMV and EBV, may increase probability of the HPV-16 integration into the host genome during cervical cancer tumorigenesis [45]. Similar mechanisms may be involved with EBV, CMV, and HPV-18 in colorectal adenocarcinomas and need to be tested in future studies. Alternatively, some of the identified viruses can also preferentially infect cancer cells, taking advantage of the impaired immune environment of the tumors.

Virus quantification

The proportion of viral transcriptome reads relative to the total number of reads in the GIA ranged from 6×10^{-9} (HHV-6B) to 2×10^{-5} (EBV). The majority of tumors did not have a sufficient number of reads to cover the whole viral genome or to allow transcript quantification (see Additional file 1: Table S1 and Additional file 2). The number of viral sequence reads detected in tumor transcriptomes varied from a single fragment to tens of thousands of fragments per sample, with a strong skew towards low counts (Figure 3). Only five or less viral sequence fragments were detected in 49% of the transcriptomes and only one fragment in 21%. However, our follow-up Basic Local Alignment Search Tool (BLAST) analysis, described in the 'Methods' section, demonstrated that even detection of a single short read may be sufficient to ensure unambiguous viral detection, confirming high specificity of sequencing alignment [8].

The estimated viral load for EBV, CMV, and HHV-6B in GIA was less than one viral copy per cell (vc/c) in all cases with a maximum of 0.72 vc/c (HHV-6B) (Additional file 1: Table S1). The latter is equivalent to one viral genome per 1.39 human cells. This data supports the hypothesis that only a small proportion of tumor cells had a virus. The viral DNA abundance for EBV and CMV correlated with the proportion of total viral RNA reads (Additional file 3). Because no genomic data was available for KSHV-positive tumor and no HPV-18 was detectable in genomic DNA from tumors or normal cells, no viral load for these viruses could be calculated. The HPV-18 genome (7,857 nt for RefSeq ID: NC_001357) is 20 to 30 times smaller than the HHV (162,114–235,646 nt). The HPV-18 DNA quantity must have been below the detection limit at the available sequencing depth. The lowest detection threshold for NGS studies is limited to one sequence read aligning to the target genome. As a result, the probability for detecting a viral sequence in the host NGS data will be proportional to the target sequence length, the viral load, and the sequencing depth. Given the HPV-18 size and average genome sequencing depth of GIA, the hypothetical average detection limit would be above 0.0047 vc/c (standard deviation (SD) = 0.0023), equivalent to 1 virus in 261 human cells (SD = 133). This estimation does not take into account possible data loss due to disproportional filtering of highly polymorphic viral sequences through an unaccepted number of mismatches and homopolymeric and repetitive regions. Thus, the viral load is most likely underestimated here. Currently, there is no clear consensus on the minimum viral load indicative for the virus causality in neoplasm. On one hand, viral genome abundance and active expression of viral oncogenes are broadly believed to indicate much greater viral involvement in disease than the silent presence of viral genome. On the other hand, according to the 'hit-and-run' mechanism, transient acquisition of viral genome may be sufficient to induce malignant conversion [46]. In the hit-and-run scenario, viruses may get partially or completely lost after they cause permanent damage to the host cell and are no longer necessary for the maintenance of the malignant state. The most reliable estimates of viral load from the literature are related to HPV-associated tumors. The quantitative PCR experiments report several HPV-18 copies per cell [8,47]. However, Yoshida et al. suggested that very early HPV-18 DNA integration may result in lower copy numbers in cervical adenosquamous carcinoma (1.50–0.89 vc/c), leading to a more aggressive transformation with greater chromosomal instabilities, higher growth rates, and rapid progression [47].

Virus association with tumors

Next, we tested if identified viruses were mostly found in tumors compared to the non-malignant matched tissue from the same individuals. One of the limitations of this study is the absence of transcriptome data for matched non-malignant tissues. Before association analysis, we explored if transcriptome and genome sequencing data can be pooled for tumors and compared to genomic data from non-malignant tissues. According to

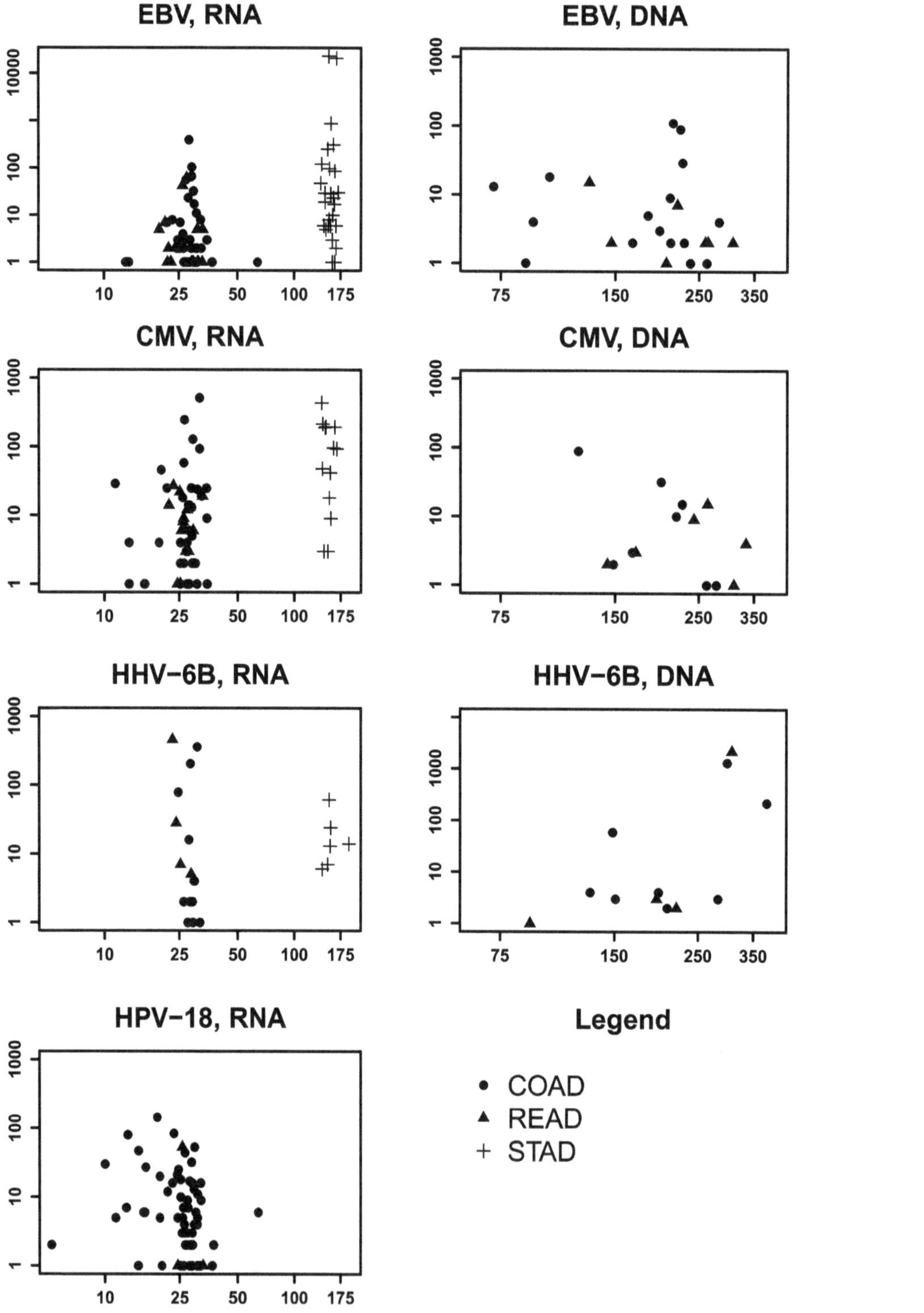

Figure 3 Number of sequencing reads mapped to virus reference versus the total number of reads. The *X*-axis shows total RNA or DNA fragments (short sequencing reads) in millions, and the *Y*-axis shows the number of fragments mapped to the particular virus, as stated in the plot subtitles. Each data point represents one tumor. HPV-18 DNA was not detectable in the whole genome sequencing data. COAD are depicted as read circles, READ as blue triangles, and STAD as black plus signs.

our results, tumor DNA and RNA did not show statistically equivalent rates of virus positivity (Table 4). For this reason, only DNA data from both tumors and non-malignant matched controls were utilized for association analysis. A sufficient number of whole genome sequencing data was available for three viruses: EBV, CMV, and HHV-6B in COAD and READ only. Since COAD and READ are genetically identical [11], we combined the two into colorectal adenocarcinomas (CRAD) to achieve a higher sample size for association analysis. Our results indicate that EBV and CMV were significantly associated with CRAD vs. matched non-malignant specimens with $p = 0.0022$ ($p_{corrected} = 0.02$) and $p = 0.0034$ ($p_{corrected} = 0.03$), respectively (Table 5). Since testing was done in three tissue types: solid tumor, solid non-malignant adjacent tissue, and whole blood, these associations may reflect tissue-specific infection. Thus, we investigated if viral rates differ between tissue types in controls. All controls positive for EBV and CMV were blood samples, and none of the tested solid tissue controls had these two viruses (Table 5). In contrary, HHV-6B was identified predominantly (80%) in solid non-malignant tissue and not blood, although association was not significant after correction for multiple testing ($p_{corrected} = 0.07$). These findings may reflect the fact that EBV and CMV are associated with tumors, while HHV-6B is associated with the colorectal tissue. EBV, CMV, and HPV-18 are capable to infect different types of skin cells, endothelium, or mucus membranes and are plausible infections in the histological context of GIA. While the oncogenic nature of CMV is still debatable [42], EBV and HPV-18 are potentially causal in GIA because both viruses encode oncoproteins, which are able to transform human cells [30,39,48]. HHV-6B is known to propagate preferentially in T lymphocytes or glial cells [49] and does not have any known oncogenes. The presence of HHV-6B in the colon and rectum may possibly originate from tissue infiltration by infected lymphocytes, although this hypothesis needs to be verified. One of the limitations of our study is the lack of availability of corresponding samples for further validation.

Virus integration into the human genome

Since no viral DNA for HPV-18 was identifiable, detection of integration sites of HPV-18 into the human genome was not possible. Nevertheless, the cumulative expression pattern of HPV-18 in CRAD supports evidence for genomic integration. The HPV episome usually becomes integrated into the host cell DNA during oncogenesis by opening the ring molecule and disrupting the *E2* gene, which normally suppresses oncogenes *E6* and *E7*. As a result, part of *E2* and *L2* and whole *E4* and *E5* genes become deleted. Expression of *E6* and *E7* downregulates p53 and pRb and promotes malignancy [50]. While three early viral genes, *E1*, *E6*, and *E7*, showed high 'cumulative expression levels' in CRAD, partial expression of *E2* and whole *L2*, *E4* and *E5* was not detected (Figure 4). Lack of expression in presumably deleted regions suggests the potentially oncogenic

Table 4 Counts of colorectal samples, positive (+) or negative (−) for identified viruses, within tumor's DNA/RNA pairs

Sample type	Virus name	Tumor DNA ($N = 117$)		CI for two one-sided hypotheses (CL = 0.975)	
Tumor RNA	EBV	+	−	0; 3.09	0.40; infinity
	+	15	9		
	−	10	83		
	CMV	+	−	0; 0.51*	0.01; infinity
	+	13	13		
	−	1	90		
	HHV-6B	+	−	0; 18.84	0.85; infinity
	+	2	3		
	−	10	102		
	HPV-18	+	−	0; 0.14*	0; infinity
	+	0	28		
	−	0	89		

N, number of matched pairs. *proportions are not equivalent at $\alpha = 0.05$ after Bonferroni correction.

Table 5 Counts of colorectal samples, positive (+) or negative (−) for identified viruses, in matched tumor/normal specimen pairs

Sample type	Virus name	Matched control DNA $N = 111$ 2 (blood:solid)		Adjusted *p* values for association: Tumors vs. all controls	Tumors vs. blood	Tumors vs. solid tissue
Tumor DNA	EBV	+	−	0.02	0.06	1
	+	3 (3:0)	21 (19:2)			
	−	5 (5:0)	82 (64:18)			
	CMV	+	−	0.03	0.06	1
	+	0	12 (11:1)			
	−	1 (1:0)	98 (79:19)			
	HHV-6B	+	−	1	0.98	0.07
	+	4 (1:3)	8 (8:0)			
	−	10 (2:8)	89 (80:9)			
	HPV-18	+	−	-	-	-
	+	0	0			
	−	0	0			

N, number of matched pairs. blood: solid, counts for the non-malignant samples by tissue type: whole blood and solid adjacent tissue, respectively.

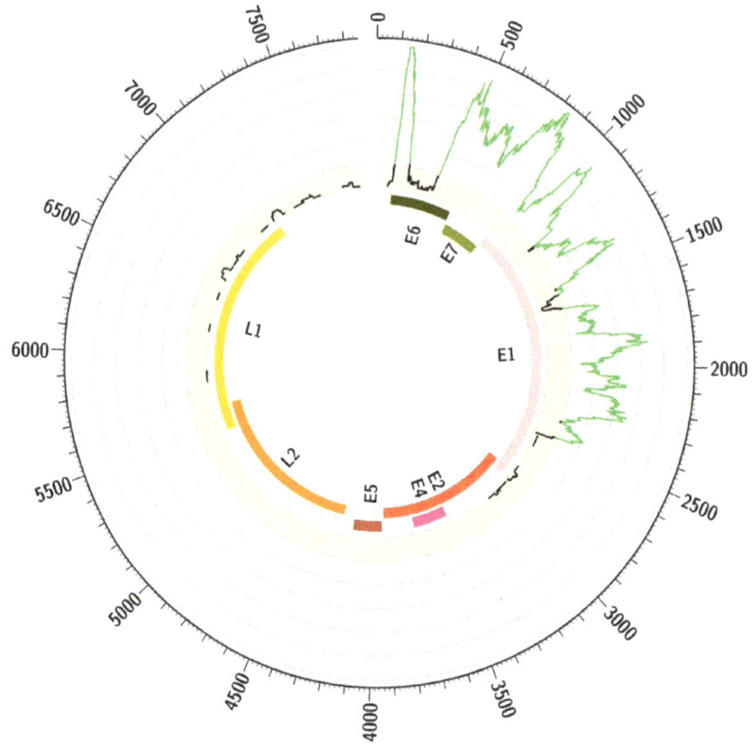

Figure 4 Circos plot for HPV-18 RNA-seq. From outside to the inside of the circle: (1) HPV-18 genomic positions; (2) number of sequencing reads mapped to the viral genome in 64 colon and rectum adenocarcinomas combined. Range from 1 to 10 shown on light yellow background as a black line, and from 11 to 61 on light green background as a green line; (3) viral genes mapped to genomic positions. While expression of genes *E6*, *E7*, and *E1* is obvious, genes *L2*, *E5*, *E4*, and part of *E2* were not detected. This pattern is expected when HPV-18 integrates in the host genome and part of the viral genome becomes deleted.

nature of HPV-18. Despite collected evidence, the temporal relationship between infection and tumorigenesis cannot be disseminated from this data. To conclusively prove a causal role of viruses in cancer, a complete chain of evidence from epidemiology, histopathology, and molecular biology is required.

For the remaining viruses detected in available genomic data, the number of identified reads was not sufficient for integration site detection (see Figure 3 and Additional file 2). Neither viral nor human genomes were covered without substantial gaps. As shown in Table 2, the median coverage of the human genome in colorectal samples was below 2x, and a great majority of the viruses with available whole genome seq data had a small fraction of the genomes covered.

Conclusions

Our results clearly demonstrate the presence of viral sequences in GIA. EBV and CMV were statistically significantly associated with CRAD. In addition, the expression pattern of HPV-18 was consistent with genomic integration typical during oncogenesis [50]. This supports the hypothesis that EBV, CMV, and HPV-18 are potentially oncogenic in GIA, although we realize that further studies are needed before a conclusion can be made about the pathophysiological role of the identified viruses in GIA. No viruses were identified in the remaining six cancer types.

Our results demonstrate the feasibility of NGS for the identification of viruses at very low levels in the human tissue. Unlike PCR-based approach, NGS data offer a unique opportunity to capture any viral nucleic acids present in the sample above the detection limit. Identification of viral infection is a first step in determining the role of viruses in cancer. Availability of comprehensive viral databases makes it possible to scan for a large number of candidates without the need for *de novo* assembly with the restriction that novel viruses will not be detected.

Finally, in this study, we established an empirical detection limit in our computational pipeline. This information can be used to calculate the required sequencing depth, as well as the amount of material needed by the given size of viral genome, and the expected viral load in similar studies.

Methods

Subjects

Whole transcriptome sequencing data for nine cancer types, comprising 1,007 patients, were obtained through TCGA (accessed on October 17, 2011). Table 1 summarizes specimen counts and abbreviations for the nine included cancer types. Additional transcriptome and whole genome sequencing data for three GIA were downloaded on November 1, 2012. Sequencing has been done using Illumina (Solexa, GAII, Illumina, Inc., San Diego, CA, USA) or SOLiD™ technology (Life Technologies, Carlsbad, CA, USA). A detailed description of the TCGA data can be found on the following TCGA websites: http://cancergenome.nih.gov/, https://tcga-data.nci.nih.gov/tcga/, as well as in two recently published studies on genomic characterization of three out of nine cancer types discussed here [10,11]. Patient enrollment and utilization of data were conducted in accordance with TCGA human subjects protection and data access policies (http://cancergenome.nih.gov/PublishedContent/Files/pdfs/6.3.1_TCGA_Human_Subjects_and_Data_Access_policies_FINAL_011211.pdf).

Cancers selected for the TCGA study were chosen based on specific criteria that included (1) poor prognosis and high public health impact, and (2) availability of human tumor and matched normal tissue that meet TCGA standards for patient consent, quality, and quantity. The proportion of 60% tumor nuclei in the specimens was found to be sufficient by TCGA project organizers to generate high-quality data, in which the tumor's signal can be distinguished from other cells' signals when using NGS. Only primary, untreated tumors were collected. Samples were frozen quickly after surgery in order to prevent degradation of the RNA and DNA.

Whole genome sequencing data was available for 37.5% of the GIA (Table 1). Blood or germ line specimens derived from the same individual as the tumor specimens were used in the TCGA study to serve as paired normal controls when available (Table 1). DNA sequencing data from the blood or adjacent healthy tissue was available for 35% of the GIA specimens.

Bioinformatics analysis

Transcriptome data (BAM files) generated by TCGA for a total of 1,007 cancer specimens were analyzed in an automated fashion on a computational cluster hosted by the High-Performance Computing core at the Center for Computational Science, University of Miami (http://ccs.miami.edu/). An IBM BladeCenter cluster was available for compute-intensive data analysis. The cluster, named *Pegasus* running under Linux operation system, was used consisting of 280 computing nodes each with 8 Xeon 2.6 GHz cores and 16 GB of memory, and 700 computing nodes each with 4 Opteron 2.2 GHz core and 4 GB of memory. These nodes are interconnected by Gigabit Ethernet and feature a 21 TB NFS file system providing an aggregate of 5,040 cores and 7.3 TB of memory. All computational tasks were submitted in parallel to the LSF job scheduler and resource management system. The computational pipeline is outlined in Figure 1. In total, 1,156 jobs were submitted to the cluster for steps I–V for DNA-seq and RNA-seq data; 25,245 CPU hours were used for data analysis. Bamtools-1.0.2 [51] and samtools-0.1.18 [52] software were employed for converting data format. Sequencing reads with phred-like quality scores $q > 30$ were utilized. TopHat (v.2.0.0) [53] was consistently used for all transcriptome mapping steps. Multiple threads were used during alignment with option –p 8. When subtracting bacterial and viral sequences, we allowed TopHat to tolerate up to four mismatches per read, instead of the default of two in the alignment step, to allow for potentially higher mismatch rates due to mutations [54] or imperfect match to the reference sequence. In addition, TopHat was instructed to use a .gtf file and not to look for novel transcript junctions by utilizing the '—no-novel-junc' flag. We combined reference fasta files into 'supergenomes' for vector sequences, bacterial genomes, and viral genomes for steps II, III, and IV, respectively (Figure 1). Each individual reference sequence in the 'supergenome' was treated as a chromosome. Reference files were indexed before alignment steps. The bacterial reference file had to be split into two parts to reduce the memory use needed for indexing and mapping steps. Even the single short read aligning to the viral reference was considered as successful detection, if following BLAST analysis [55] versus the NCBI nucleotide (nt) collection confirmed sequence similarity with the target over 98% and at least one transcriptome out of a cohort had more than 10 reads mapped to a viral genome reference. Sequences aligning to multiple organisms, known artificial (vector) sequences, or low-complexity sequences were considered false positive and removed.

Only three gastrointestinal cancer types, stomach (STAD), rectum (READ), and colon adenocarcinomas (COAD), which tested virus positive on the transcriptome level, proceeded to the whole genome analysis step (Table 1). Burrows-Wheeler Aligner (BWA, v.0.5.9) [56] with default options was consistently used for genomic data alignment. Multiple threads were used when running BWA with option –t 4. Genomic read subtraction was performed in exactly the same fashion as described above for transcriptomes (Figure 1). In order to determine computational pipeline sensitivity to single nucleotide mismatches, sequence reads on EBV and HPV-18 with different mutation/mismatch rates and lengths were simulated and run through the computational subtraction and alignment steps (see Additional files 1 and 4).

Consensus sequence for EBV

EBV reference genomes include two very similar strains HHV-4.1 (NC_007605) and HHV-4.2 (NC_009334). In order to capture as many reads as possible, we created a consensus sequence using both NC_007605 and NC_009334 genome references. We replaced the two original references for two strains with the consensus reference for computational pipeline.

Statistical analysis

Since available data comprised cases-only DNA/RNA and malignant/normal tissue pairs, a simple McNemar test implemented in R library 'exact2x2' (v1.1-1.0) was used for both equivalence and association testing [57]. Equivalence testing for virus identification in DNA and RNA was performed using two one-sided exact McNemar tests with a confidence level of 0.975 at $\alpha = 0.05$ (Bonferroni-corrected for four viruses). The null hypothesis of equivalence was rejected, when at least in one of the one-sided tests, the confidence interval (CI) did not include '1'. Association of virus with tumor vs. normal tissue was done with two-sided exact McNemar test. Since COAD and READ are genetically identical [11], we combined two cohorts for association analysis to achieve a higher sample size. Association testing of virus presence in tumor/normal tissue was done using blood and solid tissue controls in separate tests, as well as blood and solid combined. Bonferroni correction was done for nine tests (three types of control groups multiplied by three viruses identified in the whole genome data). Fisher exact test was used for association testing with clinicopathological and demographics variables. Age at initial diagnosis in virus-positive and virus-negative groups was compared using ANOVA. Bonferroni correction was applied.

Estimation of viral load

We calculated V, the number of viral copies per cell (vc/c), i.e., viral load, for each DNA sample as

$$V = C_V / C_H,$$

where C_V is the average sequencing coverage for the virus, and C_H is the average human genome coverage. Average coverage C was calculated as

$$C_i = R_i \times L / G_i,$$

where i is the species, R is the number of reads, $L = 51$ and is the average read length in nucleotides, and G is the corresponding genome length in nucleotides. For the diploid human genome, $C = C_H/2$.

Additional files

Additional file 1: Simulations and viral rate estimations. A document containing simulation methods and results, and supplementary Tables 1–12, showing summary on viral reads detected, as well as clinical and demographic data in gastrointestinal adenocarcinomas.

Additional file 2: Dot matrix. This dot matrix view shows regions of similarity based upon the BLASTN 2.2.27+ results. The viral genome positions are on the *X*-axis. The lines represent mapped reads. The *Y*-axis shows cumulative bases of the aligned reads over all GIA sorted by the percentage of the genome covered. Higher coverage yields longer lines on the plot. Viral RNA transcriptome reads, when mapped to their reference genome sequences, showed uneven distribution clustering most likely corresponding to actively transcribed genes. Genomic reads, as expected, mapped along the viral reference genome randomly and more uniformly than transcriptomic reads.

Additional file 3: Correlation of EBV and CMV load in tumor's transcriptomes and genomes. Each data point represents one tumor. The *X*-axis shows log10-transformed percentage of viral reads in tumor's transcriptome; the *Y*-axis shows log10-transformed viral load (nc/c, see methods) in tumor's whole genome. COAD are depicted as read circles, READ as blue triangles. STAD is not shown because there was not a sufficient number of tumor genomes sequenced.

Additional file 4: Simulation results. At the low mutation rate up to 2%, derived reads were not lost to any significant extent, and our pipeline still captured over 94% simulated reads by BWA (whole genome pipeline) and over 80% by Tophat v.2.0.0 (transcriptome pipeline). Our approach had highest sensitivity with the shortest reads (50 nt), being at least 80% for BWA at a mismatch rate of 0.04, and 0.05 for Tophat. Higher mutation rates greatly impacted sensitivity, especially for the longer sequence reads, consistent with the BWA and TopHat algorithms. TopHat used the bowtie2 aligner, which seems to be affected to a greater extent by the length of the reads, probably due to using a fixed number of mismatches ($N = 4$), while BWA allows a floating error rate k depending on the read length. Simulated errors were randomly distributed. The longer the read, the more likely was the inclusion of mismatches. Subtraction of non-viral reads did not affect HPV-18 alignment, and less than 1% of CMV reads were lost through this process at zero mutation rate. As expected, computational subtraction eliminates individual viral sequences to various extents, depending on the degree of homology with non-viral reference sequences included in the filters.

Abbreviations

AML: Acute myeloid leukemia; CI: Confidence interval; CMV: Cytomegalovirus; COAD: Colon adenocarcinoma; CRAD: Colorectal adenocarcinomas; EBV: Epstein-Barr virus; GIA: Gastrointestinal adenocarcinomas; HHV: Human herpes virus; HHV-6B: Roseola virus; HPV-18: Human papilloma virus type 18; KIRK: Kidney renal clear carcinoma; KIRP: Kidney renal papillary cell carcinoma; KSHV: Kaposi's sarcoma-associated human virus; LUAD: Lung adenocarcinoma; LUSK: Lung squamous cell carcinoma; NGS: Next-generation sequencing; nt: Nucleotide; READ: Rectum adenocarcinoma; SD: Standard deviation; STAD: Stomach adenocarcinoma; TCGA: The Cancer Genome Atlas; UCEC: Uterine corpus endometrioid carcinoma; vc/c: Viral copies per cell.

Competing interests

The authors declare that they have no competing interests.

Authors' contributions

DS has designed and tested the analytical pipeline, downloaded and analyzed the data, and performed results interpretation and manuscript writing. NT has been involved in drafting and revising the manuscript and has contributed to the analytical pipeline design. Both authors have given final approval of the version to be published.

Acknowledgements

We would like to thank TCGA project organizers as well as all study participants. This work was supported by the Center for Computational

Science (CCS), University of Miami and partially by a grant (1R03CA171052-01A1) from National Cancer Institute (NCI). We also thank the High-Performance Computing team at the Center for Computational Science, University of Miami, especially Joel P. Zysman, John Baringer, Pedro Davila, and Zongjun Hu for technical support, as well as Dr. Enrique A. Mesri (Microbiology and Immunology Department) and Dr. Jennifer Clarke (Epidemiology Department) for their intellectual contribution to the manuscript. Finally, we would also like to thank Camilo Valdes (CCS) for assistance with the simulations.

Author details

[1]Center for Computational Science, University of Miami, 1120 NW 14 St, Miami, FL 33136, USA. [2]Department of Medicine, Miller School of Medicine, University of Miami, 1120 NW 14 St, Miami, FL 33136, USA.

References

1. Zur Hausen H: **The search for infectious causes of human cancers: where and why.** *Virology* 2009, **392**(1):1–10.
2. Moore RA, Warren RL, Freeman JD, Gustavsen JA, Chenard C, Friedman JM, Suttle CA, Zhao YJ, Holt RA: **The sensitivity of massively parallel sequencing for detecting candidate infectious agents associated with human tissue.** *PLoS One* 2011, **6**(5):e19838.
3. Weber G, Shendure J, Tanenbaum DM, Church GM, Meyerson M: **Identification of foreign gene sequences by transcript filtering against the human genome.** *Nature genetics* 2002, **30**(2):141–142.
4. Kostic AD, Ojesina AI, Pedamallu CS, Jung J, Verhaak RG, Getz G, Meyerson M: **PathSeq: software to identify or discover microbes by deep sequencing of human tissue.** *Nature biotechnology* 2011, **29**(5):393–396.
5. Chen Y, Yao H, Thompson EJ, Tannir NM, Weinstein JN, Su X: **VirusSeq: software to identify viruses and their integration sites using next-generation sequencing of human cancer tissue.** *Bioinformatics* 2013, **29**(2):266–267.
6. Agrawal N, Frederick MJ, Pickering CR, Bettegowda C, Chang K, Li RJ, Fakhry C, Xie TX, Zhang J, Wang J, *et al*: **Exome sequencing of head and neck squamous cell carcinoma reveals inactivating mutations in NOTCH1.** *Science* 2011, **333**(6046):1154–1157.
7. Stransky N, Egloff AM, Tward AD, Kostic AD, Cibulskis K, Sivachenko A, Kryukov GV, Lawrence MS, Sougnez C, McKenna A, *et al*: **The mutational landscape of head and neck squamous cell carcinoma.** *Science* 2011, **333**(6046):1157–1160.
8. Arron ST, Ruby JG, Dybbro E, Ganem D, DeRisi JL: **Transcriptome sequencing demonstrates that human papillomavirus is not active in cutaneous squamous cell carcinoma.** *J Invest Dermatol* 2011, **131**(8):1745–1753.
9. Barzon L, Militello V, Lavezzo E, Franchin E, Peta E, Squarzon L, Trevisan M, Pagni S, Dal Bello F, Toppo S, Palù G: **Human papillomavirus genotyping by 454 next generation sequencing technology.** *J Clin Virol* 2011, **52**(2):93–97.
10. TCGARN: **Comprehensive genomic characterization of squamous cell lung cancers.** *Nature* 2012, **489**(7417):519–525.
11. TCGARN: **Comprehensive molecular characterization of human colon and rectal cancer.** *Nature* 2012, **487**(7407):330–337.
12. De Paoli P, Carbone A: **Carcinogenic viruses and solid cancers without sufficient evidence of causal association.** *International Journal of Cancer Journal International du Cancer* 2013, **133**(7):1517–1529.
13. Grulich AE, van Leeuwen MT, Falster MO, Vajdic CM: **Incidence of cancers in people with HIV/AIDS compared with immunosuppressed transplant recipients: a meta-analysis.** *Lancet* 2007, **370**(9581):59–67.
14. Khoury JD, Tannir NM, Williams MD, Chen Y, Yao H, Zhang J, Thompson EJ, Meric-Bernstam F, Medeiros LJ, Weinstein JN, Su X: **Landscape of DNA virus associations across human malignant cancers: analysis of 3,775 cases using RNA-Seq.** *Journal of Virology* 2013, **87**(16):8916–8926.
15. Takeuchi K, Tanaka-Taya K, Kazuyama Y, Ito YM, Hashimoto S, Fukayama M, Mori S: **Prevalence of Epstein-Barr virus in Japan: trends and future prediction.** *Pathol Int* 2006, **56**(3):112–116.
16. Linton MS, Kroeker K, Fedorak D, Dieleman L, Fedorak RN: **Prevalence of Epstein-Barr Virus in a population of patients with inflammatory bowel disease: a prospective cohort study.** *Aliment Pharmacol Ther* 2013, **38**:1248–1254.
17. Luzuriaga K, Sullivan JL: **Infectious mononucleosis.** *The New England Journal of Medicine* 2010, **362**(21):1993–2000.
18. Lubeck PR, Doerr HW, Rabenau HF: **Epidemiology of human cytomegalovirus (HCMV) in an urban region of Germany: what has changed?** *Med Microbiol Immunol* 2010, **199**(1):53–60.
19. Lopo S, Vinagre E, Palminha P, Paixao MT, Nogueira P, Freitas MG: **Seroprevalence to cytomegalovirus in the Portuguese population, 2002–2003.** *Euro Surveill* 2011, **16**(25):5.
20. Staras SA, Dollard SC, Radford KW, Flanders WD, Pass RF, Cannon MJ: **Seroprevalence of cytomegalovirus infection in the United States, 1988–1994.** *Clin Infect Dis* 2006, **43**(9):1143–1151.
21. Oren I, Sobel JD: **Human herpesvirus type 6: review.** *Clin Infect Dis* 1992, **14**(3):741–746.
22. Butler LM, Were WA, Balinandi S, Downing R, Dollard S, Neilands TB, Gupta S, Rutherford GW, Mermin J: **Human herpesvirus 8 infection in children and adults in a population-based study in rural Uganda.** *The Journal of Infectious Diseases* 2011, **203**(5):625–634.
23. Qu L, Jenkins F, Triulzi DJ: **Human herpesvirus 8 genomes and seroprevalence in United States blood donors.** *Transfusion* 2010, **50**(5):1050–1056.
24. Baillargeon J, Leach CT, Deng JH, Gao SJ, Jenson HB: **High prevalence of human herpesvirus 8 (HHV-8) infection in south Texas children.** *Journal of Medical Virology* 2002, **67**(4):542–548.
25. CDC: *Incidence, Prevalence, and Cost of Sexually Transmitted Infections in the United States.* Atlanta: Centers for Disease Control and Prevention; 2013.
26. Uozaki H, Fukayama M: **Epstein-Barr virus and gastric carcinoma–viral carcinogenesis through epigenetic mechanisms.** *Int J Clin Exp Pathol* 2008, **1**(3):198–216.
27. Camargo MC, Murphy G, Koriyama C, Pfeiffer RM, Kim WH, Herrera-Goepfert R, Corvalan AH, Carrascal E, Abdirad A, Anwar M, Hao Z, Kattoor J, Yoshiwara-Wakabayashi E, Eizuru Y, Rabkin CS, Akiba S: **Determinants of Epstein-Barr virus-positive gastric cancer: an international pooled analysis.** *British Journal of Cancer* 2011, **105**(1):38–43.
28. Fukayama M, Ushiku T: **Epstein-Barr virus-associated gastric carcinoma.** *Pathol Res Pract* 2011, **207**(9):529–537.
29. Marquitz AR, Mathur A, Shair KH, Raab-Traub N: **Infection of Epstein-Barr virus in a gastric carcinoma cell line induces anchorage independence and global changes in gene expression.** *Proc Natl Acad Sci U S A* 2012, **109**(24):9593–9598.
30. Ryan JL, Jones RJ, Kenney SC, Rivenbark AG, Tang W, Knight ER, Coleman WB, Gulley ML: **Epstein-Barr virus-specific methylation of human genes in gastric cancer cells.** *Infect Agent Cancer* 2010, **5**:27.
31. Yuen ST, Chung LP, Leung SY, Luk IS, Chan SY, Ho J: **In situ detection of Epstein-Barr virus in gastric and colorectal adenocarcinomas.** *The American Journal of Surgical Pathology* 1994, **18**(11):1158–1163.
32. Grinstein S, Preciado MV, Gattuso P, Chabay PA, Warren WH, De Matteo E, Gould VE: **Demonstration of Epstein-Barr virus in carcinomas of various sites.** *Cancer Research* 2002, **62**(17):4876–4878.
33. Karpinski P, Myszka A, Ramsey D, Kielan W, Sasiadek MM: **Detection of viral DNA sequences in sporadic colorectal cancers in relation to CpG island methylation and methylator phenotype.** *Tumour Biol* 2011, **32**(4):653–659.
34. Park JM, Choi MG, Kim SW, Chung IS, Yang CW, Kim YS, Jung CK, Lee KY, Kang JH: **Increased incidence of colorectal malignancies in renal transplant recipients: a case control study.** *Am J Transplant* 2010, **10**(9):2043–2050.
35. Song LB, Zhang X, Zhang CQ, Zhang Y, Pan ZZ, Liao WT, Li MZ, Zeng MS: **Infection of Epstein-Barr virus in colorectal cancer in Chinese.** *Ai Zheng* 2006, **25**(11):1356–1360.
36. Giuliani L, Ronci C, Bonifacio D, Di Bonito L, Favalli C, Perno CF, Syrjanen K, Ciotti M: **Detection of oncogenic DNA viruses in colorectal cancer.** *Anticancer Res* 2008, **28**(2B):1405–1410.
37. Chen TH, Huang CC, Yeh KT, Chang SH, Chang SW, Sung WW, Cheng YW, Lee H: **Human papilloma virus 16 E6 oncoprotein associated with p53 inactivation in colorectal cancer.** *World J Gastroenterol* 2012, **18**(30):4051–4058.
38. Salepci T, Yazici H, Dane F, Topuz E, Dalay N, Onat H, Aykan F, Seker M, Aydiner A: **Detection of human papillomavirus DNA by polymerase chain reaction and southern blot hybridization in colorectal cancer patients.** *J Buon* 2009, **14**(3):495–499.

39. Lee YM, Leu SY, Chiang H, Fung CP, Liu WT: **Human papillomavirus type 18 in colorectal cancer.** *Journal of Microbiology, Immunology, and Infection = Wei mian yu gan ran za zhi* 2001, **34**(2):87–91.
40. Bodaghi S, Yamanegi K, Xiao SY, Da Costa M, Palefsky JM, Zheng ZM: **Colorectal papillomavirus infection in patients with colorectal cancer.** *Clinical Cancer Research* 2005, **11**(8):2862–2867.
41. Damin DC, Caetano MB, Rosito MA, Schwartsmann G, Damin AS, Frazzon AP, Ruppenthal RD, Alexandre CO: **Evidence for an association of human papillomavirus infection and colorectal cancer.** *Eur J Surg Oncol* 2007, **33**(5):569–574.
42. Collins D, Hogan AM, Winter DC: **Microbial and viral pathogens in colorectal cancer.** *The Lancet Oncology* 2011, **12**(5):504–512.
43. Chen HP, Jiang JK, Chen CY, Chou TY, Chen YC, Chang YT, Lin SF, Chan CH, Yang CY, Lin CH, Lin JK, Cho WL, Chan YJ: **Human cytomegalovirus preferentially infects the neoplastic epithelium of colorectal cancer: a quantitative and histological analysis.** *J Clin Virol* 2012, **54**(3):240–244.
44. Zur Hausen H: **Oncogenic DNA viruses.** *Oncogene* 2001, **20**(54):7820–7823.
45. Szostek S, Zawilinska B, Kopec J, Kosz-Vnenchak M: **Herpesviruses as possible cofactors in HPV-16-related oncogenesis.** *Acta Biochim Pol* 2009, **56** (2):337–342.
46. Niller HH, Wolf H, Minarovits J: **Viral hit and run-oncogenesis: genetic and epigenetic scenarios.** *Cancer Letters* 2011, **305**(2):200–217.
47. Yoshida T, Sano T, Oyama T, Kanuma T, Fukuda T: **Prevalence, viral load, and physical status of HPV 16 and 18 in cervical adenosquamous carcinoma.** *Virchows Arch* 2009, **455**(3):253–259.
48. Lee JH, Kim SH, Han SH, An JS, Lee ES, Kim YS: **Clinicopathological and molecular characteristics of Epstein-Barr virus-associated gastric carcinoma: a meta-analysis.** *J Gastroenterol Hepatol* 2009, **24**(3):354–365.
49. Mori Y: **Recent topics related to human herpesvirus 6 cell tropism.** *Cell Microbiol* 2009, **11**(7):1001–1006.
50. Zur Hausen H: **Papillomaviruses and cancer: from basic studies to clinical application.** *Nature reviews Cancer* 2002, **2**(5):342–350.
51. Barnett DW, Garrison EK, Quinlan AR, Stromberg MP, Marth GT: **BamTools: a C++ API and toolkit for analyzing and managing BAM files.** *Bioinformatics* 2011, **27**(12):1691–1692.
52. Li H, Handsaker B, Wysoker A, Fennell T, Ruan J, Homer N, Marth G, Abecasis G, Durbin R: **The Sequence Alignment/Map format and SAMtools.** *Bioinformatics* 2009, **25**(16):2078–2079.
53. Trapnell C, Roberts A, Goff L, Pertea G, Kim D, Kelley DR, Pimentel H, Salzberg SL, Rinn JL, Pachter L: **Differential gene and transcript expression analysis of RNA-seq experiments with TopHat and Cufflinks.** *Nat Protoc* 2012, **7**(3):562–578.
54. Sanjuan R, Nebot MR, Chirico N, Mansky LM, Belshaw R: **Viral mutation rates.** *Journal of virology* 2010, **84**(19):9733–9748.
55. Altschul SF, Madden TL, Schaffer AA, Zhang J, Zhang Z, Miller W, Lipman DJ: **Gapped BLAST and PSI-BLAST: a new generation of protein database search programs.** *Nucleic Acids Res* 1997, **25**(17):3389–3402.
56. Li H, Durbin R: **Fast and accurate short read alignment with Burrows-Wheeler transform.** *Bioinformatics* 2009, **25**(14):1754–1760.
57. Fay MP: **Confidence intervals that match Fisher's exact or Blaker's exact tests.** *Biostatistics* 2010, **11**(2):373–374.

Permissions

All chapters in this book were first published in JNI, by BioMed Central; hereby published with permission under the Creative Commons Attribution License or equivalent. Every chapter published in this book has been scrutinized by our experts. Their significance has been extensively debated. The topics covered herein carry significant findings which will fuel the growth of the discipline. They may even be implemented as practical applications or may be referred to as a beginning point for another development.

The contributors of this book come from diverse backgrounds, making this book a truly international effort. This book will bring forth new frontiers with its revolutionizing research information and detailed analysis of the nascent developments around the world.

We would like to thank all the contributing authors for lending their expertise to make the book truly unique. They have played a crucial role in the development of this book. Without their invaluable contributions this book wouldn't have been possible. They have made vital efforts to compile up to date information on the varied aspects of this subject to make this book a valuable addition to the collection of many professionals and students.

This book was conceptualized with the vision of imparting up-to-date information and advanced data in this field. To ensure the same, a matchless editorial board was set up. Every individual on the board went through rigorous rounds of assessment to prove their worth. After which they invested a large part of their time researching and compiling the most relevant data for our readers.

The editorial board has been involved in producing this book since its inception. They have spent rigorous hours researching and exploring the diverse topics which have resulted in the successful publishing of this book. They have passed on their knowledge of decades through this book. To expedite this challenging task, the publisher supported the team at every step. A small team of assistant editors was also appointed to further simplify the editing procedure and attain best results for the readers.

Apart from the editorial board, the designing team has also invested a significant amount of their time in understanding the subject and creating the most relevant covers. They scrutinized every image to scout for the most suitable representation of the subject and create an appropriate cover for the book.

The publishing team has been an ardent support to the editorial, designing and production team. Their endless efforts to recruit the best for this project, has resulted in the accomplishment of this book. They are a veteran in the field of academics and their pool of knowledge is as vast as their experience in printing. Their expertise and guidance has proved useful at every step. Their uncompromising quality standards have made this book an exceptional effort. Their encouragement from time to time has been an inspiration for everyone.

The publisher and the editorial board hope that this book will prove to be a valuable piece of knowledge for researchers, students, practitioners and scholars across the globe.

List of Contributors

Adila Alkindy
Clinical Genetics Department, Sultan Qaboos University Hospital, Al-Khod, Muscat 123, Sultanate of Oman

Nadia Chuzhanova
School of Science and Technology, Nottingham Trent University, Clifton LaneNottingham NG11 8NS, UK

Usha Kini
Department of Clinical Genetics, Churchill Hospital, Old Road Headington, Oxford OX3 7LJ, UK

David N Cooper and Meena Upadhyaya
Institute of Medical Genetics, Cardiff University, Heath Park, Cardiff CF14 4XN, UK

Zoi Lanara
Faculty of Mathematical, Physical and Natural Sciences, Department of Biological Sciences, University of Trieste, Trieste 34128, Italy
School of Health Sciences, Department of Pharmacy, University of Patras, University Campus, Rio, Patras 26504, Greece

Evangelos Kostantinopoulos, George P Patrinos and Cristiana Pavlidis
School of Health Sciences, Department of Pharmacy, University of Patras, University Campus, Rio, Patras 26504, Greece

Efstathia Giannopoulou and Haralabos P Kalofonos
Clinical Oncology Laboratory, Division of Oncology, Department of Medicine, University of Patras, Rio, Patras 26504, Greece

Jean-Christophe Nebel and Marta Fullen
School of Computing and Information Systems, Faculty of Science, Engineering and Computing, Kingston University, London SW15 3DW, UK

Amos Toren
Department of Pediatric Hemato-Oncology, The Cancer Research Center, Sheba Medical Center, 2 Sheba Road, Ramat Gan 52621, Israel

Juergen K Reichardt
School of Pharmacy and Molecular Sciences, James Cook University, Townsville QLD 4811, Australia

Ali Andalibi
University of Connecticut, 438 Whitney Rd. Extension, Unit 1006, Storrs, CT 06269, USA

Nancy Ya-Hsuan Hsu
Quest Diagnostics Nichols Institute, 14225 Newbrook Drive, Chantilly, VA 20153, USA

Joni Doherty
Center for Neural Tumor Research, 2100 West Third Street, Los Angeles, CA 90057, USA

William Slattery
Department of Clinical Studies, House Ear Institute, Los Angeles, CA 90057, USA

Ruty Mehrian-Shai
Institute for Genetic Medicine, University of Southern California, Keck School of Medicine, Los Angeles, CA 90089, USA

Laura E Thomas, Jincy Winston, Ellie Rad, Matthew Mort, Kayleigh M Dodd, Andrew R Tee, David N Cooper and Meena Upadhyaya
Institute of Medical Genetics, School of Medicine, Cardiff University, Cardiff CF14 4XN, UK

Fionnuala McDyer and Stephen Moore
Almac Diagnostics, 19 Seagoe Industrial Estate, Craigavon, Northern Ireland BT63 5QD, UK

Ioannis Karageorgos, Cristiana Pavlidis, Zoi Zagoriti and Theodora Katsila
Department of Pharmacy, University of Patras, School of Health Sciences, University Campus, Rion GR-26504, Patras, Greece

Haralabos P. Kalofonos and Efstathia Giannopoulou
Clinical Oncology Laboratory, Division of Oncology, Department of Medicine, University of Patras, Patras, Greece

Radoje Drmanac and Brock A. Peters
Complete Genomics Inc., Mountain View, CA, USA
BGI-Shenzhen, Shenzhen 51803, China

Peter D. Stenson and David N. Cooper
Institute of Medical Genetics, School of Medicine, Cardiff University, Cardiff, UK

Konstantinos Mitropoulos
The Golden Helix Foundation, London, UK

Joseph Borg
Department of Applied Biomedical Science, Faculty of Health Sciences, University of Malta, Msida, Malta
Department of Cell Biology and Genetics, School of Medicine Karageorgos et al. Human Genomics Health Sciences, Erasmus University Medical Center, Rotterdam, The Netherlands

Andrew Stubbs and Peter van der Spek
Department of Bioinformatics, School of Medicine and Health Sciences, Erasmus University Medical Center, Rotterdam, The Netherlands

George P. Patrinos
Department of Pharmacy, University of Patras, School of Health Sciences, University Campus, Rion GR-26504, Patras, Greece
epartment of Bioinformatics, School of Medicine and Health Sciences, Erasmus University Medical Center, Rotterdam, The Netherlands

Clint Mizzi
Department of Physiology and Biochemistry, Faculty of Health Sciences, University of Malta, Msida, Malta
Department of Bioinformatics, School of Medicine and Health Sciences, Erasmus University Medical Center, Rotterdam, The Netherlands

Xiaoyu Wang and Steve Self
Vaccine and Infectious Disease Division, Fred Hutchinson Cancer Research Center, Seattle, WA, USA

James Y. Dai
Vaccine and Infectious Disease Division, Fred Hutchinson Cancer Research Center, Seattle, WA, USA
Public Health Science Division, Fred Hutchinson Cancer Research Center, Seattle, WA, USA

Xiaohong Li
Human Biology, Fred Hutchinson Cancer Research Center, Seattle, WA, USA
Public Health Science Division, Fred Hutchinson Cancer Research Center, Seattle, WA, USA

Charles Kooperberg and Yichen Cheng
Public Health Science Division, Fred Hutchinson Cancer Research Center, Seattle, WA, USA

Xin Sun
Institute of Occupational Health and Poison Control, Chinese Center for Disease Control and Prevention, Beijing, China

Xibin Sun
Henan Office for Cancer Research and Control, Henan Cancer Hospital, Zhengzhou, Henan, China

Qingxuan Song and Jun Z. Li
Department of Human Genetics, University of Michigan, Ann Arbor, MI, USA

Sofia D. Merajver
Department of Internal Medicine and Epidemiology, University of Michigan, 5789A Medical Science II, Ann Arbor, MI 48109-5618, USA

Ryan Delahanty, Xingyi Guo, Wei Zheng and Jirong Long
Division of Epidemiology, Department of Medicine, Vanderbilt University Medical Center, Nashville 37203, USA

Yanfeng Zhang
Division of Epidemiology, Department of Medicine, Vanderbilt University Medical Center, Nashville 37203, USA
HudsonAlpha Institute for Biotechnology, Huntsville 35806, USA

Xiaoya Chen, Jinjun Li and Lili Lu
Medical College, Wuhan University of Science and Technology, Wuhan 430065, China

Ling Hu
Department of Anesthesiology, Tianyou Hospital, Wuhan University of Science and Technology, Wuhan 430064, China

William Yang
Texas Advanced Computing Center, University of Texas at Austin, 10100 Burnet Road, Austin, TX 78758, USA

Hongyan Jin and Zexiong Wei
Puren Hospital, Wuhan University of Science and Technology, Wuhan 430081, China

Jack Y. Yang and Mary Qu Yang
MidSouth Bioinformatics Center, Department of Information Science, George Washington Donaghey College of Engineering and Information Technology and Joint Bioinformatics Graduate Program, University of Arkansas at Little Rock and University of Arkansas for Medical Sciences, 2801 S. University Avenue, Little Rock, AR 72204, USA

Jun S. Liu
Department of Statistics and Harvard School of Public Health, Harvard University, One Oxford St., Cambridge 02138 Massachusetts, USA

Hamid R. Arabnia
Department of Computer Science, University of Georgia, Athens, GA 30602, USA

Youping Deng
Medical College, Wuhan University of Science and Technology, Wuhan 430065, China
Department of Internal Medicine and Rush University Cancer Center, Rush University Medical Center, Chicago, IL 60612, USA

Garima Kushwaha
Christopher S. Bond Life Sciences Center, University of Missouri, Columbia, MO 65211, USA
Informatics Institute, University of Missouri, Columbia, MO 65211, USA

Mikhail Dozmorov
Department of Biostatistics, Virginia Commonwealth University, Richmond, VA 23225, USA

Jonathan D. Wren
Arthritis and Clinical Immunology Program, Oklahoma Medical Research Foundation, Oklahoma City, OK 73104, USA

Jing Qiu
Department of Applied Economics & Statistics, University of Delaware, Newark, DE 19716, USA

Huidong Shi
GRU Cancer Center, Georgia Regents University, Augusta, GA 30912, USA
Department of Biochemistry and Molecular Biology, Georgia Regents University, Augusta, GA 30912, USA

Dong Xu
Christopher S. Bond Life Sciences Center, University of Missouri, Columbia, MO 65211, USA
Informatics Institute, University of Missouri, Columbia, MO 65211, USA
Department of Computer Science, University of Missouri, Columbia, MO 65211, USA

Hong Zhou, Joseph Manthey and Ekaterina Lioutikova
Department of Mathematical Science, School of Health and Natural Sciences, University of Saint Joseph, 1678 Asylum Avenue, West Hartford, CT 06117, USA

William Yang, Kenji Yoshigoe and Mary Qu Yang
Joint Bioinformatics Ph.D. Program, University of Arkansas at Little Rock and University of Arkansas for Medical Sciences, 2801 S. University Avenue, Little Rock, AR 72204, USA

Hong Wang
Susan L. Cullman Laboratory for Cancer Research, Department of Chemical Biology and Centre for Cancer Prevention Research, Ernest Mario School of Pharmacy, Rutgers, The State University of New Jersey, 164 Frelinghuysen Road, Piscataway, NJ 08854, USA

Elisa Napolitano Ferreira, Bruna Durães Figueiredo Barros, Renan Valieris Almeida, Giovana Tardin Torrezan, Sheila Garcia, Emmanuel Dias-Neto and Dirce Maria Carraro
International Research Center/CIPE, A.C. Camargo Cancer Center, São Paulo, SP, Brazil

Jorge Estefano de Souza
Instituto Metrópole Digital, Federal University of Rio Grande do Norte, Natal, RN, Brazil

Ana Cristina Victorino Krepischi
Institute of Biosciences, University of São Paulo, São Paulo, SP, Brazil

Celso Abdon Lopes de Mello and Ademar Lopes
Departament of Abdominal Surgery, A.C. Camargo Cancer Center, São Paulo, SP, Brazil

Isabela Werneck da Cunha, Clóvis Antonio Lopes Pinto and Fernando Augusto Soares
Department of Anatomic Pathology, A.C. Camargo Cancer Center, São Paulo, SP, Brazil

Sandro José de Souza
Federal University of Rio Grande do Norte, Natal, RN, Brazil

Charlotte Philpott, Hannah Tovell, Ian M. Frayling, David N. Cooper and Meena Upadhyaya
Division of Cancer and Genetics, Institute of Medical Genetics, Cardiff University, Heath Park, Cardiff CF14 4XN, UK

Jamie K. Teer, Yonghong Zhang, Eric A. Welsh, Steven A. Eschrich and Anders E. Berglund
Department of Biostatistics and Bioinformatics, H. Lee Moffitt Cancer Center and Research Institute, Tampa, FL 33612, USA

Lu Chen and W. Douglas Cress
Department of Molecular Oncology, H. Lee Moffitt Cancer Center and Research Institute, Tampa, FL 33612, USA

Bajinder S Dhanoa and James S Friedman
Department of Ophthalmology, University of Colorado School of Medicine, Aurora, CO 80045, USA

Tiziana Cogliati and Akhila G Satish
Neurobiology-Neurodegeneration and Repair Laboratory (N-NRL), National Eye Institute, National Institutes of Health, Building 6/302, MSC 0610, 6 Center Drive, Bethesda, MD 20892, USA

Elspeth A Bruford
HUGO Gene Nomenclature Committee (HGNC), EMBL-EBI, Wellcome Trust Genome Campus, Hinxton, Cambridgeshire CB10 1SD, UK

Ashni Sedani, David N Cooper and Meena Upadhyaya
Institute of Medical Genetics, School of Medicine, Cardiff University, Heath Park, Cardiff CF14 4XN, UK

Yuhua Su
Department of Human Nutrition, Food, and Animal Sciences, University of Hawaii at Manoa, Honolulu, HI 96822, USA

Dahlia Nielsen
Bioinformatics Research Center, North Carolina State University, Raleigh, NC 27695, USA

Lei Zhu
Biomarker and Predictive Analytics, GlaxoSmithKline, 5 Moore Drive, Research Triangle Park, NC 27709, USA

Kristy Richards
Department of Genetic, University of North Carolina, Chapel Hill, NC 27599, USA

Steven Suter
Department of Clinical Sciences, Center for Comparative Medicine & Translational Research, North Carolina State University, Raleigh, NC 27695, USA

Matthew Breen
Department of Molecular Biomedical Sciences, College of Veterinary Medicine, North Carolina State University, Raleigh, NC 27695, USA

Alison Motsinger-Reif and Jason Osborne
Department of Statistics, North Carolina State University, Raleigh, NC 27695, USA

Laura Thomas, David N Cooper and Meena Upadhyaya
Institute of Medical Genetics, School of Medicine, Cardiff University, Cardiff CF14 4XN, UK

Victor-Felix Mautner
Department of Maxillofacial Surgery, University Medical Centre Hamburg-Eppendorf, Hamburg D-20246, Germany

Daria Salyakina
Center for Computational Science, University of Miami, 1120 NW 14 St, Miami, FL 33136, USA

Nicholas F Tsinoremas
Center for Computational Science, University of Miami, 1120 NW 14 St, Miami, FL 33136, USA
Department of Medicine, Miller School of Medicine, University of Miami, 1120 NW 14 St, Miami, FL 33136, USA

Index

www.ingramcontent.com/pod-product-compliance
Lightning Source LLC
LaVergne TN
LVHW080654210926
848485LV00003B/378
9781639272518